Surgery of the Thoracic Spine

Principles and Techniques

Ali A. Baaj, MD
Associate Professor
Co-Director, Spinal Deformity and Scoliosis Program
Department of Neurological Surgery
Weill Cornell Medical College
New York-Presbyterian Hospital
New York, New York, USA

U. Kumar Kakarla, MD
Director of Spinal Deformity
Department of Neurosurgery
Barrow Neurological Institute
St. Joseph's Hospital and Medical Center
Phoenix, Arizona, USA

Han Jo Kim, MD
Associate Professor
Spine Fellowship Director
Department of Orthopaedic Surgery
Hospital for Special Surgery
New York, New York, USA

147 illustrations

Thieme
New York • Stuttgart • Delhi • Rio de Janeiro

Executive Editor: Timothy Y. Hiscock
Managing Editor: Sarah Landis
Director, Editorial Services: Mary Jo Casey
Production Editor: Naamah Schwartz
International Production Director: Andreas Schabert
Editorial Director: Sue Hodgson
International Marketing Director: Fiona Henderson
International Sales Director: Louisa Turrell
Director of Institutional Sales: Adam Bernacki
Senior Vice President and Chief Operating Officer: Sarah Vanderbilt
President: Brian D. Scanlan

Library of Congress Cataloging-in-Publication Data

Names: Baaj, Ali A., editor. | Kakarla, U. Kumar, editor. | Kim, Han Jo (Orthopedic surgeon), editor.
Title: Surgery of the thoracic spine : principles and techniques / [edited by] Ali A. Baaj, U. Kumar Kakarla, Han Jo Kim.
Description: New York : Thieme, [2019] | Includes bibliographical references.
Identifiers: LCCN 2018059433| ISBN 9781626238558 (print) | ISBN 9781626238565 (eISBN)
Subjects: | MESH: Thoracic Vertebrae–surgery | Spinal Diseases–surgery
Classification: LCC RD768 | NLM WE 725 | DDC 617.4/82–dc23 LC record available at https://lccn.loc.gov/2018059433

Important note: Medicine is an ever-changing science undergoing continual development. Research and clinical experience are continually expanding our knowledge, in particular our knowledge of proper treatment and drug therapy. Insofar as this book mentions any dosage or application, readers may rest assured that the authors, editors, and publishers have made every effort to ensure that such references are in accordance with **the state of knowledge at the time of production of the book.**

Nevertheless, this does not involve, imply, or express any guarantee or responsibility on the part of the publishers in respect to any dosage instructions and forms of applications stated in the book. **Every user is requested to examine carefully** the manufacturers' leaflets accompanying each drug and to check, if necessary in consultation with a physician or specialist, whether the dosage schedules mentioned therein or the contraindications stated by the manufacturers differ from the statements made in the present book. Such examination is particularly important with drugs that are either rarely used or have been newly released on the market. Every dosage schedule or every form of application used is entirely at the user's own risk and responsibility. The authors and publishers request every user to report to the publishers any discrepancies or inaccuracies noticed. If errors in this work are found after publication, errata will be posted at www.thieme.com on the product description page.

Some of the product names, patents, and registered designs referred to in this book are in fact registered trademarks or proprietary names even though specific reference to this fact is not always made in the text. Therefore, the appearance of a name without designation as proprietary is not to be construed as a representation by the publisher that it is in the public domain.

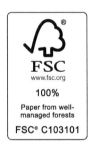

Contents

Part VII Further Topics

Foreword I

This new focused textbook on the surgical management of thoracic spinal pathology highlights the new era we have entered emphasizing the evolving specialty of spinal surgery. Throughout the 20th century, spinal surgery was performed by, and education was provided by, two distinct and separate disciplines of either Neurological Surgery or Orthopedic Surgery. Traditionally, orthopedic spinal surgery emphasized care of the spinal column/vertebrae, such as performing spinal fusion for thoracic scoliosis, while neurosurgical spine surgery focused on decompression of the spinal cord and/or cervical and lumbar nerve roots for various degenerative, traumatic and tumorous conditions. However, by the start of the 21st century, the logical collaboration between the two disciplines treating similar spinal pathology began at the societal (e.g. North American Spine Society), educational (combined Ortho/Neuro spinal surgery fellowships and various spine surgery meetings), and academic (e.g. Cleveland Clinic combined Ortho/Neuro Spine program) levels. Thus, in the current era, many surgeons from either discipline who perform surgery of the spine consider themselves "Spinal Surgeons" regardless of their prior training lineage. In addition, spinal surgery has also become subspecialized with many anatomic, pathologic, and technique-based distinctions such as Cervical Spine, Spinal Deformity, and Minimally Invasive Spinal Surgery specialists who base their practice on these focused areas.

This unique educational product is a reflection of this new brand, spinal surgery, and highlights the complex anatomy, pathology, and surgical treatments involved in the thoracic spine. With this extremely thorough and detailed approach, Baaj, Kakarla, and Kim along with a talented array of contributing authors, have taken a deep educational dive into the thoracic spinal region, which has often taken a back seat, both educationally and from a research perspective, to the mobile cervical and lumbar spine regions above and below, respectively. Although biomechanically the thoracic spinal region renders more "support" than "movement," it does provide the important structural support for the cardiopulmonary system in addition to protecting the vital thoracic spinal cord, which controls lower limb and bowel/bladder function. The 31 chapters within this book expertly describe the pathology encountered and surgical treatment options available for this intermediate region of the spinal column. Chapters covering basic Chest Wall Physiology, Biomechanics, and Anesthetic considerations are included, along with a complete list of pathologic conditions with comprehensive surgical solutions. Quality and thoroughness are accomplished with a diverse mix of spinal surgeons who truly represent the new paradigm highlighting the current symbiotic relationship of Orthopedic and Neurosurgical spinal surgery specialists. The material presented is state-of-the-art regarding the array of surgical solutions available to treat thoracic spinal pathology. Expert derived treatment algorithms are appropriately defined and illustrated.

I want to express my personal thanks to Ali Baaj, Kumar Kakarla, and Han Jo Kim and the impressive list of contributors to this textbook. I am well aware that finding time out of one's busy clinical, academic, administrative, and personal schedules to put such a comprehensive and quality book together is extremely challenging. However, this type of dedication to the profession of spinal surgery is what will be required to improve the care of our current patients while training the future generation of spinal surgeons, who will be expected to provide an even higher level of successful surgical treatments to their patients. In this manner, *Surgery of the Thoracic Spine* is an important demonstration of the new discipline of spinal surgery and should be a standard reference for all students, trainees and practicing spinal surgeons that treat patients with thoracic spine pathology. Congratulations on a job well done!

Lawrence G. Lenke, MD
Professor and Chief of Spinal Surgery
Chief of Spinal Deformity Surgery
Co-Director of the Columbia Comprehensive Adult and Pediatric Spinal Surgery Fellowship
Columbia University Vagelos College of Physicians and Surgeons
Surgeon-in-Chief
Daniel and Jane Och Spine Hospital at New York-Presbyterian/Allen
New York, New York, USA

Foreword II

Nestled between the ever-moving cervical and lumbar regions of the spine, the thoracic vertebrae lead a relatively quiet existence. Fortified by the protective rib cage and a dense network of ligaments, the thoracic region is the Fort Knox of the spinal column, designed to protect the vulnerable thoracic spinal cord from threats both external and internal. Although the thoracic spine is largely immune to the daily wear and tear experienced by its neighbors to the north and south, it is affected by pathologies unique to its location and its function as a support essential to our upright existence.

Although it harbors the greatest number of segments in the spine, the thoracic region does not garner the same amount of attention devoted to the cervical and lumbar regions. Professional societies are dedicated to the treatment of the cervical and lumbar segments of the spine, but the thoracic region has been largely ignored. This oversight has been forever changed with the publication of this book. Drs. Baaj, Kakarla, and Kim have produced a most valuable addition to the literature by assembling contributions from experienced practitioners. Their combined experience offers a wealth of knowledge in treating this region. Beginning with a thoughtful discussion on the uniqueness of this region as it relates to pulmonary function, this book covers everything from biomechanics to unique anesthetic considerations.

Many books have covered the topic of scoliosis; however, this book does so from the rarely considered perspective of the thoracic spine. Additional topics explored in this work include the diagnosis and treatment of spondylarthropathies, infections, and trauma—including spinal cord injury. The section on neoplasms encompasses primary and metastatic tumors, intradural extramedullary lesions, and intramedullary tumors. The book also addresses special topics relating to monitoring, navigation, and unusual pathologies, such as spinal cord herniation.

The authors and editors of *Surgery of the Thoracic Spine* have produced a comprehensive guide to the thoracic region of the spine, and this work will be part of a well-stocked library of any practicing spinal surgeon.

Nicholas Theodore, MD
Professor of Neurosurgery, Orthopaedic Surgery &
Biomedical Engineering
Director, Neurosurgical Spine Center
Co-Director, Carnegie Center for Surgical Innovation
Department of Neurosurgery
Johns Hopkins University
Baltimore, Maryland, USA

Preface

We are delighted to present our work, *Surgery of the Thoracic Spine*, which focuses on pathologies and surgical techniques of the thoracic spinal cord and vertebral column. As advances are gained into better understanding of the physiology, biomechanics and conditions of each segment of the spine, we have produced a unique work dedicated exclusively to the thoracic spine.

We have attempted to address the most common pathologies affecting the thoracic spine, including degenerative, traumatic, oncologic and congenital diseases. Additionally, several chapters are dedicated to idiopathic and other deformities of the thoracic spinal column, including kyphosis and scoliosis. Emphasis is placed not only on pathophysiology but also on surgical technique and reconstructive strategies.

The contributors to this work bring outstanding and diverse expertise in neurosurgery and orthopedic spine surgery. We are indebted to all of them for contributing and making this text possible. We are confident that the readers, from medical trainees to practicing surgeons, will find this work valuable as they evaluate and manage patients with complex thoracic spinal pathologies.

Ali A. Baaj, MD
U. Kumar Kakarla, MD
Han Jo Kim, MD

Contributors

A. Karim Ahmed, BS
MD Candidate
Department of Neurosurgery
Johns Hopkins School of Medicine
Baltimore, Maryland, USA

Mohammed Ali Alvi, MBBS
Post-doctoral Research Fellow
Mayo Clinic Neuro-Informatics Laboratory
Department of Neurologic Surgery
Mayo Clinic
Rochester, Minnesota, USA

Ali A. Baaj, MD
Associate Professor
Co-Director, Spinal Deformity and Scoliosis Program
Department of Neurological Surgery
Weill Cornell Medical College
New York-Presbyterian Hospital
New York, New York, USA

Lila R. Baaklini, MD
Assistant Attending Anesthesiologist
Department of Anesthesiology
Hospital for Special Surgery
New York, New York, USA

Ori Barzilai, MD
Assistant Attending
Department of Neurosurgery
Memorial Sloan Kettering Cancer Center
New York, New York, USA

Elie F. Berbari, MD, FIDSA
Consultant
Chair, Division of Infectious Diseases
Professor of Medicine
Hospital Epidemiologist
Mayo Clinic College of Medicine
Mayo Clinic
Rochester, Minnesota, USA

Mark H. Bilsky, MD
Attending Neurosurgeon
Memorial Sloan Kettering Cancer Center
Professor of Neurosurgery
Weill Medical College of Cornell University
New York, New York, USA

Srikanth R. Boddu, MSc, FRCR, MD
Assistant Professor of Radiology in Neurosurgery
Department of Neurological Surgery
Weill Cornell Medical Center
New York Presbyterian Hospital Queens
New York, New York, USA

Blake M. Bodendorfer, MD
Resident
Department of Orthopaedic Surgery
Georgetown University Medical Center
Washington, DC, USA

Michael A. Bohl, MD
Resident
Department of Neurosurgery
Barrow Neurological Institute
Phoenix, Arizona, USA

Christopher M. Bono, MD
Professor, Executive Vice Chair
Department of Orthopaedic Surgery
Harvard Medical School, Massachusetts General Hospital
Boston, Massachusetts, USA

Ian A. Buchanan, MD
Resident
Department of Neurosurgery
University of Southern California
Los Angeles, California, USA

Mohamad Bydon, MD
Associate Professor
Department of Neurologic Surgery
Mayo Clinic
Rochester, Minnesota, USA

Bridget T. Carey, MD
Assistant Professor
Department of Neurology
Weill Cornell Medical College
New York, New York, USA

Steven W. Chang, MD
Associate Professor
Department of Neurosurgery
Barrow Neurological Institute
St. Joseph's Hospital and Medical Center
Phoenix, Arizona, USA

John H. Chi, MD, MPH
Associate Professor
Department of Neurosurgery
Brigham & Women's Hospital
Harvard Medical School
Boston, Massachusetts, USA

Chad M. Craig, MD, FACP
Medical Director, Spine Service
Department of Orthopedics
Division of Spine Surgery
Hospital for Special Surgery
Assistant Professor of Medicine
Weill Medical College of Cornell University
New York, New York, USA

Peter B. Derman, MD, MBA
Spine Surgeon
Texas Back Institute
Plano, Texas, USA

Atman Desai, MD
Associate Professor
Department of Neurosurgery
Stanford University
Stanford, California, USA

Dustin J. Donnelly, MD, PhD
Resident
Department of Neurosurgery
Brigham & Women's Hospital
Harvard Medical School
Boston, Massachusetts, USA

Ronald Emerson, MD
Professor of Neurology at Hospital for Special Surgery
Department of Neurology
Weill Cornell Medical College
New York, New York, USA

Brett A. Freedman, MD
Assistant Professor
Department of Orthopedic Surgery
Mayo Clinic
Rochester, Minnesota, USA

Shashank V. Gandhi, MD
Resident
Department of Neurosurgery
Hofstra-Northwell School of Medicine
Manhasset, New York, USA

Jakub Godzik, MD
Neurosurgery Resident
Department of Neurosurgery
Barrow Neurological Institute
St. Joseph's Hospital and Medical Center
Phoenix, Arizona, USA

Sandy Goncalves, MSc
Researcher
Department of Neurologic Surgery
Mayo Clinic
Rochester, Minnesota, USA

C. Rory Goodwin, MD, PhD
Director of Metastatic Spine Tumor
Assistant Professor, Departments of Neurosurgery,
  Orthopaedic Surgery
Radiation Oncology, Medicine, Pharmacology and Cancer
  Biology
Chief of Spinal Tumor Section at Durham VA Hospital
Duke University Medical Center
Durham, North Carolina, USA

Robert Harper, MD
Resident
Department of Orthopedic Surgery
UC Davis Medical Center
Sacramento, California, USA

Roger Härtl, MD
Professor, Director of Spinal Surgery
Department of Neurological Surgery
Weill Cornell Medicine
New York, New York, USA

Randall J. Hlubek, MD
Resident
Department of Neurosurgery
Barrow Neurological Institute
St. Joseph's Hospital and Medical Center
Phoenix, Arizona, USA

Allen Ho, MD
Complex Spine Fellow
Department of Neurosurgery
Stanford University
Stanford, California, USA

Patrick C. Hsieh, MD, MSc
Professor of Neurological Surgery
Edwin M. Todd/Trent H. Wells, Jr. Professor of Neurosurgery
Department of Neurological Surgery
University of Southern California Keck School of Medicine
Los Angeles, California, USA

Kevin T. Huang, MD
Resident
Department of Neurosurgery
Harvard Medical School
Brigham and Women's Hospital
Boston, Massachusetts, USA

Ibrahim Hussain, MD
Chief Resident
Department of Neurosurgery
Weill Cornell Medical College-New York
   Presbyterian Hospital
New York, New York, USA

Trong Huynh, MD
Postdoctoral Research Fellow
Department of Neurological Surgery
Rutgers New Jersey Medical School
Newark, New Jersey, USA

Sravisht Iyer, MD
Assistant Attending
Spine Surgery
Hospital for Special Surgery
New York, New York, USA

Jacob Januszewski, DO
MIS Complex Spine Deformity Surgeon
Department of Neurosurgery
The B.A.C.K Center
Melbourne, Florida, USA

U. Kumar Kakarla, MD
Director of Spinal Deformity
Department of Neurosurgery
Barrow Neurological Institute
St. Joseph's Hospital and Medical Center
Phoenix, Arizona, USA

Panagiotis Kerezoudis, MD, MS
Resident
Department of Neurological Surgery
Mayo Clinic
Rochester, Minnesota, USA

Han Jo Kim, MD
Associate Professor
Spine Fellowship Director
Department of Orthopaedic Surgery
Hospital for Special Surgery
New York, New York, USA

Eric Klineberg, MD
Professor of Orthopaedic Surgery
Co-Director Spine Center, Spine Fellowship Director
Department of Orthopaedics
University of California, Davis
Sacramento, California, USA

Jared Knopman, MD
Assistant Professor
Department of Neurosurgery
Weill Cornell Medical College
New York, New York, USA

Ilya Laufer, MD
Associate Attending Neurosurgeon, Memorial Sloan
   Kettering Cancer
Associate Professor of Neurosurgery, Weill Cornell
   Medical College
Department of Neurosurgery
Memorial Sloan Kettering Cancer Center
New York, New York, USA

Hai Le, MD
Resident
Department of Orthopaedic Surgery
Massachusetts General Hospital
Boston, Massachusetts, USA

Ronald A. Lehman Jr., MD
Professor of Orthopedic Surgery, Tenure
Chief, Reconstructive, Robotic and Minimally
   Invasive Spine
Director, Robotic Spine Surgery
Director, Athletes Spine Center
Co-Director, Comprehensive Adult and Pediatric
   Spine Fellowship
Director, Clinical Spine Research
Co-Director, Orthopedic Clinical Research
Advanced Pediatric and Adult Deformity Service
Columbia University Medical Center
Orthopedic Spine Department
The Daniel and Jane Och Spine Hospital
New York Presbyterian/The Allen Hospital
New York, New York, USA

James D. Lin, MD, MS
Spine Surgery Fellow
The Daniel and Jane Och Spine Hospital
New York-Presbyterian/Columbia University
  Medical Center
New York, New York, USA

Thomas Link, MD, MS
Department of Neurosurgery
Weill Cornell Medical Center
New York, New York, USA

Francis Lovecchio, MD
Resident
Department of Orthopaedic Surgery
Hospital for Special Surgery
New York, New York, USA

Ana Luís, MD
Spine Fellow at Weill Cornell Brain and Spine Center
Department of Neurological Surgery
Weill Cornell Medicine
New York-Presbyterian Hospital
New York, New York, USA
Department of Neurosurgery
Hospital Egas Moniz - Centro Hospitalar de Lisboa Ocidental
Lisbon, Portugal

Maj. Patrick R. Maloney, MD
USAF, David Grant Medical Center (DGMC)
Department of Neurosurgery
Travis AFB, California, USA

Rohit Mauria, BS
Department of Neurosurgery
Barrow Neurological Institute
St. Joseph's Hospital and Medical Center
Phoenix, Arizona, USA

Ziev B. Moses, MD
Resident
Department of Neurosurgery
Brigham and Women's Hospital
Harvard Medical School
Boston, Massachusetts, USA

Gregory M. Mundis Jr., MD
Co-Director San Diego Spine Fellowship
Division of Orthopedic Surgery
Scripps Clinic
San Diego, California, USA

Jonathan Nakhla, MD
Spinal Neurosurgery Instructor
Department of Neurosurgery
Brown University / Rhode Island Hospital
Providence, Rhode Island, USA

Michael J. Nanaszko, MD
Neurosurgery Resident
Department of Neurosurgery
Barrow Neurological Institute
St. Joseph's Hospital and Medical Center
Phoenix, Arizona, USA

Ahmad Nassr, MD
Professor of Orthopedic Surgery
Professor of Neurosurgery
Associate Professor of Biomedical Engineering
Department of Orthopedic Surgery
Mayo Clinic
Rochester, Minnesota, USA

Rodrigo Navarro-Ramirez, MD, MSc
Combined Orthopedic Neurosurgery Fellowship
Department of Orthopedics
McGill University
Montreal, Quebec, Canada

Athos Patsalides, MD, MPH
Associate Professor
Department of Neurosurgery
Weill Cornell Medicine
New York, New York, USA

Arjun V. Pendharkar, MD
Resident
Department of Neurosurgery
Stanford University
Palo Alto, California, USA

Zach Pennington, BS
Medical Student
Department of Neurosurgery
Johns Hopkins School of Medicine
Baltimore, Maryland, USA

Benjamin I. Rapoport, MD, PhD
Resident
Department of Neurological Surgery
New York-Presbyterian Hospital
Weill Cornell Medicine
New York, New York, USA

Alexander E. Ropper, MD
Assistant Professor
Department of Neurosurgery
Baylor College of Medicine
Houston, Texas, USA

Daniel M. Sciubba, MD
Professor of Neurosurgery, Orthopedics and Oncology
Department of Neurosurgery
Johns Hopkins University
Baltimore, Maryland, USA

Suken A. Shah, MD
Division Chief, Spine and Scoliosis Center
Clinical Fellowship Director
Nemours/Alfred I. duPont Hospital for Children
Wilmington, Delaware
Associate Professor of Orthopaedic Surgery and Pediatrics
Sidney Kimmel Medical College of Thomas Jefferson
   University
Philadelphia, Pennsylvania, USA

Evan Sheha, MD
Resident
Department of Orthopedic Surgery
Hospital for Special Surgery
New York, New York, USA

Jamal N. Shillingford, MD
Spine Surgery Fellow
Department of Orthopaedic Surgery
Department of Neurosurgery
Norton Leatherman Spine Center
University of Louisville Medical Center
Louisville, Kentucky, USA

John H. Shin, MD
Director, Spine Oncology & Spinal Deformity
   Surgery
Massachusetts General Hospital, Harvard
   Medical School
Boston, Massachusetts, USA

Navika Shukla, BA
MD Candidate
School of Medicine
Stanford University
Stanford, California, USA

Venita M. Simpson, MD
Resident
Department of Neurosurgery
Baylor College of Medicine
Houston, Texas, USA

Laura A. Snyder, MD
Director of Neurotrauma
Department of Neurosurgery
Barrow Neurological Institute
St. Joseph's Hospital and Medical Center
Phoenix, Arizona, USA

Eric S. Sussman, MD
Resident
Department of Neurosurgery
Stanford University
Stanford, California, USA

Michael E. Steinhaus, MD
Resident
Orthopaedic Surgery
Hospital for Special Surgery
New York, New York, USA

Nicholas Theodore, MD
Professor of Neurosurgery, Orthopaedic Surgery &
   Biomedical Engineering
Director, Neurosurgical Spine Center
Co-Director, Carnegie Center for Surgical Innovation
Department of Neurosurgery
Johns Hopkins University
Baltimore, Maryland, USA

Jay D. Turner, MD, PhD
Assistant Professor
Department of Neurosurgery
Barrow Neurological Institute
St. Joseph's Hospital and Medical Center
Phoenix, Arizona, USA

Michael K. Urban, MD, PhD
Medical Director
Post Anesthesia Care Units
Hospital for Special Surgery
New York, New York, USA

Juan S. Uribe, MD
Chief, Division of Spinal Disorders
Professor and Vice Chair
Volker K. H. Sonntag Chair of Spine Research
Department of Neurological Surgery
Barrow Neurological Institute
St. Joseph's Hospital and Medical Center
Phoenix, Arizona, USA

Terence Verla, MD, MPH
Department of Neurosurgery
Baylor College of Medicine
Houston, Texas, USA

Corey T. Walker, MD
Resident
Department of Neurological Surgery
Barrow Neurological Institute
St. Joseph's Hospital and Medical Center
Phoenix, Arizona, USA

Jeffrey C. Wang, MD
Chief, Orthopaedic Spine Service
Co-Director USC Spine Center
Professor of Orthopaedic Surgery and Neurosurgery USC
 Spine Center
Los Angeles, California, USA

Joshua Weaver, MD
Assistant Professor of Clinical Neurology
Department of Neurology
Weill Cornell Medical College
New York, New York, USA

Christoph Wipplinger, MD
Neurosurgical Research Fellow
Department of Neurological Surgery
Weill Cornell Medicine
New York, New York, USA

Kyle Wu, MD
Resident
Department of Neurosurgery
Brigham and Women's Hospital
Boston, Massachusetts, USA

David S. Xu, MD
Assistant Professor
Department of Neurosurgery
Baylor College of Medicine
Houston, Texas, USA

Vijay Yanamadala, MD, MBA
Assistant Professor of Neurosurgery
Director of the Center for Surgical Optimization
Leo M. Davidoff Department of Neurological
 Surgery
Albert Einstein College of Medicine
Montefiore Medical Center
New York, New York, USA

Part I

Introduction

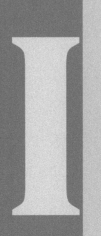

1 Pulmonary and Chest Wall Physiology

Peter B. Derman, Evan Sheha, and Chad M. Craig

Abstract

An understanding of normal and abnormal pulmonary and chest wall physiology is important for those involved in thoracic surgery. Thoracic surgery often, but not always, involves patients with significant skeletal deformities, which in turn alters the structure of the thoracic cage and influences pulmonary function. Pulmonary function tests can be useful for formally assessing baseline pulmonary lung volumes and understanding existing disease states prior to surgery, as well as in postoperative assessment of pulmonary function. Here we review scoliosis, hyperkyphosis, and ankylosing spondylitis as they relate to baseline pulmonary changes, and changes that can occur following thoracic spine surgery. Restrictive and obstructive pathologies, postoperative pulmonary function, and pulmonary complications of thoracic spine surgery in general are likewise reviewed.

Keywords: pulmonary, chest wall, thoracic wall, thoracic cage, respiratory, obstructive lung disease, restrictive lung disease, pulmonary function tests, scoliosis, ankylosing spondylitis, kyphosis

Clinical Pearls

- In patients with unexplained dyspnea, or known pulmonary or chest wall disorders, pulmonary function tests can be useful for diagnostic and prognostic purposes surrounding thoracic surgery.
- Scoliosis, age-related hyperkyphosis, and ankylosing spondylitis are all skeletal abnormalities that may be associated with significant baseline and postoperative pulmonary dysfunction.
- Restrictive lung physiology is common in patients with significant thoracic deformities.
- Preoperative assessment of restrictive and obstructive lung disease may be done through spirometry alone, or more complete lung volume measurements may be obtained through pulmonary function testing.
- The most commonly reported pulmonary complications following spine surgery include pulmonary embolism, respiratory distress, pulmonary edema, pneumothorax, pneumonia, and atelectasis.

1.1 Normal Physiology

Familiarity with normal thoracic wall and pulmonary physiology is important for understanding commonly encountered thoracic surgical issues, and for the prevention and management of associated complications. The thorax we define here as the upper portion of the trunk extending between the neck and abdomen, and includes both intrathoracic contents (heart, lungs, thymus, distal trachea, and esophagus) and the thoracic wall. The thoracic wall is a dynamic structure composed of skin, fascia, nerves, vessels, muscles, and skeletal tissue, and serves the dual function of protecting intrathoracic contents, as well as the mechanical function of respiration.[1] The primary physiological function of the lungs is to make external oxygen available for transport throughout the body, and to remove carbon dioxide that results from tissue metabolism.[2]

1.1.1 Thoracic Wall

The skeletal structure of the thoracic wall includes 12 pairs of ribs and costal cartilage, 12 thoracic vertebrae, and the sternum. The first seven of the rib pairs are vertebrocostal ribs (true ribs), attaching directly to the sternum through their own costal cartilage. Rib pairs eight through ten are vertebrochondral and are joined to the cartilage of the rib just superior to them, and have an indirect connection to the sternum. Rib pairs eleven and twelve are free floating ribs that end in the posterior abdominal musculature. Costal cartilage on anterior rib articulations provide an element of elasticity to the thoracic wall, and help prevent anterior pressure or trauma from fracturing the ribs or sternum.[1]

The 12 paired ribs collectively form a large portion of the thoracic cage structure, and contain, among other important structures, intercostal muscles that form secondary muscles of respiration. Intercostal muscle contraction leads to both superior lateral and anterior–posterior expansion of the thoracic cage. Additionally, during forced inspiration, the pectoralis major muscles may assist with expansion of the thoracic cavity, and likewise the scalene muscles that extended from the neck to the first and second ribs also function as accessory muscles to elevate these ribs during forced inspiration. These accessory muscles and intercostal muscles are *secondary* to the *primary* muscle of respiration: the diaphragm. During diaphragmatic contraction, the central portion of the diaphragm descends inferiorly, creating a negative intrathoracic pressure gradient that allows for lung expansion. During normal respiration, as well as during deep breathing, the thoracic cage moves anteriorly, superiorly, and laterally, collectively increasing intrathoracic volume. The anterior–posterior diameter of the thorax can be further increased by straightening the back. During passive expiration, the intercostal muscles and diaphragm relax, resulting in increased intrathoracic pressure, and lung tissue that was previously expanded and stretched then recoils, and collectively this results in expiration of air.[1]

The lungs sit within the thoracic cage covered by visceral pleural, and inflate and deflate in response to changes in volume of the semirigid thoracic cage in which they are suspended.[2] There are upper and lower lung lobes bilaterally, and the right lung also contains a middle lobe, whereas the left lung contains a lingula. All lung lobes are covered by visceral pleura, which abuts against either other lung tissue (where lung fissures exist), or the inner lining of the thoracic wall which is the parietal pleura. In between the visceral and parietal pleural lining exists a potential space with a normally negative pressure gradient that assists with lung expansion as the thoracic wall expands. This potential space is the pleural space and can fill (often partially) with air, fluid, and other inflammatory mediators during different pathological states. In its normal state the pleural space is thin, contains a minimal amount of fluid, and allows lung tissue to slide easily along the chest wall during lung inflation and deflation.

1.1.2 Pulmonary Function

The amount of air inspired into the bilateral lungs ranges normally from 4 L/min at rest to up to 100 L/min during maximum exercise.[2] Lung volume measurements are traditionally obtained through pulmonary function testing (PFT), and key PFT measurements to be familiar with include total lung capacity (TLC), inspiratory capacity (IC), expiratory reserve volume, residual volume (RV), forced vital capacity (FVC), forced expiratory volume in 1 second (FEV_1), and maximal voluntary ventilation (MVV). These are listed in ▸ Table 1.1 along with some other common measurements obtained during PFT that can be helpful for understanding normal versus pathological states. Note that lung capacities are composed of two or more lung volumes. PFT measurements are used often when evaluating unexplained dyspnea, severity of known pulmonary disease states, and preoperatively prior to thoracic surgery to provide baseline measurements, especially when baseline pulmonary

Table 1.1 Pulmonary function measurements

Total lung capacity (TLC)	Volume in the lungs at maximal inhalation, or the sum of VC and RV
Tidal volume (TV)	Volume of air moved into or out of the lungs during quiet breathing
Inspiratory capacity (IC)	Sum of IRV and TV
Inspiratory reserve volume (IRV)	Maximal volume of air that can be inhaled from the end-inspiratory position
Expiratory reserve volume (ERV)	Maximal volume of air that can be exhaled from the end-expiratory position
Residual volume (RV)	Volume of air remaining in the lungs after maximal exhalation
Vital capacity (VC)	Volume of air exhaled following maximal inhalation
Inspiratory vital capacity (IVC)	Maximum volume of air inhaled from the point of maximum expiration
Forced vital capacity (FVC)	Vital capacity from a maximally forced expiratory effort
Forced expiratory volume in one second (FEV1)	Volume of air exhaled at the end of the first second of forced expiration
Functional residual capacity (FRC)	Volume in the lungs at the end-expiratory position (at the end of a resting tidal breath)
Maximal voluntary ventilation (MVV)	Volume of air expired in a specified period during repetitive maximal effort
Diffusing capacity for carbon monoxide (DLCO)	Diffusing capacity of carbon monoxide from lung alveolar space into the blood, used as a proxy for assessing the extent to which oxygen passes from the alveolar space into the blood
RV/TLC%	Residual volume expressed as a percent of TLC
Peek expiratory flow (PEF)	Highest forced expiratory flow measured with a peak flow meter

dysfunction is suspected. Adequate patient effort is important when interpreting results of PFTs, and can be assessed by examining flow-volume loops that graph expiratory and inspiratory airflow against volume. Spirometry measurements, which are a subcomponent of PFTs, examine VC, FVC, FEV_1, and MVV, and can provide such flow-volume loop diagrams. Spirometry measurements are provided in actual liters of air measured, as well as given as percentages predicted of comparison population norms.

PFTs when abnormal can be broadly grouped into obstructive or restrictive processes, although many disease states involve elements of both. Reduction in TLC (< 80%) is indicative of restrictive lung disease. Such restriction can be external to the lung parenchyma, due to compression from severe obesity, scoliosis, or secondary to neuromuscular weakness. Restriction can alternatively be due to intrinsic lung pathology such as pulmonary fibrosis, among other disease states. Obstructive lung disease involves airflow obstruction (defined as FEV_1/FVC ratio of < 70%), and includes common conditions such as asthma and chronic obstructive pulmonary disease (COPD). Asthma involves reversible airflow obstruction (i.e., there is some improvement noted following inhalation of a bronchodilator) versus COPD which is generally nonreversible. Although again, even these conditions can overlap, such as with asthma–COPD overlap syndrome, where there are components of reversibility and nonreversibility.

The diffusing capacity of the lungs for carbon monoxide (DLCO) measures gas exchange at the alveolar level across the alveolar–capillary membrane. Measurement of DLCO is done during PFTs and entails inhaling a very low concentration of carbon monoxide and subsequently measuring the amount of carbon monoxide exhaled to infer the amount that was exchanged at the alveolar–capillary membrane. Disease states resulting in low DLCO measurements include vasculitis, pulmonary embolism, pulmonary hypertension, pulmonary fibrosis, and emphysema in which there is decreased alveolar surface area, and restrictive lung disease in which there is decrease in total lung area. Carbon monoxide uptake within capillaries is dependent on the presence of hemoglobin, and thus disease states with low or abnormal hemoglobin may be associated with abnormally low DLCO measurements independent of pulmonary pathology.[3]

1.2 Abnormalities Associated with Common Spinal Pathologies

1.2.1 Scoliosis

Scoliosis is the most common spinal disorder which directly impacts the thoracic cage. It is generally thought to cause a restrictive pattern of lung dysfunction with decreased TLC. However, significant reductions in lung volume do not typically manifest until spinal deformity becomes more severe (▸ Table 1.2). Other factors, such as loss of thoracic kyphosis, cephalad curve location, vertebral rotation, and greater number of involved vertebrae also contribute to diminished TLC.[4,5] These factors result in a loss of thoracic cage volume[6,7] and a chest wall that is less compliant,[8] thereby increasing the work of breathing. Pulmonary hypertension and chronic respiratory

Table 1.2 Scoliosis severity and clinical manifestations

Cobb's angle	Potential clinical findings
<10°	None
>25°	Possible pulmonary artery pressure increase on echocardiogram
>70°	Likely significant decreased pulmonary volume
>100°	Dyspnea with exertion
>120°	Likely alveolar hypoventilation, chronic respiratory failure

Source: Data from Koumbourlis.[12]

failure may develop in scoliosis patients with severe deformities.[9] Pulmonary hypertension, especially when severe, is particularly poor prognostic factor for perioperative morbidity and mortality, and is an important factor to identify preoperatively. This can be done noninvasively via echocardiogram measurements, which provides an estimation, or performed invasively for more accurate measurements via right heart catheterization. In the case of early-onset scoliosis, the presence of thoracic deformity during the time of rapid lung development may result in true pulmonary hypoplasia, further compounding respiratory deficits and potentially resulting in thoracic insufficiency syndrome (an inability of the thorax to support normal respiration and lung growth).[10,11]

The typical PFT profile of a patient with scoliosis is one of diminished TLC and IC with less of a deleterious effect on RV and functional residual capacity (FRC).[13,14] As such, the RV:TLC ratio is frequently elevated. An elevated RV:TLC ratio is traditionally viewed as evidence of obstructive airway disease; however, in patients with scoliosis this is not necessarily the case, and an elevated ratio is usually more reflective of diminished TLC specifically. Airway resistance may be increased because of distortion caused by chest wall deformity and by chronic airway inflammation due to inadequate clearance of secretions.[15,16] This predisposes patients, especially those with neuromuscular disease, to pneumonia.[13] Ventilation/perfusion mismatch has also been shown to occur with scoliosis.[17,18] This may explain the mild hypoxemia with normocapnia observed in many patients with scoliosis.[9,14] With severe deformities, however, hypercapnia develops and may limit the response to carbon dioxide,[4,19,20,21] resulting in sleep-disordered breathing.[22]

During exercise or stress, patients with significant scoliosis attempt to increase minute ventilation (the volume of gas inhaled or exhaled from the lungs per minute) via an elevated respiratory rate rather than an increased tidal volume. Work of breathing is further increased as the dead space must be exchanged with each shallow breath. This compensatory mechanism is particularly ineffective in patients with neuromuscular scoliosis as they are at an elevated risk of muscle fatigue and respiratory failure.[13] It has also been observed that exercise capacity may even be diminished in patients with milder curves.[23,24]

1.2.2 Ankylosing Spondylitis

Ankylosing spondylitis (AS) is an inflammatory condition that typically affects the sacroiliac joints first, then moves rostral along the spine, and involves the chest wall later in the course

of the disease.[13,25] It produces eventual ankyloses of the spine and sternocostal joints as well as rib cartilage calcification.[26] The spine assumes a position of rigid hyperkyphosis with the thoracic cage fixed in the inspiratory position.[27] In addition to structural abnormalities, AS may directly affect the lungs, typically via interstitial disease.[28] While it is unusual for parenchymal lung involvement to directly produce clinically significant changes in pulmonary function, it may predispose patients to infection and pneumothorax.[29]

PFT in the setting of AS reveals a restrictive pattern combined with hyperinflation. Vital capacity is diminished in proportion to the severity of disease, while FRC and RV are normal or elevated in the setting of air trapping.[29] Increased diaphragmatic and abdominal wall movements compensate for diminished thoracic cage mobility.[30,31,32,33,34] Small airway obstruction caused by interstitial lung disease may also be present.[35,36,37] Arterial blood gasses and DLCO tend to be normal unless the lung involvement is severe.[13] The literature is mixed on whether thoracic involvement in AS adversely effects exercise tolerance.[37,38,39,40,41]

1.2.3 Age-Related Hyperkyphosis

The saying "age is a kyphosing process" reflects the tendency of degenerative changes in the spine to produce increasing kyphosis over time.[42] Mean thoracic kyphosis increases from approximately 25 degrees in people age 18 to 29, to 65 degrees in those aged 75 and older,[43] with women more rapidly affected than men.[44] Between 20 and 45% of older adults exhibit hyperkyphosis,[45] typically defined as a thoracic kyphosis angle exceeding 40 degrees.[44,46] Osteoporosis-related vertebral compression fractures often play a role in the development of kyphosis—each vertebral compression fracture contributes an average of 3.8 degrees toward overall thoracic kyphosis.[47] Anterior intervertebral disc wedging from thoracic degenerative disc disease,[47,48,49,50] loss of paraspinal muscle strength,[51,52] and general deconditioning[53] are also associated with increased thoracic kyphosis.

Thoracic hyperkyphosis results in diminished chest size and impaired thoracic cage mobility.[13] Patients may exhibit moderate reductions in pulmonary function consistent with restrictive and obstructive physiology.[54,55,56,57] FVC declines with increased kyphosis.[58] In fact, patients experience an average 9% decrease in VC for each vertebral compression fracture.[55] Osteoporotic fractures of the ribs and sternum in this patient population may exacerbate these findings,[59] especially during the acute postinjury period when pain limits breathing ability. Hyperkyphotic posture, especially more severe deformities, are associated with increased pulmonary-related and all-cause mortality.[45,60,61]

1.3 Nonoperative Pulmonary Management and Considerations

No specific respiratory therapy is necessary for patients with mild-to-moderate scoliosis as their pulmonary pathology is not typically clinically significant.[12] However, pediatric patients with such curves may undergo bracing as a means of delaying or preventing surgery. These braces may iatrogenically decrease lung volume and compliance, but this is usually well tolerated by patients with relatively normal pulmonary function. Conversely, patients with baseline severe restrictive lung pathology may not tolerate the additional restriction imposed by a brace.[12,62]

Based on older studies from the 1950s to 1970s, patients with severe scoliosis and chronic respiratory failure are at increased risk of premature mortality.[63,64] Noninvasive positive pressure ventilation (NIPPV) has been shown to improve survival in these individuals.[65] Because of the tendency for sleep apnea in this patient population, sleep studies may be indicated in patients with severe scoliosis even in the setting of normal awake blood oxygen saturation.[12] Nighttime NIPPV use is typically instituted prior to daytime use. Airway clearance devices have been used with some success in the setting of neuromuscular diseases, but their effectiveness in idiopathic and degenerative scoliosis has not been well documented.[12]

Exercise, to the extent that it is safe and feasible, should be recommended to patients with spinal pathology to improve their overall cardiopulmonary status.[37,39,66,67] Preoperative respiratory therapy and incentive spirometry use have been shown to improve pulmonary function in patients with baseline deficits.[68] Smoking cessation, when applicable, should be encouraged.[29] When possible, treatment of underlying pathology (e.g., disease-modifying antirheumatic drugs for AS, and bisphosphonates or teriparatide for osteoporosis) is advisable to slow disease progression.[69,70,71,72]

1.4 Preoperative Evaluation

A detailed history should be obtained and a thorough physical examination performed on all patients undergoing thoracic spine surgery. Chest expansion can be measured in the office, and signs of hypoventilation such as finger clubbing can be easily observed.[29] Lung auscultation may suggest pulmonary fibrosis or wheezing and prompt further workup. A chest radiograph is routinely obtained, and is useful for a global assessment of chest anatomy. Inspiratory and expiratory chest radiographs can be useful if baseline unilateral diaphragmatic paralysis is suspected.[1] Advanced imaging with high-resolution noncontrast computed tomography (CT) of the chest and/or PFTs should be considered in patients with active dyspnea complaints or severe deformity. The presence of elevated hemoglobin on standard laboratory testing may alert the provider to the presence of hypoventilation and spur further workup as well.[73]

No standardized guidelines on the appropriateness of obtaining PFTs prior to surgery currently exist, especially in relation to spinal surgery. While preoperative PFTs have not consistently been shown to directly correlate with postoperative pulmonary complications in patients with scoliosis,[74] preoperative pulmonary function assessment including overnight oximetry and TLC may be considered to roughly stratify patients' pulmonary risk prior to surgery.[12,14,16] Maximum inspiratory and expiratory pressures measuring less than 30 cm H_2O and an FVC below 40% of the predicted normal value are associated with significant increases in the risk of prolonged postoperative intubation.[12] Unfortunately, pediatric patients are not always capable of participating in standard PFTs, and preoperative polysomnography and infant pulmonary function testing have not been shown to be reliable predictors of postoperative pulmonary complications in such younger patients.[75]

Identification of patients with known obstructive sleep apnea (OSA), as well as those at high risk for OSA, is important preoperatively. OSA is a chronic condition involving varying degrees of airway collapse during sleep, and is associated with higher rates of cardiopulmonary diseases in general. Interestingly, identification of such patients preoperatively and associated changes in perioperative management have not clearly been associated with improved perioperative outcomes. However, we observe that such patients often have a tenuous respiratory state in the immediate postextubation period, and in combination with thoracic surgery resulting in changes in thoracic wall and pulmonary physiology, we believe these patients warrant close observation in a monitored setting often for the first 24 hours postextubation.[76]

1.5 Complications and Postoperative Management

Pulmonary complications following spinal fusion are common. Major complications including pulmonary embolism, respiratory distress, pulmonary edema, pneumothorax, pneumonia, and atelectasis are the most commonly reported complications.[77,78,79] Large database studies have reported national rates of pulmonary complications following surgery for idiopathic scoliosis between 8 and 10% for patients of all ages.[80] In general, pulmonary embolism is a rare complication with a reported incidence of less than 1% nationally after any spine surgery, although occurs more frequently in thoracic spine surgery relative to cervical or lumbar, and more frequently following vertebral fractures or increasing number of operated levels.[81,82] Preexisting lung disease including chronic obstructive or restrictive lung disease, pulmonary arterial or venous hypertension, and thoracoplasty have been shown to be predictors of postoperative complications in general.[74] Multicenter prospective data on the incidence and risk factors for medical complications after adult spinal deformity surgery demonstrated an incidence of medical complications reaching 26.8%, half of which were cardiopulmonary in nature. Risk factors in this data set for complications included smoking, hypertension, and duration of symptoms related to a patient's spinal pathology.[83] Additionally, combined sequential anterior-posterior procedures and prolonged surgery with large blood loss have also been associated with higher rates of pulmonary complications.[79,84] Infectious complications are generally more common following posterior spinal approaches than anterior approaches.[85]

Patients with neuromuscular scoliosis often have impaired pulmonary function secondary to muscular weakness, and as such have a much higher risk of pulmonary complications following scoliosis surgery. Similar to the general population with idiopathic scoliosis, common complications include pleural effusion, pneumothorax, and pneumonia, though these have been observed to occur at much higher rates. Up to 50% of patients will experience a pulmonary complication according to one study, and 16% required prolonged intubation and mechanical ventilation.[86] PFTs in children following scoliosis surgery have been shown to decrease by as much as 60% in the immediate postoperative period; this observed postoperative decrease has been attributed to pain, immobilization, and postoperative narcotic regimens that suppress the respiratory drive.[87] Regardless of the etiology of decreased pulmonary function preoperatively, it has been observed that patients demonstrating less than 40% of the predicted value of FVC preoperatively on PFTs in the setting of neuromuscular scoliosis may require prolonged postoperative mechanical ventilation and should be considered an at-risk group for pulmonary complications.[88,89] Similarly, patients with higher intraoperative blood loss per kilogram of body weight, poor FVC, and larger curves are predisposed to pulmonary complications and should be given special consideration.[86,90]

Spinal fusion has been shown to decrease but not halt the rates of pulmonary function decline in patients with spinal muscular atrophy (SMA) and Duchenne's muscular dystrophy (DMD).[91,92] Patients with SMA II have also reported decreased rates of respiratory infection following surgery.[92] Given the relative maintenance of postoperative PFT values after spinal fusion in patients with SMA and DMD many such patients may be safely operated on even in the setting of severely decreased preoperative vital capacity if the appropriate perioperative measures are taken to ensure an optimal outcome.[93,94]

Pediatric patients undergoing spinal fusion, especially those with underlying chronic conditions, are at risk for postoperative pulmonary complications. Patients undergoing prolonged procedures with anticipated massive blood loss, large transfusion requirement, and the accompanying fluid shifts may need to remain intubated for extended periods of time, and if unable to be weaned from ventilation within a reasonable time period may occasionally require tracheostomy.[89,95] Preoperative halo gravity traction has been shown to increase preoperative vital capacity; and optimization of preoperative nutrition, including feeding tube placement where applicable, may help to improve postoperative work of breathing.[96,97] Perioperative noninvasive positive pressure ventilation training and continued use after extubation may decrease the incidence of respiratory complications in patients with underlying neuromuscular disorders.[98] Early involvement of respiratory therapists in the multidisciplinary team and teaching patients or their families simple and appropriate means of addressing postoperative atelectasis, including early ambulation, encouraging incentive spirometry, and teaching breath stacking techniques, has been shown to decrease the time on supplemental oxygen in patients with underlying chronic medical conditions.[99,100] Frequent suctioning, chest physiotherapy, and oscillating vests after surgery may also decrease the risk of pulmonary complications if able to be tolerated by the patient.[89]

1.6 Postoperative Changes

Early literature evaluating postoperative changes in pulmonary function after scoliosis surgery report a significant decrease in lung compliance, vital capacity, and the ventilation/perfusion ratio in the immediate postoperative period.[101] This has been shown to reach a nadir at approximately 3 days postoperatively.[87] Similarly, midterm results failed to reveal any demonstrable and reliable clinically significant difference in PFTs with some groups demonstrating improvement, many returning to their preoperative baseline, and others deteriorating significantly.[102,103,104] Notably, early studies were performed in an era when postoperative protocols commonly involved chest wall-restricting Risser casting for prolonged periods of time after

surgery which has been shown to impair tidal respiration.[105,106] Postoperative casting and compliance with testing in the immediate postoperative period may be confounders to the accurate measurement of true lung volume after correction of scoliosis. In one recent study measuring lung volumes using three-dimensional CT, which sought to circumvent these issues related to performing PFTs in children, patients with lower preoperative FEV$_1$ and FVC were more likely to see an increase in total lung volume postoperatively, though by and large patients' lung volumes decreased.[107] Ultimately, at long-term follow-up greater than 2 years after surgery, several studies have shown that pulmonary function approaches and even at times surpasses preoperative values, though this may also occur as early as 1 to 2 months postoperatively.[87,108,109,110,111]

1.6.1 Anterior Approach

The anterior approach during spinal fusion carries the additional morbidity of violation of the chest wall and thus patients may see an expectedly greater decrease in early PFTs and longer duration to return to preoperative values.[108] An early study comparing anterior and posterior-only approaches in adolescent idiopathic scoliosis found that while both approaches demonstrated an initial expected decrease in vital capacity, vital capacity in patients undergoing the anterior approach remained significantly decreased (45% of preoperative values) 1 week after surgery compared to patients undergoing posterior-only approaches (78%). Moreover, inspiratory muscle strength was also decreased (56% of preoperative) though not significantly compared to the posterior approach.[112] Thoracoplasty performed to free tethers of the chest wall, for autogenous bone graft, as well as for cosmetic purposes in the setting of rib hump deformity during posterior spinal fusion has not been shown to have a positive effect on short- and long-term pulmonary function in adolescents, and may in fact lead to a residual decline in adult patients at 2 years after surgery.[113] However, patients who have violation of the chest wall through thoracoplasty during posterior procedures or during anterior thoracotomy will demonstrate complete or near return to preoperative values by 2-year follow-up, though they may not demonstrate the increases in PFTs often seen in patients undergoing posterior-only fusion.[109,114] In patients undergoing anterior procedures under the age of 15, the percent predicted values for FVC, FEV$_1$, and TLC may remain persistently and significantly lower than preoperative values, and special consideration should be given to the necessity of anterior procedures in the skeletally immature patient.[109]

References

[1] Moore KL, Agur AM, eds. Essential Clinical Anatomy. 2nd ed. Baltimore, MD: Lippincott Williams & Wilkins; 2002

[2] McPhee SJ, Lingappa VR, Ganong WF, Lange JD, eds. Pathophysiology of Disease: An Introduction to Clinical Medicine. 3rd ed. New York, NY: McGraw-Hill Companies; 2000

[3] Daniels CE, Eisenstaedt RS, eds. Medical Knowledge Self-Assessment Program 16: Pulmonary and Critical Care Medicine. Philadelphia, PA: American College of Physicians; 2012

[4] Kearon C, Viviani GR, Kirkley A, Killian KJ. Factors determining pulmonary function in adolescent idiopathic thoracic scoliosis. Am Rev Respir Dis. 1993; 148(2):288–294

[5] Upadhyay SS, Mullaji AB, Luk KD, Leong JC. Evaluation of deformities and pulmonary function in adolescent idiopathic right thoracic scoliosis. Eur Spine J. 1995; 4(5):274–279

[6] Chun EM, Suh SW, Modi HN, Kang EY, Hong SJ, Song HR. The change in ratio of convex and concave lung volume in adolescent idiopathic scoliosis: a 3D CT scan based cross sectional study of effect of severity of curve on convex and concave lung volumes in 99 cases. Eur Spine J. 2008; 17(2):224–229

[7] Upadhyay SS, Mullaji AB, Luk KD, Leong JC. Relation of spinal and thoracic cage deformities and their flexibilities with altered pulmonary functions in adolescent idiopathic scoliosis. Spine. 1995; 20(22):2415–2420

[8] Kotani T, Minami S, Takahashi K, et al. An analysis of chest wall and diaphragm motions in patients with idiopathic scoliosis using dynamic breathing MRI. Spine. 2004; 29(3):298–302

[9] Kafer ER. Respiratory and cardiovascular functions in scoliosis. Bull Eur Physiopathol Respir. 1977; 13(2):299–321

[10] Campbell RM, Jr, Smith MD, Mayes TC, et al. The characteristics of thoracic insufficiency syndrome associated with fused ribs and congenital scoliosis. J Bone Joint Surg Am. 2003; 85-A(3):399–408

[11] Redding GJ, Mayer OH. Structure-respiration function relationships before and after surgical treatment of early-onset scoliosis. Clin Orthop Relat Res. 2011; 469(5):1330–1334

[12] Koumbourlis AC. Scoliosis and the respiratory system. Paediatr Respir Rev. 2006; 7(2):152–160

[13] Donath J, Miller A. Restrictive chest wall disorders. Semin Respir Crit Care Med. 2009; 30(3):275–292

[14] Tsiligiannis T, Grivas T. Pulmonary function in children with idiopathic scoliosis. Scoliosis. 2012; 7(1):7

[15] Al-Kattan K, Simonds A, Chung KF, Kaplan DK. Kyphoscoliosis and bronchial torsion. Chest. 1997; 111(4):1134–1137

[16] Borowitz D, Armstrong D, Cerny F. Relief of central airways obstruction following spinal release in a patient with idiopathic scoliosis. Pediatr Pulmonol. 2001; 31(1):86–88

[17] Secker-Walker RH, Ho JE, Gill IS. Observations on regional ventilation and perfusion in kyphoscoliosis. Respiration. 1979; 38(4):194–203

[18] Redding G, Song K, Inscore S, Effmann E, Campbell R. Lung function asymmetry in children with congenital and infantile scoliosis. Spine J. 2008; 8(4):639–644

[19] Kafer ER. Idiopathic scoliosis. Mechanical properties of the respiratory system and the ventilatory response to carbon dioxide. J Clin Invest. 1975; 55(6):1153–1163

[20] Weber B, Smith JP, Briscoe WA, Friedman SA, King TK. Pulmonary function in asymptomatic adolescents with idiopathic scoliosis. Am Rev Respir Dis. 1975; 111(4):389–397

[21] Lisboa C, Moreno R, Fava M, Ferretti R, Cruz E. Inspiratory muscle function in patients with severe kyphoscoliosis. Am Rev Respir Dis. 1985; 132(1):48–52

[22] Striegl A, Chen ML, Kifle Y, Song K, Redding G. Sleep-disordered breathing in children with thoracic insufficiency syndrome. Pediatr Pulmonol. 2010; 45(5):469–474

[23] Alves VL, Avanzi O. Objective assessment of the cardiorespiratory function of adolescents with idiopathic scoliosis through the six-minute walk test. Spine. 2009; 34(25):E926–E929

[24] Martínez-Llorens J, Ramírez M, Colomina MJ, et al. Muscle dysfunction and exercise limitation in adolescent idiopathic scoliosis. Eur Respir J. 2010; 36(2):393–400

[25] Fournié B, Boutes A, Dromer C, et al. Prospective study of anterior chest wall involvement in ankylosing spondylitis and psoriatic arthritis. Rev Rhum Engl Ed. 1997; 64(1):22–25

[26] Guglielmi G, Scalzo G, Cascavilla A, Salaffi F, Grassi W. Imaging of the seronegative anterior chest wall (ACW) syndromes. Clin Rheumatol. 2008; 27(7):815–821

[27] McCool F. Dennis. Diseases of the Diaphragm, Chest Wall, Pleura, and Mediastinum. In: Goldman L, Schaffer A, eds. Goldman-Cecil Medicine. 25th ed. Philadelphia, PA: Elsevier Saunders; 2016:613

[28] Altin R, Ozdolap S, Savranlar A, et al. Comparison of early and late pleuropulmonary findings of ankylosing spondylitis by high-resolution computed tomography and effects on patients' daily life. Clin Rheumatol. 2005; 24(1):22–28

[29] El Maghraoui A, Chaouir S, Abid A, et al. Lung findings on thoracic high-resolution computed tomography in patients with ankylosing spondylitis. Correlations with disease duration, clinical findings and pulmonary function testing. Clin Rheumatol. 2004; 23(2):123–128

[30] Grimby G, Fugl-Meyer AR, Blomstrand A. Partitioning of the contributions of rib cage and abdomen to ventilation in ankylosing spondylitis. Thorax. 1974; 29(2):179–184

[31] Romagnoli I, Gigliotti F, Galarducci A, et al. Chest wall kinematics and respiratory muscle action in ankylosing spondylitis patients. Eur Respir J. 2004; 24(3):453–460

[32] Ragnarsdottir M, Geirsson AJ, Gudbjornsson B. Rib cage motion in ankylosing spondylitis patients: a pilot study. Spine. 2008; 8(3):505–509

[33] Josenhans WT, Wang CS, Josenhans G, Woodbury JF. Diaphragmatic contribution to ventilation in patients with ankylosing spondylitis. Respiration. 1971; 28(4):331–346

[34] Ferrigno G, Carnevali P. Principal component analysis of chest wall movement in selected pathologies. Med Biol Eng Comput. 1998; 36(4):445–451

[35] Ayhan-Ardic FF, Oken O, Yorgancioglu ZR, Ustun N, Gokharman FD. Pulmonary involvement in lifelong non-smoking patients with rheumatoid arthritis and ankylosing spondylitis without respiratory symptoms. Clin Rheumatol. 2006; 25(2):213–218

[36] Feltelius N, Hedenström H, Hillerdal G, Hällgren R. Pulmonary involvement in ankylosing spondylitis. Ann Rheum Dis. 1986; 45(9):736–740

[37] Fisher LR, Cawley MI, Holgate ST. Relation between chest expansion, pulmonary function, and exercise tolerance in patients with ankylosing spondylitis. Ann Rheum Dis. 1990; 49(11):921–925

[38] Van der Esch M, van't Hul AJ, Heijmans M, Dekker J. Respiratory muscle performance as a possible determinant of exercise capacity in patients with ankylosing spondylitis. Aust J Physiother. 2004; 50(1):41–45

[39] Seçkin U, Bölükbasi N, Gürsel G, Eröz S, Sepici V, Ekim N. Relationship between pulmonary function and exercise tolerance in patients with ankylosing spondylitis. Clin Exp Rheumatol. 2000; 18(4):503–506

[40] Elliott CG, Hill TR, Adams TE, Crapo RO, Nietrzeba RM, Gardner RM. Exercise performance of subjects with ankylosing spondylitis and limited chest expansion. Bull Eur Physiopathol Respir. 1985; 21(4):363–368

[41] Carter R, Riantawan P, Banham SW, Sturrock RD. An investigation of factors limiting aerobic capacity in patients with ankylosing spondylitis. Respir Med. 1999; 93(10):700–708

[42] Milne JS, Lauder IJ. Age effects in kyphosis and lordosis in adults. Ann Hum Biol. 1974; 1(3):327–337

[43] Boyle JJ, Milne N, Singer KP. Influence of age on cervicothoracic spinal curvature: an ex vivo radiographic survey. Clin Biomech (Bristol, Avon). 2002; 17(5):361–367

[44] Fon GT, Pitt MJ, Thies AC, Jr. Thoracic kyphosis: range in normal subjects. AJR Am J Roentgenol. 1980; 134(5):979–983

[45] Kado DM, Huang MH, Karlamangla AS, Barrett-Connor E, Greendale GA. Hyperkyphotic posture predicts mortality in older community-dwelling men and women: a prospective study. J Am Geriatr Soc. 2004; 52(10):1662–1667

[46] Katzman WB, Wanek L, Shepherd JA, Sellmeyer DE. Age-related hyperkyphosis: its causes, consequences, and management. J Orthop Sports Phys Ther. 2010; 40(6):352–360

[47] Kado DM, Huang MH, Karlamangla AS, et al. Factors associated with kyphosis progression in older women: 15 years' experience in the study of osteoporotic fractures. J Bone Miner Res. 2013; 28(1):179–187

[48] Schneider DL, von Mühlen D, Barrett-Connor E, Sartoris DJ. Kyphosis does not equal vertebral fractures: the Rancho Bernardo study. J Rheumatol. 2004; 31(4):747–752

[49] Goh S, Price RI, Leedman PJ, Singer KP. The relative influence of vertebral body and intervertebral disc shape on thoracic kyphosis. Clin Biomech (Bristol, Avon). 1999; 14(7):439–448

[50] Manns RA, Haddaway MJ, McCall IW, Cassar Pullicino V, Davie MW. The relative contribution of disc and vertebral morphometry to the angle of kyphosis in asymptomatic subjects. Clin Radiol. 1996; 51(4):258–262

[51] Itoi E, Sinaki M. Effect of back-strengthening exercise on posture in healthy women 49 to 65 years of age. Mayo Clin Proc. 1994; 69(11):1054–1059

[52] Sinaki M, Itoi E, Rogers JW, Bergstralh EJ, Wahner HW. Correlation of back extensor strength with thoracic kyphosis and lumbar lordosis in estrogen-deficient women. Am J Phys Med Rehabil. 1996; 75(5):370–374

[53] Balzini L, Vannucchi L, Benvenuti F, et al. Clinical characteristics of flexed posture in elderly women. J Am Geriatr Soc. 2003; 51(10):1419–1426

[54] Lombardi I, Jr, Oliveira LM, Mayer AF, Jardim JR, Natour J. Evaluation of pulmonary function and quality of life in women with osteoporosis. Osteoporos Int. 2005; 16(10):1247–1253

[55] Harrison RA, Siminoski K, Vethanayagam D, Majumdar SR. Osteoporosis-related kyphosis and impairments in pulmonary function: a systematic review. J Bone Miner Res. 2007; 22(3):447–457

[56] Schlaich C, Minne HW, Bruckner T, et al. Reduced pulmonary function in patients with spinal osteoporotic fractures. Osteoporos Int. 1998; 8(3):261–267

[57] Di Bari M, Chiarlone M, Matteuzzi D, et al. Thoracic kyphosis and ventilatory dysfunction in unselected older persons: an epidemiological study in Dicomano, Italy. J Am Geriatr Soc. 2004; 52(6):909–915

[58] Leech JA, Dulberg C, Kellie S, Pattee L, Gay J. Relationship of lung function to severity of osteoporosis in women. Am Rev Respir Dis. 1990; 141(1):68–71

[59] Ragucci M, Vainrib A. Pulmonary rehabilitation for restrictive lung impairment secondary to osteoporotic sternal fracture: a case report. Arch Phys Med Rehabil. 2005; 86(7):1487–1488

[60] Kado DM, Browner WS, Palermo L, Nevitt MC, Genant HK, Cummings SR, Study of Osteoporotic Fractures Research Group. Vertebral fractures and mortality in older women: a prospective study. Arch Intern Med. 1999; 159 (11):1215–1220

[61] Kado DM, Lui LY, Ensrud KE, Fink HA, Karlamangla AS, Cummings SR, Study of Osteoporotic Fractures. Hyperkyphosis predicts mortality independent of vertebral osteoporosis in older women. Ann Intern Med. 2009; 150(10): 681–687

[62] Tangsrud SE, Carlsen KC, Lund-Petersen I, Carlsen KH. Lung function measurements in young children with spinal muscle atrophy; a cross sectional survey on the effect of position and bracing. Arch Dis Child. 2001; 84(6): 521–524

[63] Bergofsky EH, Turino GM, Fishman AP. Cardiorespiratory failure in kyphoscoliosis. Medicine (Baltimore). 1959; 38:263–317

[64] Zorab PA, Harrison A. Mortality in severe scoliosis. Mater Med Pol. 1978; 10 (3):177–179

[65] Buyse B, Meersseman W, Demedts M. Treatment of chronic respiratory failure in kyphoscoliosis: oxygen or ventilation? Eur Respir J. 2003; 22(3):525–528

[66] Renno ACM, Granito RN, Driusso P, et al. Effects of an exercise program on respiratory function, posture and on quality of life in osteoporotic women: a pilot study. Physiotherapy. 2005; 91(2):113–118

[67] Fuschillo S, De Felice A, Martucci M, et al. Pulmonary rehabilitation improves exercise capacity in subjects with kyphoscoliosis and severe respiratory impairment. Respir Care. 2015; 60(1):96–101

[68] Lee JW, Won YH, Kim DH, et al. Pulmonary rehabilitation to decrease perioperative risks of spinal fusion for patients with neuromuscular scoliosis and low vital capacity. Eur J Phys Rehabil Med. 2016; 52(1):28–35

[69] Maxwell LJ, Zochling J, Boonen A, et al. TNF-alpha inhibitors for ankylosing spondylitis. Cochrane Database Syst Rev. 2015; 18(4):CD005468

[70] Seo MR, Baek HL, Yoon HH, et al. Delayed diagnosis is linked to worse outcomes and unfavourable treatment responses in patients with axial spondyloarthritis. Clin Rheumatol. 2015; 34(8):1397–1405

[71] Cummings SR, Black DM, Thompson DE, et al. Effect of alendronate on risk of fracture in women with low bone density but without vertebral fractures: results from the Fracture Intervention Trial. JAMA. 1998; 280(24):2077–2082

[72] Chaudhary N, Lee JS, Wu JY, Tharin S. Evidence for use of teriparatide in spinal fusion surgery in osteoporotic patients. World Neurosurg. 2017; 100: 551–556

[73] Caubet JF, Emans JB, Smith JT, et al. Increased hemoglobin levels in patients with early onset scoliosis: prevalence and effect of a treatment with Vertical Expandable Prosthetic Titanium Rib (VEPTR). Spine(Phila Pa 1976). 2009; 34 (23):2534–2536

[74] Liang J, Qiu G, Shen J, et al. Predictive factors of postoperative pulmonary complications in scoliotic patients with moderate or severe pulmonary dysfunction. J Spinal Disord Tech. 2010; 23(6):388–392

[75] Yuan N, Skaggs DL, Davidson Ward SL, Platzker AC, Keens TG. Preoperative polysomnograms and infant pulmonary function tests do not predict prolonged postoperative mechanical ventilation in children following scoliosis repair. Pediatr Pulmonol. 2004; 38(3):256–260

[76] Urban MK. The role of the post-anesthesia care unit in the perioperative care of the orthopedic patient. In: MacKenzie CR, Cornell CN, Memtsoudis SG, eds. Perioperative Care of the Orthopedic Patient. New York, NY: Springer; 2014:91–99

[77] Cho KJ, Suk SI, Park SR, et al. Complications in posterior fusion and instrumentation for degenerative lumbar scoliosis. Spine. 2007; 32(20):2232–2237

[78] Seo HJ, Kim HJ, Ro YJ, Yang HS. Non-neurologic complications following surgery for scoliosis. Korean J Anesthesiol. 2013; 64(1):40–46

[79] Lenke LG, Newton PO, Sucato DJ, et al. Complications after 147 consecutive vertebral column resections for severe pediatric spinal deformity: a multicenter analysis. Spine. 2013; 38(2):119–132

[80] Patil CG, Santarelli J, Lad SP, Ho C, Tian W, Boakye M. Inpatient complications, mortality, and discharge disposition after surgical correction of idiopathic scoliosis: a national perspective. Spine J. 2008; 8(6):904–910

[81] Senders ZJ, Zussman BM, Maltenfort MG, Sharan AD, Ratliff JK, Harrop JS. The incidence of pulmonary embolism (PE) after spinal fusions. Clin Neurol Neurosurg. 2012; 114(7):897–901

[82] Craig CM. Pharmacologic Therapy for Venous Thromboembolism Prevention in Spine Surgery. SpineLine. 2016(May/June):19–23

[83] Soroceanu A, Burton DC, Oren JH, et al. International Spine Study Group. Medical complications after adult spinal deformity surgery: incidence, risk factors, and clinical impact. Spine. 2016; 41(22):1718–1723

[84] Urban MK, Jules-Elysee KM, Beckman JB, et al. Pulmonary injury in patients undergoing complex spine surgery. Spine J. 2005; 5(3):269–276

[85] Patel VV, Patel A, Harrop JS, eds. Spine Surgery Basics. New York, NY: Springer; 2014

[86] Kang GR, Suh SW, Lee IO. Preoperative predictors of postoperative pulmonary complications in neuromuscular scoliosis. J Orthop Sci. 2011; 16(2): 139–147

[87] Yuan N, Fraire JA, Margetis MM, Skaggs DL, Tolo VT, Keens TG. The effect of scoliosis surgery on lung function in the immediate postoperative period. Spine. 2005; 30(19):2182–2185

[88] Yuan N, Skaggs DL, Dorey F, Keens TG. Preoperative predictors of prolonged postoperative mechanical ventilation in children following scoliosis repair. Pediatr Pulmonol. 2005; 40(5):414–419

[89] Wazeka AN, DiMaio MF, Boachie-Adjei O. Outcome of pediatric patients with severe restrictive lung disease following reconstructive spine surgery. Spine. 2004; 29(5):528–534, discussion 535

[90] Shorr AF, Duh MS, Kelly KM, Kollef MH, CRIT Study Group. Red blood cell transfusion and ventilator-associated pneumonia: a potential link? Crit Care Med. 2004; 32(3):666–674

[91] Chua K, Tan CY, Chen Z, et al. Long-term follow-up of pulmonary function and scoliosis in patients with Duchenne's muscular dystrophy and spinal muscular atrophy. J Pediatr Orthop. 2016; 36(1):63–69

[92] Chou SH, Lin GT, Shen PC, et al. The effect of scoliosis surgery on pulmonary function in spinal muscular atrophy type II patients. Eur Spine J. 2017; 26 (6):1721–1731

[93] Gill I, Eagle M, Mehta JS, Gibson MJ, Bushby K, Bullock R. Correction of neuromuscular scoliosis in patients with preexisting respiratory failure. Spine. 2006; 31(21):2478–2483

[94] Chong HS, Moon ES, Kim HS, et al. Comparison between operated muscular dystrophy and spinal muscular atrophy patients in terms of radiological, pulmonary and functional outcomes. Asian Spine J. 2010; 4(2):82–88

[95] Rawlins BA, Winter RB, Lonstein JE, et al. Reconstructive spine surgery in pediatric patients with major loss in vital capacity. J Pediatr Orthop. 1996; 16 (3):284–292

[96] Bao H, Yan P, Bao M, et al. Halo-gravity traction combined with assisted ventilation: an effective pre-operative management for severe adult scoliosis complicated with respiratory dysfunction. Eur Spine J. 2016; 25(8):2416–2422

[97] Sink EL, Karol LA, Sanders J, Birch JG, Johnston CE, Herring JA. Efficacy of perioperative halo-gravity traction in the treatment of severe scoliosis in children. J Pediatr Orthop. 2001; 21(4):519–524

[98] Khirani S, Bersanini C, Aubertin G, Bachy M, Vialle R, Fauroux B. Non-invasive positive pressure ventilation to facilitate the post-operative respiratory outcome of spine surgery in neuromuscular children. Eur Spine J. 2014; 23 Suppl 4:S406–S411

[99] Shaughnessy EE, White C, Shah SS, Hubbell B, Sucharew H, Sawnani H. Implementation of postoperative respiratory care for pediatric orthopedic patients. Pediatrics. 2015; 136(2):e505–e512

[100] Cassidy MR, Rosenkranz P, McCabe K, Rosen JE, McAneny D. I COUGH: reducing postoperative pulmonary complications with a multidisciplinary patient care program. JAMA Surg. 2013; 148(8):740–745

[101] Lin HY, Nash CL, Herndon CH, Andersen NB. The effect of corrective surgery on pulmonary function in scoliosis. J Bone Joint Surg Am. 1974; 56(6):1173–1179

[102] Gagnon S, Jodoin A, Martin R. Pulmonary function test study and after spinal fusion in young idiopathic scoliosis. Spine. 1989; 14(5):486–490

[103] Gazioglu K. Pulmonary function before and after orthopaedic correction of idiopathic scoliosis. Bull Physiopathol Respir (Nancy). 1973; 9(3):711–713

[104] Upadhyay SS, Day GA, Saji MJ, Leong JC. Restrictive pattern of pulmonary functions in idiopathic and congenital scoliosis following spinal fusion. Eur Spine J. 1993; 2(1):22–28

[105] Caro CG, Dubois AB. Pulmonary function in kyphoscoliosis. Thorax. 1961; 16:282–290

[106] Kennedy JD, Robertson CF, Olinsky A, Dickens DR, Phelan PD. Pulmonary restrictive effect of bracing in mild idiopathic scoliosis. Thorax. 1987; 42(12): 959–961

[107] Lee DK, Chun EM, Suh SW, Yang JH, Shim SS. Evaluation of postoperative change in lung volume in adolescent idiopathic scoliosis: measured by computed tomography. Indian J Orthop. 2014; 48(4):360–365

[108] Kumano K, Tsuyama N. Pulmonary function before and after surgical correction of scoliosis. J Bone Joint Surg Am. 1982; 64(2):242–248

[109] Graham EJ, Lenke LG, Lowe TG, et al. Prospective pulmonary function evaluation following open thoracotomy for anterior spinal fusion in adolescent idiopathic scoliosis. Spine. 2000; 25(18):2319–2325

[110] Kim YJ, Lenke LG, Bridwell KH, Cheh G, Whorton J, Sides B. Prospective pulmonary function comparison following posterior segmental spinal instrumentation and fusion of adolescent idiopathic scoliosis: is there a relationship between major thoracic curve correction and pulmonary function test improvement? Spine. 2007; 32(24):2685–2693

[111] Izatt MT, Harvey JR, Adam CJ, Fender D, Labrom RD, Askin GN. Recovery of pulmonary function following endoscopic anterior scoliosis correction: evaluation at 3, 6, 12, and 24 months after surgery. Spine. 2006; 31(21):2469–2477

[112] Kinnear WJ, Kinnear GC, Watson L, Webb JK, Johnston ID. Pulmonary function after spinal surgery for idiopathic scoliosis. Spine. 1992; 17(6):708–713

[113] Lenke LG, Bridwell KH, Blanke K, Baldus C. Analysis of pulmonary function and chest cage dimension changes after thoracoplasty in idiopathic scoliosis. Spine. 1995; 20(12):1343–1350

[114] Vedantam R, Lenke LG, Bridwell KH, Haas J, Linville DA. A prospective evaluation of pulmonary function in patients with adolescent idiopathic scoliosis relative to the surgical approach used for spinal arthrodesis. Spine. 2000; 25(1):82–90

2 Biomechanics of the Thoracic Spinal Column

Jamal N. Shillingford, James D. Lin, and Ronald A. Lehman Jr.

Abstract

The thoracic spine is a unique load-bearing structure. It is an area of the spine that is often subject to extraphysiological forces during high energy trauma, and is often involved in spinal deformity such as scoliosis and kyphosis. The thoracic spine has unique biomechanical properties compared to other parts of the spine due to the articulations with the rib cage, the kyphotic sagittal alignment, and the transition from the stiff upper thoracic spine to the relatively mobile thoracolumbar junction. This unique anatomy comprised of articulations with the rib cage, and its overall sagittal alignment creates a distinct biomechanical environment which differs from the cervical and lumbar spine.

Keywords: thoracic, ribs, kyphosis, fourth column, costovertebral

Clinical Pearls

- The thoracic spine has unique biomechanical properties compared to other parts of the spine due to the articulations with the rib cage through the costovertebral and costotransverse joints.
- A transition zone exists between the relatively stiff upper thoracic spine and the more mobile thoracolumbar junction, creating a common area for traumatic disorders.
- Stress is defined as force applied over unit area, typically expressed as Newtons/meters^2.
- Strain is a measure of relative deformation as a result of a force, measured as change in length over original length.
- The functional spinal unit is defined as the smallest functional motion segment of the spine, and involves two adjacent vertebrae and the interposed soft tissues.
- Physiological spinal range of motion demonstrates biphasic nonlinear load displacement behavior, characterized by a neutral zone and an elastic zone.

2.1 Overview

The thoracic spine is a unique load-bearing structure in the human body. On a daily basis, it resists repeated physiological forces of axial loading, flexion and extension, lateral bending, and twisting while protecting the spinal cord and providing a foundation to the thorax. It is an area of the spine that is often subject to extraphysiological forces during high-energy trauma, and is often involved in spinal deformity such as scoliosis and kyphosis. The thoracic spine has unique biomechanical properties compared to other parts of the spine due to the articulations with the rib cage, the kyphotic sagittal alignment, and the transition from the stiff upper thoracic spine to the relatively mobile thoracolumbar junction. Thorough understanding of these biomechanical properties and the underlying anatomic structures is critical for spine surgeons who treat traumatic disorders, deformity, and degenerative conditions of the thoracic spine. A better understanding of the motion characteristics and forces transmitted through the thoracic spine will allow surgeons to elucidate the limitations of the system and the conditions that subsequently result in pain and tissue damage.

2.2 Biomechanics

2.2.1 Definitions

Spinal biomechanics builds on the basic definitions and principles of orthopaedic biomechanics and applies them to the complexity of the spinal column. It provides a quantitative tool for assessment of the forces, movements, and overall function of the spine under varying loading conditions. The bulk of biomechanical information that we have on the thoracic spine has come from in vitro studies because of the difficulty in obtaining these measures in vivo. Though biomechanical models can be utilized to predict response interactions to loads on spinal tissues of interest, these responses represent a gross estimation and likely differ from their natural occurrence in live humans.

Stress is defined as force applied over unit area, typically expressed as Newtons/meters^2. These forces can be compressive, tensile, shear, or torsional.[1] Strain is a measure of relative deformation as a result of a force, measured as change in length over original length.[1] When this deformation is temporary, it is termed elastic deformation, and when it is permanent, it is termed plastic deformation.

Every material has a unique stress–strain curve which describes how that material will respond to an external stress. The stress–strain curve typically starts with an elastic zone, where the stress and strain are proportional, and described by Young's modulus (E). At the end of this elastic point is the yield point; further deformation to the material is irreversible, until the breaking point is reached, which is the point at which the material fails.

In the realm of spinal biomechanics, the functional spinal unit (FSU) is defined as the smallest functional motion segment of the spine, and involves two adjacent vertebrae and the interposed soft tissues.[2] Each FSU can translate and/or rotate about three orthogonal axes, creating 12 possible modes of displacement. When these individual motions are combined, they result in more complex motions of flexion/extension, lateral bending, and axial rotation.

The instantaneous axis of rotation (IAR) is the imaginary line that the vertebral body will rotate about when a bending moment arm is applied to the FSU. In the thoracic spine this typically occurs in the superior end plate of the more caudal vertebral body of the two adjacent vertebrae.[3] The *neutral axis* is the line connecting the IARs in the spinal column.[2] Spinal movements are referenced on a coordinate system where rotation is described in the axial or transverse plane, lateral bending in the coronal plane, and flexion/extension in the sagittal plane.

2.2.2 Neutral and Elastic Zones

Physiological spinal range of motion (ROM) demonstrates biphasic nonlinear load displacement behavior, characterized by a neutral zone and an elastic zone. The neutral zone is the range of intervertebral motion within which physiological spinal motion is produced with minimal internal resistance. Panjabi described this as the zone of high flexibility or laxity.[4] The elastic zone is defined as the range of intervertebral motion from the end of the neutral zone to the physiological limit of motion, and is a result of internal resistance from various soft issues structures and musculature.[2,5] This is the zone of high stiffness.[4] The neutral zone represents an important functional measurement of spine stability and can be affected by muscular weakness, trauma, degeneration, and instrumentation. Muscle strengthening, osteophyte formation, and surgical fixation/fusion work to decrease the neutral zone to within a normal physiological range.[4]

2.3 Anatomy

The thoracic spine is the largest segment of the spinal column and is composed of 12 vertebrae. Although the basic structure of the vertebral body is the same, the thoracic spine is distinguished from the cervical and lumbar spine by its articulations with the ribs through the costovertebral and costotransverse joints, which contribute to the stability of the upper thoracic spine. As a result, a transition zone exists between the relatively stiff upper thoracic spine and the more mobile thoracolumbar junction, creating a common area for traumatic disorders.

2.3.1 Ribs and Sternum

The thoracic spine differs from the cervical and lumbar spine in that it articulates with the ribs through the costovertebral and costotransverse joints, and thus is ultimately stabilized by the rib cage.[6] These articulations occur from the 1st to 10th thoracic vertebrae. The costovertebral articulation occurs at the level of the thoracic disc, and is comprised of two demifacets above and below the disc bilaterally. Additionally, the ribs articulate with a concave facet on the ventral surface of the transverse process termed the costotransverse joint or costal facet of the transverse process. The 11th and 12th ribs are disconnected from the sternum and are often labeled as "floating ribs." Their respective thoracic vertebrae have unique transitional characteristics with small transverse processes that fail to buttress the last two ribs, likely contributing very little stability to that region of the spine.[7,8]

Cadaveric sequential sectioning studies have shown the ribs add stiffness to rotational and bending forces to the thoracic spine.[9] When the rib head is resected, ROM is increased from 70 to 80% in flexion, extension, and bending.[9] Watkins et al demonstrated that the rib cage increased the stability of the thoracic spine by 40% in flexion/extension, 35% in lateral bending, and 31% in axial rotation.[10] Brasiliense et al, in a cadaveric study, demonstrated that the sternum and anterior rib cage contributed most to stability in flexion/extension, the posterior rib cage was most important in lateral bending, and stability in axial rotation was directly related to the proportion of rib that remained intact.[8] Overall, they found that the ribs accounted

for 78% of mechanical thoracic stability. Given the increased stability that the rib cage and sternum confer to the thoracic spine, it has been proposed that the rib cage and sternum be considered a "fourth column" in the classic three-column model of spinal stability.[11]

2.3.2 Vertebral Body

Because of the sagittal alignment of the thoracic spine, vertebral bodies in the thoracic spine act as a buttress to compressive forces, as compared to the posterior elements which resist distractive forces. The anterior–posterior diameter of thoracic vertebral bodies increases from T1 to T12 to support increased load seen in the caudal segments. The height of the thoracic vertebral body increases posteriorly yielding the physiological thoracic kyphosis. Flattening of the left side of the anterior surface of the thoracic vertebrae can be commonly seen from its close relationship to the descending aorta. The vertebral body is the major load-bearing structure of the FSU composed of a thin but strong outer layer of cortical bone that resists bending and torsion, and an inner spongy matrix of cancellous bone which is more elastic and helps to maintain shape despite compressive forces.[7] The bony and ligamentous structures posterior to the vertebral body provide attachments for muscles and lever arms for mechanical advantage and control of the position of the vertebral body.

2.3.3 Pedicle

Compared to cervical pedicles, those in the thoracic region originate more superiorly on the dorsal surface of the vertebral body. Though pedicle height increases as one descends from T1 to T12, the pedicle width has a more unique pattern.[12,13] Cinotti et al showed that the smallest pedicle transverse diameters occurred in the region between T4 and T8 in cadaveric specimens.[14] Similarly, Scoles et al found that the smallest pedicle widths occurred in the region between T3 and T6 in human cadaveric specimens.[15] Kothe and colleagues explored the complex three-dimensional internal structure of the pedicle, demonstrating that the medial wall of the thoracic pedicle was significantly thicker than the lateral wall and that the cancellous core was more than twice as large as the cortical shell.[16]

2.3.4 Lamina

Laminae represent the medial bony projections from each pedicle, which join in the midline to form the neural arch.[7] The neural arch provides a strong bony channel that protects the spinal cord.

2.3.5 Disc

Aeby and colleagues reported that the intervertebral disc accounted for about one-fifth of the length of the thoracic spine.[17,18] The intervertebral disc in the thoracic spine is analogous to the lumbar spine, but has increased annulus thickness and decreased height. Additionally, these discs are heart-shaped, with a more centrally located nucleus pulposus. In each thoracic segment, the disc has a uniform thickness, but both disc height and width increase with the corresponding increase in vertebral body size as one progresses caudally down the thoracic spine.[7] Discs play a large role in thoracic spine stability. They act primarily as intervertebral shock absorbers, sharing and transmitting a portion of the transmitted loads between vertebral segments. The outer layer of the disc called the annulus fibrosus which is composed of circumferential collagen sheets (lamellae) which primarily withstand compressive loads while allowing bending motion. The central gelatinous nucleus pulposus expands outward when compressed increasing the tensions, and thus stiffness, of the annulus fibrosus. The system is dynamic during the day with increased stiffness as one lays flat while the disc absorbs water, and more lax when upright during the day as water is released from the disc.[7]

Directionality of the annulus fibrosus fibers determine their response to various tissue loading conditions. Lengthening of the spine and compressive loads both place fibers of the annulus fibrosus under tension in all directions. Contrastingly, both shear and torsional forces place tension on the fibers in the direction of movement while relaxing those fibers that are positioned in the opposite direction.

Takeuchi et al demonstrated through sequential sectioning studies that partial discectomy resulted in significant increases in ROM of the thoracic spine, with increased flexion/extension from 7.7 to 17.6 degrees, axial rotation from 14.8 to 21.8, left lateral bending from 11.7 to 17.2 degrees, and right lateral bending from 10.4 to 14.4 degrees.[19] Oda et al compared anterior and posterior sequential destabilization of the thoracic spine, and found that total discectomy and transection of anterior longitudinal ligament (ALL) and posterior longitudinal ligament (PLL) resulted in significant increases in ROM when compared to posterior element release, especially in flexion/extension and axial rotation.[20] The effect of the thoracic disc on spinal stability is the rationale for proponents of anterior release in thoracic deformity correction to achieve improved deformity correction. However, in the setting of using modern pedicle screw instrumentation, as compared to thoracic hook constructs, posterior-only correction may be sufficient.[21,22]

2.3.6 Sagittal Alignment

One of the hallmarks of the thoracic spine is the physiological kyphotic sagittal alignment in the upper thoracic spine which transitions through the relatively neutral thoracolumbar junction to reach the lordotic lumbar spine. On average, there is 48 degrees of kyphosis from T1 to T12, and 5 to 8 degrees of kyphosis from T10 to T12.[23] This sagittal curve is present at birth, and is closely tied to pelvic parameters of pelvic incidence, sacral slope, and pelvic tilt in creating global sagittal balance and maintaining the center of gravity. The sagittal curves of the spine are thought to improve spinal stability and increase shock absorption and improve resistance to vertical loads.[2]

2.3.7 Facet Joints (Orientation, Motion Coupling)

The facet joints (zygapophyseal joints) in the thoracic spine are oriented in an oblique plane, transitioning to a more sagittal orientation through the thoracolumbar junction. The facets are diarthrodial joints or true synovial joints with gliding type articulations and thin joint capsules that attach to the base of each respective facet. The superior articular facet originates at the junction between the pedicle and lamina, composed of a cartilaginous convex surface which projects dorsally and superolaterally in the coronal plane. The geometric orientation of the inferior articular facet is complementary to the superior facet. Facet orientation can be highly variable in the thoracolumbar junction, either being more "thoracic" and thus coronally oriented versus being more "lumbar" and sagittally oriented.[24] These joints allow for controlled motion of the spine depending on the facet orientation, and allow for coupled motion typically between axial rotation and lateral bending. Panjabi et al have shown that coupled motions can occur in all 6 degrees of freedom but that coupling in this region of the spine, however, is weaker than in the cervical spine.[3,25] In a cadaveric study, Brasiliense et al demonstrated an average of less than 0.2 degrees of coupled axial rotation per degree of lateral bending, with and without the presence of ribs.[8]

When performing posterior decompression, preservation of the lateral portion of the facet joint is thought to minimize postoperative instability and kyphosis.[20] Subtle differences in facet orientation can either permit or prevent motion in different planes along the spinal segment. Abnormal motion coupling has been associated with nociceptor stimulation and the development of low back pain with reduced movement secondary to guarding.

2.3.8 Ligaments

Spinal ligaments work in concert to provide stability to the FSU. They are able to effectively resist loads in the direction of their fibers, primarily under tension. They buckle, however, under compressive loads. Spinal ligaments serve three significant roles: they permit motion and help to orient vertebrae without muscle recruitment; they protect the spinal cord by restricting spinal motion segments to limited ranges; and they absorb energy, protecting the cord during rapid motions.[7] The ALL, the largest and strongest of the spinal ligaments, travels along the anterior vertebral bodies from the base of the skull down to the sacrum where it blends with presacral fibers.[7,26] In the thoracic spine, its fibers are firmly attached to the anterior surface at each end of the vertebrae, forming the vertebral body periosteum, but at the level of the disc, it is loosely attached to the annulus via connective tissue bands.[26] Similarly, the PLL travels from the skull down to the sacrum but within the confines of the vertebral arch. Contrastingly, the thick connective tissue does not adhere to the vertebral body, rather bowstrings across the concavity of the dorsal vertebral body and is intimately related to the vascular elements that exit the medullary sinus.[7] PLL fibers are most firmly attached at the margins of their lateral expansions, and loosely attached at the central rhomboidal area over the dorsolateral aspect of the disc. The PLL also maintains a firm attachment to the dura laterally over its dorsal surface via connective tissue, with various epidural venous connections passing between the two structures.

The remaining ligaments collectively form a syndesmosis between the vertebral arches of adjacent thoracic vertebrae. These ligaments, from deep to superficial, include the ligamentum flavum, intertransverse ligament, interspinous ligament, and the supraspinous ligament.[7] The ligamentum flavum extends laterally to the base of the facet joints and nearly join in the midline. This ligament extends from the deep ventral surface of the cephalad thoracic vertebrae superiorly, to the superior lip or upper edge of the lamina of the caudal thoracic vertebra. Moreover, the ligamentum flavum has two distinct layers, a narrow lateral portion which tapers off laterally as it attaches to the articular processes and a thick medial portion which parallels the longitudinal axis of the spine attaching to the lamina.[27] The elastic nature of this ligament keeps it taut in extension, to prevent infolding toward the ventral neurovascular structures from laxity and redundancy.[7,27]

In the thoracic spine, the intertransverse ligaments, which are comprised of the fibrous connections between adjacent transverse processes, blend with segmental muscle insertions and the intercostal ligaments. The interspinous ligaments represent a distinct layer of paired membranous fibers that attach adjacent spinous processes with a midline cleft. They are oblique in nature, connecting the base of the superior spinous process to the superior ridge of the subjacent spinous process.[7] The supraspinous ligament extends along the apices of the spinous processes with superficial fibers that extend over multiple segments, and deep fibers that bridge shorter regions composed of two to three segments.

2.4 Spinal Stability

2.4.1 Conceptual Frameworks

The spinal column is a unique structure that must provide motion for bodily movement while providing stability to protect neurovascular structures. Determining whether the pathological spine is "stable" can be a challenge. White and Panjabi defined spinal instability as the inability of the spine under physiological loads to maintain relationships between vertebrae to prevent neurological injury, deformity, or pain.[28] This instability can be caused by many factors, including trauma, degeneration, tumors, and neuromuscular disease. Panjabi proposed a conceptual framework for understanding spinal stability which consists of three subsystems: the passive subsystem, the active subsystem, and the neural control subsystem. The passive subsystem is comprised of the vertebrae, intervertebral discs, ligaments, and joint capsules, which do not provide significant stability to the spine in the neutral position. The active subsystem consists of muscles and tendons which generate forces to stabilize the spine. The neural control subsystem receives proprioceptive feedback from the passive and active subsystems to direct the active subsystem in stabilizing the spine. In most settings, the clinical determination of spinal stability is based on the passive subsystem as it is the most readily assessed with imaging modalities.

2.4.2 Classification Schemes

Holdsworth proposed a two-column theory of spinal stability, where the integrity of the posterior elements was a crucial element to stability.[29] Denis then introduced the concept of the "middle column," which consists of the PLL, posterior annulus, and the dorsal half of the vertebral column, as a crucial element to classification of thoracolumbar injuries. He observed that isolated posterior column injuries, both in trauma and

iatrogenically during posterior exposure of spinal deformity, do not create acute instability of the thoracolumbar spine. In his review of 412 thoracolumbar injuries, the mode of failure of the middle column was used to classify fractures and correlated with the risk of neurological injury. The anterior column consists of the ALL and ventral half of the vertebral body. The middle column consists of the dorsal half of the vertebral body, PLL and posterior annulus, and the posterior column consists of the posterior elements and ligamentous structures. More modern classification schemes include the Thoracolumbar Injury Classification and Severity Score, which take into account the fracture morphology, integrity of the posterior ligamentous complex, as well as the neurological status of the patient.

2.5 Conclusion

The thoracic spine is a critically important load-bearing structure in the human body that is commonly involved in traumatic disorders and spinal deformity. Its anatomy is characterized by its sagittal alignment and articulations with the rib cage that create unique biomechanical properties that differ from the cervical and lumbar spine. Thorough understanding of thoracic spine biomechanics is important for the spine surgeon treating thoracic spinal pathologies.

References

[1] Miller MD, Thompson SR, Hart J. Review of Orthopaedics. Elsevier Health Sciences; 2012

[2] Izzo R, Guarnieri G, Guglielmi G, Muto M. Biomechanics of the spine. Part I: spinal stability. Eur J Radiol. 2013; 82(1):118–126

[3] Panjabi MM, White AA 3rd. Clinical biomechanics of the spine. Clin Biomech Spine 1990

[4] Panjabi MM. The stabilizing system of the spine. Part II. Neutral zone and instability hypothesis. J Spinal Disord. 1992; 5(4):390–396, discussion 397

[5] Panjabi MM. The stabilizing system of the spine. Part I. Function, dysfunction, adaptation, and enhancement. J Spinal Disord. 1992; 5(4):383–389, discussion 397

[6] el-Khoury GY, Whitten CG. Trauma to the upper thoracic spine: anatomy, biomechanics, and unique imaging features. AJR Am J Roentgenol. 1993; 160(1): 95–102

[7] Herkowitz HN, Garfin SR, Eismont FJ, Bell GR, Balderston RA. Biomechanics of the spinal motion segment. In: Rothman-Simeone The Spine. Vol 1. 6th ed. Elsevier Health Sciences; 2011:2096

[8] Brasiliense LBC, Lazaro BCR, Reyes PM, Dogan S, Theodore N, Crawford NR. Biomechanical contribution of the rib cage to thoracic stability. Spine. 2011; 36(26):E1686–E1693

[9] Oda I, Abumi K, Lü D, Shono Y, Kaneda K. Biomechanical role of the posterior elements, costovertebral joints, and rib cage in the stability of the thoracic spine. Spine. 1996; 21(12):1423–1429

[10] Watkins R, IV, Watkins R, III, Williams L, et al. Stability provided by the sternum and rib cage in the thoracic spine. Spine. 2005; 30(11):1283–1286

[11] Berg EE. The sternal-rib complex. A possible fourth column in thoracic spine fractures. Spine. 1993; 18(13):1916–1919

[12] Banta CJ, II, King AG, Dabezies EJ, Liljeberg RL. Measurement of effective pedicle diameter in the human spine. Orthopedics. 1989; 12(7):939–942

[13] Misenhimer GR, Peek RD, Wiltse LL, Rothman SL, Widell EH, Jr. Anatomic analysis of pedicle cortical and cancellous diameter as related to screw size. Spine. 1989; 14(4):367–372

[14] Cinotti G, Gumina S, Ripani M, Postacchini F. Pedicle instrumentation in the thoracic spine. A morphometric and cadaveric study for placement of screws. Spine. 1999; 24(2):114–119

[15] Scoles PV, Linton AE, Latimer B, Levy ME, Digiovanni BF. Vertebral body and posterior element morphology: the normal spine in middle life. Spine. 1988; 13(10):1082–1086

[16] Kothe R, O'Holleran JDD, Liu W, Panjabi MMM. Internal architecture of the thoracic pedicle. An anatomic study. Spine. 1996; 21(3):264–270

[17] Aeby CT. Die Altersverschiedenheiten Der Menschlichen Wirbelsäule. Arch Anat Physiol. 1879; 10:77

[18] Taylor JR. Growth of human intervertebral discs and vertebral bodies. J Anat. 1975; 120(Pt 1):49–68

[19] Takeuchi T, Abumi K, Shono Y, Oda I, Kaneda K. Biomechanical role of the intervertebral disc and costovertebral joint in stability of the thoracic spine. A canine model study. Spine. 1999; 24(14):1414–1420

[20] Oda I, Abumi K, Cunningham BW, Kaneda K, McAfee PC. An in vitro human cadaveric study investigating the biomechanical properties of the thoracic spine. Spine. 2002; 27(3):E64–E70

[21] Luhmann SJ, Lenke LG, Kim YJ, Bridwell KH, Schootman M. Thoracic adolescent idiopathic scoliosis curves between 70° and 100°: is anterior release necessary? Spine. 2005; 30(18):2061–2067

[22] Burton DC, Sama AA, Asher MA, et al. The treatment of large (> 70°) thoracic idiopathic scoliosis curves with posterior instrumentation and arthrodesis: when is anterior release indicated? Spine. 2005; 30(17):1979–1984

[23] Gelb DE, Lenke LG, Bridwell KH, Blanke K, McEnery KW. An analysis of sagittal spinal alignment in 100 asymptomatic middle and older aged volunteers. Spine. 1995; 20(12):1351–1358

[24] Masharawi Y, Rothschild B, Dar G, et al. Facet orientation in the thoracolumbar spine: three-dimensional anatomic and biomechanical analysis. Spine. 2004; 29(16):1755–1763

[25] Panjabi MM, Brand RA, Jr, White AA, III. Three-dimensional flexibility and stiffness properties of the human thoracic spine. J Biomech. 1976; 9(4):185–192

[26] Neumann P, Keller TS, Ekström L, Perry L, Hansson TH, Spengler DM. Mechanical properties of the human lumbar anterior longitudinal ligament. J Biomech. 1992; 25(10):1185–1194

[27] Nachemson AL, Evans JH. Some mechanical properties of the third human lumbar interlaminar ligament (ligamentum flavum). J Biomech. 1968; 1(3):211–220

[28] Panjabi MM, White AA, III. Basic biomechanics of the spine. Neurosurgery. 1980; 7(1):76–93

[29] Holdsworth F. Fractures, dislocations, and fracture-dislocations of the spine. J Bone Joint Surg Am. 1970; 52(8):1534–1551

3 Anesthetic Considerations for Surgery of the Thoracic Spine

Michael K. Urban and Lila R. Baaklini

Abstract

The anesthetic considerations for surgery of the thoracic spine must include a preoperative evaluation concentrating of comorbidities which will impact surgical outcome; an intraoperative anesthetic which permits spinal cord neuromonitoring; techniques for blood conservation and preserving hemodynamic stability; and a plan for postoperative analgesia. A specifically designed total intravenous anesthesia will allow multimodal neuromonitoring such that spinal cord and nerve root injury will be detected before the development of permanent damage. In addition, hemodynamic stability and the prevention of excessive blood loss are required to prevent the devastating complications of complex thoracic surgery, spinal cord ischemia, and perioperative loss of vision. Thoracic surgery is painful, necessitating an intraoperative plan for postoperative pain management.

Keywords: total intravenous anesthesia, intraoperative neuromonitoring, postoperative visual loss, antifibrinolytics, noninvasive hemodynamic monitors, blood conservation techniques

Clinical Pearls

- The evaluation of a patient prior to thoracic spinal surgery should pay particular attention to the patient's airway, pulmonary, cardiovascular, and neurological status, as they all have the potential to be affected by the patient's surgical disease.
- Cardiovascular dysfunction can be due to a number of factors in this patient population: a direct result of the pathology requiring corrective spinal surgery, pulmonary hypertension and right ventricular hypertrophy, and/or age-related ischemic heart disease.
- All patients for thoracic spine surgery should have a neurological examination which assesses and documents any preexisting neurological deficits and under which circumstances they are exacerbated. This is essential in order to be able to identify new neurological deficits that appear postoperatively.
- For patients with unstable cervical spines and significant cervicothoracic deformities (rheumatoid arthritis, achondroplasia, ankylosing spondylitis) awake fiberoptic endotracheal intubation is the safest approach for tracheal intubation.
- The general anesthetic for these procedures is particularly challenging since it must provide analgesia, amnesia, and hemodynamic stability without compromising intraoperative neuromonitoring (IONM). This monitoring includes somatosensory, motor evoked potential, and electromyography monitoring.
- Total intravenous anesthesia is the preferred anesthetic for complex thoracic spine procedures because IONM is less affected than with inhalational anesthetics.

- Changes in IONM could be due to factors other than anesthetics, including surgical causes, hypotension, anemia, metabolic acidosis, and hypothermia.
- Blood loss and the need for homologous blood transfusions during complex spine surgery can be minimized by proper positioning of the patient to reduce intra-abdominal pressure, surgical hemostasis, deliberate controlled hypotensive anesthesia, reinfusion of salvaged blood, intraoperative normovolemic hemodilution, the use of pharmacological agents which promote clot formation, and the preoperative donation of autologous blood.
- The role of the anesthesiologists during complex spine surgery is to maintain end-organ perfusion despite large blood losses in an attempt to prevent devastating complications such as spinal cord ischemia, postoperative visual loss, renal failure, myocardial ischemia, and stroke.
- Thoracic spine patients will experience considerable postoperative pain which is best treated with a multimodality approach.

3.1 Introduction

Thoracic spinal surgeries are common procedures that are performed for a variety of different pathologies. These can range from surgical decompression for spinal stenosis, urgent procedures for trauma or infection, microsurgical techniques to excise spinal cord tumors, and large corrective procedures for deformities such as scoliosis. The procedures can be simple or involve posterior fusions at multiple levels, as well as anterior thoracotomies that result in considerable blood loss. This review will concentrate on the perioperative anesthetic management of adults undergoing thoracic spinal procedures.

3.2 Preoperative Evaluation

Regardless of the indication, all patients presenting for thoracic spinal surgery should receive a thorough preoperative evaluation with particular concern for the patient's surgical pathology and the urgency of the planned procedure. Complications after spinal surgery are associated with surgical complexity, age of the patient, and preexisting comorbidities.[1,2,3] There are specific types of patients who are more likely to have spinal surgery and are more likely to have perioperative complications. Trauma involving the spine will often involve other vital organs which must also be evaluated prior to surgery. Spinal tumors may be metastatic cancers hence compromising the function of other organs or include chemotherapeutic agents which will have an impact on the anesthetic plan. Osteoarthritis, a disease of the aging, is a significant risk factor for degenerative disc disease and spinal stenosis. Hence older patients with multiple comorbidities are more likely to have spine surgery.

Patients with orthopaedic diseases involving the axial skeleton, such as achondroplasia and ankylosing spondylitis, commonly have thoracic spine surgery and have a myriad of medical comorbidities.

The evaluation of a patient prior to thoracic spinal surgery should pay particular attention to the patient's airway, pulmonary, cardiovascular, and neurological status, as they all have the potential to be affected by the patient's surgical disease. The potential for a difficult tracheal intubation is especially pronounced in patients with cervical and upper thoracic spine disease. The patient's previous anesthetic records should also be reviewed for any history of a difficult airway. The preoperative airway evaluation involves a general assessment of cervical mobility, examination for masses, tracheal deviation, mouth opening, state of dentition, and thyromental distance. An evaluation of the patient's ability to flex and extend the neck is also performed. Comorbid conditions that may restrict mouth opening, limit cervical range of motion, and alter airway anatomy include osteoarthritis, rheumatoid arthritis, achondroplasia, ankylosing spondylitis, cerebral palsy, and other neuromuscular disorders.[4] Arthritis of the cervical spine which may result in anterior subluxation of C1 on C2 (atlantoaxial subluxation) may occur in up to 40% of patients with rheumatoid arthritis, with symptoms of progressive neck pain, headache, and myelopathy. Less common is posterior and vertical migration of the odontoid process. Flexion of the head in the presence of atlantoaxial instability could result in the displacement of the odontoid process into the cervical spine and medulla with concomitant compression of the vertebral arteries. This could precipitate quadriparesis, spinal shock, and death. In at-risk patients, preoperative cervical flexion–extension radiographs should be evaluated and if the distance from the anterior arch of the atlas to the odontoid process exceeds 3 mm, the patient should undergo awake fiberoptic tracheal intubation and the cervical spine protected with a cervical collar during the procedure. Ankylosing spondylitis is a chronic inflammatory arthritic disease that involves ossification of the axial ligaments progressing from the sacral lumbar region cranially, resulting in significant loss of spinal mobility. These patients are a significant challenge to the anesthesiologist with regard to airway management due to the reduced movement of both the cervical spine and temporomandibular joint. Assessment of the cervical spine is also crucial in trauma patients. These patients should be carefully evaluated for signs and symptoms of cervical cord compression, such as pain and neurological deficits.[5]

Pulmonary complications continue to remain common after spinal procedures.[6] Patients presenting for thoracic spine surgery frequently present with conditions that affect their pulmonary function. Patients with thoracic spinal deformities will have a reduced chest cavity with decreased chest wall compliance and restrictive lung disease. Although exercise tolerance is an important determinant of the effects of the severity of the curve on respiratory function, formal pulmonary function studies will guide decisions regarding the extent of surgery permitted and the requirement for postoperative ventilatory support. A vital capacity of less than 40% of the normal range is predictive for postoperative ventilation. Hypoxemia is a common finding, secondary to ventilation–perfusion inequalities caused by alveolar hypoventilation. This may progress to elevated pulmonary vascular resistance and ultimately cor pulmonale. An echocardiogram should be evaluated for pulmonary hypertension and right ventricular hypertrophy (RVH). Patients with severe pulmonary hypertension may not be candidates for surgical correction of the spinal deformity.[7]

Cigarette smoking not only increases the risk of postoperative pulmonary complications but has a negative impact on the success of spinal fusions.[8] Patients should be encouraged to stop smoking at least 6 to 8 weeks prior to surgery in order to reduce the risk of pulmonary complications to that of nonsmokers.[9]

Cardiovascular dysfunction can be due to a number of factors in this patient population: a direct result of the pathology requiring corrective spinal surgery, pulmonary hypertension and RVH, and/or age-related ischemic heart disease.[7,10] In addition, several studies have established an increased risk of cardiovascular morbidity and mortality in patients with rheumatic and connective diseases.[11] Since there is a significant incidence of postoperative cardiac complications after spine surgery and it is difficult to assess these patients' functional status due to the limitations imposed by their disease, many of these patients will require a preoperative pharmacological stress test.[12] There is, however, limited data available that preoperative risk stratification and/or coronary revascularization has an effect on outcome. Numerous studies have indicated that the use of perioperative β-blockers can reduce myocardial ischemia.[13,14] Recent reports have suggested that although the perioperative administration of β-blockers may prevent myocardial ischemia, they may increase the incidence of stroke and death by preventing postoperative cardiac complications, particularly in patients at intermediate risk. However, β-blockers should be continued perioperatively in those patients on chronic β-blockers and initiated in those at the highest risk with a target heart rate below 80.[15]

Patients with diabetes are not only at increased risk for perioperative complications from associated comorbidities (myocardial ischemia, vascular disease), but also have a higher incidence of postoperative infections.[16] These patients should have a preoperative HbA_{1c} less than 8% and their perioperative blood glucose levels should be maintained between 150 and 200 mg/dL.[17,18]

All patients for thoracic spine surgery should have a neurological examination which assesses and documents any preexisting neurological deficits and under which circumstances they are exacerbated. This is essential in order to be able to identify new neurological deficits that appear postoperatively. This information is also valuable in positioning the patient for surgery.

3.3 Intraoperative Management

Surgical treatment for adult spinal deformities presents multiple challenges for intraoperative management, including ventilation, hemodynamic stability, intraoperative neuromonitoring (IONM), management of blood loss, and a plan for postoperative analgesia. Success requires the collaboration between the anesthesiologist, surgeon, and IONM team.

General anesthesia with endotracheal intubation and controlled ventilation is a requirement for adult thoracic spinal surgery. Hence the initial procedure, tracheal intubation, may be a challenge in a population with preexisting arthritic conditions or cervical deformities. For many of these patients, tracheal intubation can be achieved with the aid of video-assisted laryngoscopy. However, for patients with unstable cervical spines and significant cervicothoracic deformities (rheumatoid arthritis, achondroplasia, ankylosing spondylitis) awake fiberoptic endotracheal intubation is the safest approach. In the rheumatoid arthritis patient synovitis of the temporomandibular joint may significantly limit mandibular motion and mouth opening. Arthritic damage to the cricoarytenoid joints may result in diminished movement of the vocal cords, resulting in a narrowed glottic opening which is manifested preoperatively as hoarseness and stridor. During laryngoscopy, the vocal cords may appear erythematous and edematous, and the reduced glottic opening may interfere with passage of the endotracheal tube (ETT). There also is an increased risk of cricoarytenoid dislocation with traumatic endotracheal intubations.

Surgical spinal corrections involving high anterior thoracic levels or video-assisted thoracoscopic surgery will require the isolation of one lung ventilation (OLV). OLV has been traditionally achieved with a double-lumen ETT. In single-staged anterior then posterior spinal fusions, before the postoperative procedure the double-lumen ETT should be replaced with a single-lumen ETT, to avoid trauma to the larynx from the larger double-lumen ETT. Alternatively, a single-lumen ETT with an enclosed bronchial blocker can also provide OLV and has the advantage of being left in place as a single-lumen ETT with the blocker deflated at the end of the anterior procedure.[19] In patients with restrictive lung disease, adequate oxygenation may be difficult during OLV and may require continuous positive airway pressure to the nonventilated lung and positive end-expiratory pressure (PEEP) to the ventilated lung. This, however, can only be achieved with a double-lumen ETT.

Once the airway is secured, ventilation can represent an anesthetic challenge secondary to restrictive lung disease and pulmonary hypertension. These patients should be ventilated with pressure-cycled ventilation, lower than conventional tidal volumes (6–8 mL/kg) and PEEP. Mechanical ventilation with higher, conventional tidal volumes has been shown to be contributing to the development of acute lung injury (ALI).[20] However, recently this approach has been questioned in a randomized controlled trial of patients in the prone position undergoing spinal surgery.[21] PEEP is used to prevent the collapse of recruited alveoli; however high levels of PEEP can have adverse consequences on hemodynamics and induce alveolar wall stress. Hence, PEEP levels of 5 to 7.5 mm Hg are employed with frequent assessment of oxygenation and ventilation with arterial blood gases. Both hypercarbia and hypoxia can increase pulmonary vascular resistance and exacerbate existing pulmonary hypertension. In addition, careful attention to fluid management is essential to maintain right ventricular preload and cardiac output. Nitrous oxide should be avoided in these patients since it will increase pulmonary vascular resistance in patients with preexisting pulmonary hypertension.

The general anesthetic for these procedures is particularly challenging since it must provide analgesia, amnesia, and hemodynamic stability without compromising IONM. Multimodal intraoperative monitoring has become the standard of care for complex reconstructive spinal surgery.[22,23,24,25] This monitoring includes somatosensory (SSEP), motor (MEP) evoked potential, and electromyography (EMG) monitoring. The anesthesiologist determines the quality of neuromonitoring during surgery. Successful neuromonitoring which is essential for favorable outcomes after thoracic spinal surgery depends on the careful selection of anesthetic agents, the control of critical systemic variables, and the close cooperation between the anesthesiologist, surgeon, and neuromonitoring team.[26]

EMGs are used to monitor nerve root injury during pedicle screw placement and nerve decompressions. MEPs assess the integrity of the anterior, motor, spinal cord. There are several potential adverse effects of MEP monitoring, including cognitive deficits, seizures, bite injuries, intraoperative awareness, scalp burns, and cardiac arrhythmias. It is advisable to employ a soft bite block during MEP monitoring to prevent tongue biting and dental damage. MEP monitoring should be avoided in patients with active seizures, vascular clips in the brain, and cochlear implants. The posterior sensory portion of the spinal cord is evaluated using SSEP monitoring. In SSEPs, an impulse is sent from a peripheral nerve and measured centrally. In MEPs, an impulse is triggered in the brain and monitored as movement of a specific muscle group. SSEPs and MEPs are evaluated with regard to amplitude and strength of the signal and latency, time it takes the signal to travel through the spinal cord, compared to the patient's nonsurgical control values. Although SSEP monitoring is continuous, the assessment requires temporal summation of the signals which may take several minutes to change. Spontaneous patient muscle firing will result in SSEPs which are difficult to interpret (noisy), hence the ideal environment for assessing SSEPs but not MEPs is in patients treated with muscle relaxants. MEPs are assessed intermittently but the findings are real time. A number of physiological factors will attenuate SSEP and MEP monitoring, including hypotension, hypothermia, hypocarbia, hypoxemia, anemia, and anesthetics.

The potent inhalational agents produce a dose-dependent attenuation of both SSEP and MEP monitoring. This effect, however, is nonlinear; hence for a specific patient 0.5% isoflurane may have minimal effect on IONM, while at 0.7% it may abolish the signals. The various halogenated agents are similar in action, but the less soluble inhalational agents appear to be more potent with regard to suppression of IONM. In addition, potent inhalational agents reduce systemic vascular resistance and act as negative inotropes, which can contribute to hypotension and reduced tissue perfusion. Hence, for these procedures it is best to either eliminate potent inhalational agents from the anesthetic or utilize them at a low concentration which is maintained at a constant blood concentration throughout the procedure.

Nitrous oxide is a commonly used anesthetic and a carrier gas for the more potent inhalational agents in general anesthesia, because it allows for rapid emergence and has both anxiolytic and analgesic properties. Nitrous oxide attenuates MEPs and the cortical components of SSEPs. On an effective dose equivalent basis (minimum alveolar concentration [MAC]) nitrous oxide has a greater suppressant effect on IONM than the volatile agents. In addition, nitrous oxide acts synergistically with potent inhalational agents to suppress IONM. Prolonged exposure to nitrous oxide may also promote postoperative nausea and vomiting, increase cardiovascular morbidity, and have deleterious effects on cognition.

This leaves total intravenous anesthesia (TIVA; ▶ Table 3.1) as the preferred anesthetic for complex thoracic spine procedures.

Table 3.1 Anesthetic infusion for the best intraoperative neuromonitoring during complex spine procedures

- Stable infusion of propofol 25–50 µg/kg/min
- Ketamine 2 µg/kg/min (~ 1 mg/kg/h)
- Opioid fentanyl (1–2 µg/kg/h) or remifentanil (1–2 µg/kg/min)
- Dexmedetomidine 0.5 mcg/kg/h
- +/- Lidocaine 1 mg/kg/h
- Benzodiazepines: midazolam 5 mg at induction and diazepam 10 mg

Table 3.2 Corrective measure after loss of intraoperative neuromonitoring

- Is the problem technical? Check electrodes and repeat the signals
- Is the problem related to the anesthetic?
  ○ Stop any inhalational agent
  ○ Reduce or eliminate the propofol infusion
- Is the problem spinal cord perfusion?
  ○ Raise the MAP to 90 mm Hg
  ○ Hb level ≥ 8 mg/dL
  ○ Check ABG; correct metabolic acidosis
- Is the problem the surgical correction?

Abbreviations: ABG, arterial blood gas; Hb, hemoglobin; MAP, mean arterial pressure.

IONM is the least affected by narcotics and benzodiazepines, but propofol will depress MEPs in a dose-dependent manner. Since propofol accumulates in fatty tissue, the infusion rate should be decreased during long procedures. Ketamine, an N-methyl-D-aspartate (NMDA) receptor antagonist, at subanesthetic doses, will reduce the MEP-negative effects of propofol. In addition, ketamine will reduce narcotic requirements and prevent opioid-induced hyperalgesia.[27] This is an important consideration when using remifentanil, which because of its very short half-life (metabolized by plasma esterases) and lack of MEP suppression at 20 times the usual doses, has become the opioid of choice for complex spinal procedures. However, remifentanil administration has been strongly associated with opioid-induced hyperalgesia and because of its rapid elimination, it must be supplemented with other opioids to provide analgesia upon emergence. Methadone, administered at the beginning of the procedure has the advantage of long duration of action and has both opioid and NMDA properties. Intraoperative administration of methadone has been shown to reduce postoperative opioid consumption and pain scores.[28] Postoperative analgesia can also be achieved with the administration of intraoperative intrathecal morphine.[29]

Recently, TIVA anesthesia for complex spine corrections has also included two other intravenous agents: lidocaine and dexmedetomidine. The infusion of intravenous lidocaine at 1 to 2 mg/kg/h during spine operations has been shown to reduce postoperative opioid requirements and the incidence of nausea and vomiting, as well as a faster return of bowel function.[30] Dexmedetomidine is a selective α_2 agonist with anxiolytic, sedative, and analgesic properties. When infused at 0.5 mcg/kg/h, it has minimal effect on cortical SSEPs or MEPs. During spine operations, when compared to a TIVA infusion of propofol and fentanyl, the addition of dexmedetomidine improved the quality of recovery and decreased the release of cytokines implicated in the systemic immune response syndrome.[31]

The 5th National Project Audit in Great Britain (NAP5) determined that the sole use of TIVA anesthesia was associated with accidental awareness under general anesthesia (AAGA).[32] Since the brain concentration of anesthetics required to produce loss of awareness cannot be predicted and as complex spine procedures progress anesthetic dosing is often reduced to accommodate IONM, the anesthesiologist's dilemma is how to detect consciousness. Several studies have recommended the use of depth of anesthesia monitors during TIVA anesthesia. The administration of benzodiazepines may also reduce the risk of AAGA.

If the anesthesiologist is able to provide a stable physiological environment in which IONM can be interpreted with minimal influence from the anesthetics, then changes in either the SSEPs or MEPs can be used to assess surgically induced neurological injury. An example of MEP changes during a thoracic scoliosis

correction is presented in ▶ Fig. 3.1, ▶ Fig. 3.2, ▶ Fig. 3.3, ▶ Fig. 3.4. In the presented case, a patient is undergoing a thoracic scoliosis correction under TIVA anesthesia. Nine minutes after the rods are placed and the curve is corrected, there is a loss of MEP signals in specific left-sided muscle groups. The next steps which are undertaken by all of the participants are imperative for a favorable outcome (▶ Table 3.2). If a stable TIVA anesthetic has been utilized throughout the procedure, then other causes are investigated as the cause for a change in IONM, including hypotension, anemia, metabolic acidosis, and hypothermia. Once nonsurgical causes have been eliminated, the curvature correction is released by the surgeon and the degree to which the deformity can be recorrected without neurological injury is reevaluated. In this example, the rods were replaced with less deformity correction and the procedure proceeded without any further change in IONM. If the IONM deficits had persisted, the TIVA anesthetic would have been eliminated (except possibly the dexmedetomidine) and a "wake-up" test performed. The "wake-up" test involves having the patients move their hands and feet to command during the surgical procedure. It is only feasible under circumstances where the anesthetic has been designed to provide rapid emergence with minimal chance for AAGA. Preoperatively, the potential for a "wake-up" test should be discussed with the patient. Its neurological validity is limited, as it represents one point in time and only gross movement. In addition, the complications associated with this test include AAGA, tracheal extubation, air embolization from a Valsalva maneuver, and gross movement inducing neurological injury.[33]

Complex spine surgery, particularly corrective thoracic deformity surgery, is often associated with large blood losses. Multiple factors have been suggested to influence the magnitude of this blood loss, including surgical technique, operative time, number of vertebral levels fused, anesthetics, mean arterial blood pressure, platelet abnormalities, dilutional coagulopathy, and primary fibrinolysis.[34] Several techniques have been employed to reduce this blood loss and limit the need for homologous blood transfusions (▶ Table 3.3): proper positioning of the patient to reduce intra-abdominal pressure; surgical hemostasis; deliberate controlled hypotensive anesthesia; reinfusion of salvaged blood; intraoperative normovolemic hemodilution; the use of pharmacological agents which promote clot formation; and the preoperative donation of autologous blood. The predonation of autologous blood for these procedures suffers from several disadvantages: patients often are anemic on the day of surgery; the predonation and storage of autologous

16:00 Baseline Recordings   Propofol, Precedex, Ketamine, Remifentanil

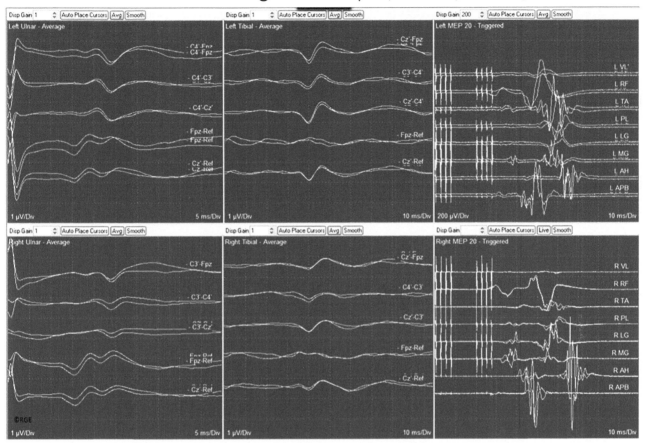

Fig. 3.1 Patient undergoing scoliosis correction under a TIVA anesthetic of propofol, Precedex, ketamine, and remifentanil. Tracing of SSEP and MEP monitoring. MEP, motor evoked potential; SSEP, somatosensory motor evoked potential; TIVA, total intravenous anesthesia.

blood is expensive; it does not eliminate the risk of a patient receiving the "wrong" unit of blood; blood is stored as packed red blood cells (RBCs), which eliminates coagulation factors; and if the surgery is rescheduled, the stored unit may expire. In patients with normal preoperative hematocrits, whole blood can be removed in the operating room prior to surgery and replaced with colloid or crystalloid such that the patient remains normovolemic.[35] This technique permits a reduction in red cell mass intraoperatively and the blood which has been removed contains platelets and coagulation factors not present in stored packed RBCs.

Several studies have demonstrated the efficacy of systemic antifibrinolytics (ε-aminocaproic acid [EACA] and tranexamic acid [TXA]) in reducing blood loss and the transfusion of homologous blood products.[36,37,38] Recently, the administration of topical TXA to reduce blood loss during spine surgery has been evaluated. Although there are no reports in the literature linking these agents with prothrombotic complications, their administration to patients with preexisting thrombophilias or pretreated with anticoagulants for coronary artery stents or prosthetic valves remains controversial.

Controlled hypotensive anesthesia has become the standard of care in limiting blood loss during idiopathic scoliosis corrections in adolescents, but must be used with caution in older patients.[39] In a young healthy patient, a mean arterial pressure (MAP) of 50 to 60 mm Hg is well tolerated, but higher pressures may be required in the adult population with cardiovascular disease. In addition, perfusion of the spinal cord during deformity correcting surgery may by exquisitely sensitive to low perfusion pressures. When employed, hypotensive anesthesia is best achieved with short-acting medications which achieve both a reduction in blood pressure and heart rate. The calcium channel blocker clevidipine reduces blood pressure by decreasing systemic vascular resistance without affecting myocardial contractility and is rapidly metabolized by plasma esterases.

The role of the anesthesiologists during complex spine surgery is to maintain end-organ perfusion despite large blood losses in an attempt to prevent devastating complications such as spinal cord ischemia, ischemic optic neuropathy (ION), renal failure, myocardial ischemia, and stroke. The best approach to achieve euvolemia and prevent end-organ ischemia and metabolic acidosis is still a dilemma. Despite the ubiquitous use of central venous pressure (CVP) monitoring during large blood loss procedures, there is a poor direct correlation between CVP and blood volume, as well as the ability of changes in CVP to predict the hemodynamic response to a fluid challenge.[40] Volume resuscitation with a pulmonary artery catheter (PAC) has been shown to be beneficial during adult reconstructive spinal

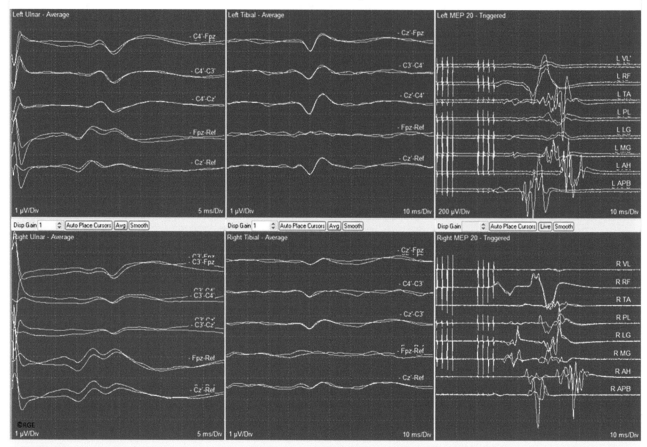

Fig. 3.2 Same patient as in ▶ Fig. 3.1, after the correction has been completed with placement of the spinal instrumentation. No change in the intraoperative neuromonitoring.

surgery.[41] However, multiple published reports have questioned the value of PAC monitoring.[42] Arterial and central venous blood gas analysis may provide information regarding tissue oxygenation requirements and perfusion. Urine output alone correlates poorly with adequate tissue perfusion, since oliguria may be a consequence of excess antidiuretic hormone release rather than hypovolemia[43] and therefore, attempts to increase urine output intraoperatively may result in excessive fluid administration.

Devices which measure arterial pulse pressure variation and provide noninvasive cardiac output measurements have been shown to be efficacious in providing goal-directed fluid therapy during complex spine procedures.[44] Several of these devices are listed in ▶ Table 3.4. Pulse contour analysis assesses ventilation-induced changes in volume loading of the heart based on the Starling curve dynamics. From this analysis these devices are able to estimate stroke volume and cardiac output.[45] The Edwards Lifesciences Vigileo/FloTrac device was used to assess and track stroke volume variation (SVV); an increase in SVV is an indicator of fluid responsiveness and hypovolemia. During a large blood loss spinal procedure, the SVV increased prior to evidence of arterial acidosis or increased oxygen utilization (decreased SVO_2) (▶ Table 3.5). Use of such monitors permits

early intervention and volume resuscitation before end-organ perfusion is compromised.

In addition to postoperative neurological deficits, postoperative visual loss (POVL) is another devastating complication of spinal surgery. POVL has been reported to be as high as 0.2% and as low as 0.028% in a large surgical population from a single hospital[46,47] after spinal surgery. The primary causes of POVL are ION, central retinal artery (CRAO) or vein occlusion, and cortical brain ischemia. CRAO has been associated with prone head positioning devices which place direct pressure on the orbit. ION has been associated with revision spine surgery, duration in the prone position, intraoperative hypotension, use of vasopressors, excessive crystalloid infusion, blood loss, anemia, and patient comorbidities including vascular disease, smoking, obesity, and diabetes.[48] However, in a retrospective case-control study of spine surgery, in patients with or without ION, anemia and hypotension were not associated factors.[49] In the American Society of Anesthesiologists (ASA) registry the patients who developed ION after spinal surgery were healthy, had a blood loss of greater than 1 L, and were positioned in the prone position for more than 6 hours. When these patients with ION were matched with spine patients who did not develop ION, the risk factors associated with ION were male

19:15
92/50

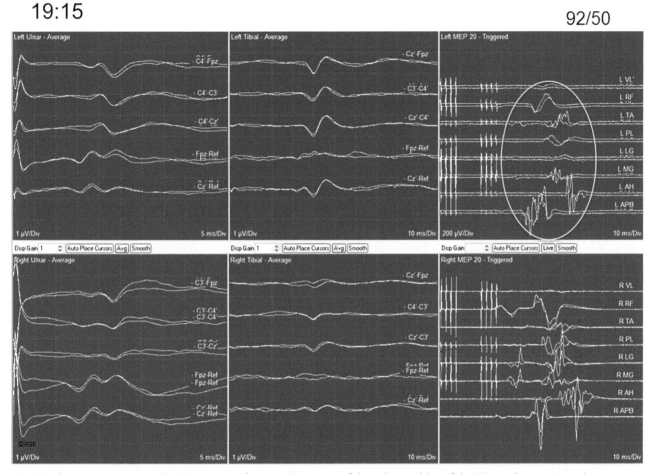

Fig. 3.3 The same patient as in ▶ Fig. 3.2, 9 minutes after surgical correction of the scoliosis with loss of the MEP signal in certain muscle groups on the left (*circle*).

sex, obesity, the use of the Wilson frame (head positioned below the heart), duration in the prone position, blood loss, and increased infusion of crystalloid as compared to colloid. These factors suggest venous congestion and interstitial edema leading to compression of the arterioles which supply the optic nerve, and ultimately ischemia to the optic nerve.

Many patients will require postoperative ventilation after thoracic spinal reconstructive surgery. Those patients with pre-existing pulmonary disease (restrictive lung disease, FEV < 50% of predicted, pulmonary hypertension), intraoperative blood loss greater than one body blood volume, intraoperative evidence of decreased perfusion (metabolic acidosis), changing ventilatory parameters (increasing peak inspiratory pressures), and evidence of impending ALI ($paO_2/FIO_2 < 300$) are candidates for postoperative ventilation. Some of these patients develop a systemic inflammatory response syndrome which manifests itself as ALI, systemic hypotension, multiple organ dysfunction, and coagulopathies. This syndrome can be quantified by the release of inflammatory cells in lung alveoli and both an increase in pulmonary and systemic cytokines.[50] The sedation goals for those patients requiring postoperative ventilation include hemodynamic stability, analgesia, and tolerance of the ventilator but awake enough for regular neurological evaluations. Dexmedetomidine has been shown to provide adequate anxiolysis, reduced narcotic requirements, and earlier extubation than propofol for postoperative ventilation.[51]

Thoracic spine patients will experience considerable postoperative pain which is best treated with a multimodality approach. Opioids will constitute a major treatment modality during the early postoperative period, but they should be administered with a patient-controlled analgesia (PCA) system. In addition, since opioids are associated with multiple deleterious side effects, they should be supplemented with intravenous and oral acetaminophen, pregabalin or gabapentin and nonsteroidal anti-inflammatory agents. When feasible, intercostal blocks can be performed with long-acting local anesthetics. In addition, as previously discussed, intrathecal morphine may be administered during the procedure.

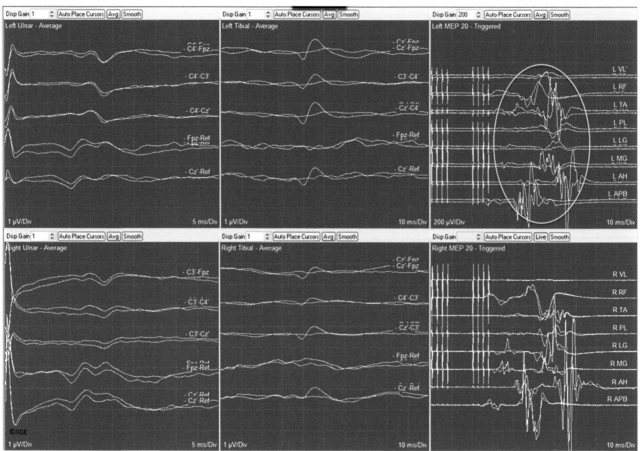

Fig. 3.4 The same patient as in ▶ Fig. 3.3, 15 minutes after a change in the surgical correction with complete restoration of all of the MEP signals (*circle*).

Table 3.3 Strategies to limit blood loss

- Autologous blood donation
- Intraoperative isovolemic hemodilution
- Antifibrinolytics
- Intraoperative scavenged blood
- Controlled hypotensive anesthesia

Table 3.4 Devices utilized for the dynamic measurements of fluid responsiveness and cardiac output

- Esophageal Doppler
- Pulse contour analysis
- Thoracic bioimpedance
- Thoracic bioreactance
- Transesophageal echocardiography

Table 3.5 Posterior thoracolumbar fusion[a]

LOS	HR	BP	CVP	CI	SVV	pH	SVO$_2$	EBL
Baseline	60	90/54	11	3.1	11	7.42	82	–
2 h	72	90/58	11	2.8	18	7.38	75	1,500
3 h	76	86/50	12	2.1	28	7.34	64	4,000
Closure	71	103/60	13	2.8	15	7.38	76	5,000[b]

Abbreviations: BP, blood pressure; CI, cardiac index; CVP, central venous pressure; EBL, estimated blood loss in milliliters; HR, heart rate; pH, arterial blood gas pH; SVO$_2$, central venous blood oxygen saturation; SVV, stroke volume variation in %, derived from the Edwards Lifesciences Vigileo/FloTrac monitor.
[a]A 55-year-old man undergoing a T3 to pelvis posterior spinal fusion for kyphoscoliosis.
[b]After resuscitation with blood and colloid.

3.4 Conclusion

The anesthetic management for thoracic spine surgery challenges the full scope of the clinician. These patients often have multiple medical comorbidities. The operative procedures have the potential for considerable blood loss. The anesthetic must provide hemodynamic stability, and match the requirement for continuous spinal cord monitoring yet provide enough depth to prevent intraoperative awareness. In addition, the operative plan must extend into the postoperative period.

References

[1] Cloyd JM, Acosta FL, Jr, Cloyd C, Ames CP. Effects of age on perioperative complications of extensive multilevel thoracolumbar spinal fusion surgery. J Neurosurg Spine. 2010; 12(4):402–408

[2] Faciszewski T, Winter RB, Lonstein JE, Denis F, Johnson L. The surgical and medical perioperative complications of anterior spinal fusion surgery in the thoracic and lumbar spine in adults. A review of 1223 procedures. Spine. 1995; 20(14):1592–1599

[3] Fujita T, Kostuik JP, Huckell CB, Sieber AN. Complications of spinal fusion in adult patients more than 60 years of age. Orthop Clin North Am. 1998; 29(4):669–678

[4] Brown MJ. Anesthesia for elective spine surgery in adults. UpToDate, 2017. https://www.uptodate.com/contents/anesthesia-for-elective-spine-surgery-in-adults/contributors. Published February 28, 2017. Accessed April 10, 2017

[5] Raw DA, Beattie JK, Hunter JM. Anaesthesia for spinal surgery in adults. Br J Anaesth. 2003; 91(6):886–904

[6] Rizzi PE, Winter RB, Lonstein JE, Denis F, Perra JH. Adult spinal deformity and respiratory failure. Surgical results in 35 patients. Spine. 1997; 22(21):2517–2530, discussion 2531

[7] Ramakrishna G, Sprung J, Ravi BS, Chandrasekaran K, McGoon MD. Impact of pulmonary hypertension on the outcomes of noncardiac surgery: predictors of perioperative morbidity and mortality. J Am Coll Cardiol. 2005; 45(10):1691–1699

[8] Glassman SD, Anagnost SC, Parker A, Burke D, Johnson JR, Dimar JR. The effect of cigarette smoking and smoking cessation on spinal fusion. Spine. 2000; 25(20):2608–2615

[9] Nakagawa M, Tanaka H, Tsukuma H, Kishi Y. Relationship between the duration of the preoperative smoke-free period and the incidence of postoperative pulmonary complications after pulmonary surgery. Chest. 2001; 120(3):705–710

[10] Memtsoudis SG, Vougioukas VI, Ma Y, Gaber-Baylis LK, Girardi FP. Perioperative morbidity and mortality after anterior, posterior, and anterior/posterior spine fusion surgery. Spine. 2011; 36(22):1867–1877

[11] Han C, Robinson DW, Jr, Hackett MV, Paramore LC, Fraeman KH, Bala MV. Cardiovascular disease and risk factors in patients with rheumatoid arthritis, psoriatic arthritis, and ankylosing spondylitis. J Rheumatol. 2006; 33(11):2167–2172

[12] Fleisher LA, Fleischmann KE, Auerbach AD et al. 2014 ACC/AHA Guideline on Perioperative Cardiovascular Evaluation and Management of Patients Undergoing Noncardiac Surgery. A Report of the American College of Cardiology/American Heart Association Task Force on Practice Guidelines 2014;64:e77–e137

[13] Devereaux PJ, Beattie WS, Choi PT, et al. How strong is the evidence for the use of perioperative beta blockers in non-cardiac surgery? Systematic review and meta-analysis of randomised controlled trials. BMJ. 2005; 331(7512):313–321

[14] Raby KE, Brull SJ, Timimi F, et al. The effect of heart rate control on myocardial ischemia among high-risk patients after vascular surgery. Anesth Analg. 1999; 88(3):477–482

[15] Devereaux PJ, Yang H, Yusuf S, et al. POISE Study Group. Effects of extended-release metoprolol succinate in patients undergoing non-cardiac surgery (POISE trial): a randomised controlled trial. Lancet. 2008; 371(9627):1839–1847

[16] Olsen MA, Nepple JJ, Riew KD, et al. Risk factors for surgical site infection following orthopaedic spinal operations. J Bone Joint Surg Am. 2008; 90(1):62–69

[17] Aldam P, Levy N, Hall GM. Perioperative management of diabetic patients: new controversies. Br J Anaesth. 2014; 113(6):906–909

[18] Kao LS, Meeks D, Moyer VA, Lally KP. Peri-operative glycaemic control regimens for preventing surgical site infections in adults. Cochrane Database Syst Rev. 2009(3):CD006806

[19] Campos JH. An update on bronchial blockers during lung separation techniques in adults. Anesth Analg. 2003; 97(5):1266–1274

[20] Determann RM, Royakkers A, Wolthuis EK, et al. Ventilation with lower tidal volumes as compared with conventional tidal volumes for patients without acute lung injury: a preventive randomized controlled trial. Crit Care. 2010; 14(1):R1

[21] Soh S, Shim JK, Ha Y, Kim YS, Lee H, Kwak YL. Ventilation with high or low tidal volume with PEEP does not influence lung function after spinal surgery in prone position: a randomized controlled trial. J Neurosurg Anesthesiol. 2018; 30(3):237–245

[22] Dormans JP. Establishing a standard of care for neuromonitoring during spinal deformity surgery. Spine. 2010; 35(25):2180–2185

[23] Eggspuehler A, Sutter MA, Grob D, Jeszenszky D, Dvorak J. Multimodal intraoperative monitoring during surgery of spinal deformities in 217 patients. Eur Spine J. 2007; 16 Suppl 2:S188–S196

[24] Rabai F, Sessions R, Seubert CN. Neurophysiological monitoring and spinal cord integrity. Best Pract Res Clin Anaesthesiol. 2016; 30(1):53–68

[25] Stecker MM. A review of intraoperative monitoring for spinal surgery. Surg Neurol Int. 2012; 3 Suppl 3:S174–S187

[26] Flynn JM, Sakai DS. Improving safety in spinal deformity surgery: advances in navigation and neurologic monitoring. Eur Spine J. 2013; 22 Suppl 2:S131–S137

[27] Gorlin AW, Rosenfeld DM, Ramakrishna H. Intravenous sub-anesthetic ketamine for perioperative analgesia. J Anaesthesiol Clin Pharmacol. 2016; 32(2):160–167

[28] Gottschalk A, Durieux ME, Nemergut EC. Intraoperative methadone improves postoperative pain control in patients undergoing complex spine surgery. Anesth Analg. 2011; 112(1):218–223

[29] Urban MK, Jules-Elysee K, Urquhart B, Cammisa FP, Boachie-Adjei O. Reduction in postoperative pain after spinal fusion with instrumentation using intrathecal morphine. Spine. 2002; 27(5):535–537

[30] Farag E, Ghobrial M, Sessler DI, et al. Effect of perioperative intravenous lidocaine administration on pain, opioid consumption, and quality of life after complex spine surgery. Anesthesiology. 2013; 119(4):932–940

[31] Bekker A, Haile M, Kline R, et al. The effect of intraoperative infusion of dexmedetomidine on the quality of recovery after major spinal surgery. J Neurosurg Anesthesiol. 2013; 25(1):16–24

[32] Pandit JJ, Andrade J, Bogod DG, et al. Royal College of Anaesthetists, Association of Anaesthetists of Great Britain and Ireland. 5th National Audit Project (NAP5) on accidental awareness during general anaesthesia: summary of main findings and risk factors. Br J Anaesth. 2014; 113(4):549–559

[33] Rodolà F, D'Avolio S, Chierichini A, Vagnoni S, Forte E, Iacobucci T. Wake-up test during major spinal surgery under remifentanil balanced anaesthesia. Eur Rev Med Pharmacol Sci. 2000; 4(3):67–70

[34] Nuttall GA, Horlocker TT, Santrach PJ, Oliver WC, Jr, Dekutoski MB, Bryant S. Predictors of blood transfusions in spinal instrumentation and fusion surgery. Spine. 2000; 25(5):596–601

[35] Murray D. Acute normovolemic hemodilution. Eur Spine J. 2004; 13 Suppl 1:S72–S75

[36] Soroceanu A, Oren JH, Smith JS, et al. Effect of antifibrinolytic therapy on complications, thromboembolic events, blood product utilization, and fusion in adult spinal deformity surgery. Spine. 2016; 41(14):E879–E886

[37] Urban MK, Beckman J, Gordon M, Urquhart B, Boachie-Adjei O. The efficacy of antifibrinolytics in the reduction of blood loss during complex adult reconstructive spine surgery. Spine. 2001; 26(10):1152–1156

[38] Verma K, Errico T, Diefenbach C, et al. The relative efficacy of antifibrinolytics in adolescent idiopathic scoliosis: a prospective randomized trial. J Bone Joint Surg Am. 2014; 96(10):e80

[39] Lyon R, Lieberman JA, Grabovac MT, Hu S. Strategies for managing decreased motor evoked potential signals while distracting the spine during correction of scoliosis. J Neurosurg Anesthesiol. 2004; 16(2):167–170

[40] Marik PE, Baram M, Vahid B. Does central venous pressure predict fluid responsiveness? A systematic review of the literature and the tale of seven mares. Chest. 2008; 134(1):172–178

[41] Urban MK, Urquhart B, Boachie-Adjei O. Evidence of lung injury during reconstructive surgery for adult spinal deformities with pulmonary artery pressure monitoring. Spine. 2001; 26(4):387–390

[42] Tuman KJ, Roizen MF. Outcome assessment and pulmonary artery catheterization: why does the debate continue? Anesth Analg. 1997; 84(1):1–4

[43] Cregg N, Mannion D, Casey W. Oliguria during corrective spinal surgery for idiopathic scoliosis: the role of antidiuretic hormone. Paediatr Anaesth. 1999; 9(6):505–514

[44] Marik PE. Noninvasive cardiac output monitors: a state-of the-art review. J Cardiothorac Vasc Anesth. 2013; 27(1):121–134

[45] Missant C, Rex S, Wouters PF. Accuracy of cardiac output measurements with pulse contour analysis (PulseCO) and Doppler echocardiography during off-pump coronary artery bypass grafting. Eur J Anaesthesiol. 2008; 25(3):243–248

[46] Chang SH, Miller NR. The incidence of vision loss due to perioperative ischemic optic neuropathy associated with spine surgery: the Johns Hopkins Hospital Experience. Spine. 2005; 30(11):1299–1302

[47] Patil CG, Lad EM, Lad SP, Ho C, Boakye M. Visual loss after spine surgery: a population-based study. Spine. 2008; 33(13):1491–1496

[48] Nickels TJ, Manlapaz MR, Farag E. Perioperative visual loss after spine surgery. World J Orthop. 2014; 5(2):100–106

[49] Lee TH, Marcantonio ER, Mangione CM, et al. Derivation and prospective validation of a simple index for prediction of cardiac risk of major noncardiac surgery. Circulation. 1999; 100(10):1043–1049

[50] Urban MK, Jules-Elysee KM, Beckman JB, et al. Pulmonary injury in patients undergoing complex spine surgery. Spine J. 2005; 5(3):269–276

[51] Turunen H, Jakob SM, Ruokonen E, et al. Dexmedetomidine versus standard care sedation with propofol or midazolam in intensive care: an economic evaluation. Crit Care. 2015; 19:67

4 Clinical Presentation of Thoracic Spinal Compression

Bridget T. Carey

Abstract

The thoracic segment of the spine has unique anatomical and neuroanatomical features that differentiate it from the cervical spine above and lumbosacral spine below. Compression of the thoracic spine may occur due to degenerative and/or spondylotic disease, traumatic injury, infection, or neoplastic disease. Neurological injury can occur on the basis of mechanical compression, and can result in clinical neurological deficits. The clinical presentation of thoracic spinal compression is varied, based on the location and the degree of compression. The clinical features of thoracic cord compression and thoracic radiculopathy are dictated by the longitudinal and cross-sectional neuroanatomy of the spine, and can be identified by characteristic features related to this neuroanatomy.

Keywords: thoracic spinal cord, thoracic myelopathy, spinal tracts, thoracic radiculopathy, spastic paraparesis, spinal cord lesion, spinal cord compression

Clinical Pearls

- Pain due to thoracic spinal compression may be radicular, axial, or claudicatory involving the lower extremities.
- Spinal cord compression due to degenerative disease is relatively rare in the thoracic segment, compared with the incidence in the lumbar and cervical segments.
- Longitudinal and cross-sectional spinal neuroanatomy allows a careful neurological examination to identify and localize neurological injury due to thoracic spinal compression.

4.1 Introduction

The thoracic segment of the spine has unique anatomical and neuroanatomical features that differentiate it from the cervical spine above and lumbosacral spine below. Compression of the thoracic spine may occur due to a number of causes, including degenerative disc disease, spondylotic disease, traumatic injury, infection, or neoplastic disease. Neurological injury can occur on the basis of mechanical compression, and can result in clinical neurological deficits. The spinal cord can be injured adjacent to the site of compression, resulting in thoracic myelopathy. Alternatively, the segmental spinal nerve roots that exit the thoracic vertebral neural foramen can be focally compressed, resulting in thoracic radiculopathy.

The clinical presentation of thoracic spinal compression is varied, based on the location and the degree of compression. The clinical features of thoracic cord compression and thoracic radiculopathy are dictated by the longitudinal and cross-sectional neuroanatomy of the spine, and can be identified by characteristic features related to this neuroanatomy.

In this chapter, anatomical considerations and pathological processes affecting the thoracic spine will be outlined to provide context for the clinical presentation of thoracic spine lesions. The reader is referred to chapters elsewhere in this text for in-depth review of anatomy and various pathological processes. Subsequently, general and specific patterns of thoracic region spinal compression are described and discussed.

4.2 Anatomical Considerations

The thoracic segment of the spine possesses anatomical features that differentiate it from the cervical and lumbosacral spine. Some of these features serve to protect the thoracic segment from injury, while others render it particularly vulnerable.

The thoracic vertebral column is relatively immobile compared with the rostral cervical and caudal lumbosacral spinal segments. The ribs and their anterior articulation with the sternum provide additional skeletal stability to the thoracic spine. Further, the extensive paraspinal and back musculature of this region, including postural muscles, longitudinal muscles, and the scapular limb-girdle musculature serves to strengthen and protect the thoracic spine from external stresses.

While the above factors serve to limit injury based on mechanical stressors, additional anatomical factors confer a greater risk of spinal cord injury when structural spine injury does occur to the thoracic spine. The diameter of the thoracic spinal canal, particularly in the rostral thoracic vertebrae, is smaller than that of the cervical and lumbar vertebrae. This increases the likelihood of neurological injury due to compression of the spinal cord within the central canal at these narrower levels.[1,2]

Additionally, the vasculature of the spinal cord is organized such that there is greater blood flow through the radicular arteries in the cervical and lumbar segments than there is through the radicular branches in the thoracic region. Further, sulcal branches off of the anterior spinal artery are least numerous in the thoracic region. As a result, the cervical and lumbar spinal cord possess a more robust anastomotic vascular network than does the thoracic segment. The thoracic spine represents a vascular watershed region, rendering it especially vulnerable to ischemic injury.[3,4]

4.3 Pathological Process of Compression

4.3.1 Mechanism of Neurological Compression Injury

The mechanism of neurological injury on the basis of compression may result from direct deformation and destruction of nervous tissue in cases of extreme compressive forces. If the compressive force is sufficient, the spinal cord can sustain contusion or crush injury, in which there is direct sheering or rupture of axonal processes. This type of injury is particularly relevant in cases of trauma. Alternatively, injuries due to milder repetitive forces, or milder forces sustained over time, may also result in direct injury to neuronal structures through direct axonal injury or by interference with the integrity of neural support cells.

The most common pathological mechanism for neurological injury on the basis of compression injury is thought to be ischemia. The spinal cord and the spinal nerve roots are highly perfused tissues. The establishment and maintenance of the action potential is energy dependent, thus nervous tissue is highly metabolic. Compression of nervous tissue in excess of capillary perfusion pressure results in ischemia, and eventually infarction.[3,4,5]

4.3.2 Degenerative Disc Disease and Spondylosis

Spinal cord compression on a degenerative basis involving the thoracic segment is relatively rare. The significantly greater motility of cervical and lumbosacral spinal segments renders these regions more vulnerable to injuries on a mechanical basis than is the thoracic spine, reinforced as it is by the thoracic cage and by the extensive paraspinal and back musculature of this region. Thoracic disc herniations comprise less than 1% of all disc prolapses that come to clinical attention.[1,6,7] Other variants of degenerative disease such as facet arthropathy, and calcification of ligaments occur more frequently. Congenital stenosis may be a contributing factor.

4.3.3 Other Compressive Pathology

In addition to degenerative and/or spondylotic disease, various pathological processes can result in spinal cord compression. Tumor and infection are the main considerations in this category. For pathological processes that affect the vertebral bodies indiscriminately, the fact that there are 12 thoracic vertebrae increases the odds that vertebral bodies belonging to this segment may become involved, simply on the basis of larger numerical representation. Bony spinal metastases involve thoracic vertebrae more frequently than they do the lumbar and cervical vertebral bodies, by a ratio of 4:2:1.[8]

4.4 Clinical Presentation of Thoracic Spinal Compression

In cases of compressive neurological injury to the thoracic spine, individual consideration is given to injuries involving the spinal roots (radiculopathy) and the spinal cord (myelopathy). Compression injuries in the thoracic spine may cause either or both. Therefore, the clinical syndromes associated with thoracic radiculopathy and myelopathy may occur separately or together. In situations resulting in the compression of both nerve root and spinal cord, one clinical syndrome may predominate, depending on the degree and exact lines of compressive force.

The neuroanatomical organization of the spinal cord allows for longitudinal as well as axial plane localization of injury in many cases. Compression of the neural structures within the thoracic spine results in specific patterns of symptoms and neurological deficits. General patterns of thoracic segment injury

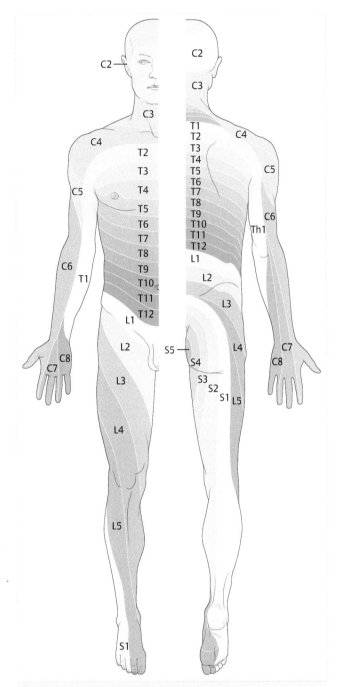

Fig. 4.1 Pattern of radicular sensory innervation. (Reproduced from Ross LM, Lamperti ED, eds. Atlas of Anatomy: General Anatomy and Musculoskeletal System. New York, NY: Thieme; 2006:66.)

are described, as are specific identifiable patterns of neurological deficits based on injury location (▶ Fig. 4.1).

4.4.1 Pain

As is true with clinically significant compression throughout all regions of the spine, pain is the common symptom of thoracic spinal compression. Pain may involve the thoracic back region, either in a radicular or axial pattern. Intermittent pain in the legs with walking or prolonged standing is common, due to neurogenic claudication.

Thoracic Radiculopathy

The spinal nerve roots are highly pain sensitive. At all levels of the spinal column, compression of the exiting spinal nerve is associated with pain. The thoracic nerve roots exit their numbered vertebral neural foramen to innervate the circumferential thoracic dermatomes, and to innervate local thoracic and abdominal musculature. Thoracic radicular pain may manifest in a classic lateralized regional pain distribution: the patient may experience pain in a region of the thoracic spine, with radiation laterally and anteriorly in a band-like distribution that reflects the territory of the affected dermatome.[6]

Of note, thoracic radicular pain is sometimes less easy to identify than is dermatomal pain in the limbs. Because of its involvement of the trunk, thoracic radicular pain may be misinterpreted as cardiac pain, costochondritis, or pleural pain.[9]

Thoracic Spinal Cord Injury

Pain is common with spinal cord compression at all levels, including in the thoracic spine. This is a consequence of the fact that the pathology that causes the compression, as well as its associated physiological processes, are frequently pain generators in their own right (e.g., trauma, bone injury, infection, inflammation). In addition, the causative mechanisms that result in spinal cord compression almost invariably compress adjacent tissues, which are pain sensitive. If the compressive lesion involves the local exiting spinal nerve root, dermatomal pain ensues. In the case of vertebral body pathology (fracture, osteomyelitis, metastatic invasion), point tenderness may be present. In some cases, pain may be vague and poorly localized, potentially perceived as originating from thoracic or abdominal viscera.

Neurogenic Claudication

Pain involving the bilateral lower extremities may occur due to thoracic spinal compression on the basis of neurogenic claudication. Characteristically, the pain develops in the setting of ambulation, and worsens as the patient continues to walk. Prolonged standing may also induce symptoms. One leg may be more affected than the other. Invariably, the pain is relieved with rest. Constant pain in the lower extremities is not a feature of thoracic segment disease; its presence would implicate lumbar root involvement, or other nonspine-related pathology.

4.4.2 Neurological Deficits

The general pattern of neurological impairment that occurs on the basis of thoracic spine compression usually involves asymmetrical spastic paraparesis, with associated asymmetrical sensory deficits in the lower extremities. The patient often presents with gait disturbance. While weakness of the legs may be endorsed, usually the patient perceives a lack of stability with walking. Gait feels poorly controlled, irregular, and erratic. Falls may be frequent. While motor weakness and spasticity may contribute to the gait dysfunction, the main pathology

likely occurs as a consequence of impaired sensory processing, motor coordination, and motor refinement, due to disruption of afferent and efferent spinal tracts resulting in sensory ataxia.[10]

On neurological examination, findings consistent with thoracic myelopathy may be present. Increased tone in the lower extremities, with normal tone in the upper extremities, may be elicited. Variable degrees of usually asymmetrical motor weakness are often seen in the legs. Changes in sensation may be present in the legs, and in some cases in the trunk, below the level of injury. Hyperreflexia in the lower extremities with normal upper extremity deep tendon reflexes is a characteristic examination finding. Ankle clonus may be present. Pathological reflexes in the lower extremities may be present, however, the absence of these does not rule out the diagnosis.[2,4,6]

4.4.3 Longitudinal Patterns of Thoracic Injury

For clinical purposes, the thoracic spine may be divided into upper and lower regions in the cranial–caudal dimension. In cross-section, the thoracic spinal cord maintains the neuroanatomical organization of the long tracts that course through the entirety of the spinal cord, from the medullary decussations in the brainstem through to the conus medullaris. Interference in the conduction of an action potential at any point along these white matter tracts will produce a neurological deficit below the level of the lesion. The longitudinal localization of an injury may thus be identified by the dermatomal and/or myotomal level above which function is preserved, and below which function is impaired.

Upper Thoracic Levels

While the cervical spine subserves the majority of afferent and efferent pathways concerning the upper limbs, clinical presentation of upper thoracic cord and/or spinal root compression may involve the upper extremities. The nerve roots that exit above and below the T1 vertebral body, the C8 and T1 nerve roots, respectively, fuse together to form the inferior trunk of the brachial plexus. The C8-T1 nerve roots predominantly comprise the medial cord of the brachial plexus. They provide the main innervation (along with a small contribution from C7) to the ulnar nerve, and contribute fibers to the median and radial nerves. Both median and ulnar intrinsic hand muscles are innervated solely by the C8-T1 roots. Therefore, interruption of neurological function at the most cephalad thoracic vertebral level may present with C8-T1 myotomal dysfunction. Clinically, this manifests as intrinsic hand muscle weakness. Subjectively, a sense of hand "clumsiness" as opposed to overt weakness may be endorsed; because function at the wrist and of the long flexors and extensors of the fingers is preserved, much of routine hand function is maintained. If the C8 level is spared, a pure T1 lesion may result only in very subtle intrinsic hand musculature dysfunction (▶ Fig. 4.2).

The sensory distribution of the medial hand (C8), medial arm (T1, T2), and axilla (T3), are additionally subserved by the upper thoracic levels. Sensory deficits involving the medial upper extremity may occur in injury involving the upper thoracic spine.

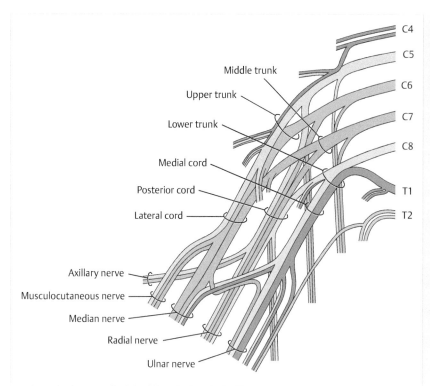

Middle trunk

Upper trunk

Lower trunk

Medial cord

Posterior cord

Lateral cord

Axillary nerve

Musculocutaneous nerve

Median nerve

Radial nerve

Ulnar nerve

C4
C5
C6
C7
C8
T1
T2

Fig. 4.2 Schematic representation of the brachial plexus. (Reproduced from Ross LM, Lamperti ED, eds. Atlas of Anatomy: General Anatomy and Musculoskeletal System. New York, NY: Thieme; 2006:314.)

In injuries superior to the T6 level, autonomic dysfunction may ensue with significant cardiovascular and thermoregulatory dysregulation, along with bowel and bladder dysfunction.[11]

Lower Thoracic Levels

In the lower regions of the thoracic spine, dermatomal deficits reflect a band-like circumferential region of sensation. Autonomic dysfunction below the level of T6 may include variable deficits of bowel, bladder, and/or sexual function.

The lower thoracic spine is the most vulnerable to degenerative injury. The T10 to T12 levels retain the greatest mobility of the thoracic column, and as such, are more likely to succumb to disc degeneration and other variants of "wear-and-tear–related" pathology.[1,6,8]

4.4.4 Cross-Sectional Patterns of Thoracic Injury

Injuries to the spinal cord due to the mechanism of compression are usually incomplete. However, complete functional spinal cord transection can occur in extreme injuries. Given the vascular watershed region in the thoracic cord, and the relatively small bony diameter of the central canal in the thoracic spine, injuries in this region can result in catastrophic neurological injury.[4,10,12]

More commonly, compression of the thoracic cord results in regional ischemia and subsequent focal demyelination. If the force of the compression is great enough, or if the duration of a lesser intensity compression goes on long for enough, axonal injury ensues.

Several classic clinical spinal cord syndromes are described, in which a regional injury to a part of the spinal cord results in a constellation of symptoms and neurological examination signs. Several of these can occur on the basis of compression injury.

Complete Cord Transection

All ascending and descending pathways are severed or functionally incapacitated. A dermatomal sensory level is typically identified one to two segments below the actual site of injury. In the acute setting, flaccid paralysis of muscles inferior to the injured level occurs (spinal shock), followed over time (weeks to months) by evolution into a spastic paralysis. Autonomic dysfunction additionally occurs below the level of the lesion, leading to dysregulation in maintenance of body temperature, loss of bowel and bladder sphincter control, orthostatic dysfunction, and other autonomic dysregulation.

Hemicord (Brown–Sequard) Syndrome

If injury of the spinal cord occurs unilaterally, or predominantly involving the right or left side of the spinal cord, a specific pattern of deficits occurs. Below the level of the lesion, ipsilateral upper motor neuron weakness will occur, along with ipsilateral loss of vibration perception and proprioception. Ipsilateral autonomic dysfunction may be present (e.g., inability to sweat on the ipsilateral side of the body below the injured level). Contralateral loss of pain and temperature sensation co-occurs. This "crossed sensory deficit" pattern occurs due to the regional spinal level decussation of the anterolateral spinal thalamic tract, which subserves the sensory modalities of pain and temperature. The dorsal column sensory tracts and the corticospinal motor tracts decussate in the medulla, superior to the level of the spinal cord lesion.

Posterior and Posterolateral Cord Syndrome

Injury affecting the posterior spinal cord will predominantly affect the posterior (dorsal) columns. The lateral corticospinal (pyramidal) tract may also be involved in posterior lesions. Loss of proprioception and discriminatory aspects of sensation in the lower extremities results from dorsal column dysfunction in the thoracic cord. Gait instability on the basis of sensory ataxia is the primary clinical manifestation of this. If the injury proceeds laterally, pyramidal tracts may be affected, resulting in ipsilateral leg weakness, most commonly with a significant degree of associated limb spasticity.

Anterior and Anterolateral Cord Syndrome

This syndrome is classically described as a consequence of vascular pathology, on the basis of anterior spinal artery territory ischemia. However, mechanical compression resulting in small vessel ischemia and demyelination may also occur. Injury to the anterior spinal cord disrupts the anterolateral spinothalamic tracts, descending autonomic pathways, anterior horn cells, and (in the case of anterior spinal artery infarction) the corticospinal tract. Anterior spinal cord injury on the basis of compression may spare the corticospinal tracts, which share the anterior spinal artery vascular distribution, but which are physically situated more laterally and posteriorly in the cord. Loss of pain and temperature below the level of injury characterize this syndrome, along with bladder incontinence, and varying degrees of additional autonomic dysregulation. Motor weakness will occur if the corticospinal tracts are sufficiently disrupted (▶ Fig. 4.3, ▶ Fig. 4.4).[5,10,12]

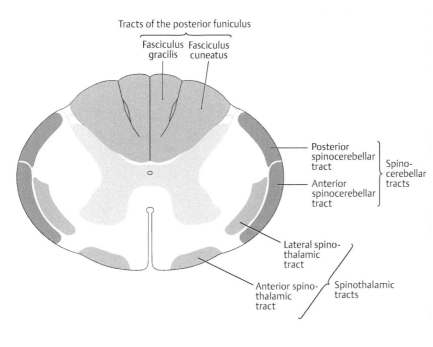

Fig. 4.3 Ascending tracts in the spinal cord. Transverse section through the spinal cord and the location of the major afferent (sensory) tracts. (Reproduced from Ross LM, Lamperti ED, Taub E, eds. Atlas of Anatomy: Head and Neuroanatomy. New York, NY: Thieme; 2007:284.)

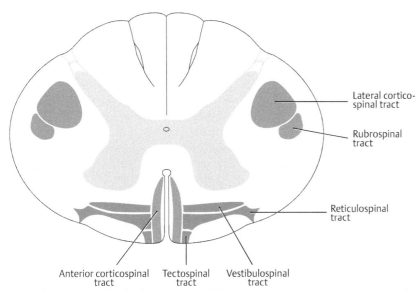

Fig. 4.4 Descending tracts in the spinal cord. Transverse section through the spinal cord and the location of the major efferent (motor) tracts. (Reproduced from Ross LM, Lamperti ED, Taub E, eds. Atlas of Anatomy: Head and Neuroanatomy. New York, NY: Thieme; 2007:285.)

4.5 Conclusions

The clinical presentation of thoracic spinal compression is varied; however, certain features are common. Pain is almost always present, to a greater or lesser extent. Pain may be radicular, axial, or may involve the lower extremities in an intermittent pattern of neurogenic claudication. Neurological deficits reflect varying degrees of impairment of the afferent and efferent spinal tracts that course through the thoracic cord. The longitudinal and cross-sectional neuroanatomy of the spinal cord should be considered in the clinical presentation. Asymmetrical upper motor neuron weakness of the legs, asymmetrical and sometimes crossed deficits in modalities of sensation, and lower extremity hyperreflexia commonly occur on the basis of thoracic segment spine compression. Careful neurological examination can often distinguish thoracic level pathology from the clinically more common cervical and lumbosacral pathological patterns.

References

[1] Byrne TN, Benzel EC, Waxman SG. Anatomy and biomechanics of the spine and spinal cord. In: Byrne TN, Benzel EC, Waxman SG, eds. Diseases of the Spine and Spinal Cord. New York, NY: Oxford University Press; 2000:3–39

[2] Fogelson JL, Krauss W. Compressive and traumatic myelopathies. American Academy of Neurology Continuum. 2008; 14(3):116–133

[3] Taylor AR. Vascular factors in the myelopathy associated with cervical spondylosis. Neurology. 1964; 14:62–68

[4] Tavee JO, Levin KH. Myelopathy due to degenerative and structural spine diseases. Continuum (Minneap Minn). 2015; 21 1 Spinal Cord Disorders: 52–66

[5] Ropper AH, Samuels MA. Diseases of the spinal cord. In: Ropper AH, Samuels MA, eds. Adams and Victor's Principles of Neurology. New York, NY: McGraw-Hill; 2008:1181–1230

[6] Raynor EM, Kleiner-Fisman G, Nardin R. Lumbosacral and thoracic radiculopathies. In: Katirji B, Kaminski HJ, Preston DC, Ruff RL, Shapiro BE, eds. Neuromuscular Disorders in Clinical Practice. Boston, MA: Butterworth Heinemann; 2002:859–883

[7] Rosenbloom SA. Thoracic disc disease and stenosis. Radiol Clin North Am. 1991; 29(4):765–775

[8] DeAngelis LM, Posner JB. Spinal metastases. In: DeAngelis LM, Posner JB, eds. Neurologic Complications of Cancer. New York, NY: Oxford University Press; 2009:194–239

[9] Shirzadi A, Drazin D, Jeswani S, Lovely L, Liu J. Atypical presentation of thoracic disc herniation: case series and review of the literature. Case Rep Orthop. 2013; 2013:621476

[10] Cho TA. Spinal cord functional anatomy. Continuum (Minneap Minn). 2015; 21 1 Spinal Cord Disorders:13–35

[11] Garstang SV, Miller-Smith SA. Autonomic nervous system dysfunction after spinal cord injury. Phys Med Rehabil Clin N Am. 2007; 18(2):275–296, vi–vii

[12] Gruener G, Biller J. Spinal cord anatomy, localization, and overview of spinal cord syndromes. Continuum: Lifelong Learning Neurol. 2008; 14(3):11–35

5 Nonoperative Neurological Diseases of the Thoracic Spinal Cord

Joshua Weaver

Abstract

This chapter provides an overview of the various nonoperative neurological diseases of the thoracic spinal cord including inflammatory, infectious, autoimmune, hereditary, and toxic/metabolic derangements. A review of the clinical features, diagnostic workup, treatment options, and prognosis is presented. Specific etiologies include multiple sclerosis, neuromyelitis optica, autoimmune disorders, sarcoidosis, paraneoplastic syndromes, infectious myelitis, vitamin deficiencies, toxic myelopathies, and hereditary myelopathies.

Keywords: thoracic cord lesions, myelopathy, inflammatory lesions, transverse myelitis, multiple sclerosis, neuromyelitis optica, B12 deficiency, copper deficiency

Clinical Pearls

- Weakness in the early phase of transverse myelitis may not be associated with the typical upper motor neuron signs of spasticity and hyperreflexia, and may be diagnostically challenging.
- Demyelinating thoracic cord lesions in multiple sclerosis may be more common than previously thought and may be correlated with more severe disability.
- Neuromyelitis optica, a demyelinating disorder similar to multiple sclerosis, is often more severe and disabling, and as such may be treated differently.
- The most common paraneoplastic antibodies associated with thoracic cord myelopathy are antiamphiphysin and collapsin response mediator protein-5 (CRMP-5).
- Myelitis may occur due to direct infection of the spinal cord or indirectly via an autoimmune reaction related to an infection elsewhere in the body.
- Copper deficiency may cause a similar clinical picture of subacute combined degeneration as B_{12} deficiency, and it is often overlooked as a possible etiology. A history of gastric surgery is a helpful clue to this diagnosis.

5.1 Introduction

There are a multitude of disease entities that can affect the thoracic spinal cord. This chapter will focus on the diseases that are treated nonoperatively. Thoracic spinal cord lesions cause sensory deficits, autonomic dysfunction, and motor weakness from the thoracic region inferiorly toward the lower extremities. A myriad of inflammatory, infectious, autoimmune, genetic, and metabolic etiologies can cause lesions in the spinal cord. First, there will be a brief review of the clinical manifestations of thoracic cord lesions in general, as many of the various etiologies can cause similar clinical presentations. Following that, specific disease entities will be briefly reviewed, detailing

the etiology, diagnosis, treatment, and prognosis of the various disorders affecting the thoracic spinal cord. Vascular and neoplastic disorders will not be discussed here as they are reviewed in other chapters.

5.2 Clinical Presentation of Thoracic Cord Lesions

A thoracic cord lesion typically presents with pain and numbness in a band-like distribution around the chest or abdomen radiating inferiorly. Muscle weakness may not be clear initially in the thoracic region due to significant overlap in the intercostal musculature. However, if the lesion involves the ascending corticospinal tracts, upper motor neuron motor deficits may affect the lower extremities causing weakness, increased tone, and hyperreflexia. Back pain and exertional leg pain are common. A spastic gait or even inability to walk may be present. If the lesion is above T6, autonomic dysfunction may occur causing cardiopulmonary, bowel, bladder, and sexual dysfunction. Patients with chronic myelopathies are at higher risk for coronary artery disease, pneumonia, deep venous thrombosis, pulmonary embolism, urinary tract infections, pressure ulcers, contractures, osteoporosis, and chronic constipation.[1]

5.3 Inflammatory Myelopathies

Inflammation of the spinal cord, known as transverse myelitis (whether involving the whole cord or only involving part of the cord), can be caused by many different disease entities or may be idiopathic. Inflammatory myelitis may occur over hours to weeks though generally reaches its peak severity in under a month if untreated.[2] Weakness in the early phase may be associated with flaccid tone and hyporeflexia; the typical upper motor neuron signs of myelopathy may occur later, and this can prove to be diagnostically challenging. Signs of inflammation can be seen on magnetic resonance imaging (MRI) with gadolinium contrast enhancement in the spinal cord and with cerebrospinal fluid (CSF) patterns of pleocytosis, elevated protein, oligoclonal bands, or elevated immunoglobulin G (IgG) index (▶ Fig. 5.1). In almost all cases of transverse myelitis, first-line treatment is high-dose intravenous (IV) methylprednisolone (1 g daily for 3–7 days) even if the cause of the inflammation is unknown. Despite the lack of studies to support this, steroids are generally used to quicken recovery and restore neurological function.[3] In general, among all cases of transverse myelitis, the prognosis is split into thirds with one-third recovering with minimal or no sequelae, one-third with moderate disability, and one-third with severe disability.[4]

5.3.1 Multiple Sclerosis

Multiple sclerosis is the most common immune-mediated inflammatory disease of the central nervous system affecting

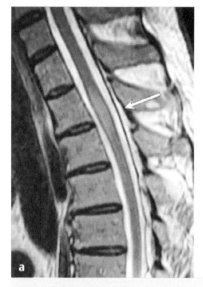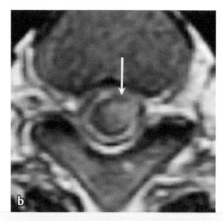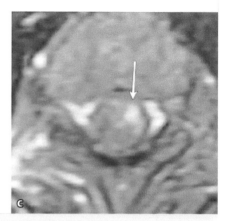

Fig. 5.1 **(a)** Sagittal and **(b)** axial images of a 51-year-old man with transverse myelitis involving the thoracic spinal cord (*arrows*) that has high signal involving more than two-thirds of the cross-sectional area of the spinal cord. **(c)** Axial fat-suppressed T1-weighted imaging shows gadolinium contrast enhancement of the actively demyelinating lesion (*arrow*). (Reproduced from Meyers SP. Differential Diagnosis in Neuroimaging: Spine. New York, NY: Thieme; 2017: 73.)

the myelin of axons within the brain, optic nerves, and spinal cord. Transverse myelitis due to multiple sclerosis commonly involves short segments of the spinal cord (spanning less than three vertebrae) and is often located dorsally[2] (▶ Fig. 5.2). Inflammation of the spinal cord tends to be partial, showing asymmetric neurological signs.[5] Involvement of the spinal cord is known to be correlated with disability outcomes.[6] Though cervical cord lesions have been more frequently studied in clinical trials of multiple sclerosis, there is growing evidence to suggest that thoracic cord lesions may be more common than previously thought, and diagnosing thoracic lesions may be important in clinical management and prognosticating on future disability.[6,7] Though the vast majority of people with acute transverse myelitis secondary to multiple sclerosis improve, only about half show complete recovery.[5] Risk factors for acute transverse myelitis as an initial event progressing into multiple sclerosis include family history of multiple sclerosis, severe impairment at onset, brain MRI lesions typical of multiple sclerosis, abnormal IgG index in the CSF, and the presence of CSF oligoclonal bands.[5] Acute treatment of transverse myelitis due to multiple sclerosis consists of IV steroids and less often plasma exchange. There are many disease-modifying treatments currently available for multiple sclerosis including injectable, oral, and IV medications that reduce the number of new lesions and number of relapses over the course of the disease.

5.3.2 Neuromyelitis Optica

Neuromyelitis optica (NMO), another demyelinating disorder, used to be considered a variant of multiple sclerosis but is now seen as a distinctly separate disease.[8] Similar to multiple sclerosis, NMO can affect many different parts of the central nervous system, though there is a predilection for the spinal cord and optic nerves. Presence of an autoantibody biomarker against

aquaporin-4 water channels is considered sufficient to make a diagnosis of NMO, though there are also NMO spectrum disorders that are aquaporin-4 seronegative.[8] Cord lesions tend to be more extensive than those seen in multiple sclerosis, often spanning more than three vertebral segments (▶ Fig. 5.3). Clinical attacks are often more severe and disabling than multiple sclerosis, and plasma exchange in addition to steroids may be necessary for better outcomes. Maintenance therapy usually consists of immunosuppressants such as rituximab, azathioprine, or mycophenolate mofetil, though data supporting their use are limited.[2,8]

5.3.3 Neurosarcoidosis

Sarcoidosis is a granulomatous disease commonly affecting the lung or lymph nodes that may also rarely (about 5%) affect the spinal cord, cranial nerves, and brain. It is often difficult to distinguish from multiple sclerosis or NMO, though the course may be more subacute, and MRI may more often show leptomeningeal enhancement (▶ Fig. 5.4).[4] Chest imaging to look for pulmonary involvement helps to aid in the diagnosis. Serum and CSF angiotensin-converting enzyme levels may also help with the diagnosis, though sensitivity tends to be poor. Acute therapy consists of steroids and antitumor necrosis factor therapy for refractory cases.[2]

5.3.4 Connective Tissue Disorders

Several connective tissue disorders can cause transverse myelitis, including systemic lupus erythematosus (SLE), Sjögren's syndrome, mixed connective tissue disorder, and systemic scleroderma.

SLE is a chronic and relapsing–remitting autoimmune disorder that may affect multiple organ systems including joints,

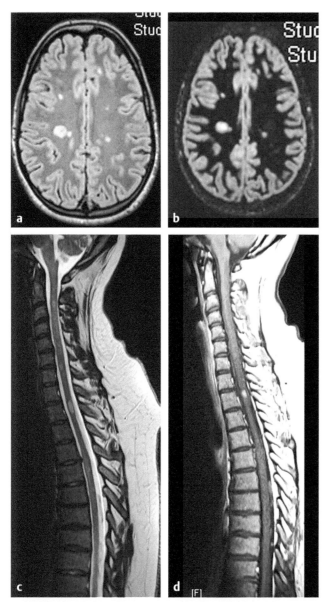

Fig. 5.2 Multiple sclerosis in a 22-year-old woman with a 6-week history of sensory disturbances in her right arm. No other symptoms were present. CSF was positive for oligoclonal bands. **(a)** Axial FLAIR sequence of the brain demonstrates multiple hyperintense lesions. **(b)** Axial DIR sequence of the brain. The lesions are depicted in higher contrast. **(c)** Sagittal T2-weighted image of the cervical spine demonstrates multiple hyperintense lesions. Each of the lesions spans no more than one vertebral body height. **(d)** Sagittal T1-weighted sequence after contrast administration. Individual lesions show marked enhancement. (Reproduced from Schlamann M. Inflammations, infections, and related diseases. In: Forsting M, Jansen O, eds. MR Neuroimaging: Brain, Spine, Peripheral Nerves. New York, NY: Thieme; 2017:519.)

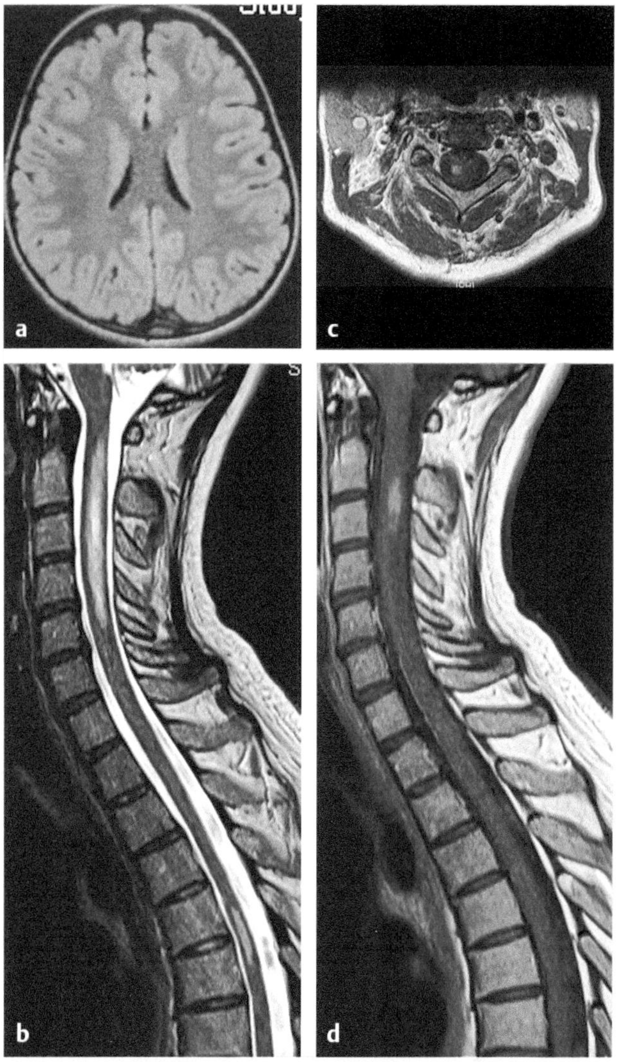

Fig. 5.3 Neuromyelitis optica in a 25-year-old woman with left-sided optic neuritis and quadriparesis. CSF examination showed pleocytosis. Serum test was positive for aquaporin antibodies. **(a)** FLAIR image of the brain shows a small, nonspecific white-matter hyperintensity in the left frontal region. **(b)** Sagittal T2-weighted image of the cervical spine shows hyperintensity extending along the spinal cord from the C1-5 levels. **(c)** Axial T1-weighted image after contrast administration shows circumscribed enhancement on the right side. **(d)** Sagittal T1-weighted image after contrast administration. The T2-weighted hyperintensity in panel **(b)** shows partial enhancement. (Reproduced from Schlamann M. Inflammations, infections, and related diseases. In: Forsting M, Jansen O, eds. MR Neuroimaging: Brain, Spine, Peripheral Nerves. New York, NY: Thieme; 2017:522.)

skin, kidneys, lungs, and heart. Neuropsychiatric involvement is seen in as many as 60% of cases and may present as seizures, stroke, or psychosis, though transverse myelitis is only seen in about 1 to 2% of people with SLE.[9] Several autoantibodies are associated with SLE including antinuclear antibody and double-stranded DNA antibody, though particularly associated with SLE myelitis is the antiphospholipid antibody.[4] Treatment with IV steroids and occasionally with cyclophosphamide and plasma exchange is generally effective, with complete recovery occurring in about 50% of patients, partial improvement in close to 30%, and no improvement or worsening seen in about 20%.[9]

Sjögren's syndrome, another chronic multisystem auto-immune disorder, typically causes sicca symptoms including dry eyes, dry mouth, and parotid gland enlargement. Anti-Sjög-

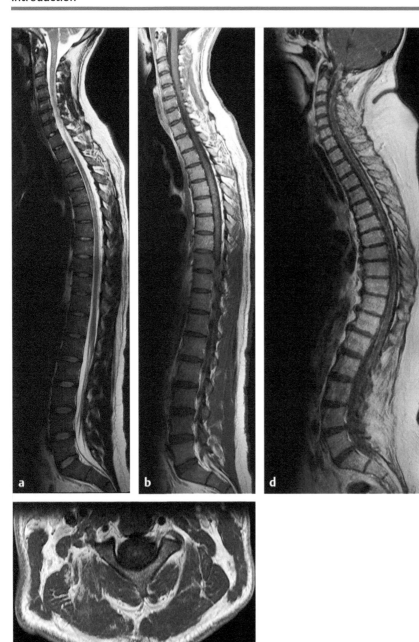

Fig. 5.4 Sarcoidosis in a 56-year-old woman with tingling paresthesias in the lower limb and a sensory level caudal to T9. She was known to have sarcoidosis. CSF examination showed lymphocytic pleocytosis with 170 cells/µL and positive oligoclonal bands. **(a)** Sagittal T1-weighted image with contrast shows a fine nodular, almost miliary pattern of intramedullary enhancement that is most pronounced in the thoracic spine. **(b)** Sagittal T2-weighted image of the spine. Some of the larger granulomas appear hyperintense in the T2-weighted sequence. **(c)** Axial T1-weighted image with contrast at the level of the C4 vertebral body shows circumscribed enhancement of a granuloma. **(d)** Fat-saturated sagittal T1-weighted image with contrast in a different patient with known neurosarcoidosis shows typical peripheral meningeal enhancement of the spinal cord. Image quality is compromised due to poor compliance. (Reproduced from Schlamann M. Inflammations, infections, and related diseases. In: Forsting M, Jansen O, eds. MR Neuroimaging: Brain, Spine, Peripheral Nerves. New York, NY: Thieme; 2017:529.)

ren's-syndrome–related antigen A (SSA/Ro) and anti-Sjögren's-syndrome–related antigen B (SSB/La) antibodies are commonly associated with this disorder. Neurological symptoms occur in about 20% of patients with Sjögren's syndrome, most commonly affecting the sensory ganglions, small fiber nerves, and spinal cord.[10] Spinal cord lesions, like NMO, tend to be longitudinally extensive (▶ Fig. 5.5). Similar to SLE, IV steroids are the mainstay of treatment with cyclophosphamide often used for refractory cases.

Transverse myelitis related to mixed connective tissue disease and systemic scleroderma is much rarer, but cases are described in the literature. Clinical presentation, treatment options, and treatment responses are similar to those described above with SLE and Sjögren's syndrome.[11,12]

5.3.5 Paraneoplastic Myelitis

Paraneoplastic myelitis is a very rare disorder associated with underlying malignancy in which it is thought that antineuronal antibodies share common antigens with the cancer and thus cause damage to neuronal tissue. The onset of symptoms is often more insidious than other inflammatory types mentioned previously, and cord involvement is often more longitudinally extensive and tract-specific.[2] The most common types of cancers involved in paraneoplastic myelitis are lung and lymphoproliferative, though it has been described in sarcoma, kidney, breast, prostate, skin, and others.[13] The most common antibodies associated are antiamphiphysin and collapsin response mediator protein-5 (CRMP-5), though many others have been described.[2,13] IV steroids, IV immunoglobulin, and plasma

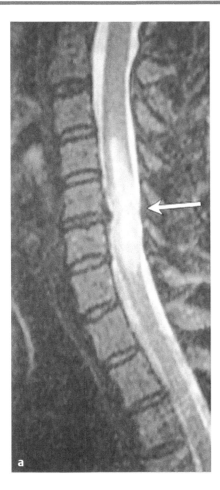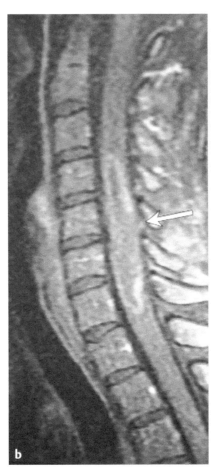

Fig. 5.5 (a) Sagittal fat-suppressed T2-weighted imaging of a 46-year-old woman with Sjögren's syndrome shows an intramedullary demyelinating lesion with high signal (*arrow*), and **(b)** a corresponding peripheral rim of gadolinium contrast enhancement on sagittal fat-suppressed T1-weighted imaging (*arrow*). (Reproduced from Meyers SP. Differential Diagnosis in Neuroimaging: Spine. New York, NY: Thieme; 2017:75.)

exchange are all potential treatments with variable response, though treating the underlying malignancy is the main goal.

5.4 Infectious Myelopathies

Transverse myelitis may also have infectious causes that include many types of viruses, bacteria, fungi, and parasites. Besides the typical myelopathic signs and symptoms, the patient may also show signs of infection including fever, rash, meningismus, or concurrent respiratory or gastrointestinal (GI) infection. Myelitis may occur due to direct infection of the spinal cord or indirectly via an autoimmune reaction related to an infection elsewhere in the body. Depending on the causative agent, the time course may vary widely from acute to chronic and the treatment is often case dependent. Particularly for viral cases, the causative agent may not be found (▶ Fig. 5.6). Specific organisms have predilections for particular areas of the spinal cord; those typically occurring in the thoracic cord will be highlighted below.

5.4.1 Herpes Viruses

Herpes simplex virus 1 (HSV-1) is most commonly known to cause cold sores, lying dormant in the trigeminal ganglion. When it involves infection of the central nervous system, it usually causes a limbic encephalitis, but myelitis (and typically thoracic cord myelitis) has been described.[14] HSV-2 more commonly causes myelitis and radiculitis than HSV-1, but tends to involve the lower cord and cauda equina.[15] Treatment consists of acyclovir, particularly in immunocompromised patients, and steroids may be considered in cases of severe inflammation.[16] Varicella-zoster virus is a herpes virus that causes myelitis much more often than other herpes viruses, though via similar mechanisms, often affecting the thoracic cord. Treatment is the same as HSV. Cytomegalovirus may cause myelopathy at the thoracolumbar region as well as rim-enhancing intramedullary lesions typically in immunocompromised patients. Pleocytosis in this case is often neutrophilic and the first-line treatment is ganciclovir.[16] Epstein–Barr virus rarely causes myelopathy but may cause this along with encephalopathy and radiculopathy. Treatment is supportive; corticosteroids may be given but evidence for this is lacking.[16]

5.4.2 Flaviviruses and Enteroviruses

Flaviviruses and enteroviruses are somewhat unique in that they can cause a flaccid paralysis instead of the typical upper motor neuron signs seen in myelopathy. Flaviviruses include West Nile virus (WNV), tick-borne encephalitis virus, Japanese encephalitis virus, St. Louis encephalitis virus, and dengue virus. WNV is a mosquito-borne disease that is usually asymp-

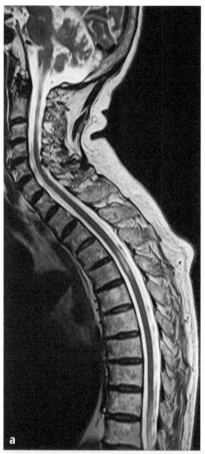
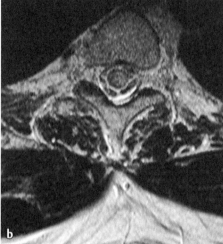
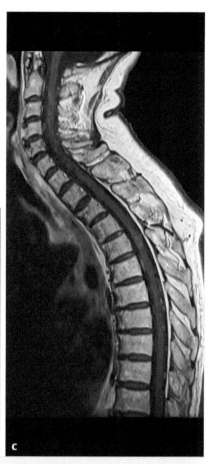

Fig. 5.6 Transverse myelitis in a 62-year-old man with acute onset of predominantly left-sided paraparesis and a thoracic sensory level at T5. **(a)** Sagittal T2-weighted image shows an intramedullary T2-weighted hyperintensity at the level of the T4 vertebral body with possible slight swelling of the affected cord segment, consistent with viral myelitis of unknown cause. The short segmental cord involvement is atypical. Symptoms improved in response to corticosteroid therapy. **(b)** Axial T2-weighted image. Intramedullary hyperintensity involves almost the entire cross-section of the spinal cord. **(c)** Sagittal T1-weighted image after contrast administration shows faint enhancement at the site of the T2-weighted hyperintensity in panel **(a)**. (Reproduced from Schlamann M. Inflammations, infections, and related diseases. In: Forsting M, Jansen O, eds. MR Neuroimaging: Brain, Spine, Peripheral Nerves. New York, NY: Thieme; 2017:523.)

tomatic but can cause neurological symptoms in about 1% of infections. Like most viral infections in the spinal cord, CSF studies usually show a lymphocytic pleocytosis and sometimes elevated protein. Steroids and intravenous immunoglobulin (IVIg) can be used to treat, though no antivirals have shown to be effective.[16] Enteroviruses include poliovirus and enterovirus 70 and 71. Poliovirus, though eradicated in the United States is still seen in some regions of the world. Poliovirus infects the anterior horn cells in the spinal cord, and this tract-specific inflammation can be seen on MRI. Treatment is supportive.[15]

5.4.3 Retroviruses

Human immunodeficiency virus (HIV), the retrovirus that causes acquired immune deficiency syndrome (AIDS), can cause many types of damage in the spine. The most common myelopathy is a vacuolar myelopathy that tends to slowly affect the dorsal columns and corticospinal tracts of the thoracic cord. This can occur in 17% of patients with AIDS, though there is no link between HIV viral load and affected site. Treatment is with antiretroviral therapy.[15,16] Direct invasion of HIV-infected mac-

rophages and microglial cells can cause an HIV myelitis, also commonly affect the posterior thoracic cord (▸ Fig. 5.7). Human T-cell lymphotropic virus type 1 is another retrovirus clearly linked to myelitis, also with an insidious onset of spastic paraparesis and neurogenic bladder. It is endemic to Central and South America as well as parts of Africa and Japan. There are no efficacious treatments available.

Treponema pallidum

Treponema pallidum, a sexually transmitted bacterium that causes syphilis, can infect the central nervous system and can cause destruction of the dorsal columns in the spine (tabes dorsalis). This can lead to vibratory and proprioceptive deficit, pain, and incoordination. Less commonly, usually in males, the infection can manifest as a meningomyelitis in the cervical or thoracic cord and can lead to lower extremity weakness, paresthesias, pain, spasticity, and autonomic dysfunction. Diagnosis is made via serum or CSF Venereal Disease Research Laboratory (VDRL) test or positive polymerase chain reaction. Treatment is with IV penicillin.

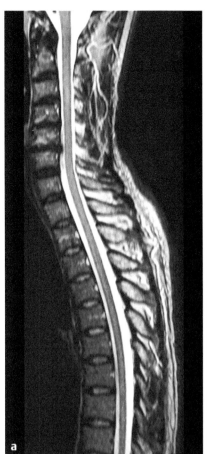
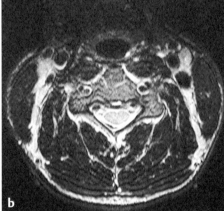
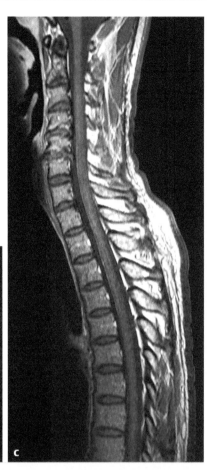

Fig. 5.7 Transverse myelitis in a 27-year-old man with known HIV infection. He presented with new onset of paraparesis and sensory level caudal to T7. **(a)** Sagittal T2-weighted image shows faint hyperintensity of the spinal cord extending from the C2 level to the lower thoracic spine, consistent with HIV myelitis. **(b)** Axial T2-weighted image shows faint hyperintensity involving the entire cross-section of the spinal cord. **(c)** Sagittal T1-weighted image after contrast administration shows no evidence of enhancement. (Reproduced from Schlamann M. Inflammations, infections, and related diseases. In: Forsting M, Jansen O, eds. MR Neuroimaging: Brain, Spine, Peripheral Nerves. New York, NY: Thieme; 2017:524.)

Mycobacterium tuberculosis

Tuberculous meningitis is the most common form of nervous system involvement of tuberculosis (TB). Spinal involvement can be found in up to 3% of patients with TB. The most common presenting symptoms are fever and paraplegia as well as bladder and bowel symptoms. The thoracic cord is predominantly affected. Tuberculous spondylitis (i.e., Pott's disease) can cause extension into and/or compression of the spinal cord. A variety of MRI findings can be seen; poor outcome is associated with cord atrophy and presence of syrinx.[17] Medical treatment usually requires up to 1 year of antibiotic therapy, and surgical decompression may be required (▶ Fig. 5.8).[15]

5.5 Metabolic and Toxic Myelopathies

5.5.1 B$_{12}$ Deficiency

Vitamin B$_{12}$ (cobalamin) is a water-soluble vitamin with a cobalt center that is involved in multiple enzymatic reactions required for DNA synthesis and the normal functioning of neurons and red blood cells. B$_{12}$ deficiency occurs most often with malabsorption syndromes (e.g., bacterial overgrowth, pernicious anemia, enteritis, gastric/ileal resection) and can occur at almost any age but is much more prevalent among the elderly population. The most common sign of B$_{12}$ deficiency is megaloblastic macrocytic anemia that can cause fatigue, pallor, and generalized weakness. Neurological manifestations may occur without hematological abnormalities and can include myelopathy, sensory ataxia, peripheral neuropathy, memory loss, and neuropsychiatric disorders.[18] Myelopathy caused by B$_{12}$ deficiency (also termed subacute combined degeneration) affects particular areas of the spinal cord including the posterior columns and lateral corticospinal tracts to cause weakness, spasticity, numbness (specifically deficits in vibration and position sense), tingling, and gait difficulty. MRI imaging shows T2 hyperintense signal in the posterior and lateral columns (▶ Fig. 5.9).[19] Though exceedingly rare, contrast enhancement, cord atrophy, and even anterior cord involvement have also been described.[20,21] Occasionally, the lesions seen on MRI may be quite extensive.[22] Low serum B$_{12}$ levels confirm the diagnosis, though elevated metabolite levels of homocysteine or

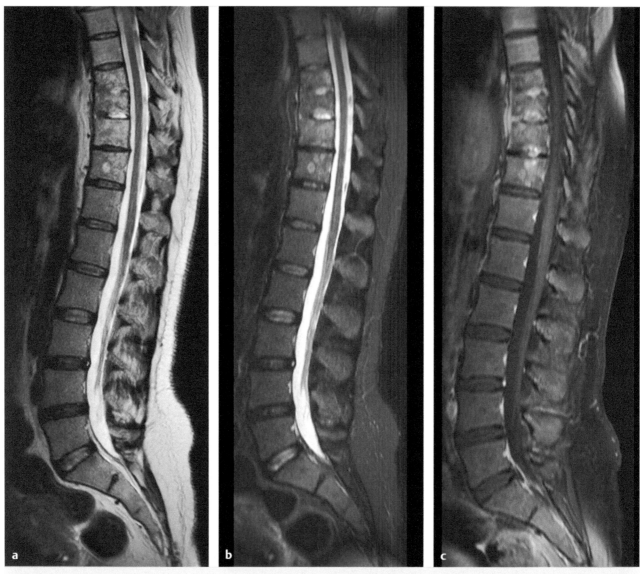

Fig. 5.8 Tuberculous spondylodiskitis in a 29-year-old woman with microbiologically confirmed tuberculosis. She had complained of chest and back pain for the past several weeks. **(a)** Sagittal T2-weighted image of the thoracic and lumbar spine. the T8-11 vertebral bodies show a patchy texture. The T8 and T9 vertebral bodies show decreased height with slight anterior wedging. the T8-9 disc space is narrowed. **(b)** STIR image corresponding to panel **(a)**. **(c)** Sagittal fat-saturated T1-weighted image of the thoracic and lumbar spine shows patchy enhancement of the T8-11 vertebral bodies. A slight concomitant epidural reaction is noted at the level of the T10 and T11 vertebral bodies. (Reproduced from Schlamann M. Inflammations, infections, and related diseases. In: Forsting M, Jansen O, eds. MR Neuroimaging: Brain, Spine, Peripheral Nerves. New York, NY: Thieme; 2017:532.)

methylmalonic acid may confirm the diagnosis in cases of borderline B_{12} levels. The condition is treatable and potentially reversible with earlier treatments leading to potentially better outcomes; as such, it is vital that B_{12} levels are tested in patients with myelopathic and neuropathic symptoms.[23]

5.5.2 Folate Deficiency

Folate deficiency may occur in the setting of chronic alcohol abuse, restricted diets, folate antagonists such as methotrexate, and various malabsorption syndromes.[18] Like B_{12} deficiency, folate deficiency can cause myelopathy, peripheral neuropathy, and cognitive changes. Treatment consists of folate repletion. It

is important to note that concurrent deficiencies in other vitamins including B_{12} are common and need to be addressed as well as the part of the treatment.[18]

5.5.3 Copper Deficiency

Copper is a trace mineral that acts as cofactor for many enzymes involved in basic cellular functioning. Copper deficiency is rare but can occur from zinc toxicity (often secondary to dental fixatives or treatment of other disorders requiring zinc repletion), malabsorption, proximal bowel resection, gastric bypass surgery, and rarely in a hereditary condition known as Menkes disease. Low copper levels can lead to anemia,

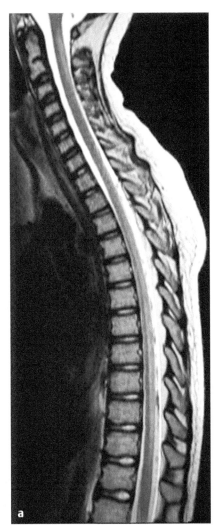

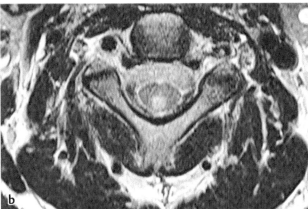

Fig. 5.9 Funicular myelosis (vitamin B_{12} deficiency) in a 39-year-old man with marked pallhypesthesia (diminished sensibility to vibrations), weakness, and pain predominantly affecting the lower extremities. He had a known history of Crohn's disease. **(a)** Sagittal T2-weighted image shows increased signal intensity of the dorsal columns in the cervical and thoracic spine. **(b)** Axial T2-weighted image at the cervical level shows marked hyperintensity of the dorsal columns. (Reproduced from Schlamann M. Inflammations, infections, and related diseases. In: Forsting M, Jansen O, eds. MR Neuroimaging: Brain, Spine, Peripheral Nerves. New York, NY: Thieme; 2017:526.)

neutropenia, and thrombocytopenia. The myelopathy that occurs is similar to the subacute combined degeneration seen in B_{12} deficiency both in terms of the neurological symptoms and MRI imaging.[24] An associated peripheral neuropathy may also be present.[18] Though the thoracic cord may be affected, cervical cord involvement is more common with the dorsal and lateral columns affected.[18,25,26] Laboratory testing to diagnose copper myelopathy includes serum copper, serum zinc, and ceruloplasmin levels, as well as 24-hour urine copper and zinc levels. Treatment includes copper supplementation and/or stopping the cause of exogenous zinc absorption. Compared to B_{12} myelopathy, copper deficiency is not as well recognized as a cause by many physicians, and the neurological deficits do not often respond as well to repletion.[18,24]

5.5.4 Vitamin E Deficiency

Vitamin E is actually a group of eight antioxidant fat-soluble molecules that are involved in free radical scavenging and other cellular processes. Deficiency of alpha-tocopherol, the most biologically active form of vitamin E, can lead to multiple medical problems including cardiomyopathy, acanthocytosis, retinitis pigmentosa, and various neurological problems including spastic ataxia, peripheral neuropathy, and myelopathy similar to the subacute combined degeneration seen in B_{12} deficiency. Vitamin E deficiency is most commonly due to malabsorption from various GI, pancreatic, or hepatic diseases; however, genetic defects in the processing of vitamin E may also cause low vitamin E levels. MRI shows increased signal in the dorsal columns.[27]

5.5.5 Myelopathies due to Toxins

Several toxins have been identified as a cause of myelopathy affecting the cervical and thoracic cords. These will be very briefly reviewed in this section.

Konzo is a well-described myelopathy causing the sudden onset of nonprogressive spastic paraparesis. Sensory and autonomic involvement is typically absent. It is caused by chronic cyanide ingestion secondary to insufficiently processed cassava root in certain parts of Africa. There is no known treatment.[28]

Lathyrism is a myelopathic disorder particularly involving the legs causing a spastic gait with sensory and autonomic dysfunction also seen to a lesser degree. It is a disorder endemic to parts of India and Bangladesh, and it is caused by a toxin in the grass pea legume known as *Lathyrus sativus*. The onset is subacute or insidious and self-limiting.[23]

Certain chemotherapeutic agents, particularly those with intrathecal administration, have been known to cause spinal cord lesions. Symptoms may range from a transient flaccid paraparesis with pain and numbness shortly after the injection, or a more progressive spastic paraparesis may occur after multiple treatments.[29] The lateral and posterior cords may enhance on MRI imaging.[30,31] It is thought that the toxicity is due to the preservatives used in the intrathecal formulations.

Hepatic myelopathy is a rare cause of progressive spastic paraparesis and is secondary to cirrhosis and portosystemic shunting. It is thought that the accumulation and circulation of various toxins including ammonia and other metabolites may lead to neurotoxicity. Sensory and autonomic involvement is generally absent. Liver transplantation is a possible treatment, but has variable results.

5.6 Hereditary Myelopathies

There are a multitude of hereditary conditions that can affect the spinal cord. Hereditary spastic paraplegias (HSP) are a group of disorders that cause gradual and progressive spastic weakness in the legs, spastic gait, and sensory/autonomic dysfunction. Other neurological signs can occur indicating involvement of the brain as well; these include ataxia, deafness, cognitive impairment, and parkinsonism. Over 50 genes have been identified and the most common mode of inheritance is autosomal dominant, though recessive and X-linked inheritance patterns have also been discovered.[27] Axonal degeneration in the pyramidal tracts and dorsal columns has been observed. MRI typically shows some degree of cervical and thoracic cord atrophy, though generally no signal abnormalities within the cord are seen. The degree of cord atrophy may differ among HSP types, but does not seem to correlate to severity of symptoms.[32] Other neurodegenerative conditions may mimic HSP in presentation, particularly milder forms of spinocerebellar ataxias such as late-onset Friedreich's ataxia, adult-onset polyglucosan body disease, some inborn errors of metabolism, women with adrenomyeloneuropathy (half of whom develop spastic paraparesis without cerebral or adrenal involvement), and adult-onset Krabbe's disease.[33]

Motor neuron disorders also predominantly affect cells in the spinal cord, causing degeneration of the anterior horns and/or descending corticospinal tracts. Amyotrophic lateral sclerosis, the most common type of motor neuron disorder, affects both types of motor neurons, causing spasticity, hyperreflexia, weakness, muscle fasciculations, and muscular atrophy. Primary lateral sclerosis, a much rarer form of motor neuron disorder, causes degeneration solely of the upper motor neurons; lower motor neuron findings of atrophy and fasciculations are not typically identified. The diagnosis is a clinical and electrodiagnostic one with the aid of electromyography. MRI is generally normal and is used more to rule out other myelopathic etiologies.[27]

References

[1] Ganguly K, Abrams GM. Management of chronic myelopathy symptoms and activities of daily living. Semin Neurol. 2012; 32(2):161–168

[2] Greenberg BM, Frohman EM. Immune-mediated myelopathies. Continuum (Minneap Minn). 2015; 21 1 Spinal Cord Disorders:121–131

[3] Scott TF, Frohman EM, De Seze J, Gronseth GS, Weinshenker BG, Therapeutics and Technology Assessment Subcommittee of American Academy of Neurology. Evidence-based guideline: clinical evaluation and treatment of transverse myelitis: report of the Therapeutics and Technology Assessment Subcommittee of the American Academy of Neurology. Neurology. 2011; 77 (24):2128–2134

[4] West TW, Hess C, Cree BAC. Acute transverse myelitis: demyelinating, inflammatory, and infectious myelopathies. Semin Neurol. 2012; 32(2):97–113

[5] Sellner J, Lüthi N, Bühler R, et al. Acute partial transverse myelitis: risk factors for conversion to multiple sclerosis. Eur J Neurol. 2008; 15(4):398–405

[6] Hua LH, Donlon SL, Sobhanian MJ, Portner SM, Okuda DT. Thoracic spinal cord lesions are influenced by the degree of cervical spine involvement in multiple sclerosis. Spinal Cord. 2015; 53(7):520–525

[7] Schlaeger R, Papinutto N, Zhu AH, et al. Association between thoracic spinal cord gray matter atrophy and disability in multiple sclerosis. JAMA Neurol. 2015; 72(8):897–904

[8] Marignier R, Cobo Calvo A, Vukusic S. Neuromyelitis optica and neuromyelitis optica spectrum disorders. Curr Opin Neurol. 2017; 30(3):208–215

[9] Kovacs B, Lafferty TL, Brent LH, DeHoratius RJ. Transverse myelopathy in systemic lupus erythematosus: an analysis of 14 cases and review of the literature. Ann Rheum Dis. 2000; 59(2):120–124

[10] Berkowitz AL, Samuels MA. The neurology of Sjogren's syndrome and the rheumatology of peripheral neuropathy and myelitis. Pract Neurol. 2014; 14 (1):14–22

[11] Bhinder S, Harbour K, Majithia V. Transverse myelitis, a rare neurological manifestation of mixed connective tissue disease—a case report and a review of literature. Clin Rheumatol. 2007; 26(3):445–447

[12] Torabi AM, Patel RK, Wolfe GI, Hughes CS, Mendelsohn DB, Trivedi JR. Transverse myelitis in systemic sclerosis. Arch Neurol. 2004; 61(1):126–128

[13] Jain RS, Gupta PK, Agrawal R, Tejwani S, Kumar S. Longitudinally extensive transverse myelitis as presenting manifestation of small cell carcinoma lung. Oxf Med Case Rep. 2015; 2015(2):208–210

[14] Anderson MD, Tummala S. Herpes myelitis after thoracic spine surgery. J Neurosurg Spine. 2013; 18(5):519–523

[15] Ho EL. Infectious etiologies of myelopathy. Semin Neurol. 2012; 32(2):154–160

[16] Lyons JL. Myelopathy associated with microorganisms. Continuum (Minneap Minn). 2015; 21 1 Spinal Cord Disorders:100–120

[17] Wasay M, Arif H, Khealani B, Ahsan H. Neuroimaging of tuberculous myelitis: analysis of ten cases and review of literature. J Neuroimaging. 2006; 16(3): 197–205

[18] Kumar N. Metabolic and toxic myelopathies. Semin Neurol. 2012; 32:123–136

[19] Locatelli ER, Laureno R, Ballard P, Mark AS. MRI in vitamin B12 deficiency myelopathy. Can J Neurol Sci. 1999; 26(1):60–63

[20] Bassi SS, Bulundwe KK, Greeff GP, Labuscagne JH, Gledhill RF. MRI of the spinal cord in myelopathy complicating vitamin B12 deficiency: two additional cases and a review of the literature. Neuroradiology. 1999; 41 (4):271–274

[21] Karantanas AH, Markonis A, Bisbiyiannis G. Subacute combined degeneration of the spinal cord with involvement of the anterior columns: a new MRI finding. Neuroradiology. 2000; 42(2):115–117

[22] de Medeiros FC, de Albuquerque LA, de Souza RB, Gomes Neto AP, Christo PP. Vitamin B12 extensive thoracic myelopathy: clinical, radiological and prognostic aspects. Two cases report and literature review. Neurol Sci. 2013; 34 (10):1857–1860

[23] Goodman BP. Metabolic and toxic causes of myelopathy. Continuum (Minneap Minn). 2015; 21 1 Spinal Cord Disorders:84–99

[24] Gabreyes AA, Abbasi HN, Forbes KP, McQuaker G, Duncan A, Morrison I. Hypocupremia associated cytopenia and myelopathy: a national retrospective review. Eur J Haematol. 2013; 90(1):1–9

[25] Kumar N, Ahlskog JE, Klein CJ, Port JD. Imaging features of copper deficiency myelopathy: a study of 25 cases. Neuroradiology. 2006; 48(2):78–83

[26] Ferrara JM, Skeen MB, Edwards NJ, Gray L, Massey EW. Subacute combined degeneration due to copper deficiency. J Neuroimaging. 2007; 17(4):375–377

[27] Hedera P. Hereditary and metabolic myelopathies. Handb Clin Neurol. 2016; 136:769–785

[28] Tshala-Katumbay D, Mumba N, Okitundu L, et al. Cassava food toxins, konzo disease, and neurodegeneration in sub-Sahara Africans. Neurology. 2013; 80 (10):949–951

[29] Hahn AF, Feasby TE, Gilbert JJ. Paraparesis following intrathecal chemotherapy. Neurology. 1983; 33(8):1032–1038

[30] McLean DR, Clink HM, Ernst P, et al. Myelopathy after intrathecal chemotherapy. A case report with unique magnetic resonance imaging changes. Cancer. 1994; 73(12):3037–3040

[31] Murata KY, Maeba A, Yamanegi M, Nakanishi I, Ito H. Methotrexate myelopathy after intrathecal chemotherapy: a case report. J Med Case Reports. 2015; 9:135

[32] Hedera P, Eldevik OP, Maly P, Rainier S, Fink JK. Spinal cord magnetic resonance imaging in autosomal dominant hereditary spastic paraplegia. Neuroradiology. 2005; 47(10):730–734

[33] Zhovtis Ryerson L, Herbert J, Howard J, Kister I. Adult-onset spastic paraparesis: an approach to diagnostic work-up. J Neurol Sci. 2014; 346(1–2):43–50

Part II

Deformity

II

6 Surgical Management of Congenital Scoliosis

Corey T. Walker, Gregory M. Mundis Jr., and Jay D. Turner

Abstract

Congenital scoliosis and kyphosis describe a spectrum of vertebral column defects that result in abnormal growth and spinal deformity. Congenital deformities range from simple, low-risk defects that can be managed nonoperatively to complex, rapidly progressive pathologies that require urgent surgical attention. In order to make proper management decisions, spine surgeons and other providers must have a clear understanding of the specific pathology involved as well as its natural history. Surgical intervention should be considered for high-risk defects, those with demonstrated progression on serial imaging, highly deforming lesions, and those causing neurological or respiratory symptoms. A host of techniques have been employed for the surgical treatment of congenital scoliosis, including in situ fusion, convex growth arrest, hemivertebra excision, posterior spinal fusion with osteotomies and growth preservation techniques. In this chapter, we describe the types of congenital scoliosis and kyphosis, the natural history, patient evaluation and work-up, and provide an expanded discussion on the most common surgical treatment strategies.

Keywords: congenital, scoliosis, kyphosis, hemivertebra, hemiepiphysiodesis, convex growth arrest, vertebral column resection, hemivertebrectomy, growing rod, vertical expandable prosthetic titanium rib

---

Clinical Pearls

- Convex growth arrest (hemiepiphysiodesis) can be an effective treatment of mild-to-moderate scoliotic lesions in young patients with growth potential; however, they must be followed closely in order to prevent uncontrolled growth.
- Hemivertebra excision corrects both the focal deformity and stops asymmetric spinal growth by removing the pathological growth plates, and can be performed safely in young patients before malignant deformity develops.
- For rigid and severe deformities, posterior correction with osteotomies and instrumentation may be required. This is often necessary in patients with multiple anomalies and large secondary curves.
- Growth preservation techniques, consisting of growing rods and vertical expandable prosthetic titanium rib (VEPTR) technology, are used to slow curve progression while allowing for thoracic expansion as patients mature.

6.1 Introduction

The term "congenital scoliosis" refers to spinal deformity that is caused by early developmental spinal anomalies. These congenital anomalies can lead to deformities that impact the coronal plane (scoliosis), sagittal plane (kyphosis), or both (mixed). Curve progression and severity varies significantly with anomaly type, number of vertebrae involved, location within the

spine, and skeletal maturity. As such, a firm understanding of the natural history of these lesions guides prognosis and management decisions. Here, we present a review of congenital vertebral anomalies, highlight the progression potential of each type, and discuss current surgical management strategies.

6.2 Congenital Vertebral Anomalies

6.2.1 Congenital Scoliosis

Embryological development of the spine occurs in the first 6 weeks of life. Patterning of the spine occurs as somites of the mesoderm segment to form vertebral bodies ventrally and neural elements dorsally. Vertebral defects most often result from either a *failure of formation* of a vertebral body or a *failure of segmentation* (▶ Fig. 6.1). Additionally, disorders during chondrification can result in fused vertebral segments with absent growth potential at the cartilaginous growth plates.

Failure of formation can be incomplete or complete. Incomplete, or partial, failures include wedge vertebrae, which have a complete lateral width with two pedicles present, but a hypoplastic vertebral body height on one side. Complete failures of formation refer to hemivertebrae, where only one of the two sides of the vertebral body forms. Hemivertebrae can be fully segmented, with a present vertebral disc and growth plate above and below the hemivertebra. In contrast, unsegmented hemivertebrae are fused rostrally and caudally to the adjacent vertebrae, and therefore, have limited growth or progression potential on that side of the vertebral body. Partial segmentation too can occur. Incarcerated hemivertebrae are those unsegmented hemivertebrae that sit within a niche of bone in the adjacent vertebrae. These defects rarely cause significant deformity.

Failure of segmentation describes the congenital lack of separation between adjacent vertebral bodies. Unlike failures of formation which produce abnormal curvature through asymmetric vertebral height and unequal rates of growth on each side of the vertebral body, failures of segmentation create deformity through a tethering effect that inhibits growth on the concave side of the scoliotic curvature. Unilateral bars are bony columns on one side of the vertebral bodies that can span multiple vertebral levels. They can have very significant effects on curve progression, particularly if they span many spinal levels. Deformity progression becomes most prominent during pediatric growth spurts when spinal growth is most rapid. Bilateral segmentation failure can occur, as well as block vertebrae, which are two fully fused completely formed vertebrae. In these instances, growth inhibition occurs on both sides of the spine, and rarely does deformity develop from such defects.

Mixed congenital anomalies can occur as well. For example, a patient may have multiple hemivertebrae, multiple unsegmented bars, or a combination of these defects. Most worrisome are those mixed cases where a unilateral bar is in association with a contralateral hemivertebrae. In this specific

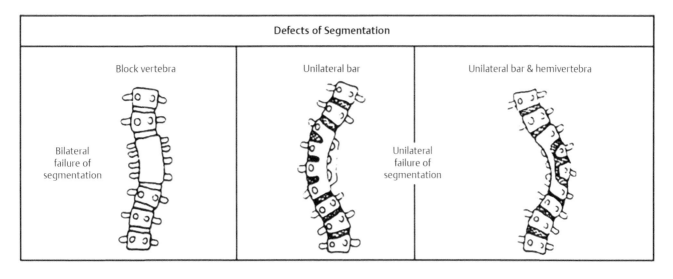

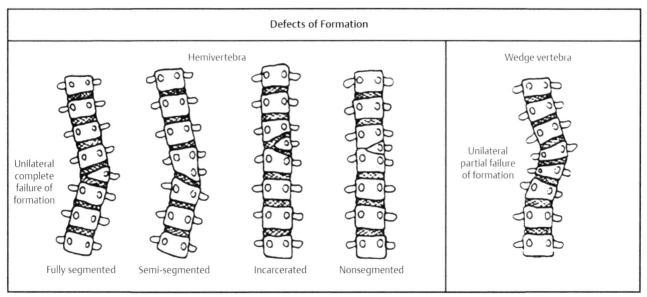

Fig. 6.1 Classification of congenital scoliosis. Bony defects are characterized as failures of segmentation and formation. (Reproduced with permission from McMaster M. Congenital scoliosis. In Weinstein S, ed. The Pediatric Spine: Principles and Practice, 2nd ed.; Lippincott Williams and Wilkins Publishers, Inc.)

scenario, there is an asymmetry from the hemivertebra itself, potential for asymmetric growth on the side of the hemivertebra (the convex side of the curve, particularly if the hemivertebra is fully segmented), and tethering of growth on the concave side of the curve because of the bar. However, in other instances, mixed defects have an opposing effect on each other and can offset one another. When two bilateral hemivertebrae exist within the same region of the spine (typically the thoracic spine), they often balance each other, and are referred to as a hemimetameric shift.

6.2.2 Congenital Kyphosis

Failures of formation and segmentation can also impact alignment in the sagittal plane. While less common than scoliosis, congenital kyphosis can cause severe deformities, and in

extreme circumstances can lead to neurological dysfunction. Large focal deformities can lead to stretching and draping of the cord across sharp angulations of the canal leading to myelopathic symptoms and even spinal cord injury.

Kyphotic failures of vertebral body formation are similar to those in scoliotic disease (▶ Fig. 6.2). Some of these defects may occur as a result of failed vascularization of the centrum during the chrondrification stage of development. A posterior hemivertebra, also referred to as a posterior hemicentrum, can exist with anterior hypoplasia of the body. Lateral hemicentrum and posterior quadrant centrum defects can also occur with aplasia of the anterolateral body. Unlike a posterior hemicentrum, which produces a pure kyphotic deformity, these two defects can also create a coronal asymmetry with consequent combined kyphoscoliotic deformity. Complete aplasia of the centrum can also occur with existing pedicles attached to no

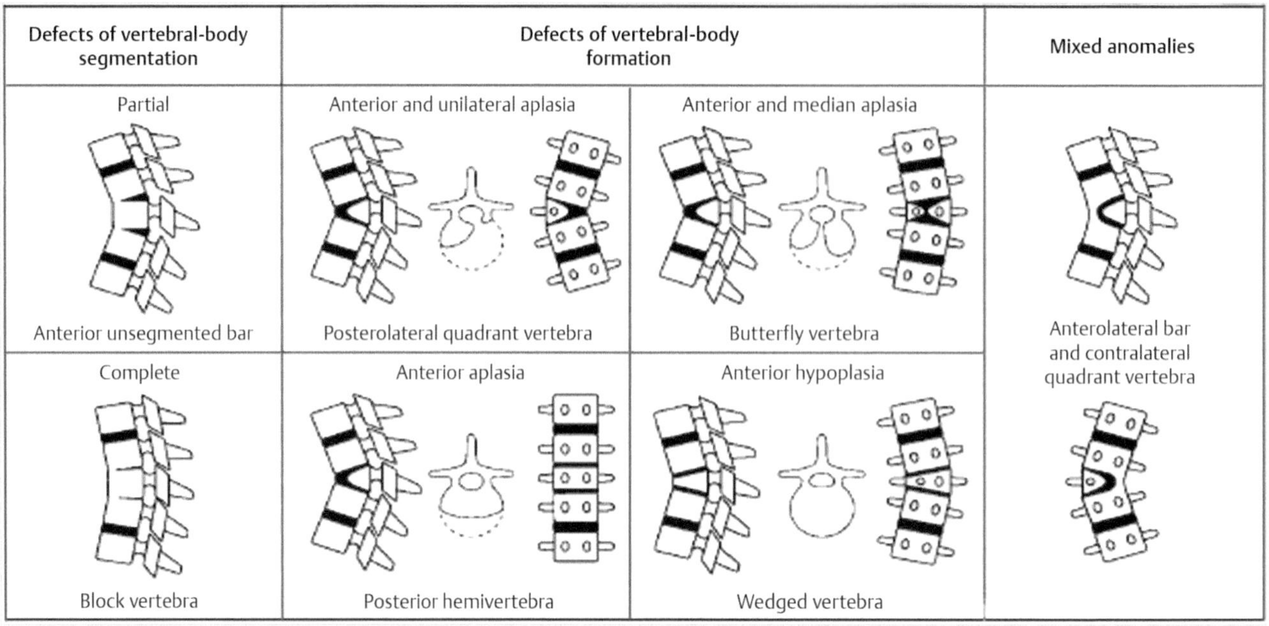

Defects of vertebral-body segmentation	Defects of vertebral-body formation		Mixed anomalies
Partial	Anterior and unilateral aplasia	Anterior and median aplasia	
Anterior unsegmented bar	Posterolateral quadrant vertebra	Butterfly vertebra	Anterolateral bar and contralateral quadrant vertebra
Complete	Anterior aplasia	Anterior hypoplasia	
Block vertebra	Posterior hemivertebra	Wedged vertebra	

Fig. 6.2 Classification of congenital kyphosis. Bony defects are similar to those seen for bony scoliotic defects, but create deformity in the sagittal plane rather than the coronal plane. These can occur in conjunction with scoliotic defects and result in kyphoscoliosis. (Reproduced with permission from aster M, Singh H. Natural history of congenital kyphosis and kyphoscoliosis. A study of one hundred and twelve patients. McMJournal of Bone 81 (10):1367-1383. Wolters Kluwer Health, Inc.)

vertebral body. As expected, these result in severe degrees of kyphotic angulation and can lead to neurological dysfunction; complete aplasia of the centrum is the most likely type to be complicated by spinal cord injury. Also, a unique sagittal cleft vertebra can occur, referred to as a butterfly vertebra, and is the result of an anteromedial and central formation failure, leaving two posterolateral fragments of bone attached to the posterior neural arch.

Failures of segmentation of the spine in the sagittal plane are similar to those bony bridging bars that occur in scoliotic disease. These can occur in the midline and produce a purely kyphotic deformity, or slightly laterally, and produce kyphoscoliosis. Such bars typically result in broad sweeping curves that worsen with growth. As with congenital scoliotic defects, mixed defects can also occur, which can either have additive effects or offset one another.

Congenital kyphotic deformities place the spinal cord at greatest risk due to focal draping and/or ventral bony compression due to the anomaly. Patients with severe focal kyphotic angulations should especially be evaluated for the presence of neurological deficits, including evidence of weakness or signs or symptoms of hyperreflexia/spasticity, both based on their history and on clinical examination. Dedicated magnetic resonance imaging (MRI) is a necessary adjunct in these cases.

6.3 Natural History

Our knowledge of the natural history of these lesions is primarily derived from exemplary studies by both Winter and McMaster.[1,2,3] Despite the rarity of these lesions, they were able to assemble a large case series, develop classification schemes, and document curve progression of the various types over time.

These studies have provided the foundation for current treatment recommendations.

Several generalizable findings can be concluded from their work. First, curve progression occurs most rapidly during the first 5 years of life and during the pubertal growth spurt. Patients with high-risk deformities, such as a hemivertebra with a contralateral bar, may require surgical intervention at a very young age to prevent progression and subsequent morbidity/deformity. For low-risk deformities, it is important that patients with congenital deformities be monitored until their growth cessation, as even stable curves can rapidly progress during puberty.

Secondly, deformities of various regions of the spine need to be evaluated differently. Deformity in some parts of the spine can yield more visible deformity and present sooner. For example, high thoracic curves often are poorly tolerated due to shoulder tilt. Listing of the head and neck occurs due to inability of secondary cervical curves to correct over this relatively short spinal region. Similarly, lumbosacral lesions can create significant pelvic obliquity, which in many instances affects not only posture, but gait. There are also regional differences noted in rates of progression. For example, junctional regions of the spine, particularly the thoracolumbar and lumbosacral regions, demonstrate high rates of progression.

Lastly, mixed deformities can be very difficult to distinguish and prognosticate. As mentioned above, their laterality with respect to one another, number, distance of separation, and location within the spine can all affect their expected rate of progression. Large heterogeneity of mixed lesions makes predictability very challenging. Since they can progress more rapidly than solitary lesions, close radiographic and clinic monitoring is recommended.

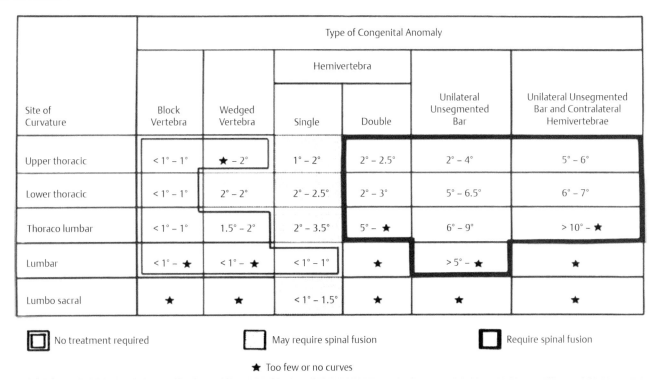

Site of Curvature	Type of Congenital Anomaly					
	Block Vertebra	Wedged Vertebra	Hemivertebra		Unilateral Unsegmented Bar	Unilateral Unsegmented Bar and Contralateral Hemivertebrae
			Single	Double		
Upper thoracic	< 1° – 1°	★ – 2°	1° – 2°	2° – 2.5°	2° – 4°	5° – 6°
Lower thoracic	< 1° – 1°	2° – 2°	2° – 2.5°	2° – 3°	5° – 6.5°	6° – 7°
Thoraco lumbar	< 1° – 1°	1.5° – 2°	2° – 3.5°	5° – ★	6° – 9°	> 10° – ★
Lumbar	< 1° – ★	< 1° – ★	< 1° – 1°	★	> 5° – ★	★
Lumbo sacral	★	★	< 1° – 1.5°	★	★	★

☐ No treatment required ☐ May require spinal fusion ☐ Require spinal fusion

★ Too few or no curves

Fig. 6.3 Annual rates of deformity progression determined by defect type and location from McMaster's original series of 251 patients. Anticipation of angular progression guides management decisions. (Reproduced with permission from McMaster M, Ohtsuka K. The natural history of congenital scoliosis. A study of two hundred and fifty-one patients. Journal of Bone 64(8):1128-1147. Wolters Kluwer Health, Inc.)

▶ Fig. 6.3 summarizes the expected annual rates of progression for congenital anomalies and is organized by anomaly type and specific location within the spine. The table is somewhat limited in that it does not account for patient age and does not include all mixed defects. Some defects follow this patterning fairly well, including unilateral bars. However, bars that span eight spinal levels may behave very differently than those that only involve two levels. Moreover, high variability can occur even among patients with a single isolated hemivertebra. Therefore, while this may serve as a guide for prognostication, it remains very difficult to predict behavior of congenital anomalies with any real precision. Close clinical and radiographic monitoring is needed to tailor the appropriate treatment to any individual patient.

6.4 Preoperative Assessment

6.4.1 Evaluation of Associated Anomalies

Embryonic malformations that result in congenital vertebral defects often are associated with insults to development of other organ systems that form at the same time. Therefore, it is important to examine all patients with a new diagnosis of congenital scoliosis for coexisting defects. These include intraspinal, musculoskeletal, genitourinary, cardiac, and gastrointestinal anomalies. The likelihood of having an associated anomaly is increased with mixed defects.

Complete neurological physical examination helps to evaluate for signs and symptoms of intraspinal disease. Neurological symptoms, including myelopathy, weakness, numbness, spasticity/contracture, or bowel or bladder dysfunction, warrant immediate work-up for underlying pathology. The most commonly associated intraspinal disorders include tethered spinal cord, diastematomyelia, syringomyelia, the Chiari malformations, Dandy–Walker malformations, or intraspinal lipomas. MRI of the spine can aid in the diagnosis, and should be performed in patients with congenital scoliosis, particularly if surgical intervention is being considered. Many of these disorders may augment the rate of deformity progression, and as such, treatment of intraspinal anomalies should precede the correction of scoliosis. Deformity correction in the presence of an untreated tethered or split cord or herniated cerebellar tonsils may cause severe neurological injury.

Skeletal anomalies can occur anywhere throughout the body, including craniofacial defects, limb or pelvic abnormalities, and rib defects. Defects of the thoracic wall, including congenital rib fusions or missing ribs are common, especially with segmentation defects, owing to the closely tied nature of vertebral and rib development. Severe rib defects can result in stunted thoracic growth, and in some cases with long segment defects of the thoracic spine, restrictive pulmonary capacity, or thoracic insufficiency syndrome.

6.4.2 Imaging Evaluation

Radiographs of the spine are essential in the evaluation of congenital defects of the spine. Standing anterior–posterior and lateral X-rays allow for visualization of vertebrae, as well as measurement of relative anatomical landmarks, Cobb's angles to evaluate curvatures, and other relative asymmetries, such as pelvic obliquity and shoulder tilt. Skeletal maturity can also be determined using the Risser Scale, which may help in prognosticating curve progression during adolescent growth spurts. Serial measurements of Cobb's angles over time may be used to determine relative rates of change over time, and help determine if the rate of progression warrants surgical treatment or continued observation. Lateral bending radiographs may also be helpful during surgical planning in determining the flexibility of curves and identifying secondary curves that may not need to be included in posterior instrumentation.

As mentioned above, MRI plays a useful role in identifying intraspinal anomalies. MRI also can be helpful in evaluating disc spaces to determine if hemivertebrae are segmented and contain growth potential. In cases of severe focal kyphotic deformities, MRI is critical for evaluation of the spinal canal and spinal cord compression.

Similarly, computed tomography (CT) imaging with three-dimensional reconstruction can be illustrative for the surgeon evaluating the vertebral and rib anomalies. This is particularly true when severe deformities create radiographic crowding on plain radiographs that limits their interpretation. As with MRI, vertebral body defects can be more precisely defined on CT reconstructions.

6.5 Nonoperative Treatment

As discussed above, the expected trajectory of the various congenital vertebral curves varies widely. A thorough understanding of the specific anomalies and their progression risk guides treatment decision making. Benign lesions such as block vertebrae and fully incarcerated hemivertebrae rarely progress to the point of warranting surgical correction. Conversely, lesions such as a unilateral bar with a contralateral hemivertebra may warrant early, and sometime prophylactic, surgical treatment before the deformity puts the patient at serious risk. Therefore, nonoperative management with close monitoring requires tailoring of the level of observation according to the risk of the lesion. Continuous documentation of neurological function and pulmonary function in cases of severe thoracic lesions is vital.

Serial radiographs every 6 to 12 months until the end of skeletal maturity are recommended to monitor deformity progression. More frequent imaging may be performed during phases of rapid growth (i.e., during the first 5 years of life and during the adolescent growth spurt). Ultimate deformity magnitude cannot be determined until after skeletal maturity.

Unlike some other types of scoliosis, bracing alone is rarely beneficial for treatment of congenital scoliosis. Curves associated with congenital vertebral defects are rigid, and consequently are rarely impacted by external forces. Moreover, in severe cases of thoracic defects where thoracic insufficiency is a concern, bracing may have deleterious effects. There is some evidence that bracing may help control severe secondary curves that can develop above or below a congenital primary curve, though bracing is rarely performed for this purpose. Likewise, bracing may be considered for postoperative stabilization after surgical fusion procedures.

6.6 Operative Intervention

6.6.1 Indications for Surgical Intervention

Decision making on the proper treatment of congenital scoliosis requires a clear understanding of the natural history of the various types of congenital defects, as discussed above. Surgical correction is necessary in patients with either severe deformity or with anomalies that are at high risk for rapid progression. In general, the goal is to surgically treat high-risk lesions before they become problematic, without treating lower-risk patients unnecessarily. The most severe curves often require aggressive surgical techniques such as three column osteotomies and thus carry a high surgical complication risk. Early treatment can minimize surgical risk and also to help to prevent secondary issues such as thoracic insufficiency and neurological deficits. Studies have demonstrated that early focal surgical correction can be performed safely and without adverse effects on patient's vertebral or thoracic growth. Surgery is also considered in patients who fail nonoperative management, for example, curves that progress beyond 60 degrees, or in cases where the curve is less than 60 degrees, but the yearly rate of progression is high and suggests that further observation is futile. Likewise, deformity of the upper thoracic and lumbosacral regions can result in visible deformity of shoulder and pelvic tilt, respectively. The disfiguring nature of these curves can be particularly distressing to patients, even with smaller curves, and therefore, surgical correction can be considered.

6.6.2 Intraoperative Considerations

All patients should be treated by surgeons with experience in treating spine deformity, and an understanding of the periprocedural risks inherent to scoliosis surgery. Specifically, attention must be paid to several key areas through the case. The first is minimizing blood loss, particularly with instrumented fusions, vertebral resections, and osteotomies, as this may result in considerable intraoperative hemorrhage. Appropriate monitoring of serial blood gases, blood hemoglobin concentrations, and replenishing of platelets and clotting factors helps to reduce the risks associated with periprocedural anemia. In general, a preoperative discussion and plan with the anesthesia and operating room team should be performed to help coordinate these efforts prior to the commencement of the case. Throughout the case, hypotension should be avoided to ensure adequate spinal cord perfusion.

Mitigating risk of neural injury during spinal manipulation is another important consideration. Intraoperative multimodal neuromonitoring, including somatosensory evoked potentials and motor evoked potentials, should be utilized. Neuromonitoring is used to detect neurological dysfunction during surgery and allows for early intervention (e.g., reversal of surgical maneuvers, elevation of systemic blood pressure to augment spinal cord perfusion, etc.) to protect against neurological injury. This is especially important in cases of severe kyphoscoliotic disease which carry a high risk of intraoperative neurological injury.

6.6.3 In situ Fusion

In situ fusion is a simple method of providing stabilization across a defect to prevent focal curve progression. This approach remains limited in its scope, as it does not provide any correction, and therefore, can only be applied to patients who have small curves (usually < 30 degrees) that are identified early in life, but are expected to progress significantly enough later in life that they warrant early prophylactic surgery. Given these limitations, this technique is not commonly employed.

If the decision to treat with in situ fusion is made, short-segment posterior instrumented fusion across the defect can be performed. Anterior fusion should also be considered in most cases to prevent a crankshaft phenomenon. This occurs when a lordotic anomaly develops in response to preserved anterior growth potential in the presence of a posteriorly fixated segment. In cases of mild, focal kyphotic disease with posterior fusion alone, this anterior growth can actually be used strategically to yield small amounts of correction with growth. Likewise, in focal lordosis, an anterior alone treatment could be performed reciprocally with the same goal.

Patients should be followed very closely after this procedure to monitor for fusion and disease progression. Early continued progression may indicate pseudoarthrosis and surgical exploration and revision may be considered. Delayed curve progression may warrant reoperation with long-segment posterior fusion (discussed below) and curve correction.

6.6.4 Convex Growth Arrest (Hemiepiphysiodesis)

Congenital scoliotic deformity is primarily caused by longitudinal growth imbalance; growth of the convexity outpaces the concavity and results in abnormal curvature. Epiphysiodesis is the process of removing the growth potential of bones to prevent progression of asymmetry. For congenital spinal disorders, this strategy is used to arrest growth on the convex side of the curve to prevent curve progression and allow for reversal of the deformity as growth continues on the concave side. This treatment option is best considered in young patients where there is the greatest potential for spontaneous correction of the scoliosis during development (► Fig. 6.4).

While the indications for convex growth arrest have been contested in the literature, the technique does seem to be well suited for specific types of patients. In general, the indications include patient age less than 5 years, a pure scoliotic curve, short-segment deformities with less than five segments involved, documented curve progression or high-risk defects with Cobb's angle less than 70 degrees, absence of cervical spine deformity, patients with anomalies due to failure of formation failure over segmentation failure, and absence of neurological deficits or other associated intraspinal/dysraphism abnormalities. Nevertheless, the application of this technique has been tested outside of these boundaries, largely with good outcomes, and these remain as loose guidelines.[4] The presence of a contralateral bar hindering concave growth limits the corrective potential of the procedure.

When hemiepiphysiodesis is indicated, it is recommended to be carried out from both anterior and posterior approaches. Most commonly, the anterior fusion targets the index levels of the congenital malformation, and the posterior fusion extends one level above and below the defect. Anteriorly, the convex lateral halves of the disc, growth plate, and bony endplate are resected. Posteriorly, facet joints are removed on the convex side with decortication of the laminae and transverse processes to promote fusion. Supplemental unilateral instrumentation may be considered and autogenous bone graft can be used anteriorly and posteriorly to augment the fusion. Patients are typically treated with a postoperative body cast for four to sixth until radiographic fusion has been confirmed. Importantly, patients should continue to be observed after treatment as a minority of patients will continue to display curve progression postoperatively.

6.6.5 Hemivertebra Excision

Hemivertebrae create both a direct angulation of the spine at the site of the deformity, and also lead to curve progression due to growth asymmetry, particularly if they are segmented. Resection of the anomalous hemivertebral body allows for immediate correction of the primary angulation, and also can help restrict the accompanying growth potential. As such, use of this technique is applied whenever it can be safely performed. Dramatic improvements in the scoliosis or kyphosis can be seen, and it is particularly effective for lumbosacral defects.[5]

Anterior–posterior combined and posterior-only approaches can be used to perform this procedure. Closure of the wedge after excision initially was accomplished with braces and casts, then subsequently by hooks and compression rods with advances in fusion instrumentation. Many surgeons now advocate for a posterior single-stage hemivertebra excision with posterior transpedicular fixation to achieve fusion. However, some surgeons still prefer an anterior and posterior two-stage strategy as they feel that this is safer and involves lower risk of neurological complication. The inclusion of an anterior approach may also be considered if there is a kyphotic defect requiring an anterior cage to maintain anterior column support or to be used as a fulcrum to restore lordosis.

Compared to other surgical treatments, hemivertebra excision has several advantages. Firstly, it can be performed in very young patients, and has been advocated for use in children ages 1 to 6 if the defect is identified early in order to prevent disease progression. This has been shown to be very safe and efficacious, and does not limit vertical growth as patients age.[6] Additionally, the number of instrumented levels required is only as few as is necessary to allow for fusion across the compressed hemivertebra excision site. In cases of a single hemivertebra without associated bars, rib synostosis or other major structural changes, this requires only the two adjacent vertebrae. If high amounts of compressive force are required to correct the deformity, particularly in instances of severe kyphoscoliosis, an additional one or two segments allow for shared loading and reduce the risk of hardware failure or pedicle fracture.

In the posterior-only approach, pedicle screws are first placed into the adjacent vertebra to be included in the fixation. Once this is complete, the posterior elements are removed, including the lamina, facet joints, transverse process, and the posterior part of the pedicle. In the thoracic spine, an extrapleural approach is required, and therefore, the rib head on the convex

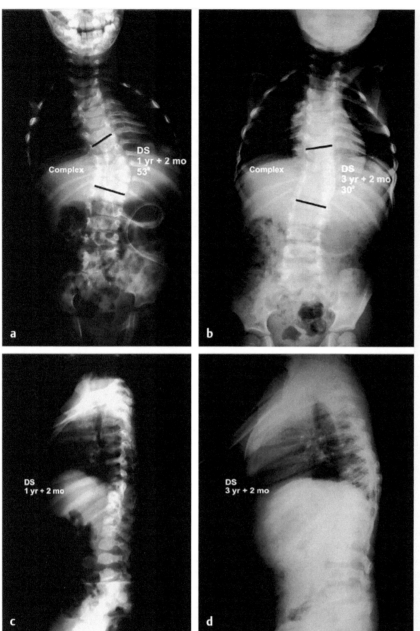

Fig. 6.4 A 14-month-old girl with complex anomaly and concomitant rib fusions who had 53 degrees of curvature pre-operatively (**a**) that improved to 30 degrees at 2 year follow-up (**b**) after a hemi-epiphysiodesis procedure. She maintained good sagittal alignment pre- and postoperatively (**c,d**, respectively). (Reproduced with permission from Uzumcugil et al. Convex growth arrest in the treatment of congenital spinal deformities, revisited. Journal of Pediatric Orthopedics. 2004; 24(6):658-666. Wolters Kluwer Health, Inc.)

side needs to be resected to gain exposure to the anterior aspect of the hemivertebra. A retroperitoneal exposure is required for lumbar hemivertebra. While protecting anterior vascular structures and associated neural structures, the defect and adjacent intervertebral disc materials need to be resected, and the adjacent growth plates rasped to enhance fusion. Screw-rod compression across the defect must be performed with direct visualization of the nerves and spinal cord to prevent neurological injury (▶ Fig. 6.5).

Hemivertebra excision can also be considered in patients with a contralateral bar. In these instances, the bar and proximal parts of the synostosed ribs, if they are present, must be cut to release the concavity. The transverse processes need to be removed and a lateral view of the fused segments incorporated in the bar must be obtained. Often a significant amount of rib needs to be removed to gain an exposure that is oblique

enough. Osteotomies of the barred segments then need to be performed to complete the release. Contralateral temporary rod placement should be performed to prevent inadvertent spinal translation which can put the neural elements at serious risk.

Given the complexity of this operation and intimacy of vertebral resection with neurological and vascular structures, there is a significant risk of complications associated with hemivertebra excision. While the rate of neurological injury reported is higher for this procedure than those mentioned above, when performed in the hands of experienced surgeons with constant attention to protecting neural structures, it can be performed safely with excellent correction and good fusion rates.

There has also been a report of a fusionless hemivertebrectomy technique.[7] After performing the hemivertebra resection from a posterior-only approach, the surgeons attached the inferior facet from the superior adjacent vertebra with the superior

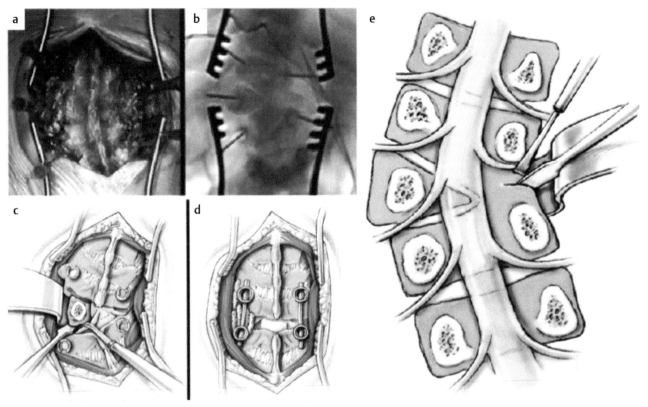

Fig. 6.5 Posterior exposure of isolated hemivertebra (**a**) with lines demarking pedicle entry points (**b**). Once the pedicle screws are placed, rostral and caudal disc spaces above the hemivertebra are removed allowing for resection (**c**). Compression across the convexity is then performed to correct the deformity (**d**). If there is a contralateral bar, exposure of the concavity is required, and osteotomies are performed to release this side of the defect for correction (**e**). (Reproduced with permission from Ruf et al. Hemivertebra resection and osteotomies in congenital spine deformity. Spine. 2009;34 (17):1791-1799. Wolters Kluwer Health, Inc.)

facet of the inferior adjacent vertebra to reconstruct a viable joint across the resected segment (▶ Fig. 6.6). The joint capsules were sutured together to create a viable joint. This was performed in the lumbar spine in an infant with unilateral convex transpedicular screw placement and wiring to create a tension band. Instrumentation was subsequently removed. Follow-up of the patient at 16 years of age demonstrated preserved motion across the disc space of the resected level. Further studies are required to investigate the viability of these approaches.

6.6.6 Instrumented Fusion and Correction of Deformity

In cases of rigid deformity encountered in older pediatric patients, posterior segmental fixation and fusion may be required to achieve correction. With this, partial correction of global spinal alignment is obtained by including the mobile vertebral segments above and below the congenital defect. Application of this technique was first applied by Winter et al using the Harrington rod instrumentation in the 1970s, and found that significantly greater correction of the deformity was seen compared to noninstrumented patients treated in a plaster jacket orthosis.[8] The introduction of pedicle screw fixation has led to biomechanically superior constructs and improved clinical and radiographic outcomes. However, screw placement may

remain technically difficult in this population secondary to distortion of anatomical reference points, particularly with congenital absences of posterior elements. Intraoperative spinal navigation may be helpful given the abnormal anatomy that is often encountered in this patient population.

In some instances, increased correction may be desired by means of anterior release with removal of the intervertebral discs. In theory, this also may help prevent crankshaft phenomenon. The extent of the crankshaft phenomenon seems to be proportional to the number of posteriorly fused segments.

For patients with more severe, rigid curves and acute angulations, vertebral osteotomies or anterior column resection can be considered (▶ Fig. 6.7). Severe truncal decompensation, pelvic obliquity, neurological deficits, and rapidly progressing disease with neurological deterioration (▶ Fig. 6.8) are all common in this patient population. Osteotomies may also be considered in patients with prior treatment or fusion that continues to progress. This can be seen in patients with progressive disease after a failed prior attempt at in situ fusion or epiphysiodesis.

An anterior–posterior or posterior-only approach can be performed to this end, each with its own advantages and disadvantages. Recent evidence suggests that an average of greater than 30 degrees of correction can be achieved of primary curves using posterior vertebral column resection (VCR) and pedicle screw fixation in congenital scoliosis patients.[5,8,9] Technically, VCR allows for both translational and rotational correction with

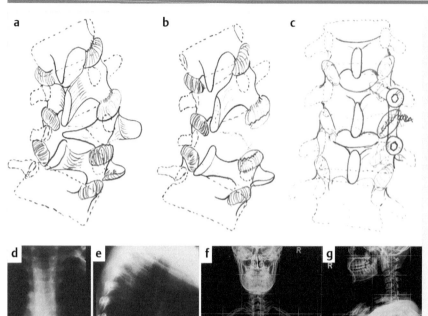

Fig. 6.6 Anatomical drawings of a lumbar hemivertebra (**a**) that has been excised (**b**) with preservation of the respective facets, reapproximation and closure of the joint capsule, and unilateral temporary pedicle screw fixation across the convexity (**c**). AP and lateral films immediately postoperatively in a patient at 18 months of age (**d,e,** respectively) and at 16 years of age (**f,g,** respectively). (Reproduced with permission from Jeszenszky D. Fusionless posterior hemivertebra resection in a 2-year-old child with 16 years follow-up. European Spine Journal. 2012; 21(8): 1471–1476. Springer, Inc.)

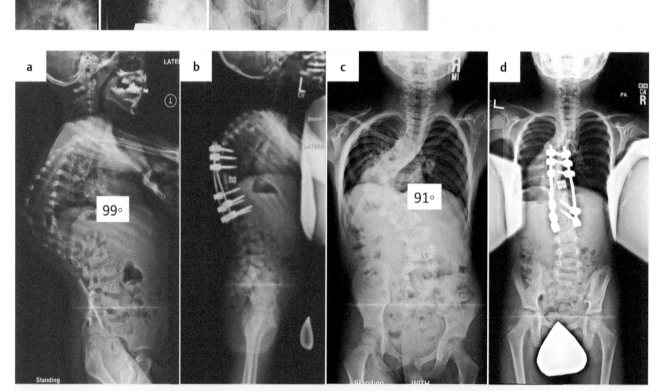

Fig. 6.7 A 5.9-year-old male with a thoracic hemivertebra and focal kyphotic (99 degrees, **a**) and scoliotic (91 degrees, **c**) curvature. The patient underwent a vertebral column resection with correction of the deformity (**b,d**). (Used with permission from Barrow Neurological Institute, Phoenix, Arizona.)

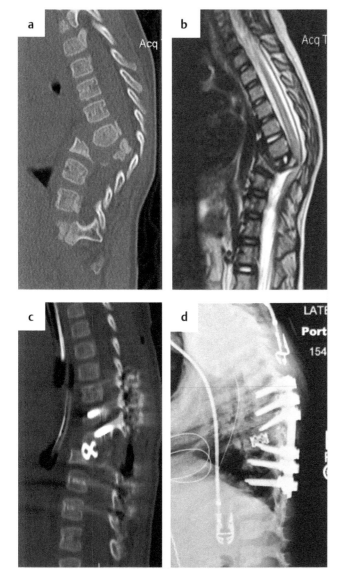

Fig. 6.8 A 25-month-old female with increasing kyphosis and progressive lower extremity weakness, bilateral lower extremity hyperreflexia and waddling gate. Image revealed a complex thoracic vertebral anomaly resulting in a severe focal kyphotic deformity **(a)** resulting in the spinal cord compression seen on MRI imaging **(b)**. Emergent surgical treatment was performed to prevent further neurological deterioration. Using a posterior-only approach, a T7-10 laminectomy was performed with vertebral column resection at T8-9, anterior strut placement and pedicle screw fixation T5-10 **(c,d)**. (Used with permission from Barrow Neurological Institute, Phoenix, Arizona.)

controlled maneuvering of anterior and posterior columns at the same time (▸ Fig. 6.9). Nevertheless, a complication rate of approximately 50% reflects the complexity of the procedure and the elevated risks of neurological injury and excessive blood loss.

Surgical technique for VCR is very similar to the technique described for hemivertebra resection. In the thoracic spine, a costotransversectomy needs to be completed on the convex side in order to appropriately remove the wall of the vertebral body on that side. Likewise, in the lumbar spine, an osteotomy

of the transverse process and facetectomy allow for complete bony removal. Pedicle screw placement above and below the defect allow for placement of a temporary rod. Wide laminectomy and gross visualization of the dura and neural elements is performed, followed by subperiosteal vertebral body resection beginning on the convex side. Constant attention should be made to protect the anterior vascular structures, and preservation of the segmental vessels should be performed if possible. Once bony removal and resection of the adjacent discs is complete on the convex side, another temporary rod can be placed on that side so that work on the concave side can be completed. Once the VCR has been completed on both sides, shorting across the temporary rods can be performed across the resected segment. Focus should be on the neural elements and dura during these maneuvers to prevent kinking or undesired distraction. Rotational and transitional realignment during this step is accomplished to achieve the desired curve correction. Once the correction has been completed, permanent rods are placed and posterolateral arthrodesis performed along the length of the construct.

6.6.7 Growth Preservation Technology

In situations where there is a severe angular deformity or a high-risk defect, definitive surgical treatment is warranted. However, in those circumstances where observation is appropriate, a growth-friendly strategy may be employed. This is especially applicable for long-segment curves over which significant growth is still expected (i.e., young children). The ultimate goals of growth-friendly approaches are to maximize spine length and mobility and mitigate growth-related negative effects on thoracic function all while correcting the deformity as patients mature.

Expandable Growing Rods

An important growth-friendly technique uses expandable growing rods. The technique involves placement of expandable distraction rod(s) across either the concave side of the deformity or bilaterally. Pedicle screws are placed at stable vertebrae above and below the primary curve to be used as the anchor points for the distractive force. Rods are then contoured in the desired sagittal conformation and proximal and distal rods are attached to a growing connector. A groove within the paravertebral muscles houses the rods, and the muscle and skin are closed over the rods. Often patients wear an external thoracolumbosacral orthosis for the first several months after surgery. After this time, patients have lengthening of the expandable rods at regular intervals (e.g., every 6 months) to allow for spinal growth (▸ Fig. 6.10).

There are several criticisms of this technique. First, the need for reoperation to repeatedly expand the rods during the child's growth increases the risk for infectious and wound complications. Recent advances in magnetically controlled growing rods have been developed to help address this issue, and greatly improve on prior technology. Other critics argue that methods of internal "bracing," which have previously been applied best to flexible idiopathic curves, should not be used for congenital scoliosis, a rigid deformity. Proponents of this technique report good results when applied to the appropriate clinical situations.

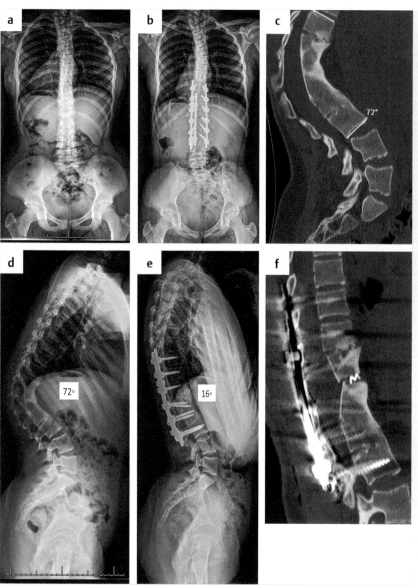

Fig. 6.9 12-year-old female with anterior unsegmented bar causing a pure congenital kyphosis with minimal scoliotic deformity (a,d). Computed tomography imaging demonstrates this deformity which spanned several vertebral levels from T10-L3 (c). She underwent surgical correction from a posterior-only approach: T12 vertebral column resection and T9 to L3 posterior fixation and fusion as seen on postoperative scoliosis radiographs (b,e) and sagittal CT imaging (f). (Used with permission from Barrow Neurological Institute, Phoenix, Arizona.)

It has been postulated that growing rods may modulate end-plate growth potential through distraction-based biomechanical forces, though this theory remains poorly understood.[10]

Expansion Thoracostomy and Vertical Expandable Prosthetic Titanium Rib

Thoracic insufficiency is an important consideration in the treatment of congenital scoliosis. Maximizing respiratory capacity is particularly important for patients with associated rib fusions and/or with thoracic restrictive disease (most often present on the concavity). Expansion thoracostomy with placement of vertical expandable prosthetic titanium rib (VEPTR) is an alternate growth-friendly treatment of congenital scoliosis that is also effective at treating thoracic insufficiency. VEPTR technology uses distracting rods on the concave ribs to maintain the correction throughout the patients' period of growth.

The most extensive experience with this technique has been on patients with fused ribs. Fused ribs have the potential to create concave tethering and exacerbate spinal deformity and lead to thoracic insufficiency.[11] While expansile thoracoplasty and VEPTR appear to be helpful for the treatment of thoracic insufficiency, these techniques appear to be less effective than growing rods for the correction of scoliosis iteself.[10] As with growing rods, skeletal immaturity with growth potential is a prerequisite to be considered for the procedure. VEPTR procedures can be coupled with growing rod techniques to achieve optimal deformity correction for simpler, more flexible congenital curves.

In performing this technique, patients are positioned in a lateral position on the operating table. Expansive thoracostomies are performed at the level of the fused rib(s), at the level of the most constricted region of the hemithorax, and at the corresponding segment of the spinal deformity. Extraperiosteal exposure helps to prevent spontaneous postoperative rib fusion. Rib-encircling anchors should also be extraperiosteal to preserve the vascular supply, and can be distracted against other caudal ribs (rib-to-rib), the insertion of caudal ribs where

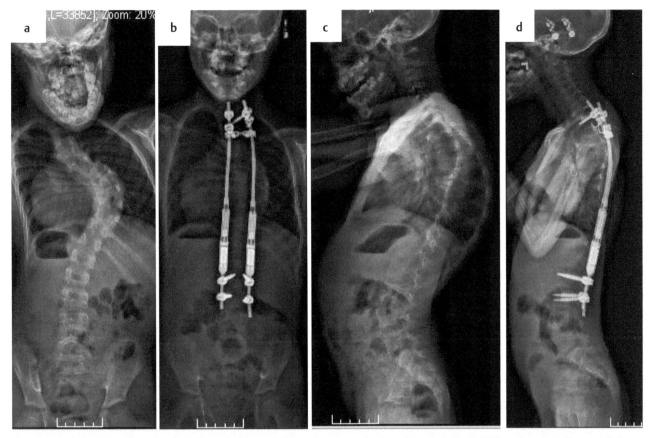

Fig. 6.10 A skeletally immature female with mixed thoracic defect causing severe kyphoscoliosis **(a,c)**. She had bilateral magnetically-controlled growing rods placed, which led to significant deformity correction after serial lengthenings **(b,d)**. (Used with permission from Barrow Neurological Institute, Phoenix, Arizona.)

they meet the spine (rib-to-spine) or to the iliac crest (rib-to-pelvis). Anchors should be carefully placed, as anchor points can migrate over time, which sometimes requires repositioning.

Wound infection remains the primary drawback to this approach, which often relates to poor soft tissue coverage over the prosthesis. With the requirement of repeat reopenings to expand the device as the patient grows, it is critical at the time of implantation that there is adequate soft tissue coverage over the implant. Careful surgical technique may help to mitigate the infection risk. Some surgeons recommend using nonaligned superficial and deep incisions when performing lengthening procedures to avoid a full-thickness exposure over the implant and minimize the risk of wound complications. Maintaining adequate patient nutrition is also essential to optimize wound healing.

It is expected that the majority of the correction will occur at the time of the index procedure and thoracostomy. Lengthening procedures are typically performed every 6 months to allow for continued growth and to prevent recurrence of the thoracic deformity. These lengthening procedures can often be performed in the outpatient setting with reopening of only a small portion of the incision. While these lengthening procedures are expected to keep up with the pace of patient's growth, rarely do they add to the extent of correction. Once the patient has completed his or her growth, the device is removed.

In addition to the concerns above, brachial plexus injury can occur with this procedure. As such, intraoperative neuromonitoring of the upper extremities should consistently be employed. Changes in signals should be addressed immediately with removal of the distraction and careful repositioning. Placement of rib anchors too cephalad or lateral may potentiate this risk. Likewise, delayed brachial plexopathy can occur if compression of the thoracic outlet occurs from scapular muscle traction during closure.

References

[1] Winter RB. Congenital scoliosis. Clin Orthop Relat Res. 1973(93):75–94
[2] McMaster MJ, Ohtsuka K. The natural history of congenital scoliosis. A study of two hundred and fifty-one patients. J Bone Joint Surg Am. 1982; 64(8): 1128–1147
[3] McMaster MJ, Singh H. Natural history of congenital kyphosis and kyphoscoliosis. A study of one hundred and twelve patients. J Bone Joint Surg Am. 1999; 81(10):1367–1383
[4] Walhout RJ, van Rhijn LW, Pruijs JE. Hemi-epiphysiodesis for unclassified congenital scoliosis: immediate results and mid-term follow-up. Eur Spine J. 2002; 11(6):543–549
[5] Yaszay B, O'Brien M, Shufflebarger HL, et al. Efficacy of hemivertebra resection for congenital scoliosis: a multicenter retrospective comparison of three surgical techniques. Spine. 2011; 36(24):2052–2060
[6] Ruf M, Jensen R, Letko L, Harms J. Hemivertebra resection and osteotomies in congenital spine deformity. Spine. 2009; 34(17):1791–1799

[7] Jeszenszky D, Fekete TF, Kleinstueck FS, Haschtmann D, Bognár L. Fusionless posterior hemivertebra resection in a 2-year-old child with 16 years follow-up. Eur Spine J. 2012; 21(8):1471–1476

[8] Hall JE, Herndon WA, Levine CR. Surgical treatment of congenital scoliosis with or without Harrington instrumentation. J Bone Joint Surg Am. 1981; 63 (4):608–619

[9] Winter RB, Moe JH, Lonstein JE. Posterior spinal arthrodesis for congenital scoliosis. An analysis of the cases of two hundred and ninety patients, five to nineteen years old. J Bone Joint Surg Am. 1984; 66(8):1188–1197

[10] Yazici M, Emans J. Fusionless instrumentation systems for congenital scoliosis: expandable spinal rods and vertical expandable prosthetic titanium rib in the management of congenital spine deformities in the growing child. Spine. 2009; 34(17):1800–1807

[11] Campbell RM, Jr, Smith MD, Mayes TC, et al. The effect of opening wedge thoracostomy on thoracic insufficiency syndrome associated with fused ribs and congenital scoliosis. J Bone Joint Surg Am. 2004; 86-A(8):1659–1674

7 Neuromuscular Scoliosis

Blake M. Bodendorfer and Suken A. Shah

Abstract

Neuromuscular scoliosis is common in children with neuropathic and myopathic disorders, the most common of which is cerebral palsy. The majority of these deformities are progressive, and can interfere with comfort, function (including ambulation, communication, transfers, sitting ability, and postural control), and allowance for daily hygienic and nutritional care. Nonoperative management and observation are reasonable for patients with curves less than 40 degrees, while operative treatment is typically recommended for patients with curves exceeding 50 degrees with concomitant development of symptoms or deterioration in function or 60 degrees with curves lacking flexibility. Curves in patients with remaining growth or flexibility can be observed at biannual intervals and surgery can be delayed until appropriate spinal height has been achieved, or the curve becomes increasingly stiff, preferably before the scoliosis exceeds 90 degrees. Since severe curves before the prepubertal growth spurt present a management dilemma, surgical intervention with growth-friendly spinal implants to control the curves may be an option. A posterior pedicle screw-based construct is the preferred method of instrumentation, as it offers a powerful mechanism of correction in both the coronal and sagittal plane. Extension of instrumentation to the pelvis is typically performed to correct pelvic obliquity and avoid distal progression of deformity. Anterior surgery, associated with increased complications and morbidity, is seldom necessary with modern instrumentation and techniques, but is reserved for large, rigid curves and may be staged when appropriate. The risk of complications in the perioperative and postoperative period is significant, but manageable, and has improved substantially with contemporary care pathways. The most common postoperative complications include infection, implant-related complications, and pulmonary issues. Caregiver satisfaction and long-term outcomes are excellent following surgery for neuromuscular scoliosis.

Keywords: neuromuscular scoliosis, cerebral palsy, pedicle screw, pelvic fixation, complications

Clinical Pearls

- The most common cause of neuromuscular scoliosis is cerebral palsy.
- The pinnacles of care for these children are to improve sitting ability, postural control, daily hygiene, and nutritional care while providing pain relief in some cases.
- Nonoperative management and observation are reasonable for select patients with curves less than 40 degrees.
- Operative treatment is typically pursued for patients with curves exceeding 50 degrees with concomitant deterioration in function or 60 degrees with curves lacking flexibility.
- Curves with remaining growth or flexibility can be observed and surgery can be delayed up to 90 degrees and still be treated with a posterior-only approach.
- Severe curves in prepubertal growth present a management dilemma, and surgical intervention with growth-friendly spinal implants to control the curves is an option.
- A posterior pedicle screw-based construct is the preferred method of instrumented fusion.
- Extension of fusion to the pelvis prevents the progression of pelvic obliquity.
- Anterior surgery is associated with increased complications and morbidity and is seldom necessary with modern instrumentation and techniques.
- The most common postoperative complications include infection, implant-related complications, and pulmonary issues (including atelectasis, prolonged ventilator support, and pneumonia).
- Caregiver satisfaction and long-term outcomes are excellent following surgery for neuromuscular scoliosis.

7.1 Introduction

Neuromuscular scoliosis is a coronal plane spinal curvature of 10 degrees or more, measured by the Cobb method, in the setting of muscle imbalance secondary to an underlying neuropathic or myopathic disease. Abnormal biomechanical loading secondary to this imbalance and spinal collapse results in asymmetric vertebral body growth in the skeletally immature patients, in accordance with the Hueter–Volkmann principle. Progression occurs as a result of progressive muscle imbalance and anatomical deformity. There are many neuropathic and myopathic disorders that may lead to neuromuscular scoliosis (▶ Table 7.1), of which cerebral palsy (CP) is the most prevalent and will be the main focus of this chapter. Cerebral palsy occurs in approximately 2 per 1,000 live births and an estimated 15 to 28% of these children will develop scoliosis, and more severe forms, such as spastic quadriplegia, have a higher incidence.[1,2]

7.2 Natural History of Neuromuscular Scoliosis in Cerebral Palsy

The rate of progression relates to the magnitude of curve. Thometz and Simon observed 0.8-degree curve progression in patients with curves less than 50 degrees, whereas 1.4 degrees per year curve progression was seen in patients with curves greater than 50 degrees.[3] During periods of rapid growth, severe progression can occur. The vast majority (85%) of patients with curves exceeding 40 degrees by 15 years of age progressed to 60 degrees, while only 13% of those with a curve less than 40 degrees by 15 years of age progressed to 60 degrees.[4] Curve progression increases the magnitude of deforming forces and leads to subsequent deformity, truncal imbalance, and pelvic decompensation. The pelvis is often the end vertebra equivalent—the most tilted component with

Table 7.1 Causes of neuromuscular scoliosis

Neuropathic	Myopathic
Upper motor neuron	Arthrogryposis
Cerebral palsy	Muscular dystrophy
Spinocerebellar degeneration	Duchenne
Friedreich's ataxia	Limb girdle
Charcot–Marie–Tooth	Facioscapulohumeral
Roussy–Levy	Fiber-type disproportion
Syringomyelia	Congenital hypotonia
Spinal cord trauma	Myotonia dystrophica
Spinal cord tumor	
Lower motor neuron	
Poliomyelitis	
Traumatic	
Spinal muscle atrophy	
Werdnig–Hoffman	
Kugelberg–Welander	
Dysautonomia	

residual axial rotation of the C curve. This was described as the pelvic vertebra by Dubousset.[5] Less frequently, pelvic obliquity presents as a compensatory fractional curve to the C curve. Pelvic obliquity alters sitting position and pressure at the typically well-distributed sitting tripod at both ischial tuberosities and pubic symphysis. Increased pressure at the ipsilateral ischial tuberosity is worsened in patients with increased pelvic tilt and can result in pressure sores.

7.3 Evaluation of Neuromuscular Scoliosis in Cerebral Palsy

Generally, neuromuscular scoliosis develops at an earlier age than adolescent idiopathic scoliosis, but can present between 3 and 20 years of age.[4] The flexible, postural curve tends to develop into a torsional, structural deformity with growth and finally into a stiff curve of considerable magnitude before growth is complete. Generally speaking, more severe forms of cerebral palsy are associated with greater degrees of deformity. Considering the physiological classification of CP, spastic quadriplegic patients have the highest incidence of scoliosis. Madigan and Wallace found a 64% incidence of scoliosis in institutionalized patients with CP.[6] The risk of scoliosis correlates with ambulatory ability as graded by the Gross Motor Function Classification System (GMFCS). Children with mild gross motor function limitation have no higher risk of developing scoliosis than the general population, whereas those with limited motor function (GMFCS levels IV and V) have approximately 50% risk of developing moderate or severe scoliosis.[1]

Depending on the dominant deforming forces and spasticity, patients may present with either kyphoscoliosis or lordoscoliosis. In kyphoscoliosis, progressive deformity with associated pelvic obliquity and retroversion may compromise the often-limited ambulatory function. Pelvic obliquity makes sitting difficult or even impossible. In lordoscoliosis, a patient may have extensor posturing. Progressive deformity makes sitting impossible. Patients may need to be nursed in a semi-reclined position in a wheelchair. These patients may have acute pain

without relief from any sitting adaptation. Significant deformity may compromise cardiopulmonary function, gastrointestinal motility, and result in rib–pelvis impingement. Upon identification of the deformity, the most important clinical determinations are flexibility of the curve and remaining growth potential. Flexibility is determined by holding the patient up at the axillae in a sitting position or side bending over a fulcrum with the child relaxed. Pelvic obliquity is assessed by positioning the patient prone with the hips and knees hanging free. Infrapelvic causes of pelvic obliquity include hip subluxation and dislocation as well as adductor contracture. Suprapelvic causes of pelvic obliquity are from scoliosis itself. Standing 36-inch posteroanterior (PA) and lateral radiographs of the entire spine should be obtained when possible. Sitting radiographs are acceptable substitutes if the patient is unable to stand, and "sitting frames" with lateral support straps are used in some centers to obtain these with minimal external support. Curve characteristics to be noted are curve type, magnitude, and progression. Sagittal and coronal balance as well as pelvic obliquity and tilt and signs of remaining growth (triradiate cartilage and Risser's sign) should be documented. Structural deformity is commonly detected by vertebral rotation, rib deformity, and wedging. Neuromuscular scoliosis secondary to CP should be monitored at a minimum of yearly follow-up examinations to determine curve progression, but 6-month follow-ups are appropriate for progressive or severe deformities, or for children in the midst of rapid growth during the onset of puberty. Magnetic resonance imaging (MRI) should be obtained if any suspicion for intraspinal pathology exists. Signs of intraspinal pathology include very rapid progression at a young age, increasing lumbar hyperlordosis, or a change in neurological status that may be expected with a tethered cord.

7.4 Classification of Neuromuscular Scoliosis in Cerebral Palsy

Lonstein and Akbarnia[7] have classified neuromuscular scoliosis secondary to CP into two groups (▶ Fig. 7.1). Group I curves are double curves with both thoracic and lumbar components, also known as "S curves." These curves tend to behave similar to idiopathic scoliotic curves and have a higher likelihood of preservation of ambulation ability. Group II curves have lumbar or thoracolumbar deformity that extend into the sacrum and have associated pelvic obliquity, also known as "C curves." The long, sweeping, and collapsing curves are more typical of neuromuscular curves in patients who are wheelchair-dependent or bedridden. The apex of these curves is centered in the thoracic spine (T2–T10) or at the thoracolumbar junction (T11–L1) and have a right-sided apex. See ▶ Fig. 7.1 for examples of groups I and II curves. The majority (94%) of patients with CP who required surgery due to pelvic obliquity, poor coronal balance, and a large magnitude of curve are categorized as group II curves.[6]

7.5 Nonoperative Treatment

Pain relief, functional preservation (including sitting ability and postural control), and allowance for daily hygienic and

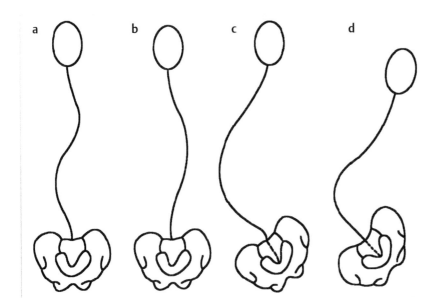

Fig. 7.1 Curve patterns in neuromuscular scoliosis secondary to cerebral palsy. Group I curves are double curves with little pelvic obliquity that may be balanced (**a**) or unbalanced (**b**). Group II curves (**c,d**) are large lumbar or thoracolumbar curves with marked pelvic obliquity. (Adapted from Lonstein and Akbarnia.[7])

nutritional care are of utmost importance when caring for these patients. A near-normal chin-brow vertical angle allows for visual and cognitive stimulations with motor response. Curves with less than 20 degrees of deformity are reasonable candidates for observation. Bracing is an option for patients that progress with observation, but this is dependent on the severity of the curve and neurological involvement. Spastic quadriplegic patients generally do not benefit long term from bracing. Rigid thoracolumbosacral orthoses (TLSOs) have been found to have little benefit on curve or rate of progression in patients that were braced 23 hours per day over greater than 5 years compared to observation alone.[8] Contrastingly, Terjesen et al[9] performed a retrospective cohort study of 86 patients with spastic quadriplegic CP and found a mean progression of 4.2 degrees per year with custom-molded TLSOs, 25% of patients less than 1 degree per year of progression per year. Soft TLSOs can assist with seating support and augment function. Improved sitting function can help with attentiveness in class, ease of care, self-image, and decreased rates of pressure ulcers. Children with flexible curves that require seating support can be fitted for offset lateral chest supports and modular seating systems on their wheelchairs. This will allow for three-point control of the coronal deformity. In ambulatory children with GMFCS I to III, rigid bracing may slow the progression of the deformity similarly to adolescent idiopathic scoliosis. Braces are commonly indicated for curves of 25 degrees or more in immature patients with significant growth remaining and should be worn for a minimum of 12 hours per day, although the optimal brace wear time is 16 to 18 hours per day. Therapeutic stretching, electrical stimulation, and botulinum toxin are lacking validity and have limited supported utility at this time.

7.6 Rationale for Operative Treatment

Interventions should always be weighted by assessing functional health gain, patient satisfaction, and technical success.[10] All decisions to proceed with operative care for these patients should be aimed at maintaining functional health against the progressive deformity and its associated morbidity, achieving reasonable patient–caregiver satisfaction, and minimizing complications. For higher functioning patients, the goal may be different. These patients may desire more normal spinal balance, preservation of function, and greater ambulatory potential. For patients with no ambulatory potential, the aim should be to maintain independence in sitting and facilitation in care. The burden of care in this group of patients with severe learning disability may change significantly.[11,12] Surgery in this group is a palliative measure that allows families to independently care for their children at home and to keep their child involved in school and community activities. Larsson et al[11] discovered that overall care burden was decreased and sitting position and vital capacity were improved in patients with neuromuscular scoliosis who underwent operative treatment in a prospective cohort study. In another study of 100 spastic CP patients who underwent spinal fusion, 85% of parents interviewed indicated that they were satisfied with the result and would opt for surgery again.[13] Caregivers believed that patients had an improved self-image. Parents and caregivers believed that surgery improved sitting ability, physical appearance, comfort, and ease of care. These results were confirmed by other studies.[14,15,16]

7.7 Surgical Treatment

Surgical intervention is considered when curve magnitude exceeds 50 degrees and there is concomitant deterioration in function.[13,17,18] Even with completion of growth, there is ample evidence that these curves will progress. For curves between 60 and 90 degrees, surgery is indicated when the deformity is rigid even with remaining growth. If flexibility remains during growth, surgery can usually be delayed until 90 degrees of deformity with a posterior-only procedure. In patients with flexible curves greater than 90 degrees, sitting may be challenging and further exacerbated by the associated pelvic obliquity. Specific considerations include the level of instrumentation, early-onset scoliosis, sagittal deformity correction, pelvic and infrapelvic coronal deformity, intraoperative neuromonitoring, necessity of anterior release, intraoperative femoral traction, and intrathecal baclofen therapy.

7.7.1 Level of Instrumentation

Patients with neuromuscular scoliosis who are indicated for surgery typically undergo long-construct fusions from T1 or T2 to the sacrum and pelvis. Increased postoperative incidence of proximal curve progression and proximal junctional kyphosis has been observed if the proximal instrumented vertebra does not extend to T2 or higher, since most of these children lack adequate head control.[19] Patients with pathological thoracic kyphosis may be better candidates for extension of the construct to C7. There is historical debate regarding extension of posterior spinal fusion to the pelvis. Pelvic obliquity has been shown to progress when fusion does not extend to the pelvis[3, 17,20]; furthermore, late revision reconstruction to the pelvis for add-on can be challenging and fraught with complications. Extension of fusion to the pelvis has been recommended in nonambulatory patients. In ambulatory patients with pelvic obliquity, extension of the fusion to the pelvis has been avoided due to concerns that it will negatively impact ambulatory function.[1,21] However, a study utilizing gait analysis at our institution demonstrated preserved ambulatory function in these patients after unit rod instrumentation to the pelvis.[22] In patients who use the gluteus maximus to propel their gait due to a weak gastrocnemius, instrumentation to L5 can be considered. McCall and Hayes investigated the results of the use of a "U rod" (a unit rod construct lacking pelvic limbs) with L5 pedicle screw fixation in patients with a stable lumbosacral articulation. the L5–S1 interspace mobility was assessed on the basis of L5 tilt. Patients with more than 15 degrees of L5 tilt were instrumented with standard unit rod construct instead. Patients had similar results in both groups.[23]

7.7.2 Early-Onset Scoliosis in Cerebral Palsy

Severe curves in prepubertal growth present a management dilemma. Continued observation, surgical intervention with growth-friendly spinal implants to control the curves, or early correction and fusion are all options. In one study of growing rods in CP patients, 27 patients at a mean 7.6 years of age had a 47% correction of the Cobb angle from a mean 85 degrees. However, 19 of these patients had complications, including 8 deep wound infections, 11 rod-related complications, and 6 anchor-related complications.[18] There have been similar complication rates utilizing the "Eiffel Tower" vertical expandable prosthetic titanium rib (VEPTR) construct.[24] In one study examining early spinal fusion in 33 patients at a mean 8.3 years of age with mean Cobb's angle of 85 degrees and minimum 5 years of follow-up with all but 2 patients being GMFCS V, there was a 28% mortality rate, with 6 patients dying between 1 and 5 years and 2 between 10 and 15 years after surgery.[25] Deep infection was reported in three patients. Although the ideal management plan has not been elucidated, the recently approved magnetically controlled growing rod systems that do not require repeat surgeries for lengthening purposes have been in use long enough for short-to-medium-term follow-up. Short-term

studies suggest minimal proximal pullout, revision surgery, and outpatient distraction complications.[26,27,28] Generally, these authors preferred the rate of revision surgeries with magnetic growing rods as compared to those experienced with traditional growing rod systems. However, the study with the longest follow-up to our knowledge (minimum 44 months) had more sobering results. Teoh et al[29] reported on eight patients (five dual-rod constructs and three single-rod constructs), of which six required eight revision surgeries. These revisions were performed for rod problems (4), proximal screw pullout (3), and development of proximal junctional kyphosis (1). These authors advised using caution for utilizing magnetically controlled growing rod systems, especially for single-rod constructs.

7.7.3 Sagittal Plane Deformities

Hyperkyphosis or lordosis may develop in patients with neuromuscular disorders, with or without scoliosis. Flexible, postural deformities may be addressed in younger patients with hamstring contractures by lengthening the posterior thigh musculature and addressing the associated posterior pelvic tilt and retroversion or by wheelchair or shoulder harness modifications. However, these adaptations may not work as well in older children. The spinal column lengthens with lumbar hyperlordosis correction and shortens with hyperkyphosis correction. Tethered cord must be evaluated prior to surgical correction of lumbar hyperlordosis. Patients who have undergone a previous dorsal rhizotomy for spasticity are at an increased risk for developing pathological hyperlordosis and associated spondylolisthesis, which impact the posterior surgical exposure. Postoperative radiculitis may develop after correction of hyperlordosis and relative lengthening of the lumbar spine from nerve root tension. Lumbar hyperlordosis and associated pelvic anteversion and obliquity alter the trajectory of pelvic fixation, which is a risk factor for pelvic fixation-related complications.[30] Bowel perforation following medial breach of the ilium by the pelvic limbs of the unit rod has been described. Modular screw-based systems are recommended to decrease morbidity with pelvic screw placement, allow customization, and afford deformity correction.[31]

7.7.4 Pelvic and Infrapelvic Coronal Plane Deformities

Compensatory scoliosis arises from coronal plane deformities of the pelvic and infrapelvic origin. Asymmetric forces of the gluteus medius and hip adductors as well as infrapelvic pathology, including hip subluxation or dislocation contribute to pelvic obliquity. Adductor and iliopsoas release may be attempted to achieve femoral head coverage and pelvic leveling in young patients. Osteotomy of the proximal femur and pelvis may be required in older age as deformities become stiff. In these cases, spinal deformity correction should be performed prior to pelvic osteotomies for femoral head coverage.

7.7.5 Intraoperative Neuromonitoring

Spinal cord monitoring with intraoperative transcranial motor evoked potentials and somatosensory evoked potentials is controversial in this population since meaningful monitoring is difficult.[32] Thirty percent of patients with severe CP may have weak or absent signals at baseline, particularly transcranial motor evoked potentials in the most severely affected children.[33,34] Intraoperative neuromonitoring changes present a management dilemma. The Stagnara wake-up test is usually not possible.[35] In patients that respond to intraoperative optimization of physiological parameters and surgical correction, it could potentially advert neurogenic bladder requiring urinary catheterization and maintain protective sensation even in the most neurologically involved patients. In patients who have lost signals despite optimization, staging the procedure versus in situ correction are both options and debatable. Involvement of the family in decision making is helpful to determine the best plan of care.

7.7.6 Anterior Release

Anterior release at the apical levels is indicated for stiff curves or curves greater than 90 degrees not reducible with a pull or fulcrum bend film to gain flexibility and allow correction. Anterior release at the lumbosacral region includes psoas muscle origin release, annulus release, and complete discectomy. These assist in correcting both pelvic obliquity and pelvic tilt.[36] Anterior surgery is associated with increased complications and morbidity. Higher rates of pulmonary and cardiovascular (coagulopathy and hypotension) complications have been reported with anterior releases.[37] Thoracoscopic anterior release is possible from the intervertebral disc of T4-5 to T11-12 and can reduce operative time and morbidity associated with open thoracotomy. When both anterior and posterior procedures are required, it is important to consider that evidence supports both staged (1–2 weeks apart) and same-day surgery. Some prefer the staged approach for patients with multiple medical comorbidities and severe CP.[38] Same-day surgery may be planned for patients with relatively good health, but may need to be reconsidered for staging with excess operative time or blood loss after the anterior release is performed. Anterior fusion to prevent crankshaft phenomenon is not necessary when rigid, segmental instrumentation with a unit rod or with pedicle screws to the pelvis is used.[39,40,41]

7.7.7 Intraoperative Halofemoral Traction

Patients with kyphoscoliosis or significant pelvic obliquity can benefit from intraoperative traction.[37,42,43] In patients with lumbar hyperlordosis, bilateral use should be avoided so as to not worsen the lordosis. Unilateral traction prior to corrective maneuvers may assist in leveling the pelvis. Traction can be applied proximally through the skull with a halo or cranial tongs and distally with femoral pins, lower extremity skin taping, or securing the feet and ankles in boots attached to the operative table.

7.7.8 Intrathecal Baclofen Pump

Intrathecal baclofen is utilized to control muscle spasticity while maintaining muscle function. Patients with intrathecal baclofen pumps must have adequate padding at the pump site for prone positioning. Concurrent pump insertion during spinal deformity surgery does not increase infection risk.[44] No significant cerebral spinal fluid leak should be encountered during the insertion of the intrathecal catheter component. The pump and connecting tubing at the intrathecal sac can be safely inserted or exchanged postspinal fusion below the conus medullaris.

7.8 Surgical Advances and Outcomes

When no other alternatives would be viable, spinal instrumentation and fusion are indicated for collapsing deformities and painful sitting.[45] Harrington rods had an unacceptably high rate of pseudarthrosis (18–27%).[7,13,46,47] Segmental instrumentation with Luque's rods and sublaminar wiring had better results than the Harrington instrumentation and obviated the need for prolonged postoperative casting.[15,48,49,50,51] Comparing cohorts who underwent posterior-only instrumentation to a combined anterior–posterior cohort, Comstock et al found a mean correction of 51 and 57%, respectively.[13]

Progression of pelvic obliquity has been noted when the fusion does not extend to the pelvis.[13,15,20] The Galveston technique to extend the fusion across the pelvis by placing each Luque's rod between the pelvic tables had acceptable fusion rates across the L5-S1 segment and provided good control of pelvic obliquity.[52] However, it was associated with a high incidence of loosening associated with micromotion at the sacroiliac joints, leading to the radiographic "windshield-wiper" effect. Impacting two Luque's rods into the pelvis with segmental fusion utilizing sublaminar wiring provides a strong construct in the sagittal plane, but a moment arm of rotation about the two rods allows for rod translation, loss of torsional control, and subsequent progression of pelvic obliquity, pseudarthrosis, and implant failure.[53] Luque's rods smaller than one-fourth of an inch in diameter may be associated with increased implant failure.[20,48,54] However, intraoperative bending of one-fourth of an inch in diameter to the ideal geometry for pelvic implantation is challenging. Lonstein et al found in a cohort of 93 patients with 50% correction of the major scoliotic curve with a mean preoperative scoliosis of 72 degrees and 40% correction of pelvic obliquity at a mean follow-up of 3.8 years using a dual Luque–Galveston technique.[55] Sanders et al found that postoperative residual curve greater than 35 degrees, preoperative curves greater than 60 degrees, crankshaft deformity, and not fusing to the pelvis were all predictive of postoperative curve progression.[20]

Bell et al developed the unit rod and this addressed some of the limitation of the dual Luque rod instrumentation.[53] The major design change was a proximally connected, precontoured rod that provided better rotational control compared to the independent rotational freedom between the dual Luque rods. Tsirikos et al observed a mean correction of 68% from a mean scoliotic curve of 76 degrees and pelvic obliquity correction of 71% at a mean follow-up of 3.9 years in 241 patients, which was more effective than the dual Luque rod instrumentation.[30] Westerlund and Dias found similar results.[39,41]

Segmental instrumentation using Cotrel–Dubousset instrumentation of hooks is limited to patients with S-shaped curves without the need to extend to the pelvis. Hybrid constructs using iliosacral screws for pelvic fixation with hooks allows for 40% correction of pelvic obliquity with a posterior approach and 47% correction using a combined anterior–posterior approach.[56,57] There is a tendency of in situ rod derotation in restoring coronal correction, which does not allow a significant biomechanical advantage in reducing pelvic obliquity over a unit rod with sublaminar wires.

Iliac screws were borne from the smooth Galveston rods and iliosacral screws. They require less dissection and have better pullout strength than Galveston's rods for pelvic fixation because they extend anteriorly beyond the pivot point of lumbosacral motion.[58] Galveston's rods may pull out and become prominent posteriorly. Segmental pedicle screw constructs have shown substantial improvement in fusion at the lumbosacral junction while correcting pelvic obliquity and addressing seating problems. The modular nature of these systems can help with the management of osteoporotic bone, three-dimensional deformity of the pelvis (e.g., rotated pelvis), and lumbar hyperlordosis which can help to avoid early hardware failure.[59] The iliac screws are offset and connected to the rods via a connector. Careful rod engagement with adequate length distal to the tulip head of the connector is required to avoid disengagement. The use of four iliac screws at the pelvis improved bony purchase but did not eliminate loosening.[60] Implant prominence can be a problem in thin patients. Placement of the screw caudad to the natural prominence of the posterior superior iliac spine (PSIS) with bony resection may avoid this problem.

Kebaish et al popularized sacral alar–iliac (S2AI) fixation, which has the advantage of an iliac screw without the prominence, since it is placed 15 mm deeper to the PSIS.[61,62] Additionally, soft-tissue dissection is less and pullout strength is similar to an iliac screw. The screw extends across the sacroiliac joint anteriorly beyond the pivot point of the lumbosacral junction and serves as an effective flexion moment against movement at the lumbosacral junction. The tulip screw head is aligned with the instrumentation array without need for an offset connector.

Lumbar pedicle screws with reduction tabs allow for effective sagittal and coronal control while allowing reduction of pelvic obliquity when used in concert with either iliac or S2AI screws. This is particularly useful for lumbar hyperlordosis and pelvic anteversion where the trajectory of the iliac anchor would be challenging. Tsirikos and Mains demonstrated 72% correction of the major curve with a mean preoperative curve of 76 degrees along with 80% correction of pelvic obliquity from a mean preoperative 22 degrees in a cohort of adolescent CP patients who underwent correction with posterior-only pedicle screw constructs.[31] Pedicle screw-based modular constructs allow for superior Cobb's correction and leveling the pelvic obliquity, but the initial cost of these systems is much greater than the unit rod. However, this is offset in the long term by less implant-related complications and a lower rate of infection as demonstrated in a multicenter series.[63] Aside from pulmonary issues, implant-related complications and infection are the two most common complications in the operative treatment of neuromuscular scoliosis.[64]

At our institution, hybrid constructs and all pedicle screw systems achieved similar results. Pedicle screws are inserted at the most caudad thoracic and lumbar vertebrae. Sacropelvic fixation is obtained with S2AI screws. A stable pelvic fixation allows a strong cantilever force to level the pelvis using dual custom rods, which are proximally connected. The reduction of the rods starts at the caudad lumbar screws and proceeds in the cephalad direction. Intervening thoracic levels are instrumented with sublaminar wiring or staggered pedicle screws. An all screw construct is used when significant correction is needed in the thoracic vertebrae.

7.9 Perioperative Management

Children with neuromuscular scoliosis tend to be medically complex and have significant preoperative risks. Risks and complications of the procedure are directly related to the severity of neurological impairment. Patients requiring nutrition through gastric or jejunal tubes, those with severe intellectual disability, lacking verbal communication and independent sitting, and epilepsy have the highest rate of complications.[65] Seizures, respiratory issues, nutritional deficiencies, gastroesophageal reflux, and gastric motility issues should be addressed preoperatively. Anesthesiologists should be made aware of children who are on ketogenic diets for seizure control, as these patients are at high risk of hypoglycemic episodes intraoperatively.

Preoperative laboratory evaluations should include a complete blood count, complete metabolic profile, urinalysis, coagulation profile, and albumin and prealbumin levels. Blood loss can be significant and a type and crossmatch of 1 to 1.5 times the patient's blood volume should be available prior to surgery.[45] Coagulation factor replacement and core body temperature should be maintained. Despite normal prothrombin time (PT) and partial thromboplastin time (PTT) values, blood loss tends to occur earlier and in larger quantity in this population.[66,67] Cell salvage and antifibrinolytics are useful adjuncts in decreasing allogenic transfusion and blood loss.[68,69] Tranexamic acid (TXA) has been shown to be more effective than epsilon–aminocaproic acid (AMICAR) with the loading dose of 100 mg/kg over 30 minutes followed by 10 mg/kg infusion until closure.[70] This infusion should be limited to 8 hours.

Intraoperatively, the surgeon should strive to constantly communicate with the anesthesia staff. Intraoperative hypothermia is the most commonly encountered issue by the anesthesiologist, reported as high as 55%.[71] This may contribute to coagulopathy, and active warming blankets with monitoring are useful to prevent hypothermia without raising the core body temperature too high. The patient is most at risk of hypothermia during induction of anesthesia and while intravenous (IV) access is being obtained prior to skin preparation and draping. Intraoperative hypotension is encountered in 15% of cases, usually related to inadequate volume replacement from chronic dehydration, increased sensitivity to anesthetic agents, and increased blood loss. Correction of kyphosis can also impede venous return to the heart and lead to hypotension, but this can be prevented by increasing the preload volume prior to the correction.[45] When hypotension during curve correction is encountered, an attempt to release pressure on the spine should be performed while increasing the rate or IV fluid and/or blood replacement. After the blood pressure has been stable for 5 to 10 minutes, it is typically safe to proceed with gradual correction after the soft tissue has creeped. If sudden hypotension with or without bradycardia occurs, anaphylaxis should be considered; unknown latex allergies are common among these patients, but reactions to colloid or blood product replacement are also possible.

Parents and caretakers are frequently not prepared for the complexity or duration of the patient's postoperative course.[13] Preoperative counseling of the family and caretakers should stress the potential or expectation of a prolonged intensive care unit (ICU) stay, as well as the significant possibility or anticipation of postoperative complications.

7.10 Surgical Technique

After intubation and induction of anesthesia, neuromonitoring lead placement, urinary catheterization, and the establishment of large-bore IV access, central venous catheterization (when necessary), and arterial line placement, the patient is positioned prone on a radiolucent table or four post frames. All bony prominences are padded to avoid skin breakdown. The abdomen should hang free and the hips can be allowed to gently flex with knee and thigh support to correct lumbar hyperlordosis. A free abdomen will decrease intraoperative blood loss by reducing inferior vena caval pressure.[72,73,74] Unilateral intraoperative skin traction can be utilized on the side with high pelvic obliquity during the corrective maneuver, if necessary.

After IV antibiotic and TXA administration, a standard posterior exposure to the spine is undertaken from T1 to the sacrum. Subperiosteal elevation is utilized out to the transverse processes with Cobb's elevators. Electrocautery is used for hemostasis. The use of bipolar sealer devices should be considered, as their use has been correlated with decreased blood loss and transfusion requirements.[75] The cephalad supra- and interspinous ligaments are preserved in an effort to prevent proximal junctional kyphosis. Aggressive posterior release with facetectomies and ligamentum flavum resection creates flexibility in the rigid apical portion of the curve. Facetectomies can be performed with a rongeur, osteotome, burr, or ultrasonic bone cutting device. This should proceed from L5 to S1 in a cephalad direction to the level below the upper instrumented vertebrae. Gelfoam soaked in thrombin or other hemostatic agents can be used to control local bleeding. If additional deformity correction is needed, posterior column osteotomies (PCOs) may be performed by removing the facet in its entirety, along with the supra- and interspinous ligament, and ligamentum flavum with a combination of a Kerrison rongeur and burr.[76] The senior author uses an ultrasonic bone cutting device for the PCO. Concave osteotomy at the apical segments may be necessary. Concave release of the taut iliolumbar ligaments at the tip of the L5 transverse process may be needed for severe, stiff pelvic obliquity.

If traditional iliac screw fixation is opted for, the PSIS is next to be exposed. To avoid screw head prominence, an osteotome is used to resect a notch 1 cm caudad to the most prominent part of the PSIS. The cancellous bone between the pelvic tables is cannulated with a drill or pedicle gearshift. Successful iliac screw fixation is possible with a miniaccess approach to avoid extensive muscle dissection of the paraspinal musculature at the lumbosacral junction and outer table of the pelvis using intraoperative fluoroscopy. The "teardrop" of the ilium is visualized by tilting the image intensifier obliquely in the plane of the

iliac wing and cephalad so that it is parallel to the cortical bone of the sciatic notch. Iliac screw placement in this area ensures excellent fixation in strong cancellous bone, adequate length to extend past the pivot point of the lumbosacral junction, and avoidance of the sciatic notch and acetabulum. The iliac screw is then connected to the thoracolumbar construct to level the pelvis.

If S2AI fixation is opted for, the exposure at the caudad incision is minimal. The starting point is at the midway of S1 and S2 foramen in line with the S1 pedicle screws. The screw traverses the sacroiliac joint and has the same endpoint as the iliac screw, pointing toward the anterior inferior iliac spine (AIIS) or greater trochanter for maximum purchase. The bony isthmus is usually at the 60-mm mark. A curved gearshift that points cephalad in relation to the plane of the ilium allows for longer screws to be inserted while gliding away from the direction of the hip joint.[77] A guidewire is then inserted prior to drill and screw insertion, with the typical screw size being 8 mm or more in diameter and at least 65 to 80 mm in length. In a neutral pelvis, 30 degrees of lateral angulation is expected, but this will need to be adjusted for rotational deformity. In hyperlordosis, a more horizontal trajectory will be needed.

Thoracic and lumbar pedicle screws are inserted with freehand technique.[78] The pars, mammillary bodies, and transverse processes are prepared. The pars interarticularis leads to the lumbar pedicle entry point at the intersection of the mid-transverse process and the mid-facet joints. A high-speed cortical burr is used to mark the starting point and penetrate the cortex. A curved gearshift is used to cannulate the entry point with the curve pointing laterally. Once 20 mm of depth is reached, the gearshift is removed to point medially. A pedicle probe is used to palpate superior, inferior, medial, lateral, and at the floor of the tract to ensure no breeches are appreciated. Polyaxial reduction pedicle screws are utilized for the lumbar vertebrae. For thoracic pedicles, a straight gearshift is used. The entry point of the thoracic pedicle screw is at the intersection of the mid-transverse process and slightly lateral to the mid-superior facet joint. Fluoroscopic guidance can be especially helpful for thoracic pedicle screw placement.

If sublaminar wire passage is to be performed, the spinous process of each thoracic level is removed to expose the ligamentum flavum. The laminae are preserved, as they are the basis of strength of fixation. The sublaminar space is exposed and sublaminar wires are passed at each level. Sixteen-gauge double Luque's wires are passed at each level from T5 to T12. Wires are passed from inferior to superior after precontouring them with a radius of curvature that approximates the width of the lamina. Avoid levering off the lamina and impinging against the cord. The wire is then contoured back over the lamina and the ends of the wire are contoured to the edges of the incision, which prevents the wire from migrating away from the undersurface of the lamina as the remaining levels are instrumented. See ▶ Fig. 7.2 for an example of a pedicle screw and rod/sublaminar wire construct.

Custom-bent 5.5-mm cobalt chrome or stainless steel rods are typically used. Recognize that correction of a thoracic hyperkyphotic deformity will shorten the spine and the correction of a lumbar hyperlordotic deformity will lengthen the spine. Rods are differentially bent and connected to S2AI or iliac screws. A cross-link is placed at the cephalad part of the rods.

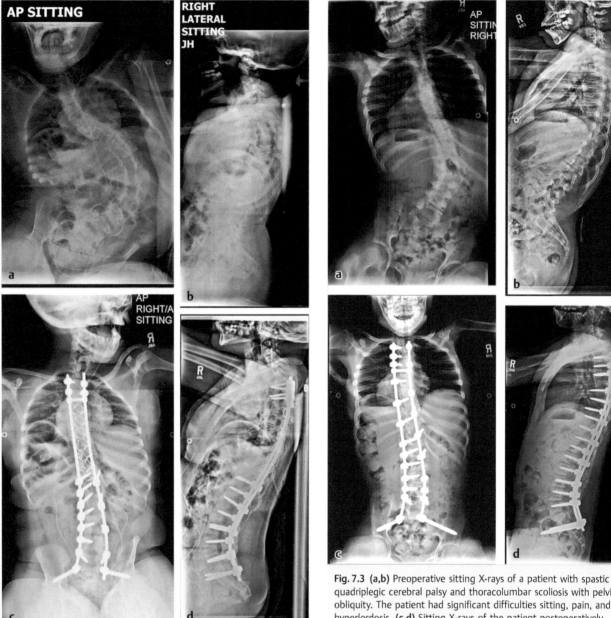

Fig. 7.2 (a,b) Preoperative sitting X-rays of a patient with spastic quadriplegic cerebral palsy and severe thoracolumbar scoliosis and pelvic obliquity. The patient had significant difficulties sitting, pain, and skin problems. **(c,d)** Postoperative sitting X-rays of the patient 2 years after posterior spinal fusion with instrumentation. Note the profound correction of pelvic obliquity and restoration of coronal decompensation and sagittal sitting balance.

Fig. 7.3 (a,b) Preoperative sitting X-rays of a patient with spastic quadriplegic cerebral palsy and thoracolumbar scoliosis with pelvic obliquity. The patient had significant difficulties sitting, pain, and hyperlordosis. **(c,d)** Sitting X-rays of the patient postoperatively demonstrating maintenance of erect alignment and sitting posture. Iliac screws were inserted via the S2AI pathway.

The reduction-tab lumbar pedicle screws allow for insetting of the rod. The spine is corrected to the rod. Pushing the rod to the spine can generate substantial force at the lever arm of pelvic fixation and should be avoided to prevent fractures. Set screws over reduction pedicle screws are tightened in a cephalad direction, as are sublaminar wires (if applicable). If sublaminar wires are utilized, they should be cut 1-cm long and bent down to the lamina to avoid implant prominence. Any additional decortication can be performed at this time, followed by copious

irrigation. Crushed autograft and allograft are packed posterolaterally. See ▶ Fig. 7.3 for an example of a pedicle screw and rod construct. Adding antibiotics such as vancomycin to bone graft is safe and effective for preventing acute deep wound infections.[79,80] Meticulous hemostasis and closure is performed. A drain may be utilized if meticulous hemostasis is not possible.

7.11 Postoperative Care

In the hemodynamically stable patient with adequate respiratory drive and pulmonary parameters, extubation in the operating room should be attempted.[81] Postoperatively, the patient should be maintained in an ICU for 24 to 48 hours for close monitoring of fluid and hemodynamic status.[82] Hemoglobin should be maintained above 7 g/dL for patients without cardiopulmonary risk factors and above 8 g/dL for patients with cardiopulmonary risk factors to maintain adequate perfusion. Coagulation parameters and platelet count should be monitored and corrected as needed. Prophylactic antibiotics are continued for 24 hours of coverage. Enteral hyperalimentation should be started early in the postoperative period either via a gastric or jejunal feeding tube for patients with poor nutritional status. After step-down from the ICU, medical comanagement with pediatric hospitalists would ideally be facilitated. Patients should be mobilized out of bed and into a wheelchair as soon as medically appropriate. The child's personal wheelchair should be readjusted. Children typically return to school within 4 weeks when sitting tolerance is attained and no postoperative restrictions or orthoses are used.

7.12 Complications

The reported range of postoperative complications varies from 18 to 68%.[13,48,49,83] Patients with curves of 70 degrees or greater, a recent history of severe medical problems, or severe intellectual disability have the highest risk of postoperative complications.[65] Atelectasis and severe respiratory issues requiring prolonged ventilatory support are common. Postoperative ileus, pancreatitis, superior mesenteric artery syndrome, pulmonary compromise, and cholelithiasis can occur and have occult presentations; thus, the orthopaedic surgeon and other consulting services should be vigilant in evaluating any clinical abnormality.[84,85,86,87] Postoperative wound infections after spine surgery tend to be most frequent in patients with neuromuscular scoliosis.[88,89] Rates of infection were as high as 90% in the 1970s, but, have fallen to between 6 and 11%,[39,50,90,91,92,93] and even less in the contemporary period of efforts to reduce infection and surgical site infection (SSI) bundles. Patients on enteral feeds, those with unit rod instrumentation, significant residual curve, skin breakdown, and implant prominence are at highest risk.[92,94] Most acute deep infections respond well to drainage and irrigation with a delayed wound closure over drains or vacuum-assisted closure with IV antibiotics and retention of instrumentation. Infection after neuromuscular scoliosis surgery is associated with worse results, pseudarthrosis, and pain at follow-up.[95] Pseudarthrosis is more common after infection, and a work-up including standard radiographs, complete blood count, inflammatory markers (erythrocyte sedimentation rate and C-reactive protein), 25-hydroxyvitamin D, and computed tomography should be undertaken if it is suspected.

7.13 Outcomes

Approximately 75 to 80% correction with leveling of the pelvis and excellent sagittal alignment should be expected when performing surgery for neuromuscular scoliosis with a pedicle screw or hybrid construct. Fusion rates are excellent and pseudarthrosis can be avoided when proper surgical techniques and rigid fixation are used. The patient and caregiver satisfaction are both very high, with over 85% of caregivers noting benefits other than sitting and facilitation of care for these children.[11,13,39] In a heterogeneous group of children with even the most

severely involved, survival rate has been predicted at 70% at 11 years following surgery.[96]

References

[1] Persson-Bunke M, Hägglund G, Lauge-Pedersen H, Wagner P, Westbom L. Scoliosis in a total population of children with cerebral palsy. Spine. 2012; 37 (12):E708–E713

[2] Weinstein SL, Flynn JM. Lovell and Winter's Pediatric Orthopaedics. Lippincott Williams & Wilkins; 2013

[3] Thometz JG, Simon SR. Progression of scoliosis after skeletal maturity in institutionalized adults who have cerebral palsy. J Bone Joint Surg Am. 1988; 70 (9):1290–1296

[4] Saito N, Ebara S, Ohotsuka K, Kumeta H, Takaoka K. Natural history of scoliosis in spastic cerebral palsy. Lancet. 1998; 351(9117):1687–1692

[5] Dubousset J, Charpak G, Dorion I, et al. [A new 2D and 3D imaging approach to musculoskeletal physiology and pathology with low-dose radiation and the standing position: the EOS system]. Bull Acad Natl Med. 2005; 189(2): 287–297, discussion 297–300

[6] Madigan RR, Wallace SL. Scoliosis in the institutionalized cerebral palsy population. Spine. 1981; 6(6):583–590

[7] Lonstein JE, Akbarnia A. Operative treatment of spinal deformities in patients with cerebral palsy or mental retardation. An analysis of one hundred and seven cases. J Bone Joint Surg Am. 1983; 65(1):43–55

[8] Miller A, Temple T, Miller F. Impact of orthoses on the rate of scoliosis progression in children with cerebral palsy. J Pediatr Orthop. 1996; 16(3):332–335

[9] Terjesen T, Lange JE, Steen H. Treatment of scoliosis with spinal bracing in quadriplegic cerebral palsy. Dev Med Child Neurol. 2000; 42(7):448–454

[10] Goldberg MJ. Measuring outcomes in cerebral palsy. J Pediatr Orthop. 1991; 11(5):682–685

[11] Larsson ELC, Aaro SI, Normelli HCM, Oberg BE. Long-term follow-up of functioning after spinal surgery in patients with neuromuscular scoliosis. Spine. 2005; 30(19):2145–2152

[12] Cassidy C, Craig CL, Perry A, Karlin LI, Goldberg MJ. A reassessment of spinal stabilization in severe cerebral palsy. J Pediatr Orthop. 1994; 14(6):731–739

[13] Comstock CP, Leach J, Wenger DR. Scoliosis in total-body-involvement cerebral palsy. Analysis of surgical treatment and patient and caregiver satisfaction. Spine. 1998; 23(12):1412–1424, discussion 1424–1425

[14] Bulman WA, Dormans JP, Ecker ML, Drummond DS. Posterior spinal fusion for scoliosis in patients with cerebral palsy: a comparison of Luque rod and Unit Rod instrumentation. J Pediatr Orthop. 1996; 16(3):314–323

[15] Sussman MD, Little D, Alley RM, McCoig JA. Posterior instrumentation and fusion of the thoracolumbar spine for treatment of neuromuscular scoliosis. J Pediatr Orthop. 1996; 16(3):304–313

[16] Watanabe K, Lenke LG, Daubs MD, et al. Is spine deformity surgery in patients with spastic cerebral palsy truly beneficial? A patient/parent evaluation. Spine. 2009; 34(20):2222–2232

[17] Dias RC, Miller F, Dabney K, Lipton GE. Revision spine surgery in children with cerebral palsy. J Spinal Disord. 1997; 10(2):132–144

[18] McElroy MJ, Sponseller PD, Dattilo JR, et al. Growing Spine Study Group. Growing rods for the treatment of scoliosis in children with cerebral palsy: a critical assessment. Spine. 2012; 37(24):E1504–E1510

[19] Cheuk DKL, Wong V, Wraige E, et al. Surgery for scoliosis in Duchenne muscular dystrophy. Cochrane Database Syst Rev. 2015 Oct 1;(10)

[20] Sanders JO, Evert M, Stanley EA, Sanders AE. Mechanisms of curve progression following sublaminar (Luque) spinal instrumentation. Spine. 1992; 17 (7):781–789

[21] McCarthy RE. Management of neuromuscular scoliosis. Orthop Clin North Am. 1999; 30(3):435–449, viii

[22] Tsirikos AI, Chang WN, Shah SA, Dabney KW, Miller F. Preserving ambulatory potential in pediatric patients with cerebral palsy who undergo spinal fusion using unit rod instrumentation. Spine. 2003; 28(5):480–483

[23] McCall RE, Hayes B. Long-term outcome in neuromuscular scoliosis fused only to lumbar 5. Spine. 2005; 30(18):2056–2060

[24] Abol Oyoun N, Stuecker R. Bilateral rib-to-pelvis Eiffel Tower VEPTR construct for children with neuromuscular scoliosis: a preliminary report. Spine J. 2014; 14(7):1183–1191

[25] Sitoula P, Holmes L, Jr, Sees J, Rogers K, Dabney K, Miller F. The long-term outcome of early spine fusion for scoliosis in children with cerebral palsy. Clin Spine Surg. 2016; 29(8):E406–E412

[26] Thompson W, Thakar C, Rolton DJ, Wilson-MacDonald J, Nnadi C. The use of magnetically-controlled growing rods to treat children with early-onset scoliosis: early radiological results in 19 children. Bone Joint J. 2016; 98-; B(9): 1240–1247

[27] La Rosa G, Oggiano L, Ruzzini L. Magnetically controlled growing rods for the management of early-onset scoliosis: a preliminary report. J Pediatr Orthop. 2017; 37(2):79–85

[28] Hickey BA, Towriss C, Baxter G, et al. Early experience of MAGEC magnetic growing rods in the treatment of early onset scoliosis. Eur Spine J. 2014; 23 Suppl 1:S61–S65

[29] Teoh KH, Winson DMG, James SH, et al. Magnetic controlled growing rods for early-onset scoliosis: a 4-year follow-up. Spine J. 2016; 16(4) Suppl:S34–S39

[30] Tsirikos AI, Lipton G, Chang WN, Dabney KW, Miller F. Surgical correction of scoliosis in pediatric patients with cerebral palsy using the unit rod instrumentation. Spine. 2008; 33(10):1133–1140

[31] Tsirikos AI, Mains E. Surgical correction of spinal deformity in patients with cerebral palsy using pedicle screw instrumentation. J Spinal Disord Tech. 2012; 25(7):401–408

[32] Miller F. Spinal deformity secondary to impaired neurologic control. J Bone Joint Surg Am. 2007; 89 Suppl 1:143–147

[33] DiCindio S, Theroux M, Shah S, et al. Multimodality monitoring of transcranial electric motor and somatosensory-evoked potentials during surgical correction of spinal deformity in patients with cerebral palsy and other neuromuscular disorders. Spine. 2003; 28(16):1851–1855, discussion 1855–1856

[34] Hammett TC, Boreham B, Quraishi NA, Mehdian SMH. Intraoperative spinal cord monitoring during the surgical correction of scoliosis due to cerebral palsy and other neuromuscular disorders. Eur Spine J. 2013; 22 Suppl 1:S38–S41

[35] Vauzelle C, Stagnara P, Jouvinroux P. Functional monitoring of spinal cord activity during spinal surgery. Clin Orthop Relat Res. 1973(93):173–178

[36] Moon ES, Nanda A, Park JO, et al. Pelvic obliquity in neuromuscular scoliosis: radiologic comparative results of single-stage posterior versus two-stage anterior and posterior approach. Spine. 2011; 36(2):146–152

[37] Keeler KA, Lenke LG, Good CR, Bridwell KH, Sides B, Luhmann SJ. Spinal fusion for spastic neuromuscular scoliosis: is anterior releasing necessary when intraoperative halo-femoral traction is used? Spine. 2010; 35(10):E427–E433

[38] Tsirikos AI, Chang WN, Dabney KW, Miller F. Comparison of one-stage versus two-stage anteroposterior spinal fusion in pediatric patients with cerebral palsy and neuromuscular scoliosis. Spine. 2003; 28(12):1300–1305

[39] Dias RC, Miller F, Dabney K, Lipton G, Temple T. Surgical correction of spinal deformity using a unit rod in children with cerebral palsy. J Pediatr Orthop. 1996; 16(6):734–740

[40] Dubousset J, Herring JA, Shufflebarger H. The crankshaft phenomenon. J Pediatr Orthop. 1989; 9(5):541–550

[41] Westerlund LE, Gill SS, Jarosz TS, Abel MF, Blanco JS. Posterior-only unit rod instrumentation and fusion for neuromuscular scoliosis. Spine. 2001; 26(18): 1984–1989

[42] Vialle R, Delecourt C, Morin C. Surgical treatment of scoliosis with pelvic obliquity in cerebral palsy: the influence of intraoperative traction. Spine. 2006; 31(13):1461–1466

[43] Huang MJ, Lenke LG. Scoliosis and severe pelvic obliquity in a patient with cerebral palsy: surgical treatment utilizing halo-femoral traction. Spine. 2001; 26(19):2168–2170

[44] Borowski A, Shah SA, Littleton AG, Dabney KW, Miller F. Baclofen pump implantation and spinal fusion in children: techniques and complications. Spine. 2008; 33(18):1995–2000

[45] Dabney KW, Miller F, Lipton GE, Letonoff EJ, McCarthy HC. Correction of sagittal plane spinal deformities with unit rod instrumentation in children with cerebral palsy. J Bone Joint Surg Am. 2004; 86-A(Pt 2) Suppl 1:156–168

[46] Bonnett C, Brown JC, Grow T. Thoracolumbar scoliosis in cerebral palsy. Results of surgical treatment. J Bone Joint Surg Am. 1976; 58(3):328–336

[47] Stanitski CL, Micheli LJ, Hall JE, Rosenthal RK. Surgical correction of spinal deformity in cerebral palsy. Spine. 1982; 7(6):563–569

[48] Broom MJ, Banta JV, Renshaw TS. Spinal fusion augmented by Luque-rod segmental instrumentation for neuromuscular scoliosis. J Bone Joint Surg Am. 1989; 71(1):32–44

[49] Boachie-Adjei O, Lonstein JE, Winter RB, Koop S, vanden Brink K, Denis F. Management of neuromuscular spinal deformities with Luque segmental instrumentation. J Bone Joint Surg Am. 1989; 71(4):548–562

[50] Gersoff WK, Renshaw TS. The treatment of scoliosis in cerebral palsy by posterior spinal fusion with Luque-rod segmental instrumentation. J Bone Joint Surg Am. 1988; 70(1):41–44

[51] Sullivan JA, Conner SB. Comparison of Harrington instrumentation and segmental spinal instrumentation in the management of neuromuscular spinal deformity. Spine. 1982; 7(3):299–304

[52] Allen BL, Jr, Ferguson RL. The Galveston technique for L rod instrumentation of the scoliotic spine. Spine. 1982; 7(3):276–284

[53] Bell DF, Moseley CF, Koreska J. Unit rod segmental spinal instrumentation in the management of patients with progressive neuromuscular spinal deformity. Spine. 1989; 14(12):1301–1307

[54] Herndon WA, Sullivan JA, Yngve DA, Gross RH, Dreher G. Segmental spinal instrumentation with sublaminar wires. A critical appraisal. J Bone Joint Surg Am. 1987; 69(6):851–859

[55] Lonstein JE, Koop SE, Novachek TF, Perra JH. Results and complications after spinal fusion for neuromuscular scoliosis in cerebral palsy and static encephalopathy using Luque Galveston instrumentation: experience in 93 patients. Spine. 2012; 37(7):583–591

[56] Piazzolla A, Solarino G, De Giorgi S, Mori CM, Moretti L, De Giorgi G. Cotrel-Dubousset instrumentation in neuromuscular scoliosis. Eur Spine J. 2011; 20 Suppl 1:S75–S84

[57] Teli MGA, Cinnella P, Vincitorio F, Lovi A, Grava G, Brayda-Bruno M. Spinal fusion with Cotrel-Dubousset instrumentation for neuropathic scoliosis in patients with cerebral palsy. Spine. 2006; 31(14):E441–E447

[58] Schwend RM, Sluyters R, Najdzionek J. The pylon concept of pelvic anchorage for spinal instrumentation in the human cadaver. Spine. 2003; 28(6):542–547

[59] Ko PS, Jameson PG, II, Chang TL, Sponseller PD. Transverse-plane pelvic asymmetry in patients with cerebral palsy and scoliosis. J Pediatr Orthop. 2011; 31 (3):277–283

[60] Phillips JH, Gutheil JP, Knapp DR, Jr. Iliac screw fixation in neuromuscular scoliosis. Spine. 2007; 32(14):1566–1570

[61] Chang TL, Sponseller PD, Kebaish KM, Fishman EK. Low profile pelvic fixation: anatomic parameters for sacral alar-iliac fixation versus traditional iliac fixation. Spine. 2009; 34(5):436–440

[62] Kebaish KM. Sacropelvic fixation: techniques and complications. Spine. 2010; 35(25):2245–2251

[63] Sponseller PD, Shah SA, Abel MF, et al. Harms Study Group. Scoliosis surgery in cerebral palsy: differences between unit rod and custom rods. Spine. 2009; 34(8):840–844

[64] Sharma S, Wu C, Andersen T, Wang Y, Hansen ES, Bünger CE. Prevalence of complications in neuromuscular scoliosis surgery: a literature meta-analysis from the past 15 years. Eur Spine J. 2013; 22(6):1230–1249

[65] Lipton GE, Miller F, Dabney KW, Altiok H, Bachrach SJ. Factors predicting postoperative complications following spinal fusions in children with cerebral palsy. J Spinal Disord. 1999; 12(3):197–205

[66] Jain A, Njoku DB, Sponseller PD. Does patient diagnosis predict blood loss during posterior spinal fusion in children? Spine. 2012; 37(19):1683–1687

[67] Brenn BR, Theroux MC, Dabney KW, Miller F. Clotting parameters and thromboelastography in children with neuromuscular and idiopathic scoliosis undergoing posterior spinal fusion. Spine. 2004; 29(15):E310–E314

[68] Bowen RE, Gardner S, Scaduto AA, Eagan M, Beckstead J. Efficacy of intraoperative cell salvage systems in pediatric idiopathic scoliosis patients undergoing posterior spinal fusion with segmental spinal instrumentation. Spine. 2010; 35(2):246–251

[69] Verma K, Errico T, Diefenbach C, et al. The relative efficacy of antifibrinolytics in adolescent idiopathic scoliosis: a prospective randomized trial. J Bone Joint Surg Am. 2014; 96(10):e80

[70] Dhawale AA, Shah SA, Sponseller PD, et al. Are antifibrinolytics helpful in decreasing blood loss and transfusions during spinal fusion surgery in children with cerebral palsy scoliosis? Spine. 2012; 37(9):E549–E555

[71] Theroux MC, DiCindio S. Major surgical procedures in children with cerebral palsy. Anesthesiol Clin. 2014; 32(1):63–81

[72] Lee TC, Yang LC, Chen HJ. Effect of patient position and hypotensive anesthesia on inferior vena caval pressure. Spine. 1998; 23(8):941–947, discussion 947–948

[73] Böstman O, Hyrkäs J, Hirvensalo E, Kallio E. Blood loss, operating time, and positioning of the patient in lumbar disc surgery. Spine. 1990; 15(5):360–363

[74] Park CK. The effect of patient positioning on intraabdominal pressure and blood loss in spinal surgery. Anesth Analg. 2000; 91(3):552–557

[75] Hardesty CK, Gordon ZL, Poe-Kochert C, Son-Hing JP, Thompson GH. Bipolar sealer devices used in posterior spinal fusion for neuromuscular scoliosis reduce blood loss and transfusion requirements. J Pediatr Orthop. 2018; 38(2): e78–e82

[76] Ponte A, Orlando G, Siccardi GL. The true Ponte osteotomy: by the one who developed it. Spine Deform. 2018; 6(1):2–11

[77] Berry JL, Stahurski T, Asher MA. Morphometry of the supra sciatic notch intrailiac implant anchor passage. Spine. 2001; 26(7):E143–E148

[78] Kim YJ, Lenke LG, Bridwell KH, Cho YS, Riew KD. Free hand pedicle screw placement in the thoracic spine: is it safe? Spine. 2004; 29(3):333–342, discussion 342

[79] Gans I, Dormans JP, Spiegel DA, et al. Adjunctive vancomycin powder in pediatric spine surgery is safe. Spine. 2013; 38(19):1703–1707

[80] Borkhuu B, Borowski A, Shah SA, Littleton AG, Dabney KW, Miller F. Antibiotic-loaded allograft decreases the rate of acute deep wound infection after spinal fusion in cerebral palsy. Spine. 2008; 33(21):2300–2304

[81] Almenrader N, Patel D. Spinal fusion surgery in children with non-idiopathic scoliosis: is there a need for routine postoperative ventilation? Br J Anaesth. 2006; 97(6):851–857

[82] Abu-Kishk I, Kozer E, Hod-Feins R, et al. Pediatric scoliosis surgery—is postoperative intensive care unit admission really necessary? Paediatr Anaesth. 2013; 23(3):271–277

[83] Benson ER, Thomson JD, Smith BG, Banta JV. Results and morbidity in a consecutive series of patients undergoing spinal fusion for neuromuscular scoliosis. Spine. 1998; 23(21):2308–2317, discussion 2318

[84] Korovessis PG, Stamatakis M, Baikousis A. Relapsing pancreatitis after combined anterior and posterior instrumentation for neuropathic scoliosis. J Spinal Disord. 1996; 9(4):347–350

[85] Leichtner AM, Banta JV, Etienne N, et al. Pancreatitis following scoliosis surgery in children and young adults. J Pediatr Orthop. 1991; 11(5):594–598

[86] Shapiro G, Green DW, Fatica NS, Boachie-Adjei O. Medical complications in scoliosis surgery. Curr Opin Pediatr. 2001; 13(1):36–41

[87] Borkhuu B, Nagaraju D, Miller F, et al. Prevalence and risk factors in postoperative pancreatitis after spine fusion in patients with cerebral palsy. J Pediatr Orthop. 2009; 29(3):256–262

[88] Mackenzie WGS, Matsumoto H, Williams BA, et al. Surgical site infection following spinal instrumentation for scoliosis: a multicenter analysis of rates, risk factors, and pathogens. J Bone Joint Surg Am. 2013; 95(9):800–806, S1–S2

[89] Sponseller PD, LaPorte DM, Hungerford MW, Eck K, Bridwell KH, Lenke LG. Deep wound infections after neuromuscular scoliosis surgery: a multicenter study of risk factors and treatment outcomes. Spine. 2000; 25(19):2461–2466

[90] Szöke G, Lipton G, Miller F, Dabney K. Wound infection after spinal fusion in children with cerebral palsy. J Pediatr Orthop. 1998; 18(6):727–733

[91] Cahill PJ, Warnick DE, Lee MJ, et al. Infection after spinal fusion for pediatric spinal deformity: thirty years of experience at a single institution. Spine. 2010; 35(12):1211–1217

[92] Mohamed Ali MH, Koutharawu DN, Miller F, et al. Operative and clinical markers of deep wound infection after spine fusion in children with cerebral palsy. J Pediatr Orthop. 2010; 30(8):851–857

[93] Sponseller PD, Jain A, Shah SA, et al. Deep wound infections after spinal fusion in children with cerebral palsy: a prospective cohort study. Spine. 2013; 38(23):2023–2027

[94] Glotzbecker MP, Riedel MD, Vitale MG, et al. What's the evidence? Systematic literature review of risk factors and preventive strategies for surgical site infection following pediatric spine surgery. J Pediatr Orthop. 2013; 33(5):479–487

[95] Sponseller PD, Shah SA, Abel MF, Newton PO, Letko L, Marks M. Infection rate after spine surgery in cerebral palsy is high and impairs results: multicenter analysis of risk factors and treatment. Clin Orthop Relat Res. 2010; 468(3):711–716

[96] Tsirikos AI, Chang WN, Dabney KW, Miller F, Glutting J. Life expectancy in pediatric patients with cerebral palsy and neuromuscular scoliosis who underwent spinal fusion. Dev Med Child Neurol. 2003; 45(10):677–682

8 Adolescent Idiopathic Scoliosis

Michael A. Bohl, Randall J. Hlubek, and U. Kumar Kakarla

Abstract

This chapter on adolescent idiopathic scoliosis (AIS) provides an in-depth review of the diagnosis, nonsurgical management, and surgical management of the disease. The most up-to-date basic science that is foundational to treating AIS is summarized and condensed for the reader. This chapter includes information on measuring curve progression, modern treatment paradigms, and criteria for observation, bracing, and surgical correction. It also covers classification systems, surgical decision making, and surgical techniques.

Keywords: adolescent idiopathic scoliosis, Lenke's classification, nonsurgical management, spinal deformity, surgical treatment, thoracolumbar spine

---

Clinical Pearls

- Curve magnitude and skeletal maturity are the major factors determining treatment of patients with adolescent idiopathic scoliosis (AIS).
- Surgical treatment is indicated for curves that are unacceptably deforming, symptomatic, or likely to progress beyond skeletal maturity.
- For patients who require surgical correction of their AIS deformity, two critical questions must be answered when developing a treatment strategy: What is the proposed upper level of instrumentation, and what is the proposed lower level of instrumentation?

8.1 Introduction

Scoliosis is the most common spinal deformity and is diagnosed when a coronal curve of 10 degrees or greater is present on a standing posteroanterior 36-inch radiograph. Identifiable etiologies of scoliosis include congenital, neuromuscular, degenerative, and iatrogenic, but when no discernible etiology exists, idiopathic scoliosis is diagnosed. Idiopathic scoliosis is the most common type of scoliosis and can be further subclassified as infantile (presenting from birth to 3 years), juvenile (age 4–10 years), adolescent (age 11–18 years), or adult (age > 18 years). Adolescent idiopathic scoliosis (AIS) is the most common type, with a prevalence of 2 to 3% for all curves greater than 10 degrees and 0.1% for curves greater than 40 degrees. The overall female-to-male ratio is 3.6:1 among those with AIS, but this ratio varies from 1:1 among those with very small curves to 10:1 among those with curves greater than 30 degrees. Although the term "idiopathic" implies that no discernible cause is known, numerous studies demonstrating familial clustering of AIS strongly suggest a genetic etiology.[1]

8.1.1 Curve Progression

Curve severity and skeletal maturity are the major factors determining treatment of patients with AIS. The progression of curve severity is primarily driven by skeletal growth, with further curve progression rare among those who have achieved skeletal maturity. Pubertal growth includes phases of both acceleration and deceleration, with the greatest rates of curve progression occurring during the growth acceleration phase (the crucial period). As such, it is important in the diagnosis and prognosis of patients with AIS to be able to accurately measure bone age.

Numerous methods have been described for identifying these pubertal phases of growth in patients with AIS. These include sequential measurements of sitting height (much more precise than standing height as it separates trunk growth from leg growth) and radiographic assessments of bone maturity. Numerous radiographic tests of bone maturity have been described, each of which grades skeletal maturity at various phases of pubertal growth. The crucial period of skeletal growth (pubertal growth acceleration) is best identified using the olecranon method. This method relies on the correlation of various phases of elbow closure, specifically of the olecranon, with stages of the pubertal acceleration phase. As the olecranon moves through phases of double ossification, semilunar, quadrangular, partial fusion, and complete fusion morphologies, the patient similarly progresses through the pubertal acceleration phase (▶ Fig. 8.1).

Another widely known method for grading skeletal maturity is the Risser grade. Risser's grading is based on the progressive fusion of the iliac apophysis from lateral to medial, with grade 0 representing no ossification, grades 1 to 4 representing quartiles of ossification, and grade 5 representing complete ossification. Risser's grading has also been shown to correlate strongly with various phases of hand maturation, with Risser 1 corresponding to ossification of the distal phalanges, Risser 2 to the metacarpal phalanges, and so forth. It is important to note that Risser grade 0 comprises the first two-thirds of all pubertal growth, including the entirety of the crucial acceleration phase. Risser grade 1 heralds the beginning of the pubertal growth deceleration phase (▶ Fig. 8.1).

Another important variable to measure is annual curve progression velocity. When curve velocity is considered against the stage of skeletal maturity, which prognosticates potential for future curve progression, one can accurately predict the probability of a patient developing a progressive curve that will require treatment. For example, 33% of patients who are in the accelerating phase of puberty with a curve velocity of less than 6 degrees per year will go on to require surgery, whereas 71% with curve velocities of 6 to 10 degrees per year and 100% with velocities greater than 10 degrees per year will require surgery.[2]

8.2 Treatment Paradigms

AIS typically causes mild or no symptoms during adolescence. However, the deformity itself can have highly negative impacts on adolescent mental health, leading to measurable detriments in quality-of-life measures that extend into adulthood. Severe curves (curves > 50 degrees) furthermore carry the risk of curve

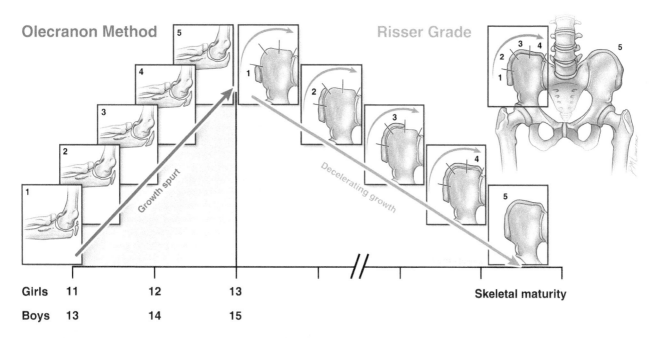

Fig. 8.1 Illustration showing pubertal growth acceleration according to the olecranon method and deceleration according to the Risser grade. Pubertal growth acceleration may be characterized by progression of ossification of the olecranon from the double to semilunar to quadrangular to partial and complete fusion morphologies in the elbow. The Risser grade is based on the progressive fusion of the iliac apophysis from lateral to medial, with grade 0 representing no ossification, grades 1 to 4 representing quartiles of ossification, and grade 5 representing complete ossification. (Used with permission from Barrow Neurological Institute, Phoenix, Arizona.)

Table 8.1 Current treatment paradigm for AIS

Curve magnitude (°)	Skeletally immature	Skeletally mature
10–25	Observe	No follow-up needed
25–45	Brace	Observe to adulthood
>45	Surgical treatment	Surgical treatment

progression into adulthood, and eventual development of pain and neurologic deficits. Very severe curves (curves > 90 degrees) also carry the risk of restricted pulmonary function. As such, treatment is indicated for curves that are unacceptably deforming, symptomatic, or statistically likely to progress beyond skeletal maturity. The goals of treatment are to correct the deformity, prevent further progression of the curve, restore trunk symmetry and balance, and minimize morbidity and pain. The treatment goals of infantile and juvenile idiopathic scoliosis are to control the curve until the patient has at least reached the age of pulmonary tree maturity (typically 10 years of age) so that fusion of the spine does not result in stunting of pulmonary maturity, which could lead to inadequate pulmonary function once adulthood is reached.

The treatment strategies available for patients with AIS can be broadly categorized as observation, bracing, or surgical correction. The choice of treatment strategy to pursue is based on both curve severity and skeletal maturity and is summarized in ▶ Table 8.1. Other indications for surgical intervention include curves that progress despite bracing and curves that are unacceptably disfiguring for the patient (especially lumbar curves).

Bracing is a treatment strategy for patients with curves of an intermediate severity who are progressing toward the surgical treatment threshold. The goal of bracing is to stabilize progressive curves, and therefore avoid the need for surgical correction. In 2013, Weinstein et al[3] published the results of the BrAIST (Bracing in Adolescent Idiopathic Scoliosis Trial), a randomized clinical trial, showing that among female AIS patients treated with bracing, 72% (105/146) stabilized and therefore avoided the need for surgical correction, whereas only 48% (46/96) of those treated without bracing avoided surgical treatment. Furthermore, brace adherence and outcome were directly correlated, with more than 90% of those who wore the brace more than 13 hours per day successfully reaching skeletal maturity without the need for surgery. These data are the highest quality of evidence currently available for bracing, and firmly establish bracing as an effective treatment strategy for patients with intermediate-severity AIS.

8.3 AIS Classification

The King classification system was originally designed in 1983 to categorize AIS and assist with surgical decision making.[4] However, the King system is limited in its utility because it fails to account for sagittal alignment and has poor intraobserver and interobserver reliability. The Lenke classification system was developed in 2001 to overcome these important limitations and help define a standardized treatment based on objective criteria.[5]

Table 8.2 Classification of the Lenke curve types

Component				Criteria
Curve type	Proximal thoracic	Main thoracic	Thoracolumbar/lumbar	Description
1	Nonstructural	Structural	Nonstructural	Main thoracic
2	Structural	Structural	Nonstructural	Double thoracic
3	Nonstructural	Structural	Structural	Double major
4	Structural	Structural	Structural	Triple major
5	Nonstructural	Nonstructural	Structural	Thoracolumbar/lumbar
6	Nonstructural	Structural	Structural	Thoracolumbar/lumbar—main thoracic
Lumbar modifier	**CSVL to lumbar apex**			
A	Between pedicles			
B	Touches apical body			
C	Completely medial			
Thoracic modifier	**Cobb's angle**			
Hypo (−)	< 10°			
Normal (N)	10–40°			
Hyper (+)	> 40°			

Abbreviation: CSVL, central sacral vertical line.

The Lenke classification system requires analysis of both the coronal and sagittal plane to characterize the curve based on three main components: (1) curve type, (2) lumbar spine modifier, and (3) sagittal thoracic modifier.

The Lenke curve type is categorized into six types (1–6) based on the characterization of the major and minor curves (▶ Table 8.2). The major curve is defined as the curve with the largest Cobb angle and is always structural in nature. However, the minor curves may be either structural or nonstructural based on flexibility on lateral bending radiographs. Structural curves are rigid and are defined as those curves with residual Cobb angles of greater than or equal to 25 degrees on lateral-bending radiographs. Nonstructural curves are flexible curves with residual Cobb angles of less than 25 degrees on side-bending radiographs. In types 1 to 4, the major curve is in the main thoracic (MT) region (apex between T6 and T11–T12 disc). An MT curve (type 1) has proximal (apex between T3 and T5) and thoracolumbar (apex between T12 and L1) curves that are nonstructural. A double thoracic curve (type 2) has a structural proximal curve and nonstructural thoracolumbar curve. A double major curve (type 3) has a nonstructural proximal curve and a structural thoracolumbar curve. A triple major curve (type 4) has both structural proximal and thoracolumbar curves. In types 5 and 6 curves, the major curve is in the thoracolumbar region. A thoracolumbar/lumbar curve (type 5) has nonstructural proximal and MT curves. A thoracolumbar/lumbar MT curve (type 6) has structural MT and nonstructural proximal thoracic (PT) curves.

The degree of lumbar coronal deformity is assessed with the lumbar spine modifier and is an important determinant of spinal balance and success of surgical treatment. Modifiers A to C describe the relationship of the apex of the lumbar curve to the central sacral vertical line (CSVL). The CSVL bisects the cranial aspect of the sacrum and is perpendicular to the true horizontal. Modifier A can only be used in patients with major curves in the MT region (types 1–4) and describes a lumbar curve in which the CSVL runs between the pedicles of the lumbar spine (L1–L4). Modifier B also can only describe types 1 to 4 curves

and represents a lumbar curve in which the CSVL passes between the medial border of the concave pedicle and the lateral border of the apical vertebral body. Modifier C can be used to describe types 1 to 6 curves and describes a lumbar curve in which the CSVL falls medial to the apical vertebra.

The sagittal thoracic modifier takes sagittal alignment into account and is another component of the Lenke classification that is imperative in surgical planning. Thoracic kyphosis is measured on a standing lateral radiograph from the superior endplate of the fifth thoracic vertebra to the inferior endplate of the twelfth thoracic vertebra. Normal kyphosis is defined as +10 to +40 degrees of thoracic kyphosis. Hypokyphosis (−) is defined as less than +10 degrees of kyphosis. Hyperkyphosis (+) is defined as greater than +40 degrees of kyphosis.

Several strengths of the Lenke classification system include excellent intraobserver and interobserver reliability, inclusiveness of all patterns of AIS, and facilitation of communication between surgeons. However, one of the biggest limitations of this classification system is the failure to address the rotational component and the three-dimensional nature of the deformity. With new technology that allows for three-dimensional analysis of the spine, the Scoliosis Research Society recognizes the need for a three-dimensional classification system to further understand and guide treatment of this complex pathology.

8.4 Surgical Decision Making

For patients who require surgical correction of their AIS deformity, two critical questions must be answered when developing a treatment strategy: What is the upper limit of instrumentation (upper instrumented vertebra [UIV])? What is the lower limit of instrumentation (lower instrumented vertebra [LIV])? A number of important considerations must be taken into account when choosing the UIV and LIV, including the types of curves present, the direction of those curves, whether those curves are structural or compensatory, and the presence of any sagittal deformity. As such, the preoperative

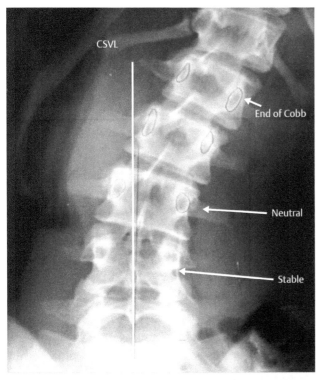

Fig. 8.2 Posteroanterior lumbar spine radiograph demonstrating the end-of-Cobb vertebra (last vertebra used in the measurement of the Cobb angle), the neutral vertebra (the first vertebra with neutral axial rotation, as indicated by the symmetric positioning of the pedicles), and the stable vertebra (the first vertebra with a spinous process that crosses the central sacral vertical line [CSVL]). (Used with permission from Miami Children's Hospital, Miami, Florida.)

radiographic work-up in AIS should include 36-inch standing posteroanterior and lateral plain radiographs, as well as lateral-bending radiographs. These radiographs can be used to identify structural and compensatory curves (curves that correct to < 25-degree Cobb angle on lateral-bending radiographs should be considered compensatory), as well as important vertebral landmarks including the end-of-Cobb vertebra (EV), neutral vertebra (NV), and stable vertebra (▶ Fig. 8.2).

The EV is the final vertebra included in the Cobb angle measurement and marks the transition point from one curve to the next. The NV is the first vertebra in a curve with a neutral axial curve (as indicated by pedicles overlying the lateral extent of the vertebral body bilaterally). The stable vertebra is the first vertebra in which the CSVL bisects the pedicles.

8.4.1 UIV Selection for Thoracic Curves

For patients with structural thoracic curves (Lenke types 1–4), selection of the UIV is dictated by three variables: presence of a structural PT curve (Lenke types 2 and 4), PT kyphosis (T2–T5 Cobb angle of ≥ 20 degrees), and shoulder height. In patients with a structural PT curve, UIV extension to higher levels (typically T1 or T2) is necessary as the PT curve will not autocorrect after surgical correction of the MT curve, potentially leaving the patient with a severe coronal imbalance. Similarly, patients with PT hyperkyphosis should be treated with a higher UIV (T1

or T2) in order to afford a UIV that is beyond the apex of the thoracic kyphosis. Finally, shoulder height is a major determiner of UIV selection. The very large majority of AIS patients have a right thoracic curve (left thoracic curves are so rare, in fact, that they should prompt further investigation for other etiologies of scoliosis), and, as such, the following explanation assumes the presence of a right thoracic curve. AIS patients with a left shoulder that is lower than the right can afford a lower UIV, as correction of the MT curve only will result in a lifting of the left shoulder back to a neutral position. Patients with a neutral or elevated left shoulder should, however, undergo fixation to a higher UIV in order to avoid further elevation of the left shoulder and creation or exacerbation of a shoulder height discrepancy. It is important to note that the presence of a sagittal plane deformity (hyperkyphosis) is the first determinant of UIV in patients with AIS, and as such should be considered first when selecting a UIV.

8.4.2 LIV Selection for Thoracic and Lumbar Curves

The critical decision in the selection of a LIV in thoracic curves is whether to perform a selective thoracic fusion or to include both the MT and thoracolumbar curves in the fixation construct. This decision is based on the presence of a structural thoracolumbar/lumbar curve, and the identification of the EV and NV (▶ Fig. 8.2).

For patients with Lenke types 1 to 4 A to C curves, selection of the LIV is determined via a similar approach. As described by Suk et al,[6] Lenke types 1 to 4 curves (including all lumbar modifiers A–C) can be further subdivided into two types based on the distance between the EV and NV. Type 1 curves are those with an NV equal to EV + 1 (▶ Fig. 8.3), whereas type 2 curves are those with an NV equal to EV + 2 or more (▶ Fig. 8.4). In type 1 curves, the LIV should equal the NV, whereas in type 2 curves the LIV should equal the NV − 1. If this rule is not followed and a gap of greater than 1 exists between the LIV and the NV, the patient is at increased risk of distal failure and persistent spinal imbalance, both of which increase the risk of requiring additional levels of fusion at the inferior adjacent segment in the future.

Lenke type 1A curves constitute a special case in that the direction of the compensatory lumbar curve dictates the LIV. The Lenke lumbar modifiers A to C are determined by the relationship of the CSVL to the apical vertebral body of the lumbar curve. This relationship does not take into account, however, the direction of the lumbar curve. Lenke 1A curves with lumbar curves to the right require lower LIV, as fixation of the right MT curve alone would result in persistent coronal imbalance (▶ Fig. 8.5). Lenke 1A curves with lumbar curves to the left, however, can afford a higher LIV as these compensatory lumbar curves will result in neutral coronal balance after correction of the MT curve (▶ Fig. 8.6).[7]

Finally, selection of LIV in patients with Lenke types 5 and 6 curves (those with major thoracolumbar/lumbar curves) is primarily dictated by the EV (the vertebra at the end of the Cobb angle measurement). This rule also generally applies to the UIV in Lenke types 5 and 6 curves.

In summary, the choice of UIV and LIV in AIS patients is dictated by the Lenke curve type, presence of sagittal hyperkyphosis,

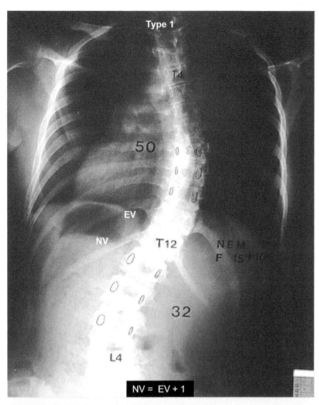

Fig. 8.3 Posteroanterior scoliosis radiograph demonstrating a type 1 curve in which the neutral vertebra (NV) is one level below the end vertebra (EV). In other words, NV = EV + 1. (Used with permission from Miami Children's Hospital, Miami, Florida.)

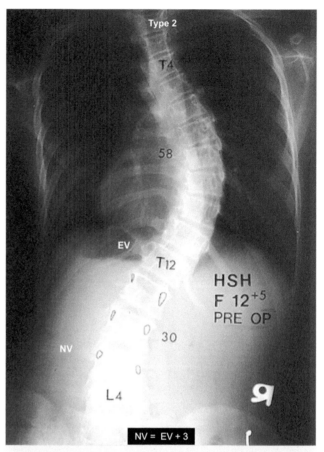

Fig. 8.4 Posteroanterior scoliosis radiograph demonstrating a type 2 curve in which the neutral vertebra (NV) is more than one level below the end vertebra (EV). In this case, the NV is three levels below the EV (NV = EV + 3). (Used with permission from Miami Children's Hospital, Miami, Florida.)

lumbar modifiers, and bending radiograph results. The Lenke classification system together with the Suk system provide comprehensive, standardized approaches to UIV and LIV selection in AIS. These approaches permit a universal diagnostic method for AIS, standardization among different surgeons and institutions treating patients with AIS, and a reliable and repeatable method for surgical planning for cases of AIS.

8.5 Surgical Technique

The positioning of the patient on the Jackson table is an important step of the operation. The pressure points should be adequately padded to prevent skin abrasions, and the abdomen should be free of restriction to decrease venous pressure and reduce intraoperative blood loss. The chest pad should be as cranial as possible while still supporting the chest, and the hip pads should be placed as caudal as possible on the iliac crests to induce lordosis of the spine.

Intraoperative monitoring with somatosensory evoked potentials and transcranial electric stimulation–motor evoked potentials (MEPs) should be performed in all patients to prevent iatrogenic spinal cord injury that may occur during correction of the deformity. Thirumala et al reported that patients with neurologic deficits after correction of idiopathic scoliosis were 250 times more likely to have changes in MEPs than a patient without a new deficit.[8] If a significant drop (not attributable to anesthetic agents or technical issues) in MEPs or somatosensory evoked potentials occurs, several steps should be undertaken by the surgical team to improve them. Mean arterial pressures should be maintained above 80 mm Hg to ensure adequate perfusion of the spinal cord. The last surgical maneuver before the drop in MEPs should be reversed. If a screw was placed immediately before the change in MEPs, then it should be removed, and the surgeon should interrogate the path of the screw to ensure that there was no spinal cord impingement. If the drop in MEPs occurred after corrective surgery, then the surgical correction should be immediately reversed. The spinal cord should be carefully inspected to ensure there is no active compression.

Pedicle screw fixation has drastically improved the surgical treatment of AIS compared to the rods and hooks originally developed by Harrington in 1962.[9] The biomechanical superiority of pedicle screws allows for improved correction in all three planes and may require fewer fusion levels to achieve this correction. Pedicle screws are placed with either freehand or fluoroscopic or computed tomography–based navigation techniques. The uniform entry site for thoracic screws is 2 mm medial from the junction of the superior border of the transverse process and the superior articulating facet. The entry site for lumbar pedicle screws is in the superior articulating facet

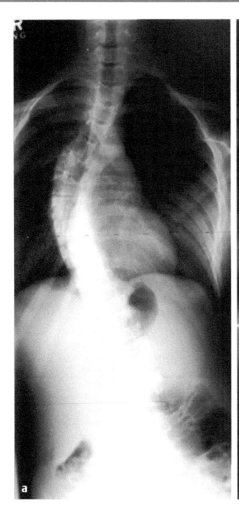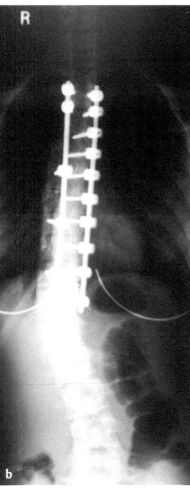

Fig. 8.5 Posteroanterior scoliosis radiograph demonstrating the Lenke type 1A scoliosis with a lumbar curve to the right before (**a**) and after (**b**) treatment. Note that the Lenke type 1A scoliosis with a right lumbar curve is not amenable to selective thoracic fusion, as demonstrated here (**b**). (Used with permission from Miami Children's Hospital, Miami, Florida.)

where the confluence of lines drawn through the middle portion of the transverse process and pars meet. The sagittal trajectory is orthogonal to the sagittal slope of the spine. Once the entry site is decorticated with the drill, the gearshift is guided down the pedicle preferentially cannulating the cancellous portion of the pedicle. The ball tip probe is then used to interrogate the path to ensure that there are no breaches. The cannulated path is tapped, and the screw is then placed. Stimulus-evoked electromyography is a neuromonitoring technique for detecting pedicle screw breaches and violations of the spinal canal. Screw stimulation thresholds below 5 mA warrant investigation for malpositioning of the screw.[10] Monoaxial screws should be placed to allow for derotation of the deformity. Polyaxial screws do not allow for significant derotation but may be necessary in severe rigid curves where full correction is not anticipated.

Progressive destabilization of the spine with osteotomies allows for increased flexibility of the deformity and more effective corrective maneuvers. The comprehensive anatomical spinal osteotomy classification consists of six anatomical grades of resection (1–6) that are related to the extent of bone resection and the destabilizing effect of the osteotomies. Grade 1 consists of removal of the inferior facet and joint capsule and, on average, 5 to 10 degrees of sagittal plane correction can be achieved. Grade 2 consists of complete removal of the facet joint. Grade 3 consists of removal of the pedicle and a portion of the vertebral

body and allows for 25 to 35 degrees of correction. Grade 4 consists of removal of the pedicle, a portion of the vertebral body, and disc. Grade 5 consists of complete removal of the vertebral body and discs. Grade 6 consists of removal of multiple adjacent vertebrae and discs.[11] Several decisions factor into which grade osteotomy is necessary, and the final treatment largely depends on the flexibility of the spine and the degree of correction desired. In general, higher-grade osteotomies should be reserved for more rigid deformities because of the blood loss and morbidity associated with these osteotomies. Osteotomies may be performed with standard osteotomes and rongeurs. The ultrasonic bone scalpel is an alternative tool that may decrease the blood loss associated with osteotomies.[12]

After the osteotomies are complete, the technique for rod placement is critical for correction of the deformity. Several different maneuvers may be utilized to achieve the correction, including rod derotation, en bloc vertebral derotation, and direct vertebral body derotation. With any of the rod-placement techniques, it is important to understand that placement of the concave rod first will induce kyphosis in the thoracic spine as distraction on the collapsed concave side will lengthen the spine. Thus, for AIS cases, which typically consist of a hypo-kyphotic thoracic curve, it is desirable to place the concave rod first to induce kyphosis. The rod should be contoured to allow for vertebral derotation. The convex portion of the curve needs

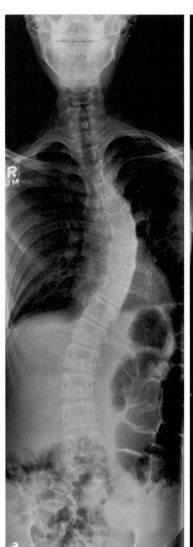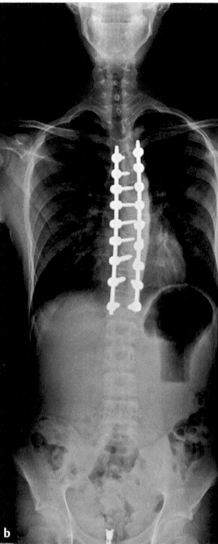

Fig. 8.6 Posteroanterior scoliosis radiograph demonstrating the Lenke type 1A scoliosis with a lumbar curve to the left before (**a**) and after (**b**) treatment. Note that the Lenke type 1A scoliosis with a left lumbar curve is amenable to selective thoracic fusion, as demonstrated here (**b**). (Used with permission from Miami Children's Hospital, Miami, Florida.)

to be rotated ventrally and the concave side needs to be displaced dorsally. Contouring the convex rod with hypokyphosis and the concave rod with hyperkyphosis will result in derotation of the vertebral body. This technique is known as differential rod bending. Once rods are in place, fine-tuning with compression on the convex rod and distraction on the concave rod will allow for further correction of the alignment.

The rod derotation technique involves placement of a rod contoured with the desired kyphosis or lordosis in the shape of the scoliotic curve. The derotation rod is placed across the scoliotic curve (typically the concave side) with the kyphotic or lordotic portions oriented in the coronal plane and loosely secured to the screw heads with set screws. The rod is then rotated in the sagittal plane toward the concave side so that the kyphosis or lordotic segments of the rod are oriented in the sagittal plane. The contralateral rod is then secured to the set screws and finally tightened. The derotation rod is then replaced with a final rod and finally tightened.

En bloc vertebral derotation is a technique that allows for rotation of the spine with the dispersion of the forces across three to four levels of pedicle screws. Derotation devices are placed on the pedicle screws at the apex after the rod is tightened to the neutral levels and the set screws left loose at the

apical levels. The devices are then linked both in the cranial–caudal and medial–lateral direction. Corrective forces are then applied across all levels with downward forces on the convex side and upward forces on the concave side. The advantage of en bloc derotation is the distribution of forces across several levels of screws, which theoretically reduces the risk of a screw pulling out and losing purchase. The disadvantage is that corrective forces are smaller at each level.

Direct vertebral body derotation has been shown to result in superior correction compared with rod derotation (42% correction vs 2.4% correction, respectively).[13] The premise is similar to en bloc vertebral derotation with the exception that the corrective forces are applied to a single vertebral segment. After the rod is in place and provisionally tightened at all levels except for the level of derotation, the derotation devices are placed bilaterally and linked medial to lateral. The derotation devices are then rotated opposite the rod derotation, and the set screws are tightened. This process is done incrementally at each level and allows for three-dimensional correction of the deformity. The disadvantage of this technique is that it places significant forces on the individual screws, which may lead to screw pullout or fracture of the pedicle.

One of the surgical goals of AIS treatment is to decrease the rib prominence that is a significant cause of cosmetic dissatisfaction and pain. Simple rod derotation techniques typically fail to induce enough axial rotation to correct rib prominence. However, the direct vertebral body derotation technique results in 50% reduction of the rib deformity due to the correction in the axial plane.[14] For those patients with a residual rib prominence after corrective maneuvers, thoracoplasty is a technique that involves subperiosteal resection of the prominent convex ribs. Suk et al reported that thoracoplasty patients showed a significantly better correction of rib hump and self-image score in the Scoliosis Research Society (Version 30) questionnaire than the nonthoracoplasty group.[6] However, there is controversy in the literature regarding whether thoracoplasty results in a decline in pulmonary function, and it should not be performed without careful consideration of the patient's pulmonary status.

References

[1] Wajchenberg M, Astur N, Kanas M, Martins DE. Adolescent idiopathic scoliosis: current concepts on neurological and muscular etiologies. Scoliosis Spinal Disord. 2016; 11:4

[2] Charles YP, Daures JP, de Rosa V, Diméglio A. Progression risk of idiopathic juvenile scoliosis during pubertal growth. Spine. 2006; 31(17):1933–1942

[3] Weinstein SL, Dolan LA, Wright JG, Dobbs MB. Effects of bracing in adolescents with idiopathic scoliosis. N Engl J Med. 2013; 369(16):1512–1521

[4] King HA, Moe JH, Bradford DS, Winter RB. The selection of fusion levels in thoracic idiopathic scoliosis. J Bone Joint Surg Am. 1983; 65(9):1302–1313

[5] Lenke LG, Betz RR, Haher TR, et al. Multisurgeon assessment of surgical decision-making in adolescent idiopathic scoliosis: curve classification, operative approach, and fusion levels. Spine. 2001; 26(21):2347–2353

[6] Suk SI, Kim JH, Kim SS, Lee JJ, Han YT. Thoracoplasty in thoracic adolescent idiopathic scoliosis. Spine. 2008; 33(10):1061–1067

[7] Miyanji F, Pawelek JB, Van Valin SE, Upasani VV, Newton PO. Is the lumbar modifier useful in surgical decision making?: defining two distinct Lenke 1A curve patterns. Spine. 2008; 33(23):2545–2551

[8] Thirumala PD, Crammond DJ, Loke YK, Cheng HL, Huang J, Balzer JR. Diagnostic accuracy of motor evoked potentials to detect neurological deficit during idiopathic scoliosis correction: a systematic review. J Neurosurg Spine. 2017; 26(3):374–383

[9] Harrington PR. Treatment of scoliosis. Correction and internal fixation by spine instrumentation. J Bone Joint Surg Am. 1962; 44-A:591–610

[10] Parker SL, Amin AG, Farber SH, et al. Ability of electromyographic monitoring to determine the presence of malpositioned pedicle screws in the lumbosacral spine: analysis of 2450 consecutively placed screws. J Neurosurg Spine. 2011; 15(2):130–135

[11] Schwab F, Blondel B, Chay E, et al. The comprehensive anatomical spinal osteotomy classification. Neurosurgery. 2015; 76 Suppl 1:S33–S41, discussion S41

[12] Bartley CE, Bastrom TP, Newton PO. Blood loss reduction during surgical correction of adolescent idiopathic scoliosis utilizing an ultrasonic bone scalpel. Spine Deform. 2014; 2(4):285–290

[13] Lee SM, Suk SI, Chung ER. Direct vertebral rotation: a new technique of three-dimensional deformity correction with segmental pedicle screw fixation in adolescent idiopathic scoliosis. Spine. 2004; 29(3):343–349

[14] Hwang SW, Samdani AF, Lonner B, et al. Impact of direct vertebral body derotation on rib prominence: are preoperative factors predictive of changes in rib prominence? Spine. 2012; 37(2):E86–E89

9 Scheuermann's Kyphosis

Francis Lovecchio, Michael E. Steinhaus, and Han Jo Kim

Abstract

Scheuermann's kyphosis was first described in 1921 in Europe and remains a relatively common condition encountered by many spine and pediatric orthopaedic surgeons. The typical presentation is an adolescent boy with back pain and concerns about his appearance. The etiology of the disease is still unknown, but is likely multifactorial. Nonsurgical treatments utilizing bracing and physical therapy are adequate at controlling symptoms in patients with mild forms of the disease, but surgical correction is often required in severe disease, adults, and rapidly progressive deformity. The goals of surgery are to reduce the kyphotic deformity by approximately one-half, fuse to the stable sagittal vertebrae, and restore sagittal balance. Achieving all three will give the surgeon the best chance at avoiding junctional kyphosis in the future. A combination of anterior and posterior techniques may be used to similar results based on the surgeon's level of comfort, though posterior-only surgery allows for sufficient correction, shorter operating times, and does not carry the associated morbidity of an anterior thoracic approach.

Keywords: Scheuermann's kyphosis, postural kyphosis, adolescent kyphosis, vertebral wedging, Scheuermann's disease

---

Clinical Pearls

- Fixed deformity upon hyperextension will distinguish Scheuermann's kyphosis from benign postural kyphosis.
- Supine imaging allows the surgeon to assess the flexibility of the curve and accurately plan for the degree of reduction and number of osteotomies needed to achieve the desired alignment.
- To avoid neurologic complications, magnetic resonance imaging (MRI) can be helpful to rule out spinal cord, dural, and nerve abnormalities before attempting surgical reduction. Neuromonitoring is mandatory in all cases.
- Correcting the deformity by approximately 50%, maintaining good sagittal balance, and fusing to the stable sacral vertebrae with symmetry of the overall construct are the best techniques to avoid proximal junctional or distal kyphosis.

9.1 Introduction

Scheuermann's disease, also known as Scheuermann's kyphosis, was first described in 1921 by Danish surgeon Holger Werfel Scheuermann. Coined "kyphosis dorsalis juvenilis," he characterized the condition after several years at the Danish Home for Crippled Children, during which he noticed a recurring pattern of painful kyphosis in many of the adolescents, especially the boys.[1] Unlike other children with "round backs," radiographs of his patients revealed compression of anterior portions of the vertebral bodies. The recent discovery of Legg–Calve–Perthes

disease led him to believe that a similar process was occurring in the spine, with compression of the vertebral bodies secondary to avascular necrosis of the ring apophysis. The modern definition, developed by Sørensen in 1964, of three contiguous vertebral bodies with anterior wedging of at least five degrees,[2] still uses vertebral body changes as the key pathological feature of the disease. The resultant thoracic hyperkyphosis is what gives patients with the disease their classic appearance. Despite advanced imaging and histopathological studies revealing that many patients have vertebral endplate irregularities ("Schmorl's nodes"), narrowing of the disc spaces, and premature disc degeneration, the original definition is still utilized today, as none of these secondary findings are necessary to diagnose the disease.

9.2 Epidemiology and Etiology

The prevalence of Scheuermann's kyphosis is believed to be somewhere between 2 and 8%.[3,4,5] Scoles examined a skeletal collection of over 1,384 spinal columns, finding that approximately 7% of the patients had vertebral changes consistent with the disease.[3] One of the most recent series by Makurthou et al[5] showed an overall rate of 4% in the Dutch population. The disease was found in 4.5% of men compared to 3.6% of women, though this difference was not significant. Despite these findings, the majority of spine surgeons would agree that the typical Scheuermann patient is an adolescent male, as originally was described. The popular belief of what comprises a "typical" Scheuermann patient—namely, an adolescent boy with a high thoracic curve—may lead clinicians to miss atypical presentations of the disease worldwide.[6]

The etiology of Scheuermann's disease is still unknown, but is postulated to be multifactorial, due to a combination of biological and mechanical factors. Examples of histopathologic findings that have been described include avascular necrosis of the annular apophysis (subsequently disproved), disorganized endochondral ossification of the wedged vertebral body endplates, and increased mucopolysaccharides in degenerated discs between these vertebrae.[3,7] However, it is impossible to know whether these findings are primary or secondary to mechanical conditions acting on the spinal column. The fact that vertebral wedging is partially reversed by bracing treatments suggests that mechanical factors play a role.[8] From the time of the initial descriptions of the disease, experts have noted mechanical differences among Scheuermann's patients. Scheuermann himself believed that children who worked heavy labor were more susceptible, and Sørensen's seminal 1964 text described children with "poor posture" who eventually progressed to having the key radiographic changes of the disease. Lambrinudi theorized that an upright posture combined with a tight anterior longitudinal ligament may contribute to the deformity.[9] Most likely, there is interplay of biological and mechanical factors, in which a biologically susceptible child is subject to mechanical forces during adolescence, progressing to disease. Discovering which are most important may prove to be an impossible task.

On the other hand, a genetic etiology is perhaps the theory with the strongest supporting evidence. Several families have shown multifactorial inheritance of the condition. In a study of one family with an autosomal dominant pattern of inheritance, McKenzie and Sillence discovered that features of Scheuermann's disease were found in untested relatives of the proband, and that other chromosomal anomalies were more likely in these family members compared with the general population.[10] The Dutch Twin Registry, a longitudinal database of all twins born in Denmark over the last 130 years, has been crucial in establishing a genetic component of the disease. Damborg et al showed that concordance of the disease was two to three times higher in monozygotic twins compared with dizygotic twins.[4] They concluded that their findings supported a multifactorial inheritance pattern with a heritability of 74%. Thus, it is most likely that children born with a genetic predisposition into the right mechanical environment are those who eventually develop the condition.

9.3 Natural History

The natural history of Scheuermann's disease is relatively benign, though many patients often find themselves with lower back pain later in life. The theory behind this observation is that to preserve sagittal balance, the hyperkyphosis of the thoracic region leads to hyperlordosis of the lumbar region, causing undue stress on the lumbar back musculature and facet joints distal to the apex of the deformity, accelerating normal degenerative changes and leading to increased back pain in middle age.[11] In a seminal study out of the University of Iowa in which 67 Scheuermann's patients were followed for 32 years, adult patients had higher rates of intense back pain, but were not significantly disabled by their condition when compared to age-matched controls.[12] In a more recent work, Ristolainen et al surveyed 80 patients with Scheuermann's after a 37-year follow-up period, comparing their responses to those from a national census survey of age-matched adults.[11] Their findings were similar to the Iowa study, in that there were no differences in employment rates, but increased rates of constant back pain and sciatic pain in the past 30 days. Adult Scheuermann's patients also found themselves having more difficulty mounting stairs and carrying 5-kg loads. Perhaps most concerning, the patients reported an overall lower quality of life (6.4 vs. 7.6 on a visual analog scale [VAS], $p < 0.001$), and a lower general health status (age-adjusted 6.4 vs. 7.3, VAS scale, $p < 0.001$). Interestingly, the degree of kyphosis did not correlate with the self-reported quality of life, back pain, or overall health. Data on whether surgery for the disease influences these outcomes is still unknown, as follow-up data through this time period using modern techniques are currently unavailable.

Given that Scheuermann's disease may present as kyphotic deformity in the thoracic, thoracolumbar, or lumbar regions, a classification system may be used to distinguish these varieties.[13] Type I disease, the typical presentation, includes thoracic kyphosis and three or more contiguous wedged vertebral bodies (▶ Fig. 9.1). Type II patients have kyphosis in the thoracolumbar/lumbar region, a more atypical form, and may only have one or two wedged vertebral bodies, though they tend to show higher rates of Schmorl's nodes and disc space narrowing on radiographs (▶ Fig. 9.2). Some authors propose that those with type II disease have a distinct natural history compared to type I patients, responding better to nonoperative treatment, though this has yet to be shown in a longitudinal series.[13]

Neurological complications as a result of the disease are rare, though rate of progression, local anatomical variations, and degree of kyphosis are all felt to be factors that increase a

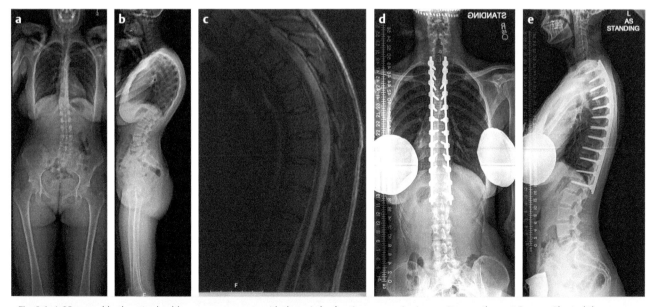

Fig. 9.1 A 22-year-old otherwise healthy woman presents with thoracic back pain, progressive in severity over the past 7 years. Physical therapy was unsuccessful in alleviating her symptoms. Preoperative imaging revealed a 92-degree thoracic kyphosis with apex at T7–T8, with a stable sagittal vertebrae at L1 (a,b). Preoperative MRI demonstrated no herniated discs or spinal cord/dural abnormalities in the region of the deformity (c). Note the relative inflexibility of curve on the supine MRI. She underwent posterior fusion from T2 to L1 with Smith–Peterson osteotomies at levels T6–9. The patient was discharged from the hospital on postoperative day 4. One month later, she developed a distal postoperative seroma that was treated with incision and drainage and a short course of oral antibiotics. Postoperative imaging 8 months later (d,e) demonstrates correction of the kyphosis to 47 degrees and good sagittal balance, with resolution of her back pain.

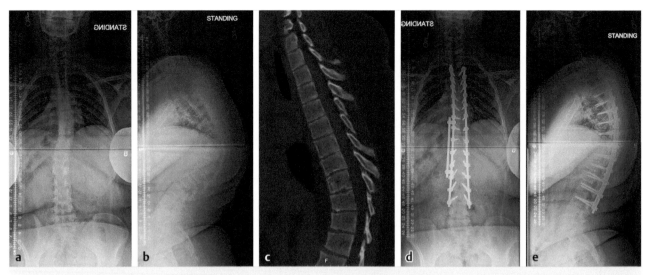

Fig. 9.2 A 15-year-old obese, otherwise healthy adolescent girl presents with progressive kyphotic deformity. The kyphosis was first noted at the onset of puberty, but quickly progressed through her growth spurt. She denies any neurologic symptoms. Preoperative imaging revealed thoracolumbar kyphosis of 100 degrees, apex at the T10–T11 disc **(a,b)**. CT imaging shows the flexibility of the curve with the patient supine **(c)**. Before surgery, she underwent pulmonary function testing given her obesity combined with the severity and age of onset of her kyphosis. Posterior spinal fusion was performed from T3 to L3, with Smith–Peterson osteotomies at T9–L1, after which the spine was flexible enough as to not require a pedicle subtraction osteotomy. A third rod using open dominoes was attached given the length of the construct and sharp angulation of the preoperative deformity. One-month postoperative imaging displays a correction to 50 degrees with good sagittal balance and no hardware complications **(d,e)**.

patients' risk. For example, a high degree of kyphosis with a sharp degree of vertebral wedging is likely a risk factor for neurologic complication, given the way the spinal cord drapes over such a deformity. On the other hand, any neurologic anomalies in the region (e.g., dural cysts) will put a patient at high risk for complication.[14] Lastly, as patients age, the accompanying disc degeneration often puts them at a higher risk of experiencing complications such as thoracic disc herniation.

9.4 Clinical Evaluation

The typical presentation of Scheuermann's kyphosis has not changed in the near century since the disease was first described. Though the majority of patients present in adolescence (typically around the time of late puberty, ages 13–17), adult presentations of the disease are also known.[15] However, whether these patients developed the disease at a later age or did not pursue treatment until adulthood remains a mystery. Often, patients seeking treatment for the disease will present with two symptoms—back pain and cosmetic concerns. If present, the characteristics of back pain should be described in detail—typically, it is present just distal to the apex of the deformity. In patients who present later in life, they may present with complaints of lumbar spondylosis, as the compensatory lumbar hyperlordosis may predispose them to this condition. Other complaints in more severe forms of the disease include difficulty maintaining horizontal gaze. Neurological complaints are atypical and should prompt further workup. Similarly, even in severe forms of the disease, cardiac and pulmonary symptoms are extremely rare and almost always associated with an alternative diagnosis. With regard to past medical history, patients are typically healthy, as Scheuer-

mann's disease is not associated with other anomalies. Some authors propose a higher rate of sex chromosome abnormalities in certain familial forms of the disease, but this has not yet been corroborated.[10]

The differential diagnosis for Scheuermann's disease is broad. Particularly, any secondary cause of vertebral wedging must be ruled out. Postural kyphosis, or "round back syndrome," must be separated as this condition is benign and will resolve with nonsurgical modalities such as physical therapy aimed at strengthening the core and paraspinal musculature. Other diagnoses that must be considered in the evaluation include tumor, vertebral body fracture, neuromuscular conditions, and congenital vertebral abnormalities. In particular, multiple anomalies should prompt thorough evaluation for other causes. With proper imaging studies and a thorough medical history, other conditions can usually be ruled out.

The physical examination is particularly helpful in distinguishing postural kyphosis from Scheuermann's disease. Though both have kyphosis while upright, the patient with postural kyphosis will have resolution of the deformity upon hyperextension. The presence of the kyphotic hump upon hyperextension is essential for the diagnosis of Scheuermann's disease, as it marks a fixed curve unlikely to resolve without intervention. The examiner should have the patient perform an Adams forward bend test, which will highlight the position of the deformity as either in the thoracic or thoracolumbar region. Furthermore, any scoliosis of the lumbar region can be appreciated, as this will be necessary later when determining the lowest instrumented vertebrae. Lastly, all patients should undergo a thorough skin evaluation to rule out neuromuscular disorders such as neurofibromatosis, which can also present with sharp thoracic deformity.

9.5 Imaging Studies

Standing long-cassette anterior–posterior (AP) and lateral radiographs are mandatory in the patient evaluation and invaluable for preoperative planning. In particular, patients should stand with the shoulders and elbows fully flexed forward so that the finger tips are resting on the clavicles. This position allows for the best visualization of the upper thoracic spine. The patient should assume a natural standing posture, with the knees fully extended. The pelvis and hips must be included in the view for calculation of pelvic parameters such as pelvic incidence, pelvic tilt, and sacral slope, which may influence the amount of correction necessary to achieve sagittal balance.[16] Supine AP, lateral, and upright flexion and extension[17] views can be helpful in evaluating the flexibility of the curve and the intervertebral discs at the most proximal and distal ends of the deformity. Though not direct correlates, the curve flexibility can be estimated on supine magnetic resonance imaging (MRI) or computed tomography (CT) imaging. Radiographs with "Cotrel's traction" are also used as a formal method to quantify the flexibility of the curve.[18]

The degree of the thoracic curve should always be measured using the Cobb method, by measuring the angle between the superior endplate of the most proximal vertebrae and the inferior endplate of the most distal vertebrae. Normal thoracic sagittal kyphosis is commonly accepted as 20 to 50 degrees of kyphosis from T2 to T12 using the Cobb method. Patients with Scheuermann's disease will show multiple abnormalities on standing plain films, especially in the sagittal plane. Radiographs must be evaluated for vertebral wedging of at least 5 degrees in three contiguous vertebrae. The patient with two or less does not qualify as having Scheuermann's disease, rather "round back" deformity (note, this does not apply in those patients with thoracolumbar kyphosis). The kyphosis in patients with round back deformity usually corrects on supine radiographs. On the other hand, a Scheuermann patient has a fixed hyperkyphosis in the thoracic or thoracolumbar region, ranging from 55 degrees to well over 100, with only partial to no correction on supine films. There is also a compensatory hyperlordosis. In a balanced sagittal spine, this hyperlordosis is expected to be approximately 10 to 30 degrees more than the thoracic kyphosis.[19] The compensatory hyperlordosis is responsible for the negative sagittal balance often seen in patients with the disease.

MRIs should be strongly considered in all patients in whom another diagnosis is suspected or in any patient undergoing surgery.[20] Cervical, thoracic, and lumbar MRIs are essential to rule out anomalies such as extradural cysts, degenerated discs about the levels of deformity, and stenosis of the thoracic canal. Dangers around the spinal cord must be identified preoperatively, as such pathology may cause neurologic compromise after surgical reduction of the deformity. A CT scan is also obtained by most experts, as the deformed vertebral bodies may require atypical pedicle screw trajectories.

9.6 Nonoperative Treatment

As with most conditions, the decision to treat should be based on the alleviation of the chief complaint—usually pain and/or cosmetic concerns. Experts vary in their decisions regarding which patients will improve with nonoperative treatment. In general, patients with flexible curves less than 75 degrees, no neurologic deficit, and minimal cosmetic complaints have the greatest chance of improving with nonoperative treatment. Asymptomatic adult patients almost always require no treatment at all. Nonoperative management is aimed at reducing the mechanical factors contributive to the pathological process. For those electing nonoperative treatment, the primary modality is bracing. Sachs followed 274 patients treated with a Milwaukee brace from the ages of 12.5 to 16 years old, and reported results up to 24 years after bracing was discontinued.[8] In patients who wore the brace consistently, 76/110 showed improvement, and 24 worsened. An initial kyphosis of 74 degrees or more universally required spinal fusion. After bracing, the kyphosis tended to correct by approximately 50%, but some of this initial correction was lost over time. Overall, at 24 years, 69% of patients showed improvement. Much like the case in adolescent idiopathic scoliosis, consistent brace wear in this age group can be difficult to achieve. The brace must be worn at least 16 hours a day. A regimen consisting of brace wear during school and at night is preferred, as this allows the patient to achieve the minimal amount of time in the brace while permitting healthy activity during free time outside of school. Of note, brace wear must be started before the child has reached skeletal maturity, as this will let the vertebral bodies to correct some of the wedging during growth. In the Sachs study, the angulation of the vertebral bodies improved from an average of 7.8 to 6.8 degrees in skeletally immature patients treated with bracing. The choice of brace is very clinician-dependent. Though the Milwaukee braces were used in the past, the impracticality and discomfort of this device has made it less favorable. The majority of Scheuermann's curves can be encompassed with a thoracic lumbar sacral orthosis (TLSO) brace, which is the choice of most physicians today.

Physical therapy is the second component of nonoperative management of the disease. Hamstring stretching should be incorporated to alleviate the increased tension in the distal part of the curve. Trunk extensor and core strengthening will also help alleviate the back pain associated with the hyperkyphosis. A series by Weiss et al of 351 Scheuermann's patients treated with physical therapy showed a reduction in pain from 16 to 32%.[21] Of note, these patients underwent daily sessions consisting of hours of physiotherapy, with multiple modalities employed, including osteopathy, manual therapy, and McKenzie exercises. Though adherence to such an intensive regimen may be impractical to accomplish in a clinical setting, the principles should be applied in any course of nonoperative treatment.

9.7 Operative Treatment

General indications for operative treatment include kyphosis greater than 75 degrees, persistent back pain not responsive to conservative measures, and unacceptable cosmesis. Of note, the decision to pursue surgical correction is not based on curve magnitude alone. In a prospective cohort study in which the decision to operate was based on surgeon and patient decision, Polly and colleagues reported that patients with higher body mass indices (BMIs) and worse pain scores were more likely to undergo operative treatment, while maximal sagittal Cobb's angle did not differ between the cohorts ($73 + 11$ degrees operative cohort vs. $70 + 12$ nonoperative cohort, $p = 0.011$).[22]

The issue of how dissatisfaction with appearance impacts decision making deserves special consideration, as many adolescents are unhappy with their appearance. The higher BMIs found in the operative cohort speak to the delicacy of determining whether an adolescent's negative self-image is normal or causing significant distress. Severe deformities may be catastrophic in their effect on a young adult's ego and subsequent personal development. Validated health-related quality-of-life forms, such as the Scoliosis Research Society questionnaires, can be particularly helpful in determining if their deformity is causing frank disability secondary to concerns over appearance. Perhaps most importantly, the adolescent or young adult who wishes to undergo surgery for Scheuermann's kyphosis, for any indication, must be able to engage in an informed discussion about the risks and benefits of the procedure. In particular, the surgeon should stress that patients may need to undergo future revision surgery. The reoperation rate for proximal or distal junctional kyphosis is much higher in this patient population compared with adolescents undergoing spinal fusion for adolescent idiopathic scoliosis.[20] Lastly, patients must understand that while surgery can greatly improve concerns over appearance, back pain is a residual complaint in many subjects.[23]

Reduction of the deformity and spinal fusion are the two basic principles on which surgery is based. Reduction is universally achieved through posterior, with or without, anterior releases. This is the key to surgical correction, as the deformity will not reduce without satisfactory release, especially posteriorly. Modern techniques almost universally employ a posterior-only approach with success. Posterior column osteotomies, performed by wide excision of the interlaminar posterior elements and facets, can achieve approximately 5 to 10 degrees of correction per level.[24] These are the workhorse of the surgical correction of Scheuermann's disease. The majority of experts are almost always able to achieve satisfactory correction with posterior column osteotomies at multiple levels, and very rarely need to use three-column osteotomies for patients with an isolated diagnosis of Scheuermann's disease.

Once reduction is achieved, solid spinal fusion is essential for maintenance of the reduction. Spinal fusion techniques used for surgery for Scheuermann's kyphosis have always correlated with those used in the treatment of adolescent idiopathic scoliosis. Harrington rods were the primary mode of instrumentation used in historical treatments of the disease, but these were plagued by high rates of pseudoarthrosis and rod breakage. Segmental instrumentation was the next wave that replaced Harrington rods. With the advent of Luque rods, surgeons had more control over the position of the vertebral bodies, but the neurological complications and difficulty associated with sublaminar wires, as well as the high rates of proximal junctional kyphosis, made this form of instrumentation fall out of favor. Cotrel–Dubousset instrumentation, first developed with a hybrid of hooks and screws, was utilized by many surgeons with good results.[23] However, the popularization and refinement of the pedicle screw allowed for a rigid form of posterior fixation with far fewer of the complications associated with earlier instrumentation (▶ Table 9.1).

In the 1990s, patients with Scheuermann's disease were treated with combined anterior and posterior fusion, the merit of which is still debated today.[28] The refinement of video-assisted thoracoscopic surgery (VATS) has allowed for anterior release of the thoracic spine without a significant increase in operation times and with a smaller number of thoracic cavity complications compared to those associated with an open anterior approach.[29] Despite this technology, there are several morbid complications associated with the anterior approach that are not present with posterior-only surgery.[25,28,29,30] Lee et al compared AP to posterior-only fixation, finding that combined techniques led to longer operation times and higher rates of complications.[25] Out of 39 patients (21 AP), 8 complications occurred in the AP group, including one spinal cord injury resulting in paraplegia. Shi et al found that patients who underwent posterior fixation with VATS anterior release had similar operating times compared to those who underwent posterior-only fixation; however, 4 out of 24 patients who underwent VATS had a complication of the thoracic cavity (two chylothorax and two hemothorax, respectively).[28] Thus, the authors' preferred technique is posterior-only fusion, as a similar degree of correction may be obtained while avoiding the complications associated with the anterior approach.[24,31]

A special note must be made regarding short-segment anterior-only fusion, a technically challenging technique first performed in 1996. Utilized by only a select number of spine surgeons worldwide, this procedure is aimed at patients with mild-to-moderate deformity whose primary complaint is pain. During the time that the procedure was pioneered, advanced imaging technologies allowed researchers to view the degenerated discs and vertebral body endplate changes for the first time, leading to the theory that these structures were the primary source of the patient's pain. Thus, proponents of this technique argue that eradicating the pain generators through discectomy and interbody fusion alleviates the patient's chief complaint. The challenging procedure involves extensive rib head resection to allow for complete discectomy and the placement of angled cages to partially correct the kyphosis. Anterior spinal instrumentation is used to stabilize the construct, which must be protected with a pleural flap or Gore–Tex membrane to prevent mediastinal injury. Thus, a vast majority of spine surgeons forgo this technique in favor of posterior-only approaches, but still obtain excellent results.

Good sagittal balance and appropriate correction of the deformity are the goals of surgical treatment. Generally, 50% correction of the kyphosis is appropriate, as any more than this has been shown to subject patients to higher rates of proximal junctional kyphosis.[23] The amount of correction necessary in each individual will vary based on the parameters that influence balance, such as the pelvic incidence. To achieve sagittal balance, the C7 plumb line should be restored so that it falls through the superior–posterior corner of the S1 body. Choosing the proper level of instrumentation is equally important in ensuring a good outcome. For most thoracic curves, T2–T3 will be the upper instrumented vertebrae, similar to patients with adolescent idiopathic scoliosis. The lowest instrumented vertebrae should be the stable sacral vertebrae (SSV), which may be determined by drawing a vertical line through the posterior–superior corner of S1.[32] The most superior vertebrae inferior to the apex of the kyphosis that touches this line is considered the SSV. Ideally, the SSV will be the lowest instrumented level (the authors' preferred technique).[32] However, similar to controversies in fusion levels in adolescent idiopathic scoliosis, some authors have been more selective with their fusion and have

Table 9.1 Contemporary and historical outcomes and complications after spinal fusion for Scheuermann's kyphosis

Authors	Year	Sample size	Surgical technique	Follow-up	Outcomes	Complications	Notes
Lonner et al[20]	2015	97	Posterior-only fusion	1 y	Reoperation in 14.4% of patients	16.5% major complication rate, 2% neurological complications, 3% related to loss of fixation	Number of levels fused was an independent predictor of complications
Koller et al[18]	2014	111	Anterior release and PSF with pedicle screws	2 y	Average preoperative Cobb's angle 68°, corrected to 37°. 86% of patients satisfied with results	12% significant revision surgery rate, 4.5% nonunion rate	Increased junctional kyphosis angle associated with revision surgery
Lonner et al[16]	2007	78	42 A/PSF; 36 posterior-only	2.9 y	Kyphosis of 78.8° corrected to 51.4°, less loss of correction in A/PSF patients despite greater preop kyphosis	23.7% complication rate in A/PSF cohort, 5.5% complications in PSF cohort	Presence of postoperative PJK correlated with degree of thoracic kyphosis and pelvic incidence
Lee et al[25]	2006	39	18 PSF, thoracic pedicle screws; 21 A/PSF, anterior discectomy, noninstrumented fusion with morselized rib graft, followed by thoracic pedicle screws	2 y	SRS-30 scores comparable in both groups	38% complication rate in the A/PSF group	SRS-30 only available for half of the A/PSF patients, most of whom did not have complications
Hosman et al[26]	2002	33	16 PSF; 17 A/PSF, H-frame posterior instrumentation with hybrid hook/rod fixation	4.5 y	Preoperative kyphosis of 78.7° corrected to 51.7°. Oswestry Disability Score improved from 21.3 to 6.6.	3 wound debridement, 4 removals of instrumentation secondary to prominence or irritation	On average the C7 plumb line was −3.1 cm posterior to sacral promontory and did not significantly shift postop
Lowe et al[23]	1994	32	Anterior release and PSF with Cotrel–Dubousset instrumentation	3.5 y	96% of patients satisfied with appearance, 65% with mild lower back pain (lumbar region)	PJK associated with >50% correction of kyphosis, DJK associated with fusions ending above first lordotic disc	Painful kyphosis >74% was the indication for surgery in 94% of patients
Bradford et al[27]	1975	22	PSF with Harrington rods	5–92 mo	16 patients lost more than 5 degrees of correction, though all patients had relief of their preoperative thoracic back pain	5 patients required reoperation for broken rods or dislodged hooks	14 patients kept supine for 2–9 mo after surgery

Abbreviations: DJK, distal junctional kyphosis; PJK, proximal junctional kyphosis; A/PSF, anterior/posterior spinal fusion.

had acceptable results by fusing to the vertebrae below the first lordotic disc (FLD), which is often one level superior to the SSV.[33] The ability of shorter fusions to lead to satisfactory results in certain cases may be explained by the concept of construct symmetry, described as an equal number of levels fused cranial and caudal to the apex of the kyphosis.[18,33] Conversely, a patient with a thoracolumbar apex may require fusion past the SSV to ensure a symmetrical construct. Kim et al, in a series of 44 patients who underwent posterior-only fusion to the SSV or FLD, found that patients who were fused to the FLD had a higher rate of revision surgery for distal junctional kyphosis compared to those fused to the SSV.[34] Since hyperkyphosis is accompanied by lumbar hyperlordosis, the surgeon may be tricked into believing a disc is lordotic when it is actually neutral or even kyphotic. Thus, fusing to the SSV is often the safer option to prevent reoperations for distal junctional kyphosis. Lastly, if a patient has lumbar scoliosis, the surgeon may need to extend the fusion distally in order to ensure a stable construct, employing the concepts described by Lenke.[35] Other factors, such as degenerated discs or inflexible segments, may also need to be taken into consideration when determining the fusion levels. For these reasons, extensive preoperative planning is mandatory.

Neurological complications during the surgery may be avoided by utilizing neuromonitoring and ensuring optimal hemodynamics. Somatosensory evoked potentials (SSEPs) and motor evoked potentials (MEPs) are mandatory. Pedicle screw stimulation may likewise be employed, though the authors do not routinely utilize this form of neuromonitoring. Likewise, hemodynamic stability through the maintenance of mean arterial blood pressure is a must. The thoracic spine is particularly vulnerable to ischemic injury due to its location along a vascular watershed (artery of Adamkiewicz). To avoid this, the authors prefer to keep mean arterial pressure above 90 throughout the case. Collaborating with an anesthesiologist familiar with the complexities of spinal surgery can be essential in ensuring optimal case hemodynamics. If no such expert is available, the time spent on preoperative planning with the surgical team will prove well worthwhile once the case is underway.

9.8 Surgical Technique

The patient is placed prone on a flat Jackson operating table. Gardner–Wells tongs are placed slightly more posterior than the usual position (approximately along a line parallel to the posterior border of the pinnae) to allow for changes in cervical lordosis or kyphosis to be made during the case if necessary. A midline incision is made, taken down through the subcutaneous tissue to expose the thoracic and lumbar spine at the desired levels. Radiographs are taken to ensure that the correct levels are exposed and correlate the preoperative alignment with the intraoperative images. Pedicle screws are placed using a freehand technique on one side at each level, and then repeated along the opposite side. Desired placement of the screws is confirmed using periodic AP and lateral radiographs, and adjustments to screw trajectories are made if needed. Next, Smith–Peterson osteotomies are performed at the planned levels. The lamina is removed to expose the ligamentum flavum,

thecal sac, and epidural fat. Portions of the spinous processes are resected to allow for closure of the osteotomy once complete. A Watson dissector is used to develop the planes of the foramen. The importance of a ensuring a wide, patent foramen cannot be underemphasized because the closure of the osteotomy risks neural root compression if the planes are underdeveloped. A no. 3 Kerrison rongeur is utilized to excise the superior articular process to complete the osteotomy and disarticulate the adjacent posterior elements.

Once the osteotomies are performed at the desired levels, the spine should be free and mobile, with chevron-shaped gaps between the posterior elements that may be closed with segmental compression along rod instrumentation. The surgical site is irrigated thoroughly to remove any bone debris from the neural canal. Rods are cut to the desired length and contour. At this point, MEPs are performed to establish a baseline before any reduction maneuvers. Proximal fixation points are locked, and sequential compression with cantilever bending is utilized to reduce the spine. Final locking is performed, and AP and lateral radiographs are taken to confirm the desired alignment. The facets are decorticated from the upper to lower instrumented vertebrae to prepare the fusion bed. After this is finished, allograft and autograft morselized bone graft is placed down into each facet. A deep drain and vancomycin powder are placed before closure of the fascia using 0 Vicryl. Subcutaneous tissues are closed using 2–0 Vicryl, with a running Monocryl suture for the skin. Patients are encouraged to ambulate on postoperative day 1. The drain is usually discontinued on postoperative day 3, and most patients are able to return home by postoperative day 4.

9.9 Conclusion

Scheuermann's kyphosis is a common condition encountered by many spinal surgeons, and usually presents in the adolescent with complaints of deformity and back pain. However, the disease can present in adults as well, and may be present in the thoracic or thoracolumbar spine. The etiology of the disease is still unknown, but is likely multifactorial. Nonsurgical treatments utilizing bracing and physical therapy are adequate at controlling symptoms in skeletally immature patients with mild forms of the disease, but surgical correction is often required in severe disease, adults, and rapidly progressive deformity. The goal of surgery is to reduce the kyphotic deformity while maintaining sagittal balance. Neurological complications, though rare, are disastrous and must be avoided through meticulous preoperative planning. A combination of anterior and posterior techniques may be used to similar results based on the surgeon's level of comfort, though posterior-only surgery allows for sufficient correction, shorter operating times, and does not carry the associated morbidity of an anterior thoracic approach. Smith–Peterson osteotomies remain the workhorse for obtaining satisfactory results.

References

[1] Scheuermann HW. The classic: kyphosis dorsalis juvenilis. Clin Orthop Relat Res. 1977(128):5–7
[2] Sørensen K. Scheuermann's Juvenile Kyphosis: Clinical Appearances, Radiography, Aetiology, and Prognosis. Munksgaard; 1964

[3] Scoles PV, Latimer BM, DiGiovanni BF, Vargo E, Bauza S, Jellema LM. Vertebral alterations in Scheuermann's kyphosis. Spine. 1991; 16(5):509–515

[4] Damborg F, Engell V, Andersen M, Kyvik KO, Thomsen K. Prevalence, concordance, and heritability of Scheuermann kyphosis based on a study of twins. J Bone Joint Surg Am. 2006; 88(10):2133–2136

[5] Makurthou AA, Oei L, El Saddy S, et al. Scheuermann disease: evaluation of radiological criteria and population prevalence. Spine. 2013; 38(19):1690–1694

[6] Lings S, Mikkelsen L. Scheuermann's disease with low localization. A problem of under-diagnosis. Scand J Rehabil Med. 1982; 14(2):77–79

[7] Ippolito E, Ponseti IV. Juvenile kyphosis: histological and histochemical studies. J Bone Joint Surg Am. 1981; 63(2):175–182

[8] Sachs B, Bradford D, Winter R, Lonstein J, Moe J, Willson S. Scheuermann kyphosis. Follow-up of Milwaukee-brace treatment. J Bone Joint Surg Am. 1987; 69(1):50–57

[9] Lambrinudi C. Adolescent and senile kyphosis. BMJ. 1934; 2(3852):800–804, 2

[10] McKenzie L, Sillence D. Familial Scheuermann disease: a genetic and linkage study. J Med Genet. 1992; 29(1):41–45

[11] Ristolainen L, Kettunen JA, Heliövaara M, Kujala UM, Heinonen A, Schlenzka D. Untreated Scheuermann's disease: a 37-year follow-up study. Eur Spine J. 2012; 21(5):819–824

[12] Murray PM, Weinstein SL, Spratt KF. The natural history and long-term follow-up of Scheuermann kyphosis. J Bone Joint Surg Am. 1993; 75(2):236–248

[13] Blumenthal SL, Roach J, Herring JA. Lumbar Scheuermann's. A clinical series and classification. Spine. 1987; 12(9):929–932

[14] Yablon JS, Kasdon DL, Levine H. Thoracic cord compression in Scheuermann's disease. Spine. 1988; 13(8):896–898

[15] Wood KB, Melikian R, Villamil F. Adult Scheuermann kyphosis: evaluation, management, and new developments. J Am Acad Orthop Surg. 2012; 20(2):113–121

[16] Lonner BS, Newton P, Betz R, et al. Operative management of Scheuermann's kyphosis in 78 patients: radiographic outcomes, complications, and technique. Spine. 2007; 32(24):2644–2652

[17] Koller H, Lenke LG, Meier O, et al. Comparison of anteroposterior to posterior-only correction of Scheuermann's kyphosis: a matched-pair radiographic analysis of 92 patients. Spine Deform. 2015; 3(2):192–198

[18] Koller H, Juliane Z, Umstaetter M, Meier O, Schmidt R, Hitzl W. Surgical treatment of Scheuermann's kyphosis using a combined antero-posterior strategy and pedicle screw constructs: efficacy, radiographic and clinical outcomes in 111 cases. Eur Spine J. 2014; 23(1):180–191

[19] Bernhardt M, Bridwell KH. Segmental analysis of the sagittal plane alignment of the normal thoracic and lumbar spines and thoracolumbar junction. Spine. 1989; 14(7):717–721

[20] Lonner BS, Toombs CS, Guss M, et al. Complications in operative Scheuermann kyphosis: do the pitfalls differ from operative adolescent idiopathic scoliosis? Spine. 2015; 40(5):305–311

[21] Weiss HR, Dieckmann J, Gerner HJ. Effect of intensive rehabilitation on pain in patients with Scheuermann's disease. Stud Health Technol Inform. 2002; 88:254–257

[22] Polly DW, Jr, Ledonio CGT, Diamond B, et al. Spinal Deformity Study Group. What are the indications for spinal fusion surgery in Scheuermann Kyphosis? J Pediatr Orthop. 2017; 0(0):1–5

[23] Lowe TG, Kasten MD. An analysis of sagittal curves and balance after Cotrel-Dubousset instrumentation for kyphosis secondary to Scheuermann's disease. A review of 32 patients. Spine. 1994; 19(15):1680–1685

[24] Geck MJ, Macagno A, Ponte A, Shufflebarger HL. The Ponte procedure: posterior only treatment of Scheuermann's kyphosis using segmental posterior shortening and pedicle screw instrumentation. J Spinal Disord Tech. 2007; 20(8):586–593

[25] Lee SS, Lenke LG, Kuklo TR, et al. Comparison of Scheuermann kyphosis correction by posterior-only thoracic pedicle screw fixation versus combined anterior/posterior fusion. Spine. 2006; 31(20):2316–2321

[26] Hosman AJ, Langeloo DD, de Kleuver M, Anderson PG, Veth RP, Slot GH. Analysis of the sagittal plane after surgical management for Scheuermann's disease: a view on overcorrection and the use of an anterior release. Spine. 2002; 27(2):167–175

[27] Bradford DS, Moe JH, Montalvo FJ, Winter RB. Scheuermann's kyphosis. Results of surgical treatment by posterior spine arthrodesis in twenty-two patients. J Bone Joint Surg Am. 1975; 57(4):439–448

[28] Shi Z, Chen J, Wang C, et al. Comparison of thoracoscopic anterior release combined with posterior spinal fusion versus posterior-only approach with an all-pedicle screw construct in the treatment of rigid thoracic adolescent idiopathic scoliosis. J Spinal Disord Tech. 2015; 28(8):E454–E459

[29] Herrera-Soto JA, Parikh SN, Al-Sayyad MJ, Crawford AH. Experience with combined video-assisted thoracoscopic surgery (VATS) anterior spinal release and posterior spinal fusion in Scheuermann's kyphosis. Spine. 2005; 30(19):2176–2181

[30] Lim M, Green DW, Billinghurst JE, et al. Scheuermann kyphosis: safe and effective surgical treatment using multisegmental instrumentation. Spine. 2004; 29(16):1789–1794

[31] Johnston CE, II, Elerson E, Dagher G. Correction of adolescent hyperkyphosis with posterior-only threaded rod compression instrumentation: is anterior spinal fusion still necessary? Spine. 2005; 30(13):1528–1534

[32] Cho KJ, Lenke LG, Bridwell KH, Kamiya M, Sides B. Selection of the optimal distal fusion level in posterior instrumentation and fusion for thoracic hyperkyphosis: the sagittal stable vertebra concept. Spine. 2009; 34(8):765–770

[33] Yanik HS, Ketenci IE, Coskun T, Ulusoy A, Erdem S. Selection of distal fusion level in posterior instrumentation and fusion of Scheuermann kyphosis: is fusion to sagittal stable vertebra necessary? Eur Spine J. 2016; 25(2):583–589

[34] Kim HJ, Nemani V, Boachie-Adjei O, et al. Distal fusion level selection in Scheuermann's kyphosis: a comparison of lordotic disc segment versus the sagittal stable vertebrae. Global Spine J. 2017; 7(3):254–259

[35] Lenke LG, Betz RR, Harms J, et al. Adolescent idiopathic scoliosis: a new classification to determine extent of spinal arthrodesis. J Bone Joint Surg Am. 2001; 83-A(8):1169–1181

10 Proximal Junctional Deformity

Michael E. Steinhaus, Francis Lovecchio, Sravisht Iyer, and Han Jo Kim

Abstract

Proximal junctional kyphosis (PJK) is a common complication following spinal fusion with an estimated incidence of 20 to 40%, and is associated with a variety of demographic, radiographic, and surgical risk factors, including age, preoperative sagittal malalignment, disruption of the posterior elements, combined anterior–posterior approach, increased construct rigidity/stiffness, choice of upper instrumented vertebra, and increased magnitude of deformity correction, among others. PJK tends to occur in the first several months postoperatively and deformity tends to progress over time. While a majority of patients exhibiting radiographic evidence of PJK remain asymptomatic, on average they may experience worse pain overall. Classification schemes have evolved to reflect this clinical reality, with initial classification attempts only accounting for radiographic evidence of disease whereas more recent work has focused on clinical manifestations in addition to radiographic severity. The most severe form of this phenomenon, proximal junctional failure, occurs in only 1 to 5% of cases, but carries significant negative consequences, with poor associated outcomes and significant cost burden. Current prevention strategies include decreasing construct rigidity and prophylactic vertebral augmentation. More research is needed to stratify patients most likely to experience symptomatic PJK and to prevent its progression.

Keywords: proximal junctional deformity, proximal junctional kyphosis, proximal junctional failure, spinal fusion, instrumentation, complications, sagittal alignment, risk factors, classification, outcomes, prevention

---

Clinical Pearls

- Proximal junctional kyphosis (PJK) has an incidence of 20 to 40%.
- PJK is defined as proximal junctional Cobb's angle greater than or equal to 10 degrees and 10 degrees greater than the preoperative measurement.
- Risk factors include age, preoperative sagittal malalignment, disruption of the posterior elements, combined anterior–posterior approach, increased construct rigidity/stiffness, choice of upper instrumented vertebra level, and increased magnitude of deformity correction.
- Proximal junctional failure is the most severe form and occurs in 1 to 5% of cases.
- Prevention strategies include decreasing construct rigidity and prophylactic vertebral augmentation.

10.1 Introduction

Proximal junctional kyphosis (PJK) is one of the most common complications associated with spinal fusions in adult spinal deformity. PJK came about with the advent of modern fusion and instrumentation techniques, when spine surgeons began to note a progressive imbalance at the junction between fused and unfused segments. First outlined by Lee et al, a case of PJK was initially defined as a patient having kyphosis of 5 degrees greater than normal from T2 to the proximal level of the instrumented fusion,[1] with the reference for "normal" angulation across segments derived from the work of Bernhardt and Bridwell.[2] Using this definition, 46% of patients with adolescent idiopathic scoliosis (AIS) were found to have developed PJK at a minimum of 2 years postoperatively. Several years later, Glattes et al made a slight modification to the definition of PJK, characterizing this phenomenon as a proximal junctional Cobb's angle in the sagittal plane greater than or equal to 10 degrees and 10 degrees greater than the preoperative measurement, measuring from the lower endplate of the uppermost instrumented vertebra (UIV) and the upper endplate of vertebra two levels above (▶ Fig. 10.1).[3] In their retrospective study of 81 adults undergoing long posterior spinal fusion for scoliosis or sagittal imbalance, these authors found that after an average follow-up of 5.3 years, 26% of patients had developed radiographic evidence of PJK.

Since this work, others have put forth a variety of definitions of PJK,[1,3,4,5,6] with no current consensus about which definition most accurately represents this process. For example, Helgeson et al defined PJK using only one segment superior to the UIV, positing that the disruption of posterior soft tissues and facet capsule at the level above are likely to play a major role, and that focusing on this superior level (rather than at two levels above) would better isolate the area of interest.[6] The reported incidence of PJK is quite varied, with the majority of studies reporting PJK incidence in the range of 20 to 40%, using the definition put forth by Kim et al.[7] Given the significant prevalence of this complication, much effort has been put forth to better understand—and to prevent the occurrence—of this phenomenon. Although the incidence of radiographic PJK following spinal fusion is significant, its clinical implications and subsequent management remain controversial. This chapter presents our current understanding of PJK, including etiology, risk factors, natural history of disease, clinical outcomes, as well as potential prevention strategies.

10.2 Etiology and Risk Factors

Though much effort has been devoted to studying PJK, its underlying etiology is not fully understood. Prior work, however, has highlighted various risk factors which make patients more susceptible to developing PJK. To better understand those variables predisposing patients to developing PJK, we break them down into demographic, radiographic, and surgical risk factors.

10.2.1 Demographic Risk Factors

Age, body mass index (BMI), and bone density have all been identified as potential risk factors for the development of PJK.

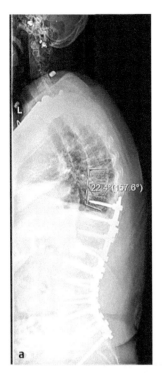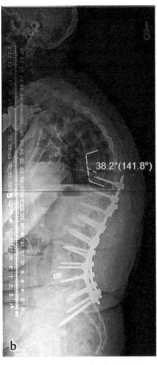

Fig. 10.1 **(a)** Lateral radiograph demonstrating the proximal junctional angle, defined as the angle between the inferior endplate of the upper instrumented vertebra and the superior endplate two levels above. **(b)** Lateral radiograph of the same patient at 2-week follow-up demonstrating proximal junctional kyphosis, as defined degrees by Glattes et al (proximal junctional angle ≥ 10 degrees and at least 10 degrees greater than the preoperative measurement).

Age is perhaps the most well-documented risk factor for PJK. In a study on adult spinal deformity by Kim et al, the authors found that those who developed PJK had a significantly older age at operation ($p = 0.007$), with 69% of patients older than 55 years in the PJK group ($p < 0.0001$).[8] Similarly, in a retrospective study of 364 patients with adult scoliosis, Kim et al found that age greater than 60 years posed a greater risk for PJK ($p = 0.021$),[9] while in a different study the same group reported significantly older age in patients demonstrating PJK requiring revision (60.1 years) compared to those without PJK (49.9 years; $p = 0.03$).[10] Finally, Bridwell et al found that patients with PJK greater than or equal to 20 degrees were older (56 vs. 46 years; $p < 0.001$).[11] Although the mechanism is not yet clear, it has been posited that age-dependent disc and facet joint degeneration and weaker spinal extensors in older patients could contribute to these differences.[8] Other studies, however, have demonstrated no significant difference in PJK with increasing age when accounting for other factors through multivariate analyses.[12,13] In a systematic review of patients undergoing surgery for scoliosis and/or kyphosis, Kim et al concluded that there was a low strength of evidence to suggest age as a potential risk factor for PJK.[7]

Whereas age is a well-studied risk factor, the association between PJK and BMI is less clear. As with age, Bridwell et al also found that PJK greater than or equal to 20 degrees was associated with significantly higher BMI ($p = 0.015$) in adult deformity patients.[11] Similarly, in their study of AIS, Helgeson

et al found that patients with a greater than 2 standard deviation increase in PJK had significantly increased BMI (26.7) compared to those without such an increase (20.9; $p = 0.013$).[6] Other studies, however, have failed to demonstrate this association between BMI and PJK.[3,8,9,10,13,14]

Similarly, equivocal results have been demonstrated for the association between low bone density and PJK development. Yagi et al found a trend in PJK development in adult scoliosis patients with low bone mineral density (BMD) (osteoporosis and/or osteopenia), though this did not reach significance ($p = 0.055$).[14] In multiple studies, Kim et al have found differing results, with one study demonstrating a significant difference between the proportion of patients with osteoporosis in a PJK versus non-PJK group (20.4 vs. 9.8%; $p = 0.016$),[9] and another study demonstrated no significant association between low bone density in PJK after performing multivariate analyses.[12] While not yet fully proven, the association between PJK and low bone density is logical, with experts suggesting that PJK could occur due to the prevalence of compression fractures and loosening of the pedicle screw at the UIV.[4,15,16,17] Indeed, biomechanical studies support the idea that bone density may play a vital role in PJK.[18,19]

10.2.2 Radiographic Risk Factors

Preoperatively, sagittal malalignment has been found to have perhaps the greatest association with PJK.[4,13,15,20,21] From a global alignment perspective, increased preoperative sagittal vertebral axis (SVA) has been demonstrated to show significant association with the development of postoperative PJK, as reported by Annis et al who found preoperative SVA greater than 5 cm to be a risk factor for acute proximal junctional failure (PJF).[20] Similarly, the association between PJK and preoperative thoracic kyphosis (TK) has been shown in several studies. Maruo et al, for example, found that preoperative TK greater than 30 degrees was a significant predictor of postoperative PJK.[15] Similarly, in a study of AIS patients, Kim et al found that increased preoperative TK (T5–T12 > 40 degrees) showed a significant association with PJK development ($p = 0.015$).[22] Finally, in their study of adult deformity, Mendoza-Lattes et al found that the average magnitude of TK was significantly larger than lumbar lordosis (LL) at baseline in the group of patients that developed PJK compared to the group that did not ($37.3° ± 19.2°$ vs. $25.9° ± 12.4°$, $p = 0.044$). Preoperatively, the PJK patients had a significantly smaller difference between LL and TK compared to the non-PJK group ($-6.6° ± 14.2°$ vs. $6.6° ± 23.2°$; $p = 0.012$), and demonstrated pelvic retroversion as well as reduced sacral slope preoperatively.[13]

More locally, proximal junctional angle (PJA) at the level of interest has also been associated with the development of PJK in AIS patients, although results are mixed. The work of Lee et al found that preoperative proximal kyphosis greater than 5 degrees from normal from T2 to the proposed UIV was indicative of the need to extend the fusion to a higher level with high sensitivity (78%) and specificity (84%).[1] Nevertheless, other reports demonstrate conflicting evidence. Hollenbeck et al studied patients with AIS and reported no difference in preoperative proximal junctional flexion in those who developed increased junctional flexion, as defined by the angle formed between the posterior wall of the UIV and that of the vertebra two levels proximal.[23] Similarly, Kim et al did not find preoperative proximal junctional flexion to be associated with increased risk in AIS patients, with the UIV level not affecting the incidence of PJK.[22]

10.2.3 Surgical Risk Factors

Surgical risk factors for the development of PJK can be broken down into approach-related risk factors, such as maintenance of soft-tissue integrity, fusion construct rigidity, UIV level selection, and overall magnitude of correction.

There is general consensus that intraoperative disruption of the posterior soft tissues is a significant risk factor for the development of PJK, with the thought that violation of the posterior tension band and other intervertebral elements are major contributors to this phenomenon.[3,7,8,11,14,24,25,26] This belief stems from cadaveric and biomechanical studies. In their study on cadavers, Anderson et al demonstrated the importance of posterior structures in adjacent segment flexion stiffness. In their study, they found incremental reductions in adjacent segment motion stiffness associated with individual procedures (supratransverse process hook, supralaminar hook, pedicle screw placement, or pedicel screw removal), with supraspinous and interspinous ligament transection adding 6.59% flexion stiffness loss alone, and transection of the remaining posterior structures, including facet joints and soft tissues, contributing 44.72% to stiffness loss. They further found that transection of all posterior structures resulted in flexion stiffness loss of 67.61%.[27] Similarly, in a biomechanical simulation of various models of adult scoliosis, Cammarata et al found that complete bilateral facetectomy, resection of the posterior ligaments, and a combination of the two predicted increase in proximal junctional kyphotic angle by 10, 28, and 53%, respectively, in addition to increasing the proximal flexion force and moment.[28] These findings suggest that disruption of these posterior stabilizing structures is important and that their preservation may reduce the risk of PJK.

In addition to the risk of posterior violation, the combined anterior–posterior approach has been reported as a significant risk factor in several studies. In a retrospective review, Kim et al reported that a combined anterior–posterior approach was the strongest risk factor for the development of PJK (▶ Fig. 10.2) with an odds ratio of 3.04 (95% confidence interval [CI] 1.56–5.93)[12]; in another retrospective review, combined anterior-posterior fusion demonstrated significantly greater rates of PJK compared to posterior fusion alone (p = 0.041).[8] Though less is known about the risk of anterior approach alone, it has been reported to be an independent risk factor for PJF.[29] Whether this is due to anterior soft tissues, or confounded by other risk factors such as larger corrections or greater construct stiffness has not been clearly delineated.

In addition to approach-related issues, construct rigidity and stiffness have been demonstrated to play an important role in PJK risk. Higher rates of PJK have been shown with pedicle screw use in long-segment instrumentation in AIS[6,22,25] and in adult deformity,[30] contributing to the risk both by increasing construct rigidity and due to the greater likelihood of facet disruption.[22] Less stiff constructs have been shown to reduce these effects. In their biomechanical simulation of adult scoliosis, Cammarata et al found that, compared with pedicle screws at

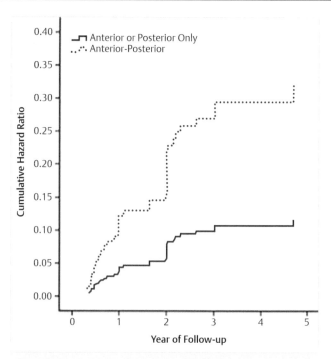

Fig. 10.2 Risk of proximal junctional kyphosis (PJK) development with combined anterior–posterior approach—cumulative hazard plot for PJK development for combined anterior–posterior approach versus anterior or posterior approach alone. (Adapted from Kim et al.[12])

the UIV, proximal transverse process hooks reduced all biomechanical indices (proximal junctional kyphotic angle, proximal flexion force and moment) by approximately 26%, while the use of reduced diameter proximal transition rods (from 5.5 to 4 mm) decreased these indices as well.[28] Thawrani et al similarly found that transverse process hooks demonstrated less stiffness and provided a more gradual transition to normal motion compared to pedicle screws.[31] Although these findings suggest instrumentation type at the UIV plays a critical role in the development of PJK, clinical studies have not been as consistent.

Finally, fusion extending to the sacrum has been associated with an increased risk of PJK, as demonstrated by Yagi et al[14] and Kim et al.[8] In further support of this idea, Bridwell et al reported that PJK greater than or equal to 20 degrees was associated with fusion to the sacrum with iliac screws (p = 0.029),[11] while Kim et al found patients with PJK requiring revision had higher rates of fusion to the pelvis (91%), compared to those with PJK not requiring revision (85%) and those without PJK (74%).[10]

In addition to construct rigidity, the choice of UIV level has been demonstrated to contribute to the risk of PJK. Studies have demonstrated a greater risk of both PJK[11] and PJF[4,21] with fusion to the lower thoracic (LT) spine, compared to the upper thoracic (UT) spine. Interestingly, Annis et al found that T10 specifically demonstrated a significantly higher risk of PJF than adjacent levels (T9, p = 0.03; T11, p = 0.01).[20] On the other hand, Kim et al reported opposite results, noting that patients with UIV to T1 through T3 were almost twice as likely to develop PJK compared to those with UIV T4 to T12 (p = 0.034).[12] Finally, equivocal results were demonstrated in a study by Fujimori et al. In patients undergoing fusion from sacrum to either UT or LT spine, at more than or equal to 2 years postoperatively the authors found no significant differences in PJK (0.9 degrees for UT, 2.8 degrees for LT; $p = 0.4$), asymptomatic PJK (32% for UT, 41% for LT; $p = 0.4$), or PJK requiring revision (6.4% for UT, 10% for LT; $p = 0.6$).[32] These authors suggest that, while UT segments are more stabilized due to the surrounding rib cage and scapulae, PJK may occur in this region due to stress being distributed over fewer proximal motion segments but that the LT region is more biomechanically vulnerable.[32] Which UIV region is more likely to result in PJK remains unclear.

Finally, the magnitude of deformity correction has been associated with PJK, with greater operative correction translating to higher rates of PJK.[10,13,14,15,20,26] Several studies have found that greater SVA correction leads to higher rates of PJK, with the thought that this may be due to either overcorrection or pelvic retroversion.[10,13,14] Indeed, adults exhibit a progressive increase in positive sagittal balance over the course of a lifetime,[33,34] so correcting postoperative sagittal balance (e.g., to 0 cm) may in fact represent overcorrection, with subsequent PJK occurring as a compensatory mechanism.[13] In support of this overcorrection theory, Mendoza-Lattes et al report that SVA is a significant predictor of PJK, with every centimeter increase in the C7 plumbline translating to a decrease in PJK by 30%.[13] Biomechanically, increased deformity correction results in increased forces in the spine. Cammarata et al report that an increase in sagittal rod curvature from 10 to 20, 30, and 40 degrees increased the proximal junctional kyphotic angle (by 6, 13, and 19%, respectively) as well as the proximal flexion force (3, 7, and 10%, respectively) and moment (9, 18, and 27%, respectively).[28] Other studies have found a lack of association between postoperative positive sagittal balance and PJK development, further lending support to this notion.[3,8] In addition to SVA, increased LL is a demonstrated risk factor for PJK. In multivariate analyses, two studies found that greater correction in LL was an independent risk factor for PJK (LL > 30 degrees)[15] and PJF.[20] Mendoza-Lattes et al found that the greater the difference between LL and TK (i.e., in cases where LL/TK mismatch was addressed), the lower the risk of developing PJK, with every 10-degree difference decreasing the risk of PJK by 140%.[13] Similarly, Kim et al noted that patients requiring revision after PJK were more likely to have a LL closer to the pelvic incidence, whereas those who did not develop PJK had a lower LL.[10] These results further support the risk associated with overcorrecting the SVA and the importance of considering global alignment when addressing sagittal imbalance. Further studies are needed to define the appropriate spinopelvic parameters to target in these deformity cases.

There are a number of strategies to address modifiable risk factors to limit the likelihood of PJK. As summarized by Lau et al, these are extending fusion to level with kyphosis greater than 5 degrees; decreasing instrumentation stiffness (including use of composite metals, fewer implants, and transverse process hooks/transition rods); preserve more soft tissues at the UIV; and attempt to achieve optimal spinal balance and alignment, taking into account the potential for overcorrection.[17] Although numerous factors have been identified as being associated with the development of PJK, it is important to remember that the vast majority of studies assessing PJK are retrospective in nature and many do not include multivariate analyses, so it is possible—and likely—that one or more of these risk factors is mistakenly identified due to the effects of confounding, which has been reported previously.[12]

10.3 Classification

As PJK is merely a radiographic finding, its existence encompasses a wide range of pathologies, from those with mild kyphosis due to soft-tissue failure to those with more severe Cobb angles from bony or implant failure. As a result, in order to better stratify these patients based on severity of disease, Yagi et al first proposed a classification scheme in 2011,[14] which has since been updated to include spondylolisthesis.[26] In their initial scheme, the authors categorized patients based on grade (amount of kyphosis) and type (underlying etiology of failure) as follows: proximal junctional increase 10 to 14 degrees (grade A), proximal junctional increase 15 to 19 degrees (grade B), proximal junctional increase greater than or equal to 20 degrees; PJK from disc/ligamentous failure (type 1), bone failure (type 2), implant/bone interface failure (type 3). According to this classification, a majority of patients were found to be grade A (56%, 18/32 patients) and type 1 (81%, 26/32).[14] While more detailed, this classification nevertheless still relies only on radiographic findings without consideration of clinical manifestations, which are similarly diverse.

Clinically speaking, many have found that a significant number of patients with PJK are asymptomatic, making a classification scheme considering only radiographic components less useful. In the study by Yagi et al, for example, only 6/32 (19%) of patients who had developed PJK were symptomatic. Perhaps to address this question, these authors further refined their scheme to stratify those with PJF, defined as symptomatic PJK requiring surgery. From their original scheme, they modified the grades (proximal junctional increase 10 to 19 degrees, grade A; proximal junctional increase 20 to 29 degrees, grade B; proximal junctional increase greater than or equal to 30 degrees, grade C) and added a component based on the presence/absence of spondylolisthesis above the UIV (▶ Table 10.1). They found that the most common form of PJF was type 2N

Table 10.1 Classification of PJK/PJF by Yagi et al[26,35]

Classification	Description
Type	
1	Disc/ligamentous failure
2	Bony failure
3	Failure at implant/bone interface
Grade	
A	PJA increase 10–19°
B	PJA increase 20–29°
C	PJA increase ≥ 30°
Spondylolisthesis	
N	No spondylolisthesis above UIV
S	Spondylolisthesis above UIV

Abbreviations: PJA, proximal junctional angle; PJF, proximal junctional failure; PJK, proximal junctional kyphosis; UIV, upper instrumented vertebra.
Source: Adapted from Kim and Iyer.[43]

(bony failure, no spondylolisthesis above UIV), whereas the most debilitating form of PJF was observed most commonly in type 2S (bony failure, spondylolisthesis above UIV).[26] While this updated classification is straightforward and better predicts which patients are likely to become symptomatic, it is neither prognostic regarding the course/severity of disease nor does it help guide treatment.[17]

In an attempt to improve upon these shortcomings, the International Spine Study Group (ISSG) put forth a new classification taking into account PJK etiology, radiographic parameters, symptoms, and disease severity. As reported by Lau et al, these authors proposed a numeric scale including six components: neurological deficit, focal pain, instrumentation problem, change in kyphosis/posterior ligament complex integrity, fracture location, and level of UIV (▶ Table 10.2). The proposed classification reportedly has good reliability and repeatability and correlates strongly with recommended treatment, with pain, kyphosis, neurological status, and instrumentation failure as the strongest predictors of the need for revision surgery.[17] Further research is needed to validate this classification scheme.

Table 10.2 Proposed PJK classification and severity scale

Component	Points
Neurological deficit	
None	0
Radicular pain	2
Myelopathy/motor deficit	4
Focal pain	
None	0
VAS ≤ 4	1
VAS ≤ 5	3
Instrumentation problem	
None	0
Partial fixation loss	1
Prominence	1
Complete fixation failure	2
Kyphosis Δ/PLC integrity	
0–10°	0
10–20°	1
> 20°	2
PLC failure	2
UIV/UIV + 1 fracture	
None	0
Compression fracture	1
Burst/chance fracture	2
Translation	3
Level of UIV	
Thoracolumbar junction	0
Upper thoracic	1

Abbreviations: PJK, proximal junctional kyphosis; PLC, posterior ligamentous complex; UIV, upper instrumented vertebra; **VAS, visual analog scale.**
Source: **Adapted from Kim and Iyer.**[43]

10.4 Natural History and Associated Clinical Outcomes

PJK typically occurs in the acute or subacute postoperative period. In a retrospective study of adult spinal deformity over a minimum of 5 years, Kim et al found that the majority (59%) of those developing PJK demonstrate a significant increase in PJA within the first 8 weeks postoperatively.[8] Similarly, Yagi et al reported that the majority (75%) of PJK is identified within 3 months postoperatively,[35] while Wang et al found that 80% would develop PJK within 18 months postoperatively.[36]

While evidence of PJK can often be seen in this acute/subacute postoperative period, it tends to progress over years. Kim et al noted that 35% of patients with PJK continued to show significant increases in PJA from 2 years postoperatively to final follow-up.[8] Similarly, Yagi et al reported that only half (53%) of the total average PJ angle increase occurred by 3 months postoperatively, with the other half occurring by 2 years postoperatively, with average PJ angle increasing from 1.2 to 14.9 (2 years) to 18.5 degrees (final follow-up, minimum 5 years) among patients with PJK[35] (▶ Fig. 10.3). While these patients tended to progress over several years, they found no patients progressing after 5 years postoperatively.

Though PJK is common and patients tend to progress postoperatively, the clinical relevance of these radiographic findings is controversial. Many studies have focused on clinical outcomes and symptoms associated with PJK and have found mixed results. Most agree that PJK does not commonly carry significant clinical consequences. In prior studies of adult deformity, Yagi and colleagues found a PJK incidence of 22%, whereas they report a rate of symptomatic PJK of only 4%,[14] and a rate of symptomatic PJK requiring surgery of only 1.4%.[26] Similarly, several studies have demonstrated that PJK has not been shown

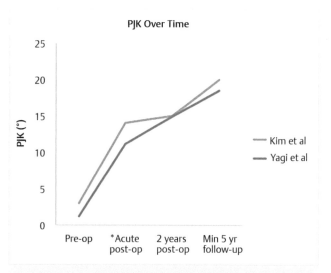

Fig. 10.3 PJK over time—development of PJK from preoperative to a minimum of 5-year follow-up, using data from Kim et al[8] and Yagi et al.[35] A majority of PJK developed in the acute postoperative period (*acute = 8 weeks postoperatively in Kim et al,[8] immediately postoperatively in Yagi et al.[35]), although PJK continued to progress over a minimum of 5 years of follow-up. PJK, proximal junctional kyphosis; pre-op, preoperative; post-op, postoperative.

to correlate with postoperative patient-reported outcomes. Glattes et al, in their study of PJK after long instrumented posterior fusion, reported no difference in Scoliosis Research Society-24 (SRS-24) scores between those with PJK and those without at a minimum of 2 years of follow-up[3]; Yagi et al studied postoperative SRS-22r and Oswestry Disability Index (ODI) in adult deformity cases and found no significant differences between the PJK and non-PJK groups[35]; and Kim et al noted similar findings in their study of patients undergoing combined anterior–posterior surgery, with no difference in SRS-22 scores between the PJK and non-PJK groups.[12]

Others have noted differences in outcomes, with PJK patients demonstrating worse functional outcomes than those without PJK.[9,10,30] Pain, in particular, has been demonstrated to be significantly greater in those with PJK. Kim et al noted greater rates of symptomatic UT pain (29.4 vs. 0.9%; $p < 0.001$), as well less improvement in SRS-22 pain subscores (0.8 vs. 1.2; $p = 0.04$) in those with PJK compared to those without at an average of 3.5 years follow-up, although no differences were seen in total or other SRS-30 subscores or in ODI.[9] In another study, Kim et al reported significantly lower SRS-22 pain subscores for PJK patients, regardless of whether they required revision surgery, compared to those without PJK.[10] Hassanzadeh et al demonstrated similarly worse outcomes, with PJK patients having significantly lower functional scores in all SRS-22 domains except satisfaction.[30]

While evidence regarding outcomes is equivocal, clearly not all patients who demonstrate radiographic evidence of PJK become symptomatic or require treatment. In order to differentiate more clinically meaningful cases of PJK, the entity PJF was described. Defined by Hart et al and the ISSG, PJF describes cases in which there is 10 degrees increase in postoperative kyphosis between UIV and UIV + 2, as well as one or more of the following: fracture of body of UIV or UIV + 1, posterior osseoligamentous disruption, or pullout of instrumentation at the UIV.[29] PJF is estimated to occur in 1 to 5% of cases, as reported in large series.[4,26] Also known as "topping-off syndrome" or "proximal junctional acute collapse," these failures tend to occur in the acute postoperative period, and may result from compensatory changes in unfused segments or from increased biomechanical loads and motion in mobile segments adjacent to the fusion construct. In a large series of adult patients, Hart et al reported that fracture was the most common cause (56%) of failure, followed by soft tissue (35%), trauma (11%), and screw pullout (9%), with both a combined anterior–posterior approach ($p = 0.001$) and greater PJK angulation ($p = 0.034$) identified as significant risk factors for revision surgery.[29] Similarly, Annis et al found that postoperative PJA greater than 5 degrees and greater correction of LL were risk factors for acute PJF,[1] while Hostin et al and Smith et al reported greater risk for those with UIV in the thoracolumbar/LT spine,[4,21] with fracture being the more common etiology for failure in the thoracolumbar region (62.2 vs. 17.4%; $p = 0.00$) and soft-tissue failure being more common in the UT region (65.2 vs. 33.3%; $p = 0.02$).[4] Unlike PJK, PJF is associated with significant morbidity and incapacitating pain, gait difficulty, inability to maintain horizontal gaze, social isolation, and neurological deterioration, including paresthesias, paresis/paralysis, radiculopathy, or myelopathy.[37] In addition to its clinical consequences, PJF carries significant economic burden, with average expense of $77,342 for revision

surgery associated with lumbar PJF.[38] Although not a significant portion of patients with PJK, due to the significant negative consequences associated with its development, PJF is a clinically important entity.

10.5 Prevention and Treatment

Currently, there is limited evidence regarding PJK prevention. Given the increased risk associated with stiffer constructs, one proposed strategy has been to decrease construct rigidity as a means to decrease PJK development. Pedicle screws have been shown to increase the risk of PJK,[6,25,30] with the thought being that they both increase construct stiffness and may destabilize the proximal junction by violating the facet joints.[17] Prior groups have attempted to decrease construct rigidity as a means to prevent PJK and have experienced success. In a study of AIS, Helgeson et al used different combinations of instrumentation and found that instrumentation with pedicle screws alone resulted in the greatest proximal level kyphosis at 2 years (8.2 degrees) compared to hybrid (5.7 degrees; $p = 0.02$) and hook (5 degrees; $p = 0.014$) constructs, as well as the greatest rate of PJK at 2 years (8.1%), compared to pedicle screws with hooks at the top level (5.6%), hybrid constructs (2.3%), and hooks alone (0%), although the differences did not reach significance.[6] Hassanzadeh et al studied the impact of hook versus pedicle screw placement at the UIV in AIS and found that those with pedicle screws developed PJK at a significantly greater rate (29.6%) than those with hooks (0%) ($p = 0.01$), and, as discussed above, showed significantly worse outcomes in all SRS-22 domains with the exception of satisfaction.[30] Kim et al found similar results in AIS, with pedicle screw constructs demonstrating the highest rate of PJK (35.1%) compared to hybrid (proximal hooks with distal pedicle screws, 29.1%) and hook-only constructs (24.1%).[25] Finally, in a study on patients with Scheuermann's kyphosis, Yanik et al found that leaving two screw threads proud for the pedicle screws at the UIV significantly decreased the rate of PJK (0%) compared to controls (17%) ($p = 0.02$).[39] Although these studies were performed in heterogeneous patient populations and across different pathologies, biomechanically these results lend support to the notion that reducing construct stiffness at the UIV may reduce the risk of PJK.

Given the prevalence of vertebral compression fracture leading to PJK, another logical strategy to prevent this phenomenon is prophylactic vertebral augmentation, which has been reported by several groups. Kebaish et al performed a biomechanical study in which they performed prophylactic vertebroplasty both at the UIV (one group) and at the UIV and UIV + 1 (another group) prior to T10 to L5 posterior instrumented fusions and subsequently compressed the constructs through eccentric axial load until failure. They found significant differences in the fracture rate, with 5/6 fractures in the control group, 6/6 in the UIV group, and 1/6 in the UIV/UIV + 1 group.[19] In a clinical study, Martin et al performed two-level prophylactic vertebroplasty on adult deformity patients and reported lower rates of PJK (13% total) than has been reported in the literature, although there was no control group in this study.[40] In another biomechanical study, Kayanja et al studied the effects of augmenting different number of vertebral levels and found that stiffness and strength were not dependent on the number of augmented levels rather varied significantly by BMD, suggesting that augmentation should especially target weaker levels at higher risk of fracture.[18]

In addition to its potential clinical efficacy for the prevention of PJK, prophylactic augmentation may be cost-effective as well. In their study of women over the age of 60 undergoing fusions from L5 to S1 to the thoracolumbar junction, Hart et al found a significant reduction in instances of proximal junctional acute collapse requiring revision surgery in those treated with prophylactic two-level vertebroplasty (0%) versus those without prophylaxis (15%), with vertebroplasty associated with an estimated cost of $46,240 compared to an average cost of $77,432 for a revision instrumented fusion.[38] Nevertheless, there remain risks associated with cement augmentation, including accelerating degenerative disc disease[41] as well as load transfer and provoking fractures in adjacent segments,[42] the impact of which on a prophylaxis strategy is currently unknown.

Although there are limited studies testing prevention strategies in PJK, Lau et al in their review on PJK recommend numerous potential strategies based on our current understanding of this phenomenon.[17] These strategies include fusion extension to include levels with baseline segmental kyphosis greater than 5 degrees; decreased instrument stiffness; use of composite materials; use of fewer implants; more distal osteotomies; less destruction of the soft tissues at the UIV; attempt to achieve optimal spinal balance; use of transition rods; and optimizing postoperative alignment. ▶ Table 10.3 summarizes our current

understanding of risk factors for PJK and potential prevention strategies, as adapted from Kim and Iyer.[43]

10.6 Conclusions

PJK is a common entity that commonly occurs in the acute postoperative period. PJK includes a broad spectrum of clinical manifestations, including many who are asymptomatic, as well as 1 to 5% of patients who experience the more severe form, PJF requiring revision surgery. Prevention strategies include limiting exposure to known risk factors, with decreasing construct rigidity and prophylactic vertebral augmentation showing some success. Future research should focus on better identifying those patients who are likely to become symptomatic as well as on strategies to prevent PJK before it develops.

References

[1] Lee GA, Betz RR, Clements DH, III, Huss GK. Proximal kyphosis after posterior spinal fusion in patients with idiopathic scoliosis. Spine. 1999; 24(8):795–799

[2] Bernhardt M, Bridwell KH. Segmental analysis of the sagittal plane alignment of the normal thoracic and lumbar spines and thoracolumbar junction. Spine. 1989; 14(7):717–721

[3] Glattes RC, Bridwell KH, Lenke LG, Kim YJ, Rinella A, Edwards C, II. Proximal junctional kyphosis in adult spinal deformity following long instrumented posterior spinal fusion: incidence, outcomes, and risk factor analysis. Spine. 2005; 30(14):1643–1649

[4] Hostin R, McCarthy I, O'Brien M, et al. International Spine Study Group. Incidence, mode, and location of acute proximal junctional failures after surgical treatment of adult spinal deformity. Spine. 2013; 38(12):1008–1015

[5] O'Shaughnessy BA, Bridwell KH, Lenke LG, et al. Does a long-fusion "T3-sacrum" portend a worse outcome than a short-fusion "T10-sacrum" in primary surgery for adult scoliosis? Spine. 2012; 37(10):884–890

[6] Helgeson MD, Shah SA, Newton PO, et al. Harms Study Group. Evaluation of proximal junctional kyphosis in adolescent idiopathic scoliosis following pedicle screw, hook, or hybrid instrumentation. Spine. 2010; 35(2):177–181

[7] Kim HJ, Lenke LG, Shaffrey CI, Van Alstyne EM, Skelly AC. Proximal junctional kyphosis as a distinct form of adjacent segment pathology after spinal deformity surgery: a systematic review. Spine. 2012; 37(22) Suppl:S144–S164

[8] Kim YJ, Bridwell KH, Lenke LG, Glattes CR, Rhim S, Cheh G. Proximal junctional kyphosis in adult spinal deformity after segmental posterior spinal instrumentation and fusion: minimum five-year follow-up. Spine. 2008; 33(20): 2179–2184

[9] Kim HJ, Bridwell KH, Lenke LG, et al. Proximal junctional kyphosis results in inferior SRS pain subscores in adult deformity patients. Spine. 2013; 38(11): 896–901

[10] Kim HJ, Bridwell KH, Lenke LG, et al. Patients with proximal junctional kyphosis requiring revision surgery have higher postoperative lumbar lordosis and larger sagittal balance corrections. Spine. 2014; 39(9):E576–E580

[11] Bridwell KH, Lenke LG, Cho SK, et al. Proximal junctional kyphosis in primary adult deformity surgery: evaluation of 20 degrees as a critical angle. Neurosurgery. 2013; 72(6):899–906

[12] Kim HJ, Yagi M, Nyugen J, Cunningham ME, Boachie-Adjei O. Combined anterior-posterior surgery is the most important risk factor for developing proximal junctional kyphosis in idiopathic scoliosis. Clin Orthop Relat Res. 2012; 470(6):1633–1639

[13] Mendoza-Lattes S, Ries Z, Gao Y, Weinstein SL. Proximal junctional kyphosis in adult reconstructive spine surgery results from incomplete restoration of the lumbar lordosis relative to the magnitude of the thoracic kyphosis. Iowa Orthop J. 2011; 31:199–206

[14] Yagi M, Akilah KB, Boachie-Adjei O. Incidence, risk factors and classification of proximal junctional kyphosis: surgical outcomes review of adult idiopathic scoliosis. Spine. 2011; 36(1):E60–E68

[15] Maruo K, Ha Y, Inoue S, et al. Predictive factors for proximal junctional kyphosis in long fusions to the sacrum in adult spinal deformity. Spine. 2013; 38(23):E1469–E1476

Table 10.3 Risk factors/prevention techniques for PJK/PJF

Risk factor	Prevention measure
Surgical	
Posterior soft-tissue disruption	Meticulous dissection and protect facet at UIV
Instrumentation rigidity/stiffness	Use of hooks, transition rods, leaving proximal screw threads proud
Choice of vertebral levels	Risks of both UIV in lower/upper thoracic spine; avoid fusion to sacrum/pelvis
Choice of approach	Avoid combined anterior–posterior approach
SVA overcorrection/increased LL correction	Consider norms for age, optimize global sagittal alignment, avoid SVA 0 cm
Radiographic	
Increased preoperative TK	Nonmodifiable
Increased preoperative PJA	Include levels with PJA > 5°
Demographic	
Advanced age (> 55 years)	Nonmodifiable
BMI	Weight loss, lifestyle modifications
Low bone density	Prophylactic vertebral augmentation, optimize medical management

Abbreviations: BMI, body mass index; **LL, lumbar lordosis; PJA, proximal junctional angle**; PJF, proximal junctional failure; PJK, proximal junctional kyphosis; **SVA, sagittal vertebral axis; TK, thoracic kyphosis;** UIV, upper instrumented vertebra.
Source: **Adapted from Kim and Iyer.**[43]

[16] Lee J, Park YS. Proximal junctional kyphosis: diagnosis, pathogenesis, and treatment. Asian Spine J. 2016; 10(3):593–600

[17] Lau D, Clark AJ, Scheer JK, et al. SRS Adult Spinal Deformity Committee. Proximal junctional kyphosis and failure after spinal deformity surgery: a systematic review of the literature as a background to classification development. Spine. 2014; 39(25):2093–2102

[18] Kayanja MM, Schlenk R, Togawa D, Ferrara L, Lieberman I. The biomechanics of 1, 2, and 3 levels of vertebral augmentation with polymethylmethacrylate in multilevel spinal segments. Spine. 2006; 31(7):769–774

[19] Kebaish KM, Martin CT, O'Brien JR, LaMotta IE, Voros GD, Belkoff SM. Use of vertebroplasty to prevent proximal junctional fractures in adult deformity surgery: a biomechanical cadaveric study. Spine J. 2013; 13(12):1897–1903

[20] Annis P, Lawrence BD, Spiker WR, et al. Predictive factors for acute proximal junctional failure after adult deformity surgery with upper instrumented vertebrae in the thoracolumbar spine. Evid Based Spine Care J. 2014; 5(2):160–162

[21] Smith MW, Annis P, Lawrence BD, Daubs MD, Brodke DS. Early proximal junctional failure in patients with preoperative sagittal imbalance. Evid Based Spine Care J. 2013; 4(2):163–164

[22] Kim YJ, Bridwell KH, Lenke LG, Kim J, Cho SK. Proximal junctional kyphosis in adolescent idiopathic scoliosis following segmental posterior spinal instrumentation and fusion: minimum 5-year follow-up. Spine. 2005; 30(18):2045–2050

[23] Hollenbeck SM, Glattes RC, Asher MA, Lai SM, Burton DC. The prevalence of increased proximal junctional flexion following posterior instrumentation and arthrodesis for adolescent idiopathic scoliosis. Spine. 2008; 33(15):1675–1681

[24] Denis F, Sun EC, Winter RB. Incidence and risk factors for proximal and distal junctional kyphosis following surgical treatment for Scheuermann kyphosis: minimum five-year follow-up. Spine. 2009; 34(20):E729–E734

[25] Kim YJ, Lenke LG, Bridwell KH, et al. Proximal junctional kyphosis in adolescent idiopathic scoliosis after 3 different types of posterior segmental spinal instrumentation and fusions: incidence and risk factor analysis of 410 cases. Spine. 2007; 32(24):2731–2738

[26] Yagi M, Rahm M, Gaines R, et al. Complex Spine Study Group. Characterization and surgical outcomes of proximal junctional failure in surgically treated patients with adult spinal deformity. Spine. 2014; 39(10):E607–E614

[27] Anderson AL, McIff TE, Asher MA, Burton DC, Glattes RC. The effect of posterior thoracic spine anatomical structures on motion segment flexion stiffness. Spine. 2009; 34(5):441–446

[28] Cammarata M, Aubin CE, Wang X, Mac-Thiong JM. Biomechanical risk factors for proximal junctional kyphosis: a detailed numerical analysis of surgical instrumentation variables. Spine. 2014; 39(8):E500–E507

[29] Hart R, McCarthy I, O'brien M, et al. International Spine Study Group. Identification of decision criteria for revision surgery among patients with proximal

junctional failure after surgical treatment of spinal deformity. Spine. 2013; 38(19):E1223–E1227

[30] Hassanzadeh H, Gupta S, Jain A, El Dafrawy MH, Skolasky RL, Kebaish KM. Type of anchor at the proximal fusion level has a significant effect on the incidence of proximal junctional kyphosis and outcome in adults after long posterior spinal fusion. Spine Deform. 2013; 1(4):299–305

[31] Thawrani DP, Glos DL, Coombs MT, Bylski-Austrow DI, Sturm PF. Transverse process hooks at upper instrumented vertebra provide more gradual motion transition than pedicle screws. Spine. 2014; 39(14):E826–E832

[32] Fujimori T, Inoue S, Le H, et al. Long fusion from sacrum to thoracic spine for adult spinal deformity with sagittal imbalance: upper versus lower thoracic spine as site of upper instrumented vertebra. Neurosurg Focus. 2014; 36(5):E9

[33] Vedantam R, Lenke LG, Keeney JA, Bridwell KH. Comparison of standing sagittal spinal alignment in asymptomatic adolescents and adults. Spine. 1998; 23(2):211–215

[34] Gelb DE, Lenke LG, Bridwell KH, Blanke K, McEnery KW. An analysis of sagittal spinal alignment in 100 asymptomatic middle and older aged volunteers. Spine. 1995; 20(12):1351–1358

[35] Yagi M, King AB, Boachie-Adjei O. Incidence, risk factors, and natural course of proximal junctional kyphosis: surgical outcomes review of adult idiopathic scoliosis. Minimum 5 years of follow-up. Spine. 2012; 37(17):1479–1489

[36] Wang J, Zhao Y, Shen B, Wang C, Li M. Risk factor analysis of proximal junctional kyphosis after posterior fusion in patients with idiopathic scoliosis. Injury. 2010; 41(4):415–420

[37] McClendon J, Jr, O'Shaughnessy BA, Sugrue PA, et al. Techniques for operative correction of proximal junctional kyphosis of the upper thoracic spine. Spine. 2012; 37(4):292–303

[38] Hart RA, Prendergast MA, Roberts WG, Nesbit GM, Barnwell SL. Proximal junctional acute collapse cranial to multi-level lumbar fusion: a cost analysis of prophylactic vertebral augmentation. Spine J. 2008; 8(6):875–881

[39] Yanik HS, Ketenci IE, Polat A, et al. Prevention of proximal junctional kyphosis after posterior surgery of Scheuermann kyphosis: an operative technique. J Spinal Disord Tech. 2015; 28(2):E101–E105

[40] Martin CT, Skolasky RL, Mohamed AS, Kebaish KM. Preliminary results of the effect of prophylactic vertebroplasty on the incidence of proximal junctional complications after posterior spinal fusion to the low thoracic spine. Spine Deform. 2013; 1(2):132–138

[41] Verlaan JJ, Oner FC, Slootweg PJ, Verbout AJ, Dhert WJ. Histologic changes after vertebroplasty. J Bone Joint Surg Am. 2004; 86-A(6):1230–1238

[42] Watanabe K, Lenke LG, Bridwell KH, Kim YJ, Koester L, Hensley M. Proximal junctional vertebral fracture in adults after spinal deformity surgery using pedicle screw constructs: analysis of morphological features. Spine. 2010; 35(2):138–145

[43] Kim HJ, Iyer S. Proximal junctional kyphosis. J Am Acad Orthop Surg. 2016; 24(5):318–326

11 Posttraumatic Deformity

A. Karim Ahmed, Randall J. Hlubek, and Nicholas Theodore

Abstract

The thoracic spine is particularly susceptible to ischemia and life-threatening complications after traumatic injury because of its poor collateralization of vasculature and its proximity to vital structures. Traumatic injuries of the thoracic spine are classified as flexion, distraction, or torsional injuries. The most common presenting symptoms of posttraumatic deformity are pain and neurological deficit. An assessment of focal deformity, as well as global balance, is critical in these patients. Surgical management for posttraumatic deformity may be indicated if the patient has increasing back pain, increasing neurological deficit, instability, and severe or progressive deformity.

Keywords: deformity, ischemia, kyphosis, laminectomy, neurological deficit, thoracic spine, trauma

Clinical Pearls

- Imaging for posttraumatic deformity is multimodal and should include an assessment of osseous structures, interosseous spaces, soft tissue ligamentous structures, neural element compression, spinal instability, global balance parameters, and flexibility of the deformity.
- Surgical indications are increasing back pain, increasing neurological deficit, instability, and severe or progressive deformity.
- Surgical approaches for the treatment for posttraumatic deformity include an anterior approach, a posterior approach, or a combination of the two.
- The thoracolumbar junction serves as a transition zone between the semirigid thoracic spine and the mobile lumbar spine, requiring special consideration to prevent aberrant motion and iatrogenic deformity.
- Osteotomies may be necessary for a patient with rigid deformities including Smith–Petersen osteotomy, pedicle subtraction osteotomy, or vertebral column resection, listed by increasing angle of correction.

11.1 Thoracic Spinal Anatomy

The thoracic spine is relatively immobile and does not impart significant range of motion during activity. The 12 thoracic spine segments are caudal to the cervical spine. The thoracic vertebrae have vertically oriented articulating facets that connect with adjacent vertebrae. The posterolateral surface of the vertebral body in the thoracic spine has two demifacets. The cranial demifacet articulates with the head of the corresponding numbered rib, and the caudal demifacet articulates with the head of the rib below. An additional facet on the lateral aspect of the transverse process articulates with the tubercle of the rib; T1, T11, and T12 are exceptions to this rule. T1 has a single facet that articulates with the head of the first rib and an inferior demifacet that articulates with the head of the second rib.

T11 and T12 do not contain costal facets on their transverse processes, but they do contain singular facets on their pedicles that articulate with the 11th and 12th ribs, respectively.[1,2]

The anterior and posterior aspects of the vertebral bodies and discs are enclosed by the anterior and posterior longitudinal ligaments. The ligamentum flavum forms the posterior aspect of the central canal, connecting adjacent laminae. The interspinous ligament travels in between the spinous processes, draped superficially by the supraspinous ligament.[1,2,3]

The intervertebral discs between the vertebral bodies are composed of an outer annulus fibrosis and an inner nucleus pulposus. Composed primarily of type I collagen fibers, the annulus fibrosis is the fibrocartilaginous portion that resists motion and restricts the nucleus pulposus. The nucleus pulposus, as the primary shock absorber, is abundant in proteoglycan for water retention. The high water content of the nucleus pulposus creates hydrostatic pressure that resists compressive forces on the spinal column. Compared to the intervertebral discs in the cervical or lumbar spine, those in the thoracic spine are relatively thin and narrow, maintaining the immobility of this region.[4,5]

The blood supply to the spinal cord is composed of two systems: the central system and the peripheral system. The central system, arising from the anterior spinal artery, supplies the anterior two-thirds of the spinal cord, which consists of the anterior gray matter, the anterior portion of the posterior gray matter, the anterior portion of the posterior white columns, the inner half of the anterior and lateral white columns, and the base of the posterior white columns. The peripheral system, arising from the posterior spinal arteries and pial arterial plexus, supplies the outer portion of the anterior and lateral white columns and the remainder of the posterior gray matter and posterior white columns.[6,7,8] In the thoracic spine, posterior intercostal arteries from the aorta and subclavian artery give rise to segmental arteries. Branches of the segmental spinal arteries (the anterior and posterior radicular arteries) supply the anterior and posterior nerve roots. The segmental spinal arteries further branch into radiculomedullary arteries, which contribute to the anterior spinal artery and radiculopial arteries, which contribute to the posterior spinal arteries and pial network.[9] The largest radiculomedullary artery, arising around T9 to T10, is the artery of Adamkiewicz. Compared to the cervical or lumbar spinal cord, the thoracic cord has a particularly inadequate collateralization of vasculature and is especially susceptible to ischemia.[9,10]

The thoracic spine innervates somatic muscles in the chest and abdomen below T1. Of note, the only preganglionic sympathetic neurons originate from T1 to L2, in the lateral horns of the spinal gray matter. Central (first-order) neurons from the hypothalamus synapse at C8-T2, at the ciliospinal center of Budge. Preganglionic (second-order) neurons exit the spinal cord and synapse at the superior cervical ganglion.

Splanchnic nerves arise from the sympathetic trunk and contain efferent preganglionic sympathetic and visceral sensory afferent nerve fibers. The thoracic splanchnic nerves are from T1 to T4, the greater splanchnic nerves are from T5 to T9, the lesser splanchnic nerves are from T9 to T11, and the least splanchnic nerve is T12; however, there is variation regarding the spinal nerve that contributes to each splanchnic nerve.[1,2]

Trauma to the thoracic spine can be potentially devastating because of the close proximity of many vital structures. The sternal angle (i.e., the angle of Louis), at the level of T4 divides the superior and inferior mediastinum. Additionally, the carina of the trachea and the inner concavity of the aortic arch are located at T4. The inferior vena cava, esophagus, and aorta pass through the diaphragm at the level of T8, T10, and T12, respectively—each representing a potential site of injury.

11.2 Mechanisms of Injury

The thoracolumbar junction, at the inflection point of T12-L1, is the most frequent site of spine fractures, comprising about 64% of all spinal column fractures.[11] Traumatic fractures of the thoracic spine are due primarily to high-energy impact, most commonly motor vehicle collisions and falls from a height.[11,12,13,14,15] Posttraumatic deformity is a late complication of spinal column fractures. Traumatic thoracic spine fractures are best described using the AOSpine classification system,[16,17] which is based on the three resistive forces of the spine (i.e., flexion, distraction, and torsion)[18] and which replaces the previous Denis classification.[19]

11.2.1 Flexion Injuries (Type A)

The flexion fracture pattern encompasses injuries due to vertebral body axial loading. Compression fractures (type A1) represent the most common spinal fracture. In type A1 injuries, the anterior column is the first to fail; the resulting fracture is known as a wedge fracture. Posterior element involvement follows, with greater compressive force. Subgroups of the type A1 injury, in increasing severity, include endplate impaction (A1.1), wedge fracture (A1.2), and vertebral body collapse (A1.3).

Type A2 injuries are split fractures of the vertebral body. These consist of a sagittal split (A2.1), a coronal split (A2.2), and a pincer fracture (A2.3). Pincer fractures often contain intervertebral disc material impacted within the vertebral body defect, leading to possible pseudarthrosis.[16,17,20]

The most severe compression injury is a burst fracture (type A3), which may include fragment retropulsion into the spinal canal. Subtypes of burst fractures are classified by increasing severity as incomplete (A3.1), complete (A3.2), or burst split fractures (A3.3).

11.2.2 Distraction Injuries (Type B)

Type B injuries are primarily due to a failure of the posterior column. The posterior ligamentous complex, often referred to as the *tension band*, plays a critical role in spinal column stabilization. The posterior ligamentous complex, which resists distraction, consists of the supraspinous ligament, interspinous ligaments, articular facet capsules, and ligamentum flavum.[12,16,17,21]

Type B1 injuries are due to flexion–distraction and are predominantly posterior ligamentous injuries. Posterior disruption with predominantly osseous involvement is classified as a type B2 injury, also known as a Chance or seat belt fracture. However,

a hyperextension-shear injury, denoted as a type B3 injury, results in a combined anterior column disruption through the disc.

11.2.3 Torsional Injuries (Type C)

Type C injuries are attributed to axial rotation and are characterized by dual-column involvement and rotational displacement. Type C injuries may be present concomitantly with other fracture patterns such as a type A fracture with rotation (C1), a type B fracture with rotation (C2), or a rotation-shear injury (C3). Type C injuries have the potential for translational displacement and have the greatest association with posttraumatic neurological deficits.[16,17]

In accordance with the AOSpine classification,[16,17] the increasing severity of injury is indicated by type (i.e., A–C) and respective subtype (e.g., A1.1–A1.3). However, with respect to severity, a comparison cannot be made between subtypes of different groups (e.g., B1.3 vs. C1.1). The AO classification system indicates severity of bony involvement, ligamentous involvement, neurological deficit, and mechanical instability.

Most posttraumatic deformities occur as a direct result of a traumatic insult, but they may also be the result of treatment. Kyphosis is the most common posttraumatic deformity of the thoracic spine. However, injuries such as lateral compression fractures or torsional injuries may lead to coronal deformity and should be carefully evaluated.

Injuries affecting the anterior, middle, and posterior columns are more likely to result in instability. As such, a stable compression fracture confined to the anterior column with minimal focal kyphosis (< 20 degrees) is unlikely to progress and will be compensated to maintain sagittal alignment. However, it should be noted that compensation from adjacent levels is biomechanically unfavorable and accelerates degenerative changes. Injuries with a focal kyphosis greater than 20 degrees may indicate posterior ligamentous involvement from a distraction injury, and they have a significantly greater chance of progressing to posttraumatic deformity.[22,23,24] The sagittal index, as will be described later in this chapter, is a useful tool for guiding the management of posttraumatic deformity. An injury that affects all columns, such as a complete burst fracture, has a greater likelihood of progression. Moreover, the potential for posttraumatic deformity is exacerbated with lower thoracic injury to the thoracolumbar junction, which is devoid of rib cage support.[22,23,24,25,26]

Posttraumatic deformity that occurs after surgical treatment may be caused by pseudarthrosis, hardware failure, short fusions, and iatrogenic instability. Pseudarthrosis, or nonunion, may be due to various factors such as deep infections and inadequate bone mineralization, resulting in progressive deformity and adjacent segment instability.[27] Hardware failure is a potential risk for any patient undergoing instrumented surgery. Young's modulus (the modulus of elasticity) is a measure of the resistance, or stiffness, of a material under tension and is a fixed property equal to the ratio of stress over strain. For a given stress, or force, a material has a finite capacity to deform; this capacity is defined as *strain*. Hardware failure occurs when the force placed on either the implanted hardware or the bone exceeds the material's capacity for strain. Such failure may include hardware migration, rod fracture, screw fracture, and screw pullout, often necessitating larger surgical revisions.[28,29] Both laminectomy and short fusion constructs (less than five levels), particularly at the thoracolumbar junction, have been associated with progressive posttraumatic deformity and are generally not advised.[22,23,24,30]

Rarely, neuropathic spinal arthropathy (Charcot's spine) or vertebral body osteonecrosis (Kümmell's disease) may occur after trauma. Charcot's spinal arthropathy may occur after spinal cord injury and is characterized by a sequence of sensory feedback loss, atypical joint motion, microtrauma, bone resorption, joint destruction, and adjacent segment pseudarthrosis.[31,32,33,34] In Kümmell's disease, avascular osteonecrosis and nonunion lead to vertebral body collapse and progressive deformity.[35,36]

Although most traumatic fractures of the thoracic spine occur because of high-energy impact, patients with poor bone quality may sustain traumatic injury and progress more easily to posttraumatic deformity or hardware failure. Conditions associated with poor bone quality include osteoporosis, ankylosing spondylitis, osteogenesis imperfecta, and other endocrine disorders.[22,23,24,37] Osteoporosis is the condition of having bone mineral density 2.5 standard deviations or more below that of young adults (t-score $\leq$ –2.5); patients with osteoporosis are at high risk for spinal compression fractures.[38] A single compression fracture in a patient with osteoporosis substantially increases the risk for subsequent compression fractures, propagating kyphosis and sagittal imbalance.[39,40]

Patients with ankylosing spondylitis require special attention after trauma because of the altered spinal biomechanics present in this population. Bridging ossification leads to a rigid kyphotic deformity and atypical fracture patterns. Most often caused by extension–distraction injuries, these fractures are transverse through the anterior column of ossified discs or vertebral bodies. The fractures result in substantial instability between two adjacent segments and may lead to translational displacement and deformity.[41,42]

Pediatric patients with traumatic thoracic spine injury are a unique population due to their skeletal immaturity and growth potential. In children, ligament laxity and a large head size make trauma of the cervical spine more common than trauma of the thoracic spine. When injury of the pediatric thoracic spine does occur, it can result in posttraumatic kyphosis and paralytic scoliosis with rates as high as 64 and 96%, respectively.[43,44,45,46] Various mechanisms exist for posttraumatic spinal deformity in pediatric patients. Muscle spasticity from spinal cord injury, joint surface abnormality from misalignment, and asymmetric physeal closure can all facilitate the development of progressive deformity in children who sustain thoracic spine trauma.[47,48,49,50,51,52]

11.3 Clinical Features of Posttraumatic Deformity

In acute situations, the appropriate identification and management of thoracic spine trauma are essential. Traumatic injury to the upper thoracic cord (above T6) may result in life-threatening autonomic dysreflexia, neurogenic shock, or spinal shock. Poor collateralization makes the thoracic spine especially susceptible to ischemia. Mean arterial blood pressure elevation, decompression, and stabilization are critical components in acute management.[8,53,54]

After trauma, patients who develop a posttraumatic deformity may have a noticeable curvature with or without compensation. Although kyphosis is the most common posttraumatic deformity, lateral compression fractures or burst fractures may cause focal scoliosis and trunk shift in the coronal plane. Common symptoms of deformity include back pain, a loss in height, neurological deficit, and difficulty standing. Pain is the most common presenting symptom of patients with posttraumatic deformity, and a localized kyphotic deformity greater than or equal to 30 degrees has been shown to significantly increase the risk for chronic pain in that region.[24,55,56,57]

Patients with posttraumatic deformity may also experience new or progressive neurological deficits. In a study by Malcolm et al[56] of 48 patients with posttraumatic deformity, 27% experienced increasing neurological deficit. New or worsening neurological deficits may be due to posttraumatic cystic myelopathy, spinal cord tethering, and progression of deformity, but they are most commonly due to posttraumatic syringomyelia. Posttraumatic syringomyelia comprises 25% of all diagnosed syringomyelia cases.[58,59,60] Syringomyelia may also be closely associated with the underlying deformity. In a study of 207 cases of traumatic paraplegia with fully healed fractures, Abel et al[61] demonstrated that posttraumatic kyphosis greater than 15 degrees and canal stenosis greater than 25% doubled the likelihood of syringomyelia. Interestingly, there was significant correlation between the extent of spinal stenosis and the amount of deformity.

Severe posttraumatic deformity can also have an impact on the overall health of these patients. They may experience premature gastrointestinal satiety, difficulty breathing, or cardiac abnormalities secondary to compression of the abdomen and thoracic cavity.[22]

11.4 Sagittal and Coronal Balance

A spinal deformity is an aberrant curvature of the spinal column that may be congenital, iatrogenic, idiopathic, degenerative, or traumatic. Nonetheless, it is necessary to define a few key terms relating to coronal and sagittal balance parameters when assessing spinal deformity. Each of these measurements is best appreciated using standing 36-inch cassette plain films.

11.4.1 C7 Plumb Line (C7PL)

On the lateral view, the C7 plumb line is a line drawn caudally from the C7 vertebrae to the sacrum. In normal sagittal alignment, the C7 plumb line should be within 2.5 cm of the posterior aspect on the sacral endplate—also known as the *sagittal vertebral axis* (SVA). An SVA value greater than 2.5 cm may indicate positive sagittal balance, whereas an SVA value less than 2.5 cm may indicate negative sagittal balance. However, these values should be considered along with other parameters, as the SVA becomes more positive as individuals age.[62]

On the standing anteroposterior view, a line drawn caudally from the center of the C7 vertebrae should overlap a corresponding line drawn cephalad from the center of the sacral promontory. This is known as the *central sacral vertical line*. Trunk shift in the coronal plane may be suspected if these two lines do not overlap.[63,64]

11.4.2 Cervical Lordosis

Cervical lordosis is the angle between the inferior endplate of C2 and the inferior endplate of C7. Lordosis of the cervical spine is typically 40 ± 9.7 degrees and is primarily determined by the T1 slope.[34,62] The magnitude of cervical lordosis is highly variable and responds to changes in alignment in the thoracolumbar spine.

11.4.3 Thoracic Kyphosis

Thoracic kyphosis, measured from the superior endplate of the T5 vertebral body to the inferior endplate of the T12 vertebral body, is normally between 20 and 50 degrees. The degree of thoracic kyphosis is greatly influenced both by the position of C7 cephalad and by the extent of lumbar lordosis caudal.[65,66,67] Focal kyphosis of a single-level fracture is most appropriately measured as the angle formed by the superior endplate and the inferior endplate of the adjacent cephalad and caudal vertebra, respectively.[22,23,24]

11.4.4 Lumbar Lordosis

Lumbar lordosis is the angle formed from the superior endplate of L1 and the superior endplate of S1, and it is typically 30 to 60 degrees. The ideal amount of lumbar lordosis is determined by the pelvic incidence and should be within 10 degrees of that value. In general, thoracic kyphosis and lumbar lordosis are proportional in order to maintain balance in the sagittal plane. As such, increasing lumbar lordosis is positively associated with an increase in thoracic kyphosis.[62,67,68,69]

11.4.5 Pelvic Incidence

The pelvic incidence is measured with a line drawn from the midpoint of the femoral head to the center of the sacral endplate. A second line, drawn inferiorly and perpendicular to the sacral endplate, forms the angle of the pelvic incidence. Spinopelvic parameters dictate the attachment of the spinal column to the pelvis and are fundamental components of global deformity and spinal biomechanics.

As a general rule, the pelvic incidence should be within 10 degrees of the lumbar lordosis. It is influenced by multiple factors such as the sacral slope, pelvic tilt, and shape of the pelvis. The pelvic tilt, or rotation of the pelvis about the femoral heads, is the angle formed between a vertical line and a second line reaching the center of the sacral endplate, both originating from the midpoint of the femoral heads. Moreover, the sacral slope is the downward angle formed from the sacral endplate, relative to the horizontal. Although the pelvic tilt and sacral slope are influenced by posture, the sum of the two values yields the pelvic incidence and highlights both the associations among numerous spinal alignment parameters and the compensation that occurs to maintain upright posture and balance.[62,70,71,72,73,74,75] Moreover, the vertebral loading forces that result from thoracic hyperkyphosis may be compensated for by an increase in lumbar lordosis or pelvic tilt, with the former achieving the more biomechanically favorable vertebral loading.[68]

11.4.6 Sagittal Index

The sagittal index is a measure of segmental kyphotic deformity. It is calculated by subtracting the baseline values for contours of the spine from the kyphotic angle of the involved level. Instrumented arthrodesis is indicated for a sagittal index greater than 15 degrees.[76,77]

11.4.7 Apex

In patients with coronal deformity, the apex is the disc or vertebra that is deviated farthest from the vertebral column.[63]

11.4.8 Neutral Vertebra

Vertebral rotation in the axial plane often accompanies coronal deformity. Neutral vertebrae are those that are not rotated in the axial plane. They are characterized by clearly visible pedicles and a spinous process in the center of each vertebra.[63]

11.4.9 Stable Vertebra

In coronal deformity, stable vertebrae are the most cephalad. They are bisected, or nearly bisected, by the central sacral vertical line.

11.4.10 End Vertebra

The end vertebrae in patients with coronal deformity are those that are the most tilted cranially and caudally that surround the curve.

11.4.11 Cobb's Angle

The Cobb angle is the angle formed by the cranial and caudal end vertebrae.

11.5 Imaging

Imaging is the mainstay for diagnosing a posttraumatic deformity, and it will dictate clinical decision making. As described previously, standing 36-inch plain films are essential in evaluating sagittal deformity, coronal deformity, and global balance. Flexion–extension (anteroposterior) and bending radiographs (lateral) shed light on the flexibility of a deformity.[24,78,79,80]

Computed tomography (CT) is unparalleled in the evaluation of bony structures, as well as of the interosseous spaces. After acute trauma, many patients undergo a CT scan of the chest, abdomen, and pelvis (CT/CAP, chest abdomen pelvis). In a study by Hauser et al,[81] 215 patients with high-risk thoracolumbar spine trauma were evaluated using CT/CAP and thoracolumbar radiographs. The accuracy of CT compared to radiography for identifying acute thoracolumbar fractures was found to be 99 and 87%, respectively. Similarly, McAfee et al[82] demonstrated that CT was the most sensitive imaging modality for the diagnosis of posterior element defects and unstable burst fractures.

Soft tissue structures and neural elements are best visualized by magnetic resonance imaging. Posttraumatic cystic myelopathy, spinal cord tethering, and syringomyelia are also best visualized on magnetic resonance imaging. Moreover, serial imaging can be used to monitor the progression of posttraumatic deformity.[58,83,84,85,86]

11.6 Surgical Treatment

Surgery for posttraumatic deformity may be indicated for increasing back pain, increasing neurological deficit, instability, and severe or progressive deformity.[22,23,24] Patients with posttraumatic deformity may experience debilitating pain related to degeneration and compensation for global alignment. Results of studies on pain related to fixed sagittal imbalance and canal compromise have been promising, with most reports indicating that patients achieved clinically significant pain relief.[87,88,89,90,91] However, patients with degenerative sagittal imbalance had less pain relief and more postoperative complications.[90,91] Nonetheless, the pain level after surgery is difficult to predict and should be assessed along with other symptoms, the extent of surgery, and possible complications.

New or worsening neurological deficit, such as myelopathy and radiculopathy, after posttraumatic deformity is an indication for surgery. Surgery should be aimed both at decompression, often in the anterior column, and at stabilization. An anterior approach and a corpectomy can be used to address neurological deficits related to posttraumatic kyphosis. The anterior approach has demonstrated greater effectiveness than the posterolateral approach in improving neurological deficits, and it allows for anterior column reconstruction.[22,23,24,61,92,93,94] While the anterior approach historically demonstrated efficacy for the treatment of thoracolumbar burst fractures, newer instrumentation and posterior techniques have made both approaches highly effective.[95,96,97,98] A meta-analysis comparing anterior and posterior approaches, consisting of seven clinical trials, found no differences in neurological recovery, return to work, complications, and Cobb's angle between the two approaches. The anterior approach, however, was associated with increased operative duration, blood loss, and cost.[99] The decision of surgical approach should be taken on a case-by-case basis, with careful consideration of clinical characteristics and operative goals.[95,96,97,98,99]

Surgical approaches for the treatment of posttraumatic deformity include anterior, posterior, or combined approaches, and they vary based on symptoms and the nature and extent of the deformity. The anterior approach may be useful for extensive decompression (i.e., retropulsed fragments in the canal), spinal mobilization, or anterior reconstruction.[95,96,97,98,99] Attempts at stabilization must consider iatrogenic instability and posterior element instability, potentially requiring a combined posterior instrumented fixation.[22,23,24,57,92,93,94]

Osteotomies may be necessary in cases of rigid deformity and should be planned based on the amount and nature of correction. The Smith–Petersen osteotomy allows for a mean correction of 10 to 15 degrees through shortening of the posterior column.[22,97] Pedicle subtraction osteotomy allows 30 to 35 degrees of sagittal correction at a given level and avoids destabilization of the anterior column. Vertebral column resection is the most extensive procedure, and it involves the removal of one or more vertebral segments.[100,101,102,103] Decisions about surgeries, including osteotomies, for rigid posttraumatic thoracic deformity are outlined well by Buchowski et al[103] and are based on sagittal balance or imbalance. For normal sagittal balance, smooth thoracic kyphosis may be best treated using the Smith–Petersen osteotomy, whereas sharp angular kyphosis may be best treated using pedicle subtraction osteotomy or vertebral column resection. For patients with global imbalance, both smooth and sharp angular kyphosis can be used based on the extent of imbalance. With smooth thoracic kyphosis, both minor sagittal imbalance (SVA < 2.5–5 cm) and major imbalance (SVA > 5 cm) can be treated by Smith–Petersen osteotomies. However, cases of anterior column fusion or sharp angular kyphosis, with sagittal deformity, may require a more extensive pedicle subtraction osteotomy or vertebral column resection. The posterior vertebral column resection and pedicle subtraction osteotomies are performed from a posterior approach and provide adequate deformity correction, in addition to canal decompression, in such cases. However, the benefits of these technically involved osteotomies should be weighed against risks of blood loss and iatrogenic neurological injury.[104,105]

11.7 Case Illustration

A 30-year-old woman from Greece presented with progressive kyphosis, worsening neurological function, and a painful gibbus deformity at the thoracolumbar junction. She had sustained a fall 14 years previously that resulted in a T12 burst fracture. She was originally treated with posterior instrumentation consisting of a Luque rectangle. Upon presentation at our institute, she underwent a physical examination, which revealed a Brown–Séquard–type injury. Her strength was assessed as 1 to 2 of 5 in the proximal right lower extremity, and she had good sensation in the left lower extremity. Imaging demonstrated posttraumatic kyphosis at the thoracolumbar junction with spinal cord compression (▶ Fig. 11.1). Surgery was performed in three stages to prevent further neurological decline and to stabilize the spinal column. In stage 1, the Luque rectangle was removed, and pedicle screws were placed at T10, T11, L1, and L2 (▶ Fig. 11.2). Osteotomies were performed at the fracture site to allow for reduction of the deformity. In stage 2, a left-sided thoracotomy and a T12 corpectomy were performed to reduce the kyphotic deformity. Then an expandable titanium cage and plating were placed from T11 to L1 (▶ Fig. 11.3). In stage 3, rods were secured in the previously placed pedicle screws (▶ Fig. 11.4). Postoperative imaging demonstrated correction of the posttraumatic deformity (▶ Fig. 11.5). After surgery, the patient experienced no immediate change in neurological function and began working with the neurorehabilitation team.

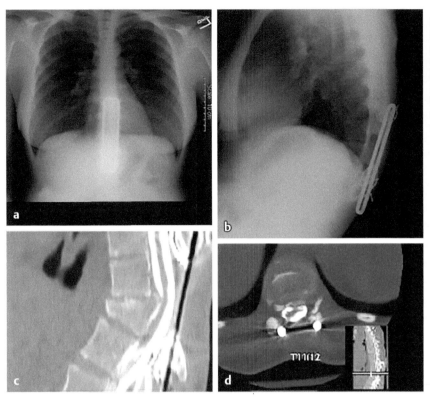

Fig. 11.1 Imaging of a posttraumatic deformity from a previously treated T12 burst fracture; the patient presented to our institute with worsening neurological function and thoracolumbar kyphosis. (a) Anteroposterior radiograph with the Luque rectangle. (b) Lateral radiograph. (c) Sagittal computed tomography myelogram showing spinal cord compression. (d) Axial computed tomography myelogram.

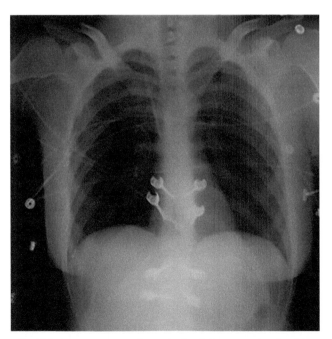

Fig. 11.2 Anteroposterior radiograph of pedicle screws placed at T10, T11, L1, and L2 with osteotomies performed at the fracture site.

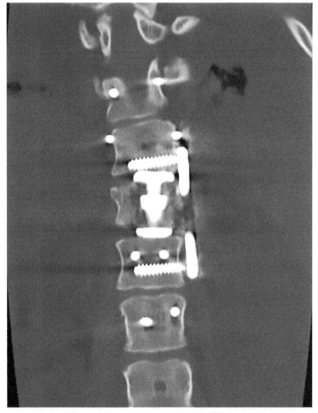

Fig. 11.3 Coronal computed tomography following left thoracotomy, T12 corpectomy, expandable cage placement, and plating from T11 to L1.

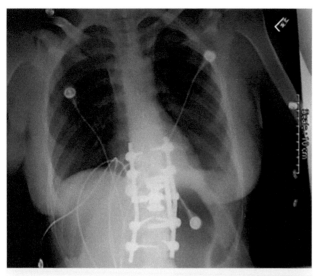

Fig. 11.4 Postoperative anteroposterior radiograph showing posterior rod placement.

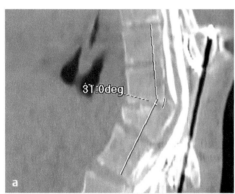
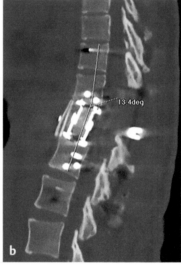

Fig. 11.5 Posttraumatic deformity correction. **(a)** Preoperative sagittal computed tomography myelogram showing the extent of the deformity. **(b)** Postoperative sagittal computed tomography showing the final construct and correction of the deformity.

References

[1] Drake RL, Vogl AW, Mitchell AWM. Gray's Anatomy for Students. 3rd ed. Philadelphia, PA: Elsevier Churchill Livingstone; 2013

[2] Vanderah TW, Gould DJ. Nolte's the Human Brain. 7th ed. Philadelphia, PA: Elsevier; 2015

[3] Akdemir G. Thoracic and lumbar intraforaminal ligaments. J Neurosurg Spine. 2010; 13(3):351–355

[4] Martirosyan NL, Patel AA, Carotenuto A, et al. Genetic alterations in intervertebral disc disease. Front Surg. 2016; 3:59

[5] Kalb S, Martirosyan NL, Kalani MY, Broc GG, Theodore N. Genetics of the degenerated intervertebral disc. World Neurosurg. 2012; 77(3–4):491–501

[6] Turnbull IM. Chapter 5. Blood supply of the spinal cord: normal and pathological considerations. Clin Neurosurg. 1973; 20:56–84

[7] Tveten L. Spinal cord vascularity. III. The spinal cord arteries in man. Acta Radiol Diagn (Stockh). 1976; 17(3):257–273

[8] Martirosyan NL, Feuerstein JS, Theodore N, Cavalcanti DD, Spetzler RF, Preul MC. Blood supply and vascular reactivity of the spinal cord under normal and pathological conditions. J Neurosurg Spine. 2011; 15(3):238–251

[9] Miyasaka K, Asano T, Ushikoshi S, Hida K, Koyanagi I. Vascular anatomy of the spinal cord and classification of spinal arteriovenous malformations. Interv Neuroradiol. 2000; 6 Suppl 1:195–198

[10] Tator CH, Koyanagi I. Vascular mechanisms in the pathophysiology of human spinal cord injury. J Neurosurg. 1997; 86(3):483–492

[11] Freidberg SR, Maggie SN. Trauma to the spine and spinal cord. In: Jones HR, Srinivasan J, Allam GJ, Baker RA, eds. Netter's Neurology. Philadelphia, PA: Saunders Elsevier; 2012:562–574

[12] Khurana B, Sheehan SE, Sodickson A, Bono CM, Harris MB. Traumatic thoracolumbar spine injuries: what the spine surgeon wants to know. Radiographics. 2013; 33(7):2031–2046

[13] Leucht P, Fischer K, Muhr G, Mueller EJ. Epidemiology of traumatic spine fractures. Injury. 2009; 40(2):166–172

[14] Sekhon LH, Fehlings MG. Epidemiology, demographics, and pathophysiology of acute spinal cord injury. Spine. 2001; 26(24) Suppl:S2–S12

[15] Jackson AB, Dijkers M, Devivo MJ, Poczatek RB. A demographic profile of new traumatic spinal cord injuries: change and stability over 30 years. Arch Phys Med Rehabil. 2004; 85(11):1740–1748

[16] Magerl F, Aebi M, Gertzbein SD, Harms J, Nazarian S. A comprehensive classification of thoracic and lumbar injuries. Eur Spine J. 1994; 3(4):184–201

[17] Aebi M. Classification of thoracolumbar fractures and dislocations. Eur Spine J. 2010; 19 Suppl 1:S2–S7

[18] Whitesides TE, Jr. Traumatic kyphosis of the thoracolumbar spine. Clin Orthop Relat Res. 1977(128):78–92

[19] Denis F. The three column spine and its significance in the classification of acute thoracolumbar spinal injuries. Spine. 1983; 8(8):817–831

[20] Marchesi DG. Classification of thoracic and lumbar fractures. In: Vaccaro AR, ed. Fractures of the cervical, thoracic, and lumbar spine. Boca Raton, FL: CRC Press Taylor & Francis Group; 2002:385–398

[21] Barcelos AC, Joaquim AF, Botelho RV. Reliability of the evaluation of posterior ligamentous complex injury in thoracolumbar spine trauma with the use of computed tomography scan. Eur Spine J. 2016; 25(4):1135–1143

[22] Wilson J, Buchowski JM. Post-traumatic deformity: prevention and management. Handb Clin Neurol. 2012; 109:369–384

[23] Polly DW, Jr, Klemme WR, Shawen S. Management options for the treatment of posttraumatic thoracic kyphosis. Semin Spine Surg. 2000; 12:110–116

[24] Vaccaro AR, Silber JS. Post-traumatic spinal deformity. Spine. 2001; 26(24) Suppl:S111–S118

[25] Bohlman HH. Treatment of fractures and dislocations of the thoracic and lumbar spine. J Bone Joint Surg Am. 1985; 67(1):165–169

[26] Bohlman HH, Freehafer A, Dejak J. The results of treatment of acute injuries of the upper thoracic spine with paralysis. J Bone Joint Surg Am. 1985; 67 (3):360–369

[27] Raizman NM, O'Brien JR, Poehling-Monaghan KL, Yu WD. Pseudarthrosis of the spine. J Am Acad Orthop Surg. 2009; 17(8):494–503

[28] Amankulor NM, Xu R, Iorgulescu JB, et al. The incidence and patterns of hardware failure after separation surgery in patients with spinal metastatic tumors. Spine J. 2014; 14(9):1850–1859

[29] Parmar V, Li Yiping L, Kutlauy U, Resnick DK. Posterior thoracic and lumbar universal spinal instrumentation. In: Steinmetz MP, Benzel EC, eds. Benzel's spine surgery: techniques, complications, avoidance, and management. Philadelphia, PA: Elsevier; 2016:729–741

[30] Keene JS, Lash EG, Kling TF, Jr. Undetected posttraumatic instability of "stable" thoracolumbar fractures. J Orthop Trauma. 1988; 2(3):202–211

[31] Sobel JW, Bohlman HH, Freehafer AA. Charcot's arthropathy of the spine following spinal cord injury. A report of five cases. J Bone Joint Surg Am. 1985; 67(5):771–776

[32] Standaert C, Cardenas DD, Anderson P. Charcot spine as a late complication of traumatic spinal cord injury. Arch Phys Med Rehabil. 1997; 78(2):221–225

[33] Goodwin CR, Ahmed AK, Abu-Bonsrah N, De la Garza-Ramos R, Petteys RJ, Sciubba DM. Charcot spinal arthropathy after spinal cord injury. Spine J. 2016; 16(8):e545–e546

[34] Aebli N, Pötzel T, Krebs J. Characteristics and surgical management of neuropathic (Charcot) spinal arthropathy after spinal cord injury. Spine J. 2014; 14 (6):884–891

[35] Chou LH, Knight RQ. Idiopathic avascular necrosis of a vertebral body. Case report and literature review. Spine. 1997; 22(16):1928–1932

[36] Young WF, Brown D, Kendler A, Clements D. Delayed post-traumatic osteonecrosis of a vertebral body (Kummell's disease). Acta Orthop Belg. 2002; 68 (1):13–19

[37] Wekre LL, Kjensli A, Aasand K, Falch JA, Eriksen EF. Spinal deformities and lung function in adults with osteogenesis imperfecta. Clin Respir J. 2014; 8 (4):437–443

[38] Cosman F, Krege JH, Looker AC, et al. Spine fracture prevalence in a nationally representative sample of US women and men aged ≥ 40 years: results from the National Health and Nutrition Examination Survey (NHANES) 2013–2014. Osteoporos Int. 2017; 28(6):1857–1866

[39] Organization WH. Prevention and management of osteoporosis. World Health Organ Tech Rep Ser. 2003; 921:1–164

[40] Roux C, Fechtenbaum J, Kolta S, Said-Nahal R, Briot K, Benhamou CL. Prospective assessment of thoracic kyphosis in postmenopausal women with osteoporosis. J Bone Miner Res. 2010; 25(2):362–368

[41] Kubiak EN, Moskovich R, Errico TJ, Di Cesare PE. Orthopaedic management of ankylosing spondylitis. J Am Acad Orthop Surg. 2005; 13(4):267–278

[42] Werner BC, Samartzis D, Shen FH. Spinal fractures in patients with ankylosing spondylitis: etiology, diagnosis, and management. J Am Acad Orthop Surg. 2016; 24(4):241–249

[43] Mayfield JK, Erkkila JC, Winter RB. Spine deformity subsequent to acquired childhood spinal cord injury. J Bone Joint Surg Am. 1981; 63(9):1401–1411

[44] Dearolf WW, III, Betz RR, Vogel LC, Levin J, Clancy M, Steel HH. Scoliosis in pediatric spinal cord-injured patients. J Pediatr Orthop. 1990; 10(2):214–218

[45] Bedbrook GM. Correction of scoliosis due to paraplegia sustained in paediatric age-group [proceedings]. Paraplegia. 1977; 15(1):90–96

[46] Been HD, Poolman RW, Ubags LH. Clinical outcome and radiographic results after surgical treatment of post-traumatic thoracolumbar kyphosis following simple type A fractures. Eur Spine J. 2004; 13(2):101–107

[47] Lancourt JE, Dickson JH, Carter RE. Paralytic spinal deformity following traumatic spinal-cord injury in children and adolescents. J Bone Joint Surg Am. 1981; 63(1):47–53

[48] Slotkin JR, Lu Y, Wood KB. Thoracolumbar spinal trauma in children. Neurosurg Clin N Am. 2007; 18(4):621–630

[49] Hamilton MG, Myles ST. Pediatric spinal injury: review of 174 hospital admissions. J Neurosurg. 1992; 77(5):700–704

[50] Cirak B, Ziegfeld S, Knight VM, Chang D, Avellino AM, Paidas CN. Spinal injuries in children. J Pediatr Surg. 2004; 39(4):607–612

[51] Daniels AH, Sobel AD, Eberson CP. Pediatric thoracolumbar spine trauma. J Am Acad Orthop Surg. 2013; 21(12):707–716

[52] Srinivasan V, Jea A. Pediatric thoracolumbar spine trauma. Neurosurg Clin N Am. 2017; 28(1):103–114

[53] Hagen EM. Acute complications of spinal cord injuries. World J Orthop. 2015; 6(1):17–23

[54] Sezer N, Akkuş S, Uğurlu FG. Chronic complications of spinal cord injury. World J Orthop. 2015; 6(1):24–33

[55] Gertzbein SD. Scoliosis Research Society. Multicenter spine fracture study. Spine. 1992; 17(5):528–540

[56] Malcolm BW, Bradford DS, Winter RB, Chou SN. Post-traumatic kyphosis. A review of forty-eight surgically treated patients. J Bone Joint Surg Am. 1981; 63(6):891–899

[57] Roberson JR, Whitesides TE, Jr. Surgical reconstruction of late post-traumatic thoracolumbar kyphosis. Spine. 1985; 10(4):307–312

[58] Lee TT, Alameda GJ, Gromelski EB, Green BA. Outcome after surgical treatment of progressive posttraumatic cystic myelopathy. J Neurosurg. 2000; 92 (2) Suppl:149–154

[59] Batzdorf U, Klekamp J, Johnson JP. A critical appraisal of syrinx cavity shunting procedures. J Neurosurg. 1998; 89(3):382–388

[60] Brodbelt AR, Stoodley MA. Post-traumatic syringomyelia: a review. J Clin Neurosci. 2003; 10(4):401–408

[61] Abel R, Gerner HJ, Smit C, Meiners T. Residual deformity of the spinal canal in patients with traumatic paraplegia and secondary changes of the spinal cord. Spinal Cord. 1999; 37(1):14–19

[62] Roussouly P, Nnadi C. Sagittal plane deformity: an overview of interpretation and management. Eur Spine J. 2010; 19(11):1824–1836

[63] Kim H, Kim HS, Moon ES, et al. Scoliosis imaging: what radiologists should know. Radiographics. 2010; 30(7):1823–1842

[64] Vieira RLR, Arora R, Schweitzer ME. Radiologic imaging of spinal deformities. In: Errico TJ, Lonner BS, Moulton AW, eds. Surgical Management of Spinal Deformities. Philadelphia, PA: Saunders Elsevier; 2009:45–59

[65] Djurasovic M, Glassman SD. Correlation of radiographic and clinical findings in spinal deformities. Neurosurg Clin N Am. 2007; 18(2):223–227

[66] Bernhardt M, Bridwell KH. Segmental analysis of the sagittal plane alignment of the normal thoracic and lumbar spines and thoracolumbar junction. Spine. 1989; 14(7):717–721

[67] Boseker EH, Moe JH, Winter RB, Koop SE. Determination of "normal" thoracic kyphosis: a roentgenographic study of 121 "normal" children. J Pediatr Orthop. 2000; 20(6):796–798

[68] Bruno AG, Anderson DE, D'Agostino J, Bouxsein ML. The effect of thoracic kyphosis and sagittal plane alignment on vertebral compressive loading. J Bone Miner Res. 2012; 27(10):2144–2151

[69] Qian J, Qiu Y, Qian BP, Zhu ZZ, Wang B, Yu Y. Compensatory modulation for severe global sagittal imbalance: significance of cervical compensation on quality of life in thoracolumbar kyphosis secondary to ankylosing spondylitis. Eur Spine J. 2016; 25(11):3715–3722

[70] Van Royen BJ, Toussaint HM, Kingma I, et al. Accuracy of the sagittal vertical axis in a standing lateral radiograph as a measurement of balance in spinal deformities. Eur Spine J. 1998; 7(5):408–412

[71] Berthonnaud E, Dimnet J, Roussouly P, Labelle H. Analysis of the sagittal balance of the spine and pelvis using shape and orientation parameters. J Spinal Disord Tech. 2005; 18(1):40–47

[72] Lafage V, Schwab F, Patel A, Hawkinson N, Farcy JP. Pelvic tilt and truncal inclination: two key radiographic parameters in the setting of adults with spinal deformity. Spine. 2009; 34(17):E599–E606

[73] Roussouly P, Pinheiro-Franco JL. Sagittal parameters of the spine: biomechanical approach. Eur Spine J. 2011; 20 Suppl 5:578–585

[74] Savage JW, Patel AA. Fixed sagittal plane imbalance. Global Spine J. 2014; 4(4):287–296

[75] Glassman SD, Bridwell K, Dimar JR, Horton W, Berven S, Schwab F. The impact of positive sagittal balance in adult spinal deformity. Spine. 2005; 30(18):2024–2029

[76] Farcy JP, Weidenbaum M, Glassman SD. Sagittal index in management of thoracolumbar burst fractures. Spine. 1990; 15(9):958–965

[77] Kang SK, Lee CW, Park NK, et al. Predictive risk factors for refracture after percutaneous vertebroplasty. Ann Rehabil Med. 2011; 35(6):844–851

[78] Parizel PM, van der Zijden T, Gaudino S, et al. Trauma of the spine and spinal cord: imaging strategies. Eur Spine J. 2010; 19 Suppl 1:S8–S17

[79] Tsou PM, Wang J, Khoo L, Shamie AN, Holly L. A thoracic and lumbar spine injury severity classification based on neurologic function grade, spinal canal deformity, and spinal biomechanical stability. Spine J. 2006; 6(6):636–647

[80] Bagley LJ. Imaging of spinal trauma. Radiol Clin North Am. 2006; 44(1):1–12, vii

[81] Hauser CJ, Visvikis G, Hinrichs C, et al. Prospective validation of computed tomographic screening of the thoracolumbar spine in trauma. J Trauma. 2003; 55(2):228–234, discussion 234–235

[82] McAfee PC, Yuan HA, Fredrickson BE, Lubicky JP. The value of computed tomography in thoracolumbar fractures. An analysis of one hundred consecutive cases and a new classification. J Bone Joint Surg Am. 1983; 65(4):461–473

[83] Van Goethem JW, Maes M, Ozsarlak O, van den Hauwe L, Parizel PM. Imaging in spinal trauma. Eur Radiol. 2005; 15(3):582–590

[84] Connolly PJ, Abitbol JJ, Martin RJ. Spine: trauma. In: Garfin SR, Vaccaro AR, eds. Orthopaedic Knowledge Update: Spine. Rosemont, IL: American Academy of Orthopaedic Surgeons; 1997:197–217

[85] Shen H, Tang Y, Huang L, et al. Applications of diffusion-weighted MRI in thoracic spinal cord injury without radiographic abnormality. Int Orthop. 2007; 31(3):375–383

[86] Curati WL, Kingsley DP, Kendall BE, Moseley IF. MRI in chronic spinal cord trauma. Neuroradiology. 1992; 35(1):30–35

[87] Bohlman HH, Kirkpatrick JS, Delamarter RB, Leventhal M. Anterior decompression for late pain and paralysis after fractures of the thoracolumbar spine. Clin Orthop Relat Res. 1994(300):24–29

[88] Kostuik JP, Matsusaki H. Anterior stabilization, instrumentation, and decompression for post-traumatic kyphosis. Spine. 1989; 14(4):379–386

[89] Ahn UM, Ahn NU, Buchowski JM, et al. Functional outcome and radiographic correction after spinal osteotomy. Spine. 2002; 27(12):1303–1311

[90] Bridwell KH, Lewis SJ, Edwards C, et al. Complications and outcomes of pedicle subtraction osteotomies for fixed sagittal imbalance. Spine. 2003; 28(18):2093–2101

[91] Bridwell KH, Lewis SJ, Lenke LG, Baldus C, Blanke K. Pedicle subtraction osteotomy for the treatment of fixed sagittal imbalance. J Bone Joint Surg Am. 2003; 85-A(3):454–463

[92] Transfeldt EE, White D, Bradford DS, Roche B. Delayed anterior decompression in patients with spinal cord and cauda equina injuries of the thoracolumbar spine. Spine. 1990; 15(9):953–957

[93] Anderson PA, Bohlman HH. Late anterior decompression of thoracolumbar spine fractures. Semin Spine Surg. 1990; 2:54–62

[94] Bradford DS, McBride GG. Surgical management of thoracolumbar spine fractures with incomplete neurologic deficits. Clin Orthop Relat Res. 1987(218):201–216

[95] Danisa OA, Shaffrey CI, Jane JA, et al. Surgical approaches for the correction of unstable thoracolumbar burst fractures: a retrospective analysis of treatment outcomes. J Neurosurg. 1995; 83(6):977–983

[96] Hitchon PW, Torner J, Eichholz KM, Beeler SN. Comparison of anterolateral and posterior approaches in the management of thoracolumbar burst fractures. J Neurosurg Spine. 2006; 5(2):117–125

[97] Wood KB, Bohn D, Mehbod A. Anterior versus posterior treatment of stable thoracolumbar burst fractures without neurologic deficit: a prospective, randomized study. J Spinal Disord Tech. 2005; 18 Suppl:S15–S23

[98] Hitchon PW, Torner J, Eichholz KM, Beeler SN. Comparison of anterolateral and posterior approaches in the management of thoracolumbar burst fractures. J Neurosurg Spine. 2006; 5(2):117–125

[99] Xu GJ, Li ZJ, Ma JX, Zhang T, Fu X, Ma XL. Anterior versus posterior approach for treatment of thoracolumbar burst fractures: a meta-analysis. Eur Spine J. 2013; 22(10):2176–2183

[100] McLain RF, Burkus JK, Benson DR. Segmental instrumentation for thoracic and thoracolumbar fractures: prospective analysis of construct survival and five-year follow-up. Spine J. 2001; 1(5):310–323

[101] Shen WJ, Liu TJ, Shen YS. Nonoperative treatment versus posterior fixation for thoracolumbar junction burst fractures without neurologic deficit. Spine. 2001; 26(9):1038–1045

[102] Smith-Petersen MN, Larson CB, Aufranc OE. Osteotomy of the spine for correction of flexion deformity in rheumatoid arthritis. Clin Orthop Relat Res. 1969; 66(66):6–9

[103] Buchowski JM, Kuhns CA, Bridwell KH, Lenke LG. Surgical management of posttraumatic thoracolumbar kyphosis. Spine J. 2008; 8(4):666–677

[104] Wang Y, Lenke LG. Vertebral column decancellation for the management of sharp angular spinal deformity. Eur Spine J. 2011; 20(10):1703–1710

[105] Brayda-Bruno M, Luca A, Lovi A, Zambotti M, Sinigaglia A, Lamartina C. Posttraumatic high thoracic angular kyphosis: posterior approach with correction and fusion in two steps. Eur Spine J. 2012; 21(12):2724–2726

Part III

Degenerative Disease

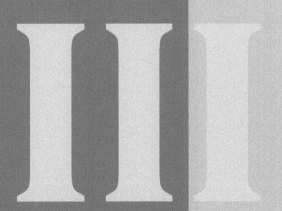

12 Thoracic Spinal Stenosis

Ian A. Buchanan, Jeffrey C. Wang, and Patrick C. Hsieh

Abstract

Thoracic spinal stenosis (TSS) is relatively uncommon compared to its cervical and lumbar counterparts. Perhaps as a consequence, it is an underrecognized cause of neurological sequelae and frequently misdiagnosed on account of the vague nature of its presentation and similarity in symptomatology to cervical and lumbar disorders. There are no standardized criteria for diagnosing TSS and no formal guidelines exist for management. However, surgical decompression is a mainstay in management and the treatment of choice once symptoms have progressed or become progressive. Considerable variation exists in the surgical approach for addressing thoracic stenosis, but the corridor employed is of little import, so long as there is adequate decompression of neural elements without introduction of iatrogenic instability. Several factors have been shown to influence treatment outcomes, most notably the shorter the duration from symptom onset to diagnosis. Timely decompression is therefore imperative to ensuring optimal neurological recovery. As the world's population ages and life expectancy continues to rise, so too will the incidence of TSS and other degenerative spine pathologies. Thorough understanding of the nuances of TSS presentation and management will prove fundamental to successfully navigating a spine surgery practice in the years to come.

Keywords: thoracic myelopathy, thoracic stenosis, thoracic spine, facet hypertrophy, spondylosis, degenerative spine disease, ossification of ligamentum flavum, ossification of posterior longitudinal ligament

---

Clinical Pearls

- Thoracic stenosis is a rare occurrence in the everyday practice of spine surgeons.
- Symptoms can be vague and easily attributed to cervical and lumbar pathologies, hence there is a tendency for delayed diagnosis.
- Identification of thoracic stenosis should prompt an investigation for other stenotic regions due to the high rates of tandem stenosis.
- The shorter the interval from symptom onset to surgery, the higher the likelihood for optimal neurological recovery.
- Surgical decompression is an effective treatment for thoracic stenosis.
- Long-term follow-up is recommended because of the possibility for delayed neurological decline from recurrent or new areas of stenosis.

12.1 Introduction

Thoracic spinal stenosis (TSS) is a rare clinical entity when considered vis-à-vis cervical and lumbar degenerative spine pathologies. Of individuals suffering from spinal stenosis, thoracic disease is estimated to account for less than 1% of cases.[1] Because of its rarity, and close presenting symptomatology to cervical and lumbar variants, TSS is often missed or misdiagnosed, which leads to delayed treatment and, perhaps as a consequence, suboptimal outcomes. As the U.S. population ages, however, the number of individuals aged 65 and above is expected to double by the year 2050.[2] Such a demographic shift heralds increased societal burden from spinal disorders in which there is chronological deterioration with advancing age. Intimate knowledge of the operative and perioperative management of patients with TSS will therefore prove increasingly valuable in a surgeon's armamentarium, as the field of spine surgery evolves around changing demographics.

12.2 Definition of Thoracic Spinal Stenosis

The term "spinal stenosis" can be used broadly to encompass any anatomical narrowing of the spinal canal irrespective of neurological sequelae. Nonetheless, it more commonly denotes a reduced canal dimension that results in cord or nerve root impingement with resulting neurological deterioration as well as detriment to daily functions and overall quality of life.[3] Various TSS cutoffs have been reported in the literature, including an absolute anteroposterior diameter of 10 mm or less.[1,4] In a study of 700 adult cadaveric specimens, detailed sagittal canal diameter and interpedicular distances were determined throughout the thoracic spine and the respective values falling two or more standard deviations below the mean equated with thoracic stenosis. It was discovered that an anteroposterior diameter of 15 mm and an interpedicular distance of 18.5 mm were predictive of congenital stenosis at all levels throughout the thoracic spine with a sensitivity and specificity of 80 and 100%, respectively.[1] Despite such attempts at standardization, no universally accepted quantitative or radiographic criteria have been adopted to date. A formal diagnosis of TSS is therefore dependent on overlap between clinical presentation and radiographic evidence of canal compromise.

By definition, TSS excludes compressive etiologies from thoracic malignancy (primary or metastatic), infection, kyphosis, scoliosis, and trauma.[5] TSS can be classified as primary or secondary in origin. Primary stenosis constitutes a congenitally narrowed canal that over time encroaches on neural elements owing to one or more degenerative precipitants. Causative factors include namely disc extrusion, ossification of the ligamentum flavum (OLF), ossification of the posterior longitudinal ligament (OPLL), facet joint hypertrophy, and osteophytes at the posterior aspect of the vertebral endplates.[5] Conversely, secondary stenosis occurs in the wake of rheumatological, metabolic, or orthopaedic disorders that narrow the spinal canal globally. Conditions commonly implicated include Paget's disease, acromegaly, achondroplasia, rheumatoid arthritis, renal osteodystrophy, diffuse idiopathic skeletal hyperostosis (DISH), ankylosing spondylitis, osteofluorosis, osteochondrodystrophy, familial hypophosphatemic vitamin D–refractory rickets, and Scheuermann's disease.[6,7,8,9]

12.3 Pathophysiology

The spine is subjected to repetitive stresses, over and above routine wear-and-tear, which accumulate throughout one's lifetime and can result in spinal degeneration.[10] The underlying pathophysiological events that account for this breakdown have been termed the *degenerative cascade* and were first proposed by Kirkaldy-Willis et al in the 1970s.[11] It was postulated that repetitive microtrauma to mobile components of the axial spine (i.e., facet joints and intervertebral disc) led to disc tears, synovial reaction, osteophyte formation, and other spondylotic changes that culminated in mechanical deterioration and central stenosis. The original theory was devised with the lumbar spine in mind and has less implications for the thoracic region, which is relatively limited in motion and stable on account of the surrounding rib cage. However, as mobility increases toward the thoracolumbar junction so too does the predilection for TSS,[12,13] underscoring the idea that recurring motion and microtrauma are at least contributory, if not causal, in the pathogenesis of thoracic stenosis as well.

While TSS can exist anywhere along the thoracic spine, a disproportionate number of cases involve caudal segments, namely T10 to T12.[14,15] This is especially true when ossification of the OLF is responsible for TSS.[16,17] Higher incidence of spinal degeneration at the thoracolumbar junction is presumably related to increased mobility as aforementioned. Two factors account for this: first, there is gradual enlargement of the spinal canal in the vicinity of T10 to T12 with transition to floating ribs that lack thoracic articulation ventrally and, second, there is increased axial rotation due to orientation of the zygapophyseal joints.[4] Apropos to the latter, Maigne et al demonstrated that the caudal thoracic spine constituted somewhat of a transitional zone in which vertebrae could take on either a lumbar or thoracic configuration. Those that were more thoracic in anatomical structure permitted greater degrees of rotational freedom and an increased likelihood for TSS from OLF. Conversely, those that were more lumbar-like in shape restricted rotation and were associated with decreased rates of TSS secondary to OLF degeneration.[13] Similar reports detailing differential vertebral configuration in the distal thoracic spine have been confirmed by others albeit with different results: three-dimensional studies of cadaveric thoracic vertebrae by Punjabi et al determined that T10 to T12 vertebrae exhibiting a lumbar phenotype were more predisposed to spondylosis than their thoracic counterparts.[4,12]

OPLL and OLF are two of the most common causes of TSS. Whereas OPLL predominates in the mid- to upper thoracic spine, OLF and disc herniation account for the majority of cases in the lower thoracic spine.[18,19] The genetic factors and cellular processes at play in spinal degeneration and abnormal ossification of spinal ligaments remain obscure, but there have been advances over the years. Recent work has identified bone morphogenetic protein-2 and tissue transglutaminase-2 as key regulators in heterotopic ossification of ligaments.[20] Other key players in chondrogenesis, osteogenesis, and bone mineralization have also been implicated.[21] In addition, roles for various

proinflammatory cytokines, such as TGF-beta, IL-6, IL-12, IL-18, TNF, and VEGF[22] have been established. Polymorphisms for various genes (vitamin D receptor and hyaluronan and proteoglycan link protein 1/HAPLN1) have been linked to intervertebral disc failure and spine degeneration.[23,24]

The finding that tensile train was shown to modulate expression of ossification signaling factors (beta-catenin, Runx2, Sox9, and osteopontin) in cultured human ligamentum flavum cells[25] underscores this idea that biomechanical changes within the spine can, in and of themselves, lead to an overhaul of molecular expression at a cellular level. It is conceivable then that repetitive microtrauma, height loss from intervertebral disc deterioration, or some other precipitant could create perturbations in the strain experienced by facet joints and intraspinal ligaments, ultimately serving as a catalyst for their hypertrophy or ossification and overall spine degradation.

12.4 Clinical Presentation

The average age of presentation for thoracic stenosis is in the 50 s and prevalence is known to increase with age.[18,26,27,28,29] TSS is more common in the male gender (~ 2:1) and people of Japanese or East Asian descent.[18,27,28,30] Presenting symptoms vary with the anatomical level of compression and degree of canal compromise: some present acutely with paraplegia, whereas others exhibit myelopathy with a more insidious onset with vague symptoms persisting for months to years. Such diversity in presentation, coupled with the fact that neurological manifestations are not entirely dissimilar from symptoms encountered in cervical or lumbar disease, makes correct identification of TSS challenging and explains the tendency toward delayed diagnosis or misdiagnosis.[31] Lesions in the upper thoracic spine can present with upper motor neuron symptoms, anywhere along a spectrum from radiculopathy, to myelopathy, to complete motor and sensory loss below the affected level. Conversely, lower thoracic involvement can produce a hybrid picture of both upper and lower motor neuron signs due to impingement on the conus medullaris and upper aspect of the cauda equina.[32,33]

General complaints in TSS include but are not limited to back pain, neurogenic claudication, torso and abdominal radiculopathy, lower extremity sensory and motor disturbance, gait abnormalities, bowel, bladder, and sexual dysfunction. Of these, lower extremity motor and sensory deficits are the most frequently reported on initial presentation.[18,33] In one of the largest retrospective studies of a TSS cohort to date, 81% of patients exhibited motor dysfunction, followed closely by sensory disturbance in 64%.[18] Sphincter dysfunction is evident in only a small proportion of patients and is not a prototypical feature of this disorder.[34,35] However, sphincter dysfunction and saddle anesthesia are more likely when there is involvement of the conus medullaris.[36]

On physical examination, patients may exhibit upper motor neuron signs in the lower extremities, including increased spasticity, hyperactive knee and ankle reflexes, and pathological responses (e.g., Babinski, Chaddock signs). In fact, patellar and Achilles reflex changes have been observed in the majority of patients (70–85%) in some series.[18,28] If stenosis involves the T10 to T12 segment, the physical examination may be complicated by a mixed picture in which there are both upper and lower motor neuron signs in which patients may exhibit patellar tendon hyperreflexia and concomitant Achilles' tendon hyporeflexia.[5]

TSS symptoms can be intermittent if there is dynamic instability at a compressive segment.[37] Several theories have been proposed to explain symptomatology: neurogenic compression theory and vascular compression theory. The former states that symptoms are the direct consequence of mechanical compression of neural elements, while the latter posits that impaired vascular flow at the stenotic level is the root cause.[38] The higher incidence of severe motor rather than sensory deficits reported in the literature lends credence to a vascular hypothesis; the robust vasculature supplying posterior columns more readily resists compression than the tenuous network of anterior and lateral spinal artery perforators which create a watershed zone in the vicinity of anterior gray matter.[4] Although there is no objective data to support one theory over another, it is plausible that both contribute to the eventual neurological decline seen in TSS.

12.5 Diagnostic Modalities

The advent of widely available imaging modalities like magnetic resonance (MR) and computed tomography (CT) have increased the detection rates for spinal stenosis. A diagnosis of TSS can thus be readily rendered so long as clinical suspicion prompts further imaging. Stenotic patterns vary from single to multiple, contiguous or remote, levels throughout the thoracic spine. While TSS can occur in isolation, it is usually accompanied by stenosis in other areas (▶ Fig. 12.1). In a recent retrospective analysis of 427 cases of thoracic stenosis, coexisting disease was identified in the cervical and lumbar regions in 15 and 11% of patients, respectively.[18] High clinical suspicion should therefore

be maintained for tandem pathologies, particularly when the presenting symptoms that led to a diagnosis of TSS are not entirely explained by available radiographic evidence.

Plain radiographs of the thoracic spine with anteroposterior and lateral views can generally be obtained with relative ease and at low cost in a clinic setting and are useful as a screening test. Although somewhat limited in their visualization of the spinal canal because of obstruction from the shoulders and overlying ribs, lateral views can reveal changes that intimate underlying degeneration and stenosis, including disc height loss, shortened pedicles, exuberant hyperostosis, or abnormal ossification (▶ Fig. 12.2). If clinical symptoms are sufficiently concerning, the clinician may forego plain radiographs in favor of more comprehensive imaging modalities.

CT is the preferred technique for depicting osseous anatomy and calcific changes. OPLL, OLF, and calcified discs are accordingly readily identified (▶ Fig. 12.1, ▶ Fig. 12.3a, b). Image acquisition is fast and multiplanar reformats can greatly aid surgical planning. CT is particularly helpful in distinguishing ligament hypertrophy from ossification. Use of intravenous contrast enhancement can also facilitate a diagnosis of disc herniation if there is sufficient thoracic stenosis to impair flow within the epidural venous plexus. However, because compression of neural elements is inferred from reduced canal or neuroforaminal cross-sectional areas, and not directly visualized, it makes CT an unreliable modality for detecting neural impingement. Moreover, it carries the unwanted risks of exposure to ionizing radiation. As a result, it is not ideal for diagnosing TSS and is reserved for scenarios in which MR is contraindicated or where images would otherwise be too degraded from susceptibility artifact caused by implanted hardware.

MR remains the gold standard for diagnosing spinal stenosis because of its high sensitivity, noninvasive functionality, and clear delineation of canal contents, disc pathology, and marrow abnormalities. Additionally, assessment for the attendant

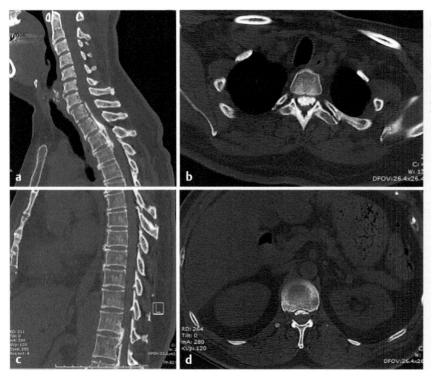

Fig. 12.1 CT images from a patient with tandem thoracic and lumbar ossification of the posterior longitudinal ligament (OPLL). **(a)** Sagittal reconstruction of OPLL extending from T1 to T4. **(b)** There is evidence of severe thoracic stenosis as seen on this axial section. **(c, d)** OPLL is also evident at the thoracolumbar junction bridging T12 to L2 with concomitant narrowing of the lumbar canal.

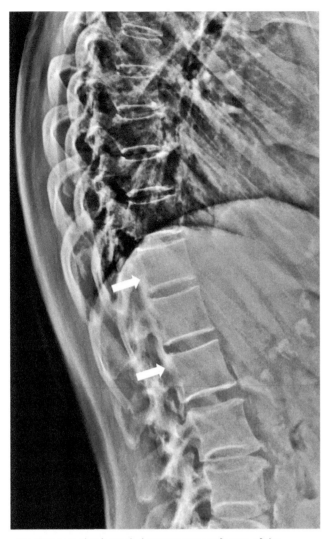

Fig. 12.2 Lateral radiograph demonstrating ossification of the posterior longitudinal ligament at the thoracolumbar junction. Note the ossified segments along the posterior aspect of the vertebral body extending from T12 through L2 (*yellow arrows*).

consequences of compression, such as cord edema or volume loss, allows for predictions regarding the significance of canal narrowing and informs the timing of any surgical interventions. Evaluation for thoracic stenosis is best conducted by systematically reviewing axial and sagittal T2-weighted MR images level by level. Radiographic findings vary with the underlying process at play and degree of neurovascular compression, which spans the gamut from mild deformation of the thecal sac to severe cerebrospinal fluid (CSF) effacement, cord signal change, and myelomalacia. Osteophytes, calcified discs, and calcified ligaments are recognizably hypointense on T1- and T2-weighted fast spin-echo sequences (▶ Fig. 12.3c, d, ▶ Fig. 12.4). Because the facet joints are oriented coronally in the thoracic spine, hypertrophy produces posterolateral compression of the thecal sac which can lead to a trefoil-shaped canal.[32] Finally, gadolinium-enhanced T1 sequences are particularly useful in the detection of infection and neoplasm.

CT myelogram is a viable alternative for cases where MR is inconclusive or simply cannot be performed. It is an invasive technique and subjects the patient to the discomfort and risks that accompany dural puncture for instillation of intrathecal contrast. Despite these risks, it appears to have comparable efficacy to MR in detecting stenosis in other areas of the spine.[39] While myelographic block of contrast can be diagnostic for cord compression, it does not delineate the source of the obstruction as well as MR imaging.

Another diagnostic adjunct worth mentioning is electroneurophysiology. Electromyography and nerve conduction studies are widely used in the preoperative evaluation of cervical and lumbar disorders, but they are seldom employed in thoracic stenosis seeing that the majority of thoracic levels do not have easily testable motor groups. There is, however, a role for somatosensory and motor evoked potentials (SSEP, MEP) in the intraoperative setting where it has proven to be a valid and reliable method for improving spine surgery through early identification of neural damage.[40] Given the potential for neurological deterioration during surgery, multimodality neurophysiological monitoring with SSEP and MEP can provide high sensitivity and specificity for detecting compromise of spinal cord long tracts and preventing irreversible intraoperative neurological injuries.

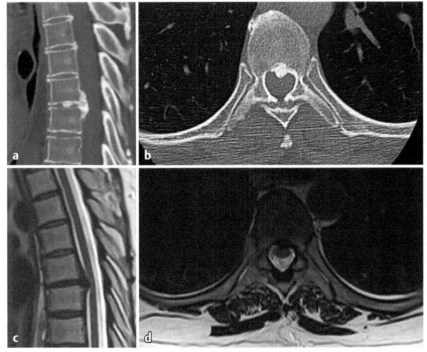

Fig. 12.3 T6-7 spinal stenosis from disc calcification. (a,b) Sagittal and axial CT cuts demonstrating dense calcification of disc space with canal encroachment. (c,d) Ventral compression of thecal sac with intramedullary T2 hyperintensity at level of stenosis indicating cord edema.

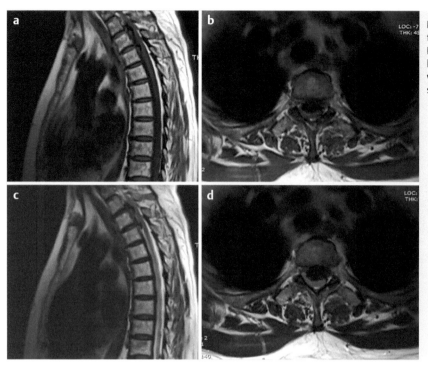

Fig. 12.4 Typical MR findings in ossification of the posterior longitudinal ligament. **(a,b)** Ligament ossification is visualized as a hypointense signal on sagittal and axial T1-weighted sequences and **(c,d)** T2-weighted sequences as well.

12.6 Surgical Management

The caliber of the spinal cord is smallest in the thoracic spine, as is the bony enclave that surrounds it. Compressive pathologies can therefore result in severe neurological manifestations and poor outcomes if not addressed in a timely manner. The problem is further compounded by the tenuous nature of the blood supply to the thoracic cord, and surgery for TSS is decidedly at higher risk than it would be for the cervical or lumbar regions.[36] In the early stages when patients have mild clinical sequelae, nonsteroidal anti-inflammatory drugs, physical therapy, and close follow-up can be pursued. However, once neurological symptoms have progressed or become progressive, surgical interventions are warranted.

Symptomatic TSS is notorious for failing conservative measures,[41,42,43,44] hence surgical decompression is a mainstay in patient management. The optimal surgical approach is dependent on a multitude of factors, namely patient function, underlying comorbidities, number of stenotic levels, and their location within the spinal canal. As a rule of thumb, predominantly dorsal compression is best addressed by laminectomy and medial partial facetectomy. Consistent with the basic tenets of spine surgery, this may be supplemented with posterior instrumentation in cases where there is instability or suspected instability. On the other hand, primarily ventral compression is ideally tackled along a corridor that provides access to the anterior canal and disc space, which include, but are not limited to, anterolateral (transthoracic), lateral (extracavitary), posterolateral (costotransversectomy), and posterior (transpedicular) approaches.[45] These procedures can be performed in conjunction with subtotal corpectomy and are sufficiently destabilizing to the spine so as to require concomitant instrumented fusion. If there is evidence of circumferential compression, then a combination of both anterior and posterior approaches may become necessary (see ▶ Fig. 12.5, ▶ Fig. 12.6).[5,15,46]

Although ventral lesions have been known to be treated with posterior decompression, caution is advised especially in the mid- to lower thoracic spine where physiological kyphosis limits the extent of decompression since the cord cannot migrate backward away from the stenotic site. Additionally, instability can arise and lead to worsening kyphosis, further draping the spinal cord over an already compressive ventral lesion and increasing the likelihood for unfavorable outcomes.[32,47]

Another important operative consideration is the issue of multilevel stenosis. In cases where multiple contiguous segments are involved, the transthoracic approach readily provides access to the vertebral bodies and their respective disc spaces from T4 to the thoracolumbar junction.[45] Additionally, it is well suited to midline lesions and is amenable to repair of ventral dural lacerations. However, TSS is an affliction of the elderly and a transthoracic approach incurs substantial chest and cardiopulmonary morbidity that may at times be deemed unacceptable. In such a situation, posterior decompression may be preferred in high-risk surgical candidates to obviate these risks.

If multiple noncontiguous segments are involved, as is the case with tandem disease in the cervical or lumbar spine, it is important to weigh the severity of clinical symptoms attributable to either in order to address the most offending pathology first. If the stenosis is equally severe in the cervical or lumbar region as in the thoracic spine, then cervical decompression is warranted first to mitigate the risks of quadriplegia in lieu of paraplegia.[48]

12.7 Treatment Outcomes

It is difficult to draw conclusions from the literature in its current form because of the rarity of TSS, small sample sizes of published reports, and considerable variation in patient-related factors (i.e., presentation, location of stenosis, and underlying

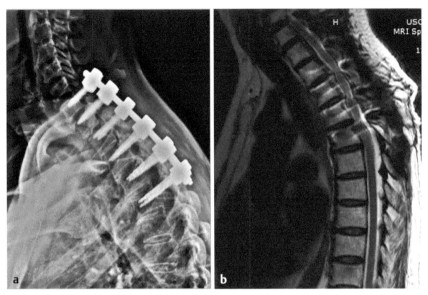

Fig. 12.5 Postoperative images of the patient with thoracic ossification of the posterior longitudinal ligament depicted in ▶ Fig. 12.1a, b, ▶ Fig. 12.4. **(a)** The patient underwent C7-T5 laminectomy and concomitant fusion. **(b)** Postoperative MRI confirms decompression of the thoracic canal with return of cerebrospinal fluid dorsally and ventrally.

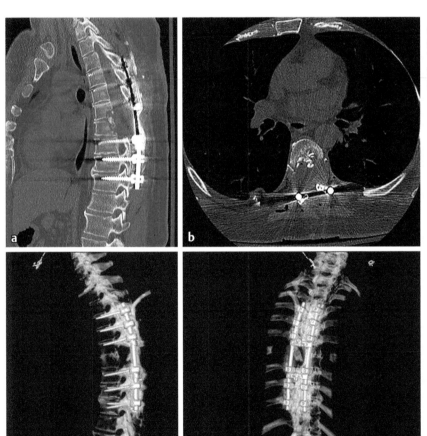

Fig. 12.6 (a-d) Postoperative CT scans of the patient depicted in ▶ Fig. 12.3, who underwent T7 costotransversectomies, resection of and subtotal corpectomies at T6-7 along with T4-10 posterior spinal fusion.

etiology). Moreover, immense differences in surgical management and length of long-term follow-up limit statistical comparison across studies and make distillation of any guidelines premature at best. Several case series and literature reports chronicle outcomes after TSS treatment,[4,9,26,34,46,49] but the long-term consequences of these interventions remain unknown. Based on the few studies that offer evidence for long-term follow-up, surgical results appear durable. However, there can be late progression of symptoms owing to recurrence of stenosis or new instability at junctional segments.[14,15,35,47] These data are instructive in that they emphasize the importance of long-term follow-up and advocate for concomitant fusion in cases where adequate decompression places the patient at risk for destabilization.

In one of the largest series on treatment outcomes featuring 132 patients, Aizawa et al found that length of clinical prodrome correlated with likelihood for improvement postoperatively, with milder symptoms and shorter duration to decompression being significant predictors of a positive outcome.[46] Similar findings have been reported by various groups,[28,32,50] emphasizing early diagnosis and timely decompression as core principles in management. Other notable predictors of outcome include intraoperative blood loss, low intraoperative mean arterial pressures, and tandem stenosis.[32,51,52,53]

Surgical complications after thoracic stenosis surgery can include postoperative hematoma and surgical site infection. Nerve root injury is infrequent, of little import, and tends to occur during posterior approaches to the ventral canal when there is excessive traction on the nerve.[54] CSF leakage from dural violation is a known occurrence and is more common with OPLL and OLF where dural adhesions are expected.[46] Perhaps the most dreaded of complications is acute neurological deterioration (AND), up to and including motor paraplegia. This can occur after a seemingly uneventful course with incidence as high as 33% in published reports.[55,56,57,58] In some cases, the source of demise was treatable (e.g., postoperative hematoma) but in others the etiology remained elusive.[46,55] Cautionary measures have been suggested against AND,[51] but they are no different than would be adhered to at all times: adequate hemostasis, maintenance of mean arterial pressures at or above normal levels, use of high-speed drill to thin hypertrophied or ossified elements, and limiting use of foot-plated instruments like the Kerrison rongeurs against the thoracic dura.

12.8 Conclusions

Lumbar and cervical stenosis are relatively common diagnoses in the daily practice of spine surgeons. By comparison, thoracic stenosis is rarely encountered. As the population ages and life expectancy continues to rise, so too is the projected burden from spinal ailments, TSS included. Due to close similarity in presentation between TSS and other spine pathologies, there is often a delay in diagnosis with detriment to clinical outcomes. There are currently no established diagnostic or treatment guidelines for TSS. Consequently, there is immense variation in operative and postoperative management. It is generally accepted, however, that once there is myelopathy or symptoms become progressive that surgical interventions be pursued. Decompression, be it posterior, anterior or any variation thereof, is an effective treatment so long as mass effect is eliminated from neural elements and iatrogenic instability is not introduced. Although neurological deficits are reversible with surgery, outcomes are influenced by the initial symptom duration, adequacy of decompression, and presence of tandem stenosis. Timely interventions are therefore warranted to halt clinical deterioration and increase likelihood for meaningful functional recovery. Long-term follow-up is also recommended given the tendency for remote neurological decline despite immediate postoperative improvement.

References

[1] Bajwa NS, Toy JO, Ahn NU. Establishment of parameters for congenital thoracic stenosis: a study of 700 postmortem specimens. Clin Orthop Relat Res. 2012; 470(11):3195–3201

[2] Ortman JM, Velkoff VA, Hogan H. An Aging Nation: The Older Population in the United States. Available at: https://www.census.gov/prod/2014pubs/p25–1140.pdf. 2014 Accessed July 9, 2017

[3] Melancia JL, Francisco AF, Antunes JL. Spinal stenosis. Handb Clin Neurol. 2014; 119:541–549

[4] Epstein NE, Schwall G. Thoracic spinal stenosis: diagnostic and treatment challenges. J Spinal Disord. 1994; 7(3):259–269

[5] Chen ZQ, Sun CG, Spine Surgery Group of Chinese Orthopedic Association. Clinical guideline for treatment of symptomatic thoracic spinal stenosis. Orthop Surg. 2015; 7(3):208–212

[6] Fortuna A, Ferrante L, Acqui M, Santoro A, Mastronardi L. Narrowing of thoraco-lumbar spinal canal in achondroplasia. J Neurosurg Sci. 1989; 33(2):185–196

[7] Wagle VG, Rossi AJ, Roberts MP, Goldman R, Ziter F, Clark WE. Thoracic spinal stenosis associated with renal osteodystrophy. Diagnosis based on magnetic resonance imaging and computed tomography. Spine. 1993; 18(10):1373–1375

[8] Wilson FM, Jaspan T. Thoracic spinal cord compression caused by diffuse idiopathic skeletal hyperostosis (DISH). Clin Radiol. 1990; 42(2):133–135

[9] Barnett GH, Hardy RW, Jr, Little JR, Bay JW, Sypert GW. Thoracic spinal canal stenosis. J Neurosurg. 1987; 66(3):338–344

[10] Ha SB, Corriveau M, Strayer A, Trost GR. Geriatric spine. In: Steinmetz MP, Benzel EC, eds. Benzel's Spine Surgery. Techniques, Complication, Avoidance and Management. 4th ed. Philadelphia, PA: Elsevier; 2017

[11] Kirkaldy-Willis WH, Wedge JH, Yong-Hing K, Reilly J. Pathology and pathogenesis of lumbar spondylosis and stenosis. Spine. 1978; 3(4):319–328

[12] Panjabi MM, Takata K, Goel V, et al. Thoracic human vertebrae. Quantitative three-dimensional anatomy. Spine. 1991; 16(8):888–901

[13] Maigne JY, Ayral X, Guérin-Surville H. Frequency and size of ossifications in the caudal attachments of the ligamentum flavum of the thoracic spine. Role of rotatory strains in their development. An anatomic study of 121 spines. Surg Radiol Anat. 1992; 14(2):119–124

[14] Okada K, Oka S, Tohge K, Ono K, Yonenobu K, Hosoya T. Thoracic myelopathy caused by ossification of the ligamentum flavum. Clinicopathologic study and surgical treatment. Spine. 1991; 16(3):280–287

[15] Palumbo MA, Hilibrand AS, Hart RA, Bohlman HH. Surgical treatment of thoracic spinal stenosis: a 2- to 9-year follow-up. Spine. 2001; 26(5):558–566

[16] Guo JJ, Luk KD, Karppinen J, Yang H, Cheung KM. Prevalence, distribution, and morphology of ossification of the ligamentum flavum: a population study of one thousand seven hundred thirty-six magnetic resonance imaging scans. Spine. 2010; 35(1):51–56

[17] Lang N, Yuan HS, Wang HL, et al. Epidemiological survey of ossification of the ligamentum flavum in thoracic spine: CT imaging observation of 993 cases. Eur Spine J. 2013; 22(4):857–862

[18] Hou X, Sun C, Liu X, et al. Clinical features of thoracic spinal stenosis-associated myelopathy: a retrospective analysis of 427 cases. Clin Spine Surg. 2016; 29(2):86–89

[19] Matsumoto M, Toyama Y, Chikuda H, et al. Outcomes of fusion surgery for ossification of the posterior longitudinal ligament of the thoracic spine: a multicenter retrospective survey: clinical article. J Neurosurg Spine. 2011; 15(4):380–385

[20] Yin X, Chen Z, Guo Z, Liu X, Yu H. Tissue transglutaminase expression and activity in human ligamentum flavum cells derived from thoracic ossification of ligamentum flavum. Spine. 2010; 35(20):E1018–E1024

[21] Stapleton CJ, Pham MH, Attenello FJ, Hsieh PC. Ossification of the posterior longitudinal ligament: genetics and pathophysiology. Neurosurg Focus. 2011; 30(3):E6

[22] Ren L, Hu H, Sun X, Li F, Zhou JJ, Wang YM. The roles of inflammatory cytokines in the pathogenesis of ossification of ligamentum flavum. Am J Transl Res. 2013; 5(6):582–585

[23] Videman T, Leppävuori J, Kaprio J, et al. Intragenic polymorphisms of the vitamin D receptor gene associated with intervertebral disc degeneration. Spine. 1998; 23(23):2477–2485

[24] Urano T, Narusawa K, Shiraki M, et al. Single-nucleotide polymorphism in the hyaluronan and proteoglycan link protein 1 (HAPLN1) gene is associated with spinal osteophyte formation and disc degeneration in Japanese women. Eur Spine J. 2011; 20(4):572–577

[25] Cai HX, Yayama T, Uchida K, et al. Cyclic tensile strain facilitates the ossification of ligamentum flavum through β-catenin signaling pathway: in vitro analysis. Spine. 2012; 37(11):E639–E646

[26] Hitchon PW, Abode-Iyamah K, Dahdaleh NS, et al. Risk factors and outcomes in thoracic stenosis with myelopathy: a single center experience. Clin Neurol Neurosurg. 2016; 147:84–89

[27] Aizawa T, Sato T, Sasaki H, Kusakabe T, Morozumi N, Kokubun S. Thoracic myelopathy caused by ossification of the ligamentum flavum: clinical features and surgical results in the Japanese population. J Neurosurg Spine. 2006; 5(6):514–519

[28] Kang KC, Lee CS, Shin SK, Park SJ, Chung CH, Chung SS. Ossification of the ligamentum flavum of the thoracic spine in the Korean population. J Neurosurg Spine. 2011; 14(4):513–519

[29] Fehlings MG, Tetreault L, Nater A, et al. The aging of the global population: the changing epidemiology of disease and spinal disorders. Neurosurgery. 2015; 77 Suppl 4:S1–S5

[30] Yang Z, Xue Y, Dai Q, et al. Upper facet joint en bloc resection for the treatment of thoracic myelopathy caused by ossification of the ligamentum flavum. J Neurosurg Spine. 2013; 19(1):81–89

[31] Toribatake Y, Baba H, Kawahara N, Mizuno K, Tomita K. The epiconus syndrome presenting with radicular-type neurological features. Spinal Cord. 1997; 35(3):163–170

[32] Chang UK, Choe WJ, Chung CK, Kim HJ. Surgical treatment for thoracic spinal stenosis. Spinal Cord. 2001; 39(7):362–369

[33] Takenaka S, Kaito T, Hosono N, et al. Neurological manifestations of thoracic myelopathy. Arch Orthop Trauma Surg. 2014; 134(7):903–912

[34] Marzluff JM, Hungerford GD, Kempe LG, Rawe SE, Trevor R, Perot PL, Jr. Thoracic myelopathy caused by osteophytes of the articular processes: thoracic spondylosis. J Neurosurg. 1979; 50(6):779–783

[35] Yamamoto I, Matsumae M, Ikeda A, Shibuya N, Sato O, Nakamura K. Thoracic spinal stenosis: experience with seven cases. J Neurosurg. 1988; 68(1):37–40

[36] Feng FB, Sun CG, Chen ZQ. Progress on clinical characteristics and identification of location of thoracic ossification of the ligamentum flavum. Orthop Surg. 2015; 7(2):87–96

[37] Kikuchi S, Watanabe E, Hasue M. Spinal intermittent claudication due to cervical and thoracic degenerative spine disease. Spine. 1996; 21(3):313–318

[38] Rosenbloom SA. Thoracic disc disease and stenosis. Radiol Clin North Am. 1991; 29(4):765–775

[39] Kreiner DS, Shaffer WO, Baisden JL, et al. North American Spine Society. An evidence-based clinical guideline for the diagnosis and treatment of degenerative lumbar spinal stenosis (update). Spine J. 2013; 13(7):734–743

[40] Eggspuehler A, Sutter MA, Grob D, Porchet F, Jeszenszky D, Dvorak J. Multimodal intraoperative monitoring (MIOM) during surgical decompression of thoracic spinal stenosis in 36 patients. Eur Spine J. 2007; 16 Suppl 2:S216–S220

[41] Kuh SU, Kim YS, Cho YE, et al. Contributing factors affecting the prognosis surgical outcome for thoracic OLF. Eur Spine J. 2006; 15(4):485–491

[42] Hirabayashi H, Ebara S, Takahashi J, et al. Surgery for thoracic myelopathy caused by ossification of the ligamentum flavum. Surg Neurol. 2008; 69(2):114–116, discussion 116

[43] Ando K, Imagama S, Ito Z, et al. Predictive factors for a poor surgical outcome with thoracic ossification of the ligamentum flavum by multivariate analysis: a multicenter study. Spine. 2013; 38(12):E748–E754

[44] Park BC, Min WK, Oh CW, et al. Surgical outcome of thoracic myelopathy secondary to ossification of ligamentum flavum. Joint Bone Spine. 2007; 74(6):600–605

[45] Kojima T, Waga S, Kubo Y, Matsubara T. Surgical treatment of ossification of the posterior longitudinal ligament in the thoracic spine. Neurosurgery. 1994; 34(5):854–858, discussion 858

[46] Aizawa T, Sato T, Sasaki H, et al. Results of surgical treatment for thoracic myelopathy: minimum 2-year follow-up study in 132 patients. J Neurosurg Spine. 2007; 7(1):13–20

[47] Fujimura Y, Nishi Y, Nakamura M, Toyama Y, Suzuki N. Long-term follow-up study of anterior decompression and fusion for thoracic myelopathy resulting from ossification of the posterior longitudinal ligament. Spine. 1997; 22(3):305–311

[48] Matsumoto Y, Harimaya K, Doi T, et al. Clinical characteristics and surgical outcome of the symptomatic ossification of ligamentum flavum at the thoracic level with combined lumbar spinal stenosis. Arch Orthop Trauma Surg. 2012; 132(4):465–470

[49] Smith DE, Godersky JC. Thoracic spondylosis: an unusual cause of myelopathy. Neurosurgery. 1987; 20(4):589–593

[50] Inamasu J, Guiot BH. A review of factors predictive of surgical outcome for ossification of the ligamentum flavum of the thoracic spine. J Neurosurg Spine. 2006; 5(2):133–139

[51] Wang H, Ma L, Xue R, et al. The incidence and risk factors of postoperative neurological deterioration after posterior decompression with or without instrumented fusion for thoracic myelopathy. Medicine (Baltimore). 2016; 95 (49):e5519

[52] Onishi E, Yasuda T, Yamamoto H, Iwaki K, Ota S. Outcomes of surgical treatment for thoracic myelopathy: a single-institutional study of 73 patients. Spine. 2016; 41(22):E1356–E1363

[53] Fushimi K, Miyamoto K, Hioki A, Hosoe H, Takeuchi A, Shimizu K. Neurological deterioration due to missed thoracic spinal stenosis after decompressive lumbar surgery: A report of six cases of tandem thoracic and lumbar spinal stenosis. Bone Joint J. 2013; 95-B(10):1388–1391

[54] He B, Yan L, Xu Z, Guo H, Liu T, Hao D. Treatment strategies for the surgical complications of thoracic spinal stenosis: a retrospective analysis of two hundred and eighty three cases. Int Orthop. 2014; 38(1):117–122

[55] Young WF, Baron E. Acute neurologic deterioration after surgical treatment for thoracic spinal stenosis. J Clin Neurosci. 2001; 8(2):129–132

[56] Takahata M, Ito M, Abumi K, Kotani Y, Sudo H, Minami A. Clinical results and complications of circumferential spinal cord decompression through a single posterior approach for thoracic myelopathy caused by ossification of posterior longitudinal ligament. Spine. 2008; 33(11):1199–1208

[57] Li M, Meng H, Du J, Tao H, Luo Z, Wang Z. Management of thoracic myelopathy caused by ossification of the posterior longitudinal ligament combined with ossification of the ligamentum flavum—a retrospective study. Spine J. 2012; 12(12):1093–1102

[58] Yamazaki M, Mochizuki M, Ikeda Y, et al. Clinical results of surgery for thoracic myelopathy caused by ossification of the posterior longitudinal ligament: operative indication of posterior decompression with instrumented fusion. Spine. 2006; 31(13):1452–1460

13 Paracentral Disc Herniations of the Thoracic Spine

David S. Xu and Laura A. Snyder

Abstract

Paracentral disc herniations of the thoracic spine are uncommon pathological entities. Patients have diverse clinical presentations and require surgical therapy to treat motor deficits or intractable sensory disturbances caused by the condition. Although anterior surgical approaches are frequently employed for both central and paracentral thoracic disc herniations, posterior approaches are a common viable option for the latter. Multiple approach options exist, and careful selection of the appropriate treatment strategy must take into account the anatomy of the disc herniation, patient habitus, and surgeon comfort.

Keywords: back pain, discectomy, myelopathy, radiculopathy, thoracic disc herniation

Clinical Pearls

- Thoracic disc herniations are uncommon and patients can present with expected symptoms, such as radicular pain and myelopathy, as well as atypical symptoms, such as dysesthetic chest and abdominal pain.
- Preoperative workup should include magnetic resonance imaging and computed tomography to identify the degree of disc calcification.
- Adequate preoperative imaging to determine landmarks for identification of correct spinal levels is critical, and surgeons should consider placement of an intraosseous fiducial.
- Aside from anterior approaches, multiple posterior approaches can be used for discectomy, and approach selection should focus on how oblique a trajectory is needed to access the disc space and the herniated disc fragment.
- A transdural approach can be used successfully to reduce the obliquity of the surgical trajectory needed for discectomy.
- Pedicle screw instrumentation should be used in most cases to allow early postoperative mobility and facilitate greater intraoperative removal of bony elements.

13.1 Introduction

Thoracic disc herniations are uncommon, comprising less than 1% of all symptomatic disc herniations with an incidence of approximately 1 in 1 million persons.[1,2] On the basis of the limited evidence in the medical literature, the natural history of thoracic disc herniations is unclear. Approximately 75% of patients with small disc herniations or asymptomatic individuals with an incidental diagnosis can remain clinically stable on follow-up and may not require further treatment.[3,4] Those who become symptomatic or who have radiographic evidence of spinal cord compression require surgical intervention. This chapter focuses on surgical strategies for paracentral thoracic disc herniations, with a focus on posterior approaches. Anterior approaches, either through an open transthoracic approach or with a thorascope port access technique, are suitable for paracentral discs, but are used more frequently to treat midline or giant disc herniations; these approaches are discussed elsewhere in this book.

13.2 Preoperative Considerations

13.2.1 Clinical Presentation

Symptoms of thoracic disc herniation are varied and include multiple sensory and motor manifestations that depend on the anatomical configuration of the disc herniation.[2] Paracentral disc herniations may impinge on exiting or passing thoracic nerve roots, causing radicular or dysesthetic pain along the back, chest wall, abdomen, or viscera.[5,6] Larger disc herniations that cause mass effect on the thecal sac can result in motor deficits and myelopathy.

13.2.2 Preoperative Workup

Patients with suspected thoracic disc disease initially should undergo magnetic resonance imaging (MRI) (▶ Fig. 13.1a) followed by computed tomography (CT) if a herniated disc is confirmed and the patient is deemed to require surgical intervention. The addition of CT-based imaging allows the extent of disc calcification to be visualized, which can guide selection of the surgical approach (▶ Fig. 13.1b, c). Disc calcification is common and was found in 65% of cases (53 of 82 discs) in a large clinical series.[7] Extensive, densely calcified discs are more difficult to mobilize intraoperatively or may be fused to the dura and thus require a larger exposure and potentially an anterior approach to resect and repair the thecal sac.

Additional preoperative imaging should also be pursued to aid intraoperative verification of the correct surgical level. Misidentification of the surgical level is a devastating complication in thoracic disc surgery, and it is a common cause of patients requiring reoperation.[8] Full visualization of landmark anatomy, such as rib heads, must be obtained preoperatively. For obese patients or those with variant anatomy, intraoperative fluoroscopic image quality is likely to be poor, so a preoperative intraosseous CT-guided radiographic fiducial can be placed in the pedicle or transverse process adjacent to the disc herniation. The fiducial allows easy confirmation of the appropriate level during surgery (▶ Fig. 13.1d). Unfortunately, this tool is frequently underutilized.

13.3 Surgical Technique

13.3.1 Selection of Approach

The earliest surgical experience with resection of herniated thoracic discs relied on laminectomy alone and resulted in major morbidity rates ranging from 18 to 75%.[1,9] Several explanations may account for these poor results, but the most widely accepted is that a laminectomy by itself does not provide

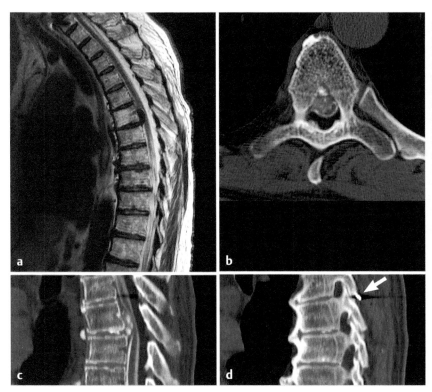

Fig. 13.1 **(a)** Sagittal T2-weighted magnetic resonance image (MRI) shows a large disc herniation at the T6-7 interspace with cranial migration behind the T6 vertebral body. **(b)** Axial and **(c)** sagittal thoracic computed tomography (CT) images show mixed calcification within the herniated disc with a right paracentral location. **(d)** Sagittal CT shows an intraosseous fiducial (*arrow*) that was placed within the left T6 transverse process at the level of the pedicle. (Used with permission from Barrow Neurological Institute, Phoenix, Arizona.)

enough lateral exposure of the underlying disc space, necessitating manipulation of the thecal sac, which may cause mechanical injury. Consequently, a myriad of alternative surgical approaches with progressive degrees of removal of bony elements has been developed and described to facilitate safe discectomy. Commonly referenced approaches include transfacet pedicle-sparing,[10] transpedicular,[11] costo-transversectomy,[12] lateral extracavitary,[13] and, more recently, transdural approaches.[14,15]

Choosing an appropriate approach can initially be daunting because of the number of options, their technical nuances, and the comfort level of the surgeon. To simplify the decision-making process, we recommend a cognitive framework centered on how much bone must be removed to adequately access and visualize the disc herniation. ▶ Fig. 13.2a shows an axial view of the bony elements that must be removed to visualize the thecal sac and underlying disc herniation, as well as the corresponding trajectories that can be used after removal. As seen in ▶ Fig. 13.2b, proceeding from midline to lateral requires the incremental removal of the bony elements (i.e., lamina, facet, pedicle, transverse process, and rib heads) that must be removed to allow increasingly more oblique access to the disc space. Factors that favor limiting the removal of bony elements to only the lamina and facet include disc herniations located more laterally, limited disc calcifications, and thin patients, as these factors allow a shorter working distance and consequently require a less oblique approach to visualize the disc space. More extensive removal of bony elements that encompasses the pedicle, transverse process, rib head, and varying degrees of the rib body is needed to visualize medially located discs, to access the disc in obese patients with a longer working distance, and to remove heavily calcified discs.

13.3.2 Instrumentation

Considerable discussion exists on whether instrumented fusion should be performed with thoracic discectomy.[16] In general, aside from situations in which only limited unilateral facet removal is performed in a healthy patient without abnormal curvature or preoperative back pain, we recommend concurrent placement of pedicle screw instrumentation and arthrodesis during discectomy for several reasons. The first is that pedicle screw placement allows for more aggressive removal of bony elements without concern for causing spinal instability, and it removes the psychological barrier, especially for less experienced surgeons, to achieving greater exposure when it is needed intraoperatively. Second, pedicle screws allow safe intervertebral distraction, facilitating dissection and mobilization of the herniated disc. Lastly, segmental arthrodesis secures physiological thoracic alignment, and in theory facilitates postoperative mobilization by reducing increased motion across the operative segment.

13.3.3 Extradural Discectomy

After the appropriate approach is selected, surgery proceeds in the following stepwise fashion at our institution. Patients are positioned prone on a Jackson table (Mizuho OSI, Union City, CA), and the incision is planned using anteroposterior and lateral fluoroscopy. A midline incision and dissection are adequate for the majority of patients, but a paramedian incision 2 cm off midline, ipsilateral to the side of disc herniation, may be used if an extremely oblique surgical trajectory is planned. The exposure of bony elements encompasses the medial facet border on

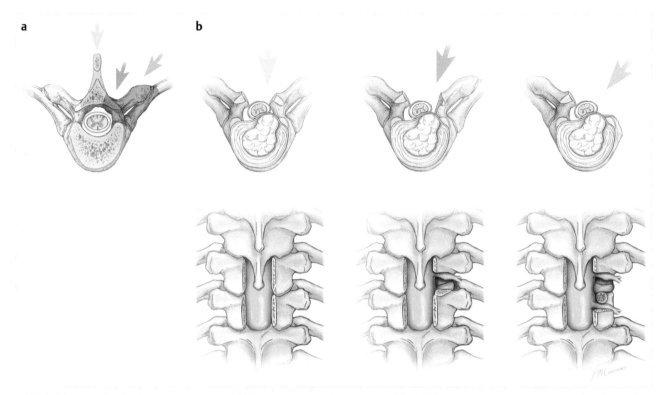

Fig. 13.2 Artist's illustrations of thoracic vertebra. **(a)** Axial view demonstrates the areas of bone that can be removed; color coding corresponds to the angle of obliquity attained during surgical dissection. **(b)** Three columns of axial (*top*) and coronal (*bottom*) overhead views further demonstrate the extent of exposure gained with incremental removal of bony elements. The green region corresponds to the lamina, which requires a straight-on angle of approach, with little visualization beyond the lateral margin of the thecal sac that necessitates manipulation of the neural elements to access the disc. The blue region corresponds to the facet complex that, when removed, allows visualization beyond the lateral margin of the thecal sac and the lateral disc annulus. The red region represents the lateral bony elements, including the pedicle, transverse process, rib head, and rib body. When the lateral bony elements are removed, their absence allows a very oblique angle of surgical approach, suitable for medially located discs and for patients with a large body habitus. (Used with permission from Barrow Neurological Institute, Phoenix, Arizona.)

the contralateral side to the ipsilateral transverse process or farther along the rib head.

The removal of bony elements then proceeds with bilateral laminectomies. In patients in whom conservative removal without instrumentation is planned, laminotomies may be performed instead of laminectomies, thereby preserving the dorsal interspinous ligaments. Facetectomies are then performed with either a Kerrison rongeur aimed out of the neuroforamen or a high-speed drill in patients with severe spinal stenosis in order to minimize manipulation of the thecal sac by surgical instruments. The pedicle is resected next, by using either an osteotome cut from the medial pedicle border directed laterally or by drilling down the cancellous interior with a high-speed drill followed by removal of the cortical bone with a rongeur. If additional rib head and body resection is needed, it is achieved by dissecting the ventral parietal pleura off the ventral rib with a rib periosteal elevator or a Cobb elevator, followed by resection of the rib with rongeurs.

After adequate exposure is achieved, discectomy proceeds under high-loupe or operative-microscope magnification. The next and most important step is to make a large working "cavity" within either the disc space or vertebral body to allow mobilization of the herniated disc. This is achieved by first incising the posterior longitudinal ligament and the disc

annulus. Then the disc space is cleared by curettes, and the vertebral body is cleared by drilling. After a large working cavity is made, the ventral surface of the thecal sac is dissected free from the herniated disc with a flat dissector, such as a dental tool, and is pushed ventrally into the cavity. If the disc herniation is large, medially located, or its interface with the thecal sac is difficult to visualize, the nerve root may be tied off, cut, and gently retracted in the contralateral direction to allow additional medial visualization of the disc herniation. Sacrifice of the nerve root should not be done in the territory of the artery of Adamkiewicz, which is found on the left side from T9 to T12 in 70% of patients.[17]

Case Example: Extradural Transpedicular Approach

A 70-year-old man presented with progressive immobility due to lower extremity weakness, myelopathy, and left chest pain. MRI demonstrated a large disc herniation at T6-7, with upward migration causing frank mass effect on the thecal sac and displacing it leftward (▶ Fig. 13.1a, b). Additional CT imaging demonstrated minimal calcification, and a fiducial was placed above the T6 pedicle (▶ Fig. 13.1c, d). The patient underwent a right transpedicular approach with resection of the right T6 pedicle, pedicle screw fixation from T6 to T9, and partial corpectomy of the T6 body to create a working cavity (▶ Fig. 13.3a). Intraoperatively, multiple large disc fragments were pushed into the working cavity and removed (▶ Fig. 13.3b). The patient remained neurologically stable postoperatively and at follow-up 1 year later had recovered his full strength and was ambulatory. Repeat MRI at the 1-year follow-up showed full decompression of the spinal cord with mild myelomalacia (▶ Fig. 13.3d).

13.3.4 Transdural Discectomy

Initially described in 2010, the resection of paracentral herniated thoracic discs can be performed in a transdural fashion,

which confers two advantages.[14,15] First, by dividing the dentate ligaments that support the spinal cord and using them as a source of retraction, the surgeon can gently yet substantially roll the spinal cord laterally. Displacement of the spinal cord allows better visualization of medial herniated discs, permits a less oblique surgical trajectory that aids surgery in obese patients, and reduces the need for aggressive lateral removal of bony elements in thin patients (▶ Fig. 13.4). Second, division of the dentate ligaments reduces the tautness of the spinal cord and, in theory, may dampen forces inadvertently transmitted to the cord during discectomy.[18]

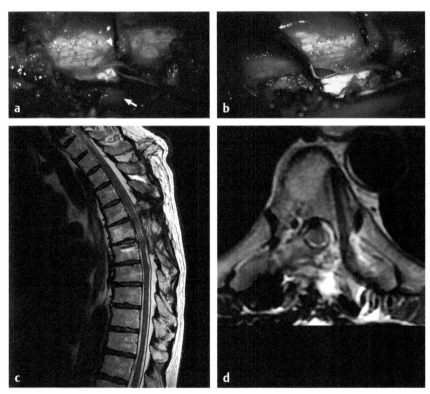

Fig. 13.3 **(a)** Intraoperative photograph from a right transpedicular approach to a T6-7 disc demonstrates the creation of a large working cavity (*arrow*) after removal of the T6 pedicle and part of the vertebral body. The T6 nerve root is sutured and ligated, and the stump is used for gentle medial retraction (*arrowhead*) to facilitate exposure and dissection of the underlying disc fragment. **(b)** Intraoperative photograph shows dissection of the ventral epidural plane with a dental tool, which frees the herniated disc fragment and allows it to be pushed ventrally into the working cavity away from the thecal sac. **(c)** Sagittal T2-weighted magnetic resonance image (MRI) obtained 1 year postoperatively reveals full decompression of the thecal sac at the index level of surgery with mild myelomalacia. **(d)** An axial T2-weighted MRI at the level just below the T6 pedicles reveals full decompression of the spinal canal and absence of the right T6 pedicle. (Used with permission from Barrow Neurological Institute, Phoenix, Arizona.)

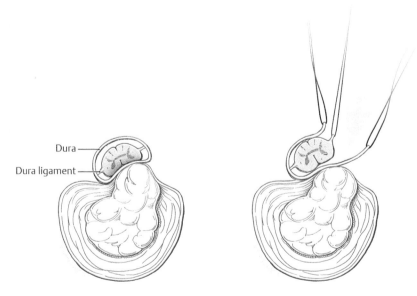

Fig. 13.4 Artist's illustration of an axial view of a paracentral thoracic herniated disc before (*left*) and after (*right*) a transdural approach demonstrates lateral mobilization and rolling of the spinal cord away from and off the herniated disc after resection of the dentate ligament and use of it as a point for mild retraction. This procedure permits a less oblique surgical approach angle to be used safely for performance of the discectomy. (Used with permission from Barrow Neurological Institute, Phoenix, Arizona.)

Dura

Dura ligament

A transdural approach is performed by making a longitudinal incision in the thecal sac approximately 1 cm off midline ipsilateral to the disc herniation. The dura is tacked up, and the dentate ligaments are identified and divided. Additional tack-up sutures can be applied to the divided dentate ligament or to the nerve root to allow contralateral mobilization of the spinal cord. The ventral dura is then incised, and a discectomy is performed. Closure of the ventral dura is performed with an onlay graft, with or without microsutures, and the dorsal longitudinal dural incision is closed with direct repair and biological sealant.

Case Example: Intradural Facetectomy with a Pedicle-Sparing Approach

A 68-year-old woman presented to our institution with progressive loss of ambulation due to severe atypical chest pain involving her right side that occasionally radiated from her back. A thoracic MRI demonstrated a disc herniation at T6-7, impinging the thecal sac, as well as a smaller disc bulge at T7-8 abutting the dura (▶ Fig. 13.5a). CT imaging further demonstrated the T6-7 disc to be partially calcified and eccentric to

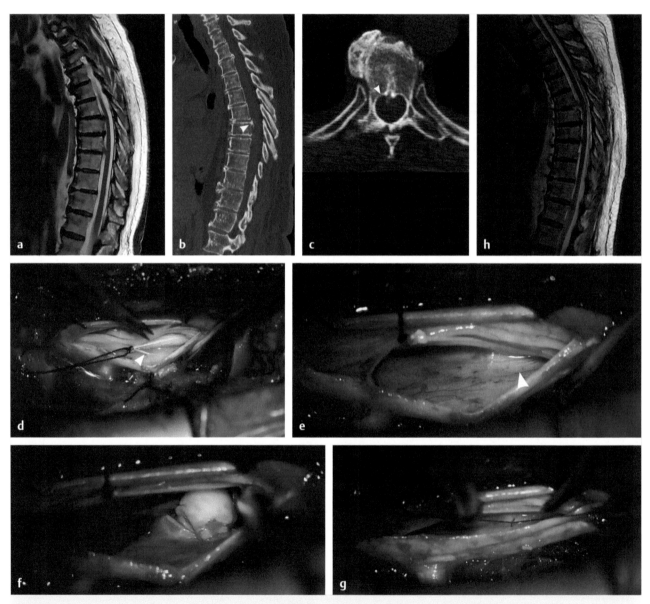

Fig. 13.5 (a) Sagittal T2-weighted magnetic resonance imaging (MRI) demonstrates a disc herniation at T6-7 impinging on the spinal cord, as well as a small disc bulge at T7-8. (b) Sagittal computed tomogram (CT) reveals speckles of calcification in the herniated disc (arrowhead), whereas (c) axial CT shows speckles of calcification in a right paracentral location (arrowhead). (d) Intraoperative view of a right-sided transdural transfacet approach to the herniated disc shows the initial exposure after opening the dura with the leaflets tacked up and the dentate ligament sutured. The attachment of the dentate ligament to the dura is identified (arrowhead), which when severed will allow contralateral mobilization of the spinal cord. (e) After the dentate ligament is cut and used to gently retract the spinal cord laterally, much of the medial ventral intradural space can be seen, as well as a bulge corresponding to the location of the disc herniation (arrowhead). (f) The ventral dura is opened along with the posterior longitudinal ligament, revealing a calcified piece of herniated disc that is freely mobilized and removed. (g) After completion of the discectomy, the ventral dural opening can be reapproximated with interrupted microsutures. (h) Immediate postoperative sagittal T2-weighted MRI shows adequate discectomy and decompression of the T6-7 level. (Used with permission from Barrow Neurological Institute, Phoenix, Arizona.)

the right (▶ Fig. 13.5b, c). The more medial location of the herniated disc in this patient required a transdural transfacet approach, with sparing of the pedicle (▶ Fig. 13.5d–g). Postoperatively, the patient reported relief of chest pain and was able to ambulate independently. An immediate postoperative MRI showed adequate discectomy and decompression of the thecal sac (▶ Fig. 13.5h).

13.3.5 Complications and Outcomes

Literature reviews of reported morbidity and mortality associated with posterior approaches to herniated thoracic discs have demonstrated consistently low rates of adverse events for specific approaches, ranging from 1.4 to 5.5% for neurological deterioration; only one incidence of mortality has been reported for a patient who died due to postoperative pulmonary embolism after undergoing a lateral extracavitary approach.[1,9,19] The limitations of these studies must be considered when trying to infer and stratify risk indices for individual approaches because published cases only represent a small fraction of the total number of cases that are performed. Furthermore, outcome studies are not direct representations of the surgical approach alone, rather reflect the underlying disc pathology that guides surgical planning. Each approach has its own advantages and disadvantages, and the overall low rates of reported complication suggest that when posterior thoracic discectomies are thoughtfully planned, the surgery can be performed in a safe manner with relatively low risk to the patient.

13.4 Postoperative Care

Postoperative care is provided in the intensive care unit for the first 24 hours after surgery. Antibiotic prophylaxis should not be routinely used postoperatively; however, when used, antibiotic prophylaxis should be limited to less than 24 hours of care.[20] Early patient mobilization is essential to prevent pulmonary complications, regardless of whether an intradural approach or an inadvertent durotomy was encountered. In terms of additional imaging, CT can be performed to verify the correct level of surgery and additional MRI or CT myelogram should be pursued if the patient has unexpected or worsening neurological deficits.

13.5 Conclusion

Paracentral thoracic disc herniations are uncommon entities that frequently do not require further treatment. Patients with motor deficits or intractable sensory symptoms require surgical discectomy, which can be successfully achieved through a variety of anterior and posterior approaches. When deciding on a posterior approach, the selection process should center on the anatomical configuration of the herniated disc, with particular attention paid to the surgical trajectory required to access the disc that minimizes the need for manipulation of the thecal sac and spinal cord.

References

[1] McCormick WE, Will SF, Benzel EC. Surgery for thoracic disc disease. Complication avoidance: overview and management. Neurosurg Focus. 2000; 9(4): e13

[2] Dietze DD, Jr, Fessler RG. Thoracic disc herniations. Neurosurg Clin N Am. 1993; 4(1):75–90

[3] Brown CW, Deffer PA, Jr, Akmakjian J, Donaldson DH, Brugman JL. The natural history of thoracic disc herniation. Spine. 1992; 17(6) Suppl:S97–S102

[4] Wood KB, Blair JM, Aepple DM, et al. The natural history of asymptomatic thoracic disc herniations. Spine. 1997; 22(5):525–529, discussion 529–530

[5] Lara FJP, Berges AF, Quesada JQ, Ramiro JAM, Toledo RB, Muñoz HO. Thoracic disk herniation, a not infrequent cause of chronic abdominal pain. Int Surg. 2012; 97(1):27–33

[6] Shirzadi A, Drazin D, Jeswani S, Lovely L, Liu J. Atypical presentation of thoracic disc herniation: case series and review of the literature. Case Rep Orthop. 2013; 2013:621476

[7] Stillerman CB, Chen TC, Couldwell WT, Zhang W, Weiss MH. Experience in the surgical management of 82 symptomatic herniated thoracic discs and review of the literature. J Neurosurg. 1998; 88(4):623–633

[8] Dickman CA, Rosenthal D, Regan JJ. Reoperation for herniated thoracic discs. J Neurosurg. 1999; 91(2) Suppl:157–162

[9] Fessler RG, Sturgill M. Review: complications of surgery for thoracic disc disease. Surg Neurol. 1998; 49(6):609–618

[10] Bransford R, Zhang F, Bellabarba C, Konodi M, Chapman JR. Early experience treating thoracic disc herniations using a modified transfacet pedicle-sparing decompression and fusion. J Neurosurg Spine. 2010; 12(2):221–231

[11] Le Roux PD, Haglund MM, Harris AB. Thoracic disc disease: experience with the transpedicular approach in twenty consecutive patients. Neurosurgery. 1993; 33(1):58–66

[12] Simpson JM, Silveri CP, Simeone FA, Balderston RA, An HS. Thoracic disc herniation. Re-evaluation of the posterior approach using a modified costotransversectomy. Spine. 1993; 18(13):1872–1877

[13] Maiman DJ, Larson SJ, Luck E, El-Ghatit A. Lateral extracavitary approach to the spine for thoracic disc herniation: report of 23 cases. Neurosurgery. 1984; 14(2):178–182

[14] Moon SJ, Lee JK, Jang JW, Hur H, Lee JH, Kim SH. The transdural approach for thoracic disc herniations: a technical note. Eur Spine J. 2010; 19(7):1206–1211

[15] Coppes MH, Bakker NA, Metzemaekers JD, Groen RJ. Posterior transdural discectomy: a new approach for the removal of a central thoracic disc herniation. Eur Spine J. 2012; 21(4):623–628

[16] Wakefield AE, Steinmetz MP, Benzel EC. Biomechanics of thoracic discectomy. Neurosurg Focus. 2001; 11(3):E6

[17] Yoshioka K, Niinuma H, Ehara S, Nakajima T, Nakamura M, Kawazoe K. MR angiography and CT angiography of the artery of Adamkiewicz: state of the art. Radiographics. 2006; 26 Suppl 1:S63–S73

[18] Tubbs RS, Salter G, Grabb PA, Oakes WJ. The denticulate ligament: anatomy and functional significance. J Neurosurg. 2001; 94(2) Suppl:271–275

[19] Ridenour TR, Haddad SF, Hitchon PW, Piper J, Traynelis VC, Van Gilder JC. Herniated thoracic disks: treatment and outcome. J Spinal Disord. 1993; 6(3):218–224

[20] Bratzler DW, Dellinger EP, Olsen KM, et al. American Society of Health-System Pharmacists, Infectious Disease Society of America, Surgical Infection Society, Society for Healthcare Epidemiology of America. Clinical practice guidelines for antimicrobial prophylaxis in surgery. Am J Health Syst Pharm. 2013; 70 (3):195–283

14 Midline Disc Herniations of the Thoracic Spine

Shashank V. Gandhi, Jacob Januszewski, and Juan S. Uribe

Abstract

Symptomatic midline thoracic disc herniations (TDHs) are uncommon. Typically, TDHs are degenerative in nature, presenting with back pain progressing to myelopathy. Thorough physical examination and proper diagnostic imaging are vital as symptomatology can initially be difficult to isolate to the thoracic spine. The majority of cases can be treated conservatively; however, early surgery is key in the presence of neurological compromise or unremitting pain. Calcification and location must be evaluated, as preoperative planning is dependent on these characteristics. Posterior decompressive laminectomies are not recommended due to a high risk of neurological deterioration. Ideal surgical approaches to thoracic spine for midline disc herniations allow direct exposure of the herniation with minimal to no spinal cord manipulation. The majority of patients improve with timely and appropriate surgical intervention; however, there is a real risk of neurological deficits with surgery.

Keywords: midline, thoracic, disc herniation, calcified, transpedicular, costotransversectomy, lateral extracavitary, myelopathy

---

Clinical Pearls

- The majority of midline thoracic disc herniations (TDHs) are asymptomatic. Of the symptomatic cases, approximately 63% may be treated with conservative management.
- Midline TDHs are more likely to cause myelopathy than lateral TDHs.
- Early surgical management in patients with myelopathy is recommended to avoid rapid deterioration.
- About 70% of TDHs are calcified, requiring appropriate preoperative planning to gain optimal midline and ventral exposure.
- Confirmation of spinal level with intraoperative fluoroscopy or preoperative radiographic tagging/marking and correlation to preoperative imaging is vital.
- Laminectomy for access to midline disc is not recommended due to high risk of neurological deterioration.
- Minimally invasive lateral and anterior transthoracic approaches have lower risk of new postoperative neurological deficits and are best for calcified midline TDH.
- Instrumented fusion should be considered when extensive bone resection is conducted and instability is suspected.

14.1 Epidemiology

The true incidence of thoracic disc herniations (TDHs) is difficult to ascertain as many tend to be asymptomatic; however, it is estimated that 1 in 1 million people per year develop symptoms at some point.[1] In stark contrast to the cervical and lumbar regions, the thoracic spine accounts for 0.25 to 0.75% of all symptomatic disc herniations, representing 0.15 to 4% of all disc surgeries.[1,2,3] The lower incidence of TDH is likely due to the rigidity of the thoracic spine afforded by the stabilizing ribs. For this reason, 75% occur below T8, mostly at T11–T12—the more mobile region of the thoracic spine. The majority of TDHs occur in the midline (94%).[3,4,5,6]

14.2 Pathogenesis

Most (80%) TDHs occur in the third to fifth decades and tend to be a result of degenerative disc disease in the thoracolumbar spine.[2,4] These disc herniations are more likely to be calcified, which occur in up to 70% of all TDHs.[7] Calcified disc herniations can become adherent to the ventral dura (44%) and may be associated with an intradural component in up to 17% of cases.[8] Younger patients typically have soft disc herniations and often have a history of trauma.[9] These patients have acute onset of symptoms.

There are two beliefs on the pathogenesis of neurological symptoms from thoracic disc herniations: direct spinal cord compression and vascular compromise. The thoracic spinal cord anatomy lends itself to be more vulnerable to direct compression than the cervical and lumbar spine. The central canal diameter is smaller with shorter pedicles, accounting for 40% of the canal being occupied by the spinal cord, whereas the cervical cord occupies 25% of the central canal.[10] The thoracic kyphosis places the spinal cord more anteriorly in the canal, in near proximity to the posterior longitudinal ligament and intervertebral disc. When a central TDH occurs, posterior migration of the spinal cord is limited by the dentate ligaments, which anchor the cord to the dura increasing the effects of spinal cord compression.

The spinal cord is fed by a single midline anterior spinal artery and paired posterior spinal arteries. The anterior spinal artery supplies the majority of the spinal cord, except the dorsal columns. Midline thoracic disc herniations may cause compression of the anterior spinal artery, leading to vascular insufficiency and even thrombosis. Vascular insufficiency may explain instances where symptomatology is localized to higher spinal levels than that of the thoracic disc herniation. Abrupt neurological decline may also be explained by vascular compromise, especially in the setting of chronic disc herniations.

14.3 Clinical Presentation

Thoracic disc herniations can present in various ways. Initially, most patients have axial thoracic back pain (57%) which later progresses to a combination of both motor and sensory symptoms (61%). Pain is typically in a band-like distribution radiating ventrally along thoracic dermatomes.[4] The sensory and radicular pain pattern on physical examination can provide vital detail into localization of the herniated thoracic disc to a specific level. Because of pain anteriorly on the chest and abdomen, the clinical presentation may be confused with cardiac, pulmonary, or abdominal etiologies. Bladder dysfunction occurs in 30% of cases.[4] Signs of myelopathy, including increased deep tendon reflexes of the lower extremities, clonus, and positive Babinski sign, are worrisome. Midline herniations are more likely to be associated with cord compression and myelopathy than lateral disc herniations, which cause radicular symptoms.

14.4 Diagnostic Evaluation

As with all spinal pathologies complete and thorough physical examination is required. Diagnostic imaging has now become the mainstay in evaluation for spinal pathology with the use of magnetic resonance imaging (MRI), computed tomography (CT), and myelography. Imaging findings should be correlated with symptoms and physical examination findings, especially in cases with multiple thoracic disc herniations.

MRI can provide information on soft tissue, particularly the intervertebral disc and spinal cord. The degree of ventral compression can be assessed by evaluating surrounding cerebrospinal fluid (CSF) and deformation of the spinal cord, however, disc herniations may be exaggerated on T2 sequences. Spinal cord edema noted by the T2 signal changes can shed light onto the severity of compression. MRI has the potential to distinguish intradural disc herniations. Although difficult to ascertain, calcifications in a disc are hypointense on T1 and T2.

Thoracic CT is vital to assess bony anatomy and evaluate for calcified discs, which impacts surgical planning. CT myelography is an option when an MRI is contraindicated or cannot be obtained. A focal disruption in contrast in the CSF can indicate a herniated disc; however, a complete block is only found in 10 to 15% of cases.[11] Nerve roots, bone anatomy, and calcified disc can be characterized with myelography, but information about the spinal cord parenchyma cannot be assessed.

Spinal radiographs may aid in identification and localization of calcified discs; however, because of more specific and detailed imaging modalities, it has a limited use in diagnosis of TDH. Spinal radiographs can provide information on global alignment, regional kyphosis or lordosis, and signs of instability on dynamic imaging—all of which can impact surgical planning and indications for possible fusion and instrumentation.

14.5 Nonsurgical Management

Nonsurgical management of thoracic disc herniations is the first course of treatment when pain is the only symptom. Brown et al found that 63% of patients notice an improvement in pain with conservative management, which includes nonsteroidal anti-inflammatory drugs, oral pain medications, oral steroids, epidural steroid injections, physical therapy, and bracing.[12] When sensory changes or radiculopathy in dermatomal distribution are the only symptoms, all measures of conservative therapy should be first exhausted before attempting any surgical options. Radiofrequency ablation, facet injections/blocks, nerve root rhizotomies, and transforaminal epidural steroid injections are all preferred methods of treatment in patients who have no neurological compromise. Patients should be referred for pain management for further treatment options.

14.6 Surgical Management

14.6.1 Indications for Surgery and Preoperative Planning

Although few thoracic disc herniations require intervention, indications for surgical treatment of thoracic disc herniations include (1) pain that is refractory to conservative management and (2) signs of myelopathy, including hyperreflexia of patellar and Achilles reflexes, Babinski sign, clonus, ataxic gait, lower extremity weakness, and bowel or bladder dysfunction.

Surgical treatment of midline thoracic disc herniations requires detailed preoperative planning tailored to each case. Localization of the correct disc space is vital on intraoperative fluoroscopy by counting up from the sacrum, and must be confirmed with preoperative imaging studies. Simply assuming the most caudal rib as T12 may lead to miscounting and arrival at the incorrect level due to inconsistency of lower ribs from patient to patient. Unique morphological characteristics that are also seen on preoperative imaging studies can be utilized to further confirm correct level. Alternatively, patients can be referred to interventional radiology to mark specific thoracic level prior to surgical intervention. Calcified discs should be identified preoperatively and evaluated for potential intradural components. These discs are more likely to be adherent to the ventral dura, leading to higher risks of durotomy. Calcified discs require a more extensive resection of the surrounding bony structures to safely remove the disc without retraction on the spinal cord. Typically, in order to avoid a durotomy and neurological injury, a thin shell of calcified disc is left if it is severely adherent to the ventral dura (▸ Fig. 14.1).

14.6.2 Surgical Approaches

Historically, a posterior approach with a decompressive laminectomy was the treatment for TDH. However, this has been abandoned due to high risk of neurological compromise, as excessive spinal cord retraction is needed to remove a central disc. As shown in ▸ Fig. 14.2, an appropriate surgical approach must be utilized to obtain adequate access to the midline of the disc bilaterally and the ventral dura, with minimal to no retraction and manipulation of the spinal cord. A laminectomy or transpedicular approach does not accomplish this goal. ▸ Table 14.1 summarizes the advantages and disadvantages of each approach for midline TDH.

Costotransversectomy and Lateral Extracavitary

The lateral surgical corridor comprises the costotransversectomy approach, developed by Menard in 1894, and later revised by Larson in 1976 as the lateral extracavitary approach.[13,14] Both require resection of the ipsilateral transverse process, rib head, and pedicle to obtain exposure to the disc space. The corridor remains in the retropleural space, reducing pulmonary complications and without the need for a chest tube. Midline exposure is limited with a costotransversectomy—reserving this approach as best for paracentral disc herniations. However, with further lateral resection of the rib the midline can be accessed with a lateral extracavitary approach. A rhizotomy is

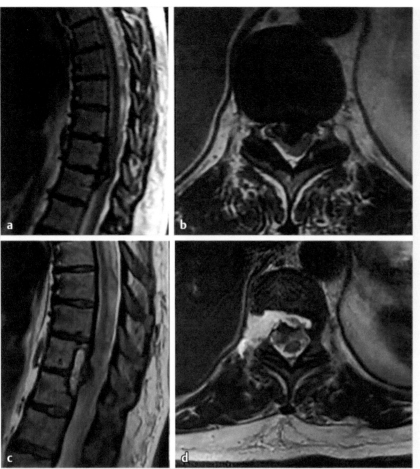

Fig. 14.1 Preoperative sagittal MRI (a) and axial (b) giant calcified thoracic midline disc herniation at T7–T8 in a patient who underwent lateral, retropleural partial corpectomy. In this case, the calcified portion was intradural. In order to avoid a CSF leak, the calcified intradural portion was left intact as a "floating" portion, detached from the disc space and the posterior longitudinal ligament. Postoperative sagittal (c) and axial (d) MRI showing the residual "free-floating" intradural disc is detached from the disc space with the spinal cord decompressed.

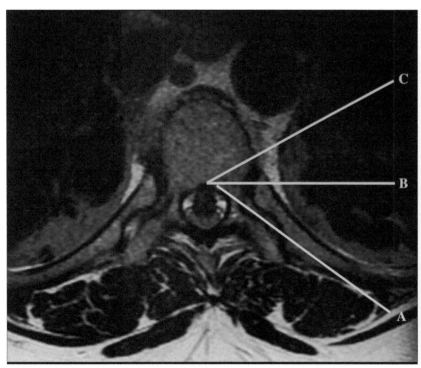

Fig. 14.2 Surgical corridors to midline thoracic disc herniation. Axial MRI of a giant calcified thoracic disc herniation is shown—large hypointensity in central canal. Line A demonstrates a costotransversectomy approach. There is a limitation of medial access and the contralateral side cannot be reached. Line B is the trajectory in a mini-open or minimally invasive surgery (MIS) lateral transthoracic/retropleural approach. Line C is the anterior transthoracic approach. There is no retraction of the spinal cord required to reach the midline, ventral dura, and the contralateral disc in both the lateral (B) and anterior (C) approaches.

Table 14.1 Advantages and disadvantages of surgical approaches to midline thoracic disc herniations

Approach	Advantage	Disadvantage
Laminectomy	For lesions dorsal to spinal cord	No midline exposure No ventral dura exposure High risk of neurological deficits
Costotrans-versectomy	Fair midline disc exposure Good for lateral or paracentral disc Intact pleura	No access to contralateral disc Limited ventral dura exposure Rhizotomy required
Lateral extracavitary	More midline exposure Intact pleura can access multiple levels	No access to contralateral disc Limited ventral dura exposure Rhizotomy required More boney resection needed
Minimally invasive lateral transthoracic/retropleural	Good midline disc exposure Good ventral dura exposure Can have intact pleura—may not require chest tube Can access contralateral disc Can access multiple levels	Limited view working through retractors Steep learning curve
Anterior transthoracic and thoracoscopic	Best midline disc exposure Great best ventral dura exposure Can access contralateral disc	Requires cardiothoracic surgeon Steep learning curve Painful Requires chest tube Pulmonary complications

conducted to further open a corridor toward the midline. However, both approaches have limited exposure of the ventral dura, making resection of a calcified midline TDH difficult. If a durotomy is encountered, repair of a ventral tear is usually not possible. The segmental artery is typically ligated when exposing the lateral vertebral body. There is a risk of vascular compromise to the spinal cord if the artery of Adamkiewicz, a major medullary feeder, is injured.

Minimally Invasive Lateral

With advances in technology, minimally invasive surgery (MIS) approaches are becoming more prevalent. The mini-open or MIS lateral approach utilizes a small dilated corridor between the ribs while the patient is in a lateral decubitus position. This approach can be either transthoracic or retropleural by sweeping the pleura and lung anteriorly and docking on the lateral spine, obviating the need for postoperative chest tube or single-lung ventilation. Rib resection is necessary, however, to access the thoracic disc space. This approach does not involve extra bony resection, except that of the ipsilateral rib head, ipsilateral pedicle, and posterior margin of the vertebral body (▶ Fig. 14.3). With a lateral trajectory, the midline, contralateral disc extension, and ventral dura can all be accessed without manipulation of the spinal cord (▶ Fig. 14.4). With a smaller incision and less retraction, there is less postoperative pain, shorter length of stay, and reduced pulmonary complications.[15] In a multicenter series, Uribe et al[16] demonstrated 80% improvement in symptoms, 5% poor outcome, and no paraplegia or death.

Anterior Transthoracic

The anterior transthoracic approach has been widely utilized for midline TDH, as direct exposure of the midline and ventral dura can be obtained without any manipulation of the spinal

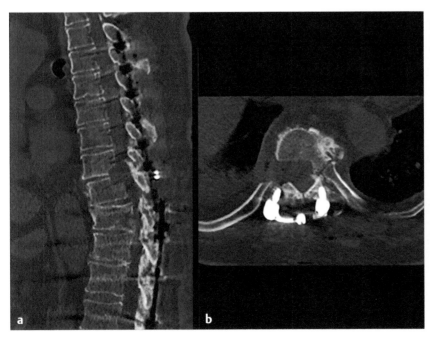

Fig. 14.3 Sagittal (a) and axial (b) thoracic spine CT representing the amount of bone resection through a lateral retropleural T8–T9 discectomy. Only ipsilateral rib head, pedicle, and posterior margin of the vertebral body are removed.

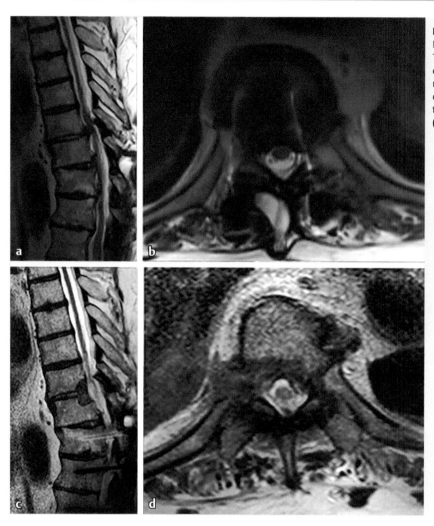

Fig. 14.4 Preoperative sagittal **(a)** and axial **(b)** MRI thoracic spine without contrast showing T8–T9 midline disc herniation with spinal cord compression. With a lateral trajectory, the midline, contralateral disc extension, and ventral dura can all be accessed without manipulation of the spinal cord as seen in postoperative sagittal **(c)** and axial **(d)** MRI thoracic spine images.

cord. The posterior elements remain intact, reducing the risk of instability. With wide exposure, a large graft can be placed when necessary. However, a cardiothoracic surgeon and thorough knowledge of the thoracic anatomy is required. The postoperative complication rates (other than neurological compromise) are highest with the anterior approach due to larger opening and greater retraction. This is due to a need for postoperative chest tube, increased risk of pneumonia, and risk of long-term chest wall neuralgia occurring in 30% of patients at 4 to 5 years postoperatively.[17] Video-assisted thoracoscopic surgery (VATS) has been shown to reduce many of these complications. Regan et al[18] compared VATS to open transthoracic approach and found a reduction in intensive care unit stay, days with chest tube in place, and quicker return to work. However, there is a steep learning curve with this technology. Durotomies can be difficult to repair via VATS.

14.6.3 Necessity for Fusion

The necessity for fusion after thoracic discectomy is still controversial. Clear indications of fusions include kyphosis, scoliosis, severe mechanical back pain, extensive bony resection of the vertebral body or posterior elements, extensive discectomy, multiple thoracic discectomies, or presence of Scheuermann's disease. Numerous studies have shown that instrumented fusion is not necessary with thoracoscopic or transthoracic discectomies—which involved the removal of the ipsilateral rib head, ipsilateral pedicle, and posterior vertebral body.[19,20,21,22] Approximately 1.8 to 10.1% of patients develop postoperative spinal instability.[23,24] Instrumented fusion may be necessary in cases of giant TDH or calcified disc herniations that require significant bone resection for safe access. However, fusion can be generally avoided if less than 50% of vertebral body is resected. Ultimately, the decision for fusion is up to the surgeon's discretion after weighing all patient-specific risk factors for developing spinal instability.

References

[1] Carson J, Gumpert J, Jefferson A. Diagnosis and treatment of thoracic intervertebral disc protrusions. J Neurol Neurosurg Psychiatry. 1971; 34(1):68–77

[2] el-Kalliny M, Tew JMJ, Jr, van Loveren H, Dunsker S. Surgical approaches to thoracic disc herniations. Acta Neurochir (Wien). 1991; 111(1–2):22–32

[3] Stillerman CB, Chen TC, Couldwell WT, Zhang W, Weiss MH. Experience in the surgical management of 82 symptomatic herniated thoracic discs and review of the literature. J Neurosurg. 1998; 88(4):623–633

[4] Arce CA, Dohrmann GJ. Herniated thoracic disks. Neurol Clin. 1985; 3(2):383–392

[5] Videman T, Battié MC, Gill K, Manninen H, Gibbons LE, Fisher LD. Magnetic resonance imaging findings and their relationships in the thoracic and lumbar spine. Insights into the etiopathogenesis of spinal degeneration. Spine. 1995; 20(8):928–935

[6] Awwad EE, Martin DS, Smith KRJ, Jr, Baker BK. Asymptomatic versus symptomatic herniated thoracic discs: their frequency and characteristics as detected by computed tomography after myelography. Neurosurgery. 1991; 28(2):180–186

[7] Logue V. Thoracic intervertebral disc prolapse with spinal cord compression. J Neurol Neurosurg Psychiatry. 1952; 15(4):227–241

[8] Gille O, Soderlund C, Razafimahandri HJC, Mangione P, Vital JM. Analysis of hard thoracic herniated discs: review of 18 cases operated by thoracoscopy. Eur Spine J. 2006; 15(5):537–542

[9] Arseni C, Nash F. Thoracic intervertebral disc protrusion: a clinical study. J Neurosurg. 1960; 17(3):418–430

[10] Newton TH, Potts DG, Rizzoli HV. Modern Neuroradiology, Volume I: Computed Tomography of the Spine and Spinal Cord. 1984

[11] Tovi D, Strang RR. Thoracic intervertebral disk protrusions. Acta Chir Scand Suppl. 1960 Suppl 267:1–41

[12] Brown CW, Deffer PAJ, Jr, Akmakjian J, Donaldson DH, Brugman JL. The natural history of thoracic disc herniation. Spine. 1992; 17(6) Suppl:S97–S102

[13] Lifshutz J, Lidar Z, Maiman D. Evolution of the lateral extracavitary approach to the spine. Neurosurg Focus. 2004; 16(1):E12

[14] Larson SJ, Holst RA, Hemmy DC, Sances A, Jr. Lateral extracavitary approach to traumatic lesions of the thoracic and lumbar spine. J Neurosurg. 1976; 45(6):628–637

[15] Angevin PD, McCormick PC. Retropleural thoracotomy. Technical note. Neurosurg Focus. 2001; 10(1):ecp1

[16] Uribe JS, Smith WD, Pimenta L, et al. Minimally invasive lateral approach for symptomatic thoracic disc herniation: initial multicenter clinical experience. J Neurosurg Spine. 2012; 16(3):264–279

[17] Karmakar MK, Ho AMH. Postthoracotomy pain syndrome. Thorac Surg Clin. 2004; 14(3):345–352

[18] Regan JJ. Percutaneous endoscopic thoracic discectomy. Neurosurg Clin N Am. 1996; 7(1):87–98

[19] Krauss WE, Edwards DA, Cohen-Gadol AA. Transthoracic discectomy without interbody fusion. Surg Neurol. 2005; 63(5):403–408, discussion 408–409

[20] Broc GG, Crawford NR, Sonntag VK, Dickman CA. Biomechanical effects of transthoracic microdiscectomy. Spine. 1997; 22(6):605–612

[21] Anand N, Regan JJ. Video-assisted thoracoscopic surgery for thoracic disc disease: Classification and outcome study of 100 consecutive cases with a 2-year minimum follow-up period. Spine. 2002; 27(8):871–879

[22] Feiertag MA, Horton WC, Norman JT, Proctor FC, Hutton WC. The effect of different surgical releases on thoracic spinal motion. A cadaveric study. Spine. 1995; 20(14):1604–1611

[23] Quint U, Bordon G, Preissl I, Sanner C, Rosenthal D. Thoracoscopic treatment for single level symptomatic thoracic disc herniation: a prospective followed cohort study in a group of 167 consecutive cases. Eur Spine J. 2012; 21(4):637–645

[24] Wait SD, Fox DJ, Kenny KJ, Dickman CA. Thoracoscopic resection of symptomatic herniated thoracic discs: clinical results in 121 patients. Spine. 2012; 37(1):35–40

15 Spondyloarthropathies

Navika Shukla, Allen Ho, Arjun V. Pendharkar, Eric S. Sussman, and Atman Desai

Abstract

Ankylosing spondylitis is a spondyloarthropathy consisting of degenerative and inflammatory changes of the spinal column. It is most often associated with spinal cord injury due to poor bone quality and cervical kyphosis. Ankylosing spondylitis remains a challenging condition for surgical intervention and outcomes tend to be poor in comparison to the general trauma population. When surgery is indicated, it is important to consider the increased risk of intraoperative blood loss as well as the increased difficulty in performing imaging studies, intubating the patient, and adequately positioning the patient to prevent further injury. Techniques including minimally invasive stabilization, pedicle screw fixation, and spinal instrumentation may help tackle some of the challenges of operating on a patient with ankylosing spondylitis.

Keywords: spondyloarthropathies, ankylosing spondylitis, MIS, pedicle screw fixation, spinal instrumentation

Clinical Pearls

- Surgical interventions should only be utilized when conservative nonsurgical alternatives have been exhausted or there is significant instability or deformity causing neurological deficit.
- If surgery is indicated, continual neurological and neurophysiological monitoring is essential.
- Risk of blood loss and iatrogenic fractures during surgery is high within the ankylosing spondylitis patient population.
- Intraoperative computed tomography guidance is recommended over standard intraoperative fluoroscopy.
- Use of preoperative planning, minimally invasive stabilization, pedicle screw fixation, and spinal instrumentation may provide modest improvements in surgical outcomes.

15.1 Introduction

Spondyloarthropathies (SpA) are a family of chronic, inflammatory rheumatic diseases involving axial or peripheral arthritis. Progression of SpA is often associated with enthesitis, dactylitis, as well as extra-articular symptoms such as uveitis and skin rash. The hallmark of diagnosis is radiographic evidence of sacrolitis.[1] The family of SpA includes ankylosing spondylitis (AS), psoriatic arthritis, juvenile-onset spondyloarthritis, reactive arthritis, SpA associated with inflammatory bowel disease, and undifferentiated SpA. This chapter will focus specifically on axial SpA, or SpA of the spine. The most common presentation of axial SpA is AS.

15.2 Background

15.2.1 Ankylosing Spondylitis

Ankylosing spondylitis is a slowly progressive inflammatory disease that mainly affects the spinal column and sacroiliac joints. As inflammation of the vertebral column progresses, peripheral arthritis, enthesitis, and anterior uveitis also become common. Patients typically present with chronic inflammatory back pain at a mean age of onset of less than 30 years.[2] Men are affected twice as often as women and the prevalence rate of AS is between 0.1 and 1.4%.[2,3] Incidence is highest among Caucasian patients.[4]

There is a known genetic predisposition toward AS associated with the major histocompatibility complex (MHC) group of molecules—specifically the HLA-B27 allele. Over 90% of AS patients are HLA-B27 +, but only 5% of HLA-B27 + individuals go on to develop AS.[2,5] This discrepancy is not yet fully understood, but might be accounted for by the variety in HLA-B27 subtypes that exist. Certain subtypes such as the most common parent subtype, *B*2705*, are more closely linked to AS than others.[3,5] Another explanation for the discrepancy in AS susceptibility might be attributable to differences in expression levels. The antigen-presenting cells of patients with AS tend to more heavily express HLA-B27 than the cells of unaffected HLA-B27 + patients.[5]

The exact mechanism by which the HLA-B27 allele confers disease susceptibility is also not yet known. It may be that the allele may uniquely bind and present arthritogenic peptides leading to CD8 + T-cell–directed responses against self-antigens. Alternatively, it may be that HLA-B27 is more likely to fold aberrantly in a manner that has been shown to lead to increased, unnecessary binding and recognition by KIR3DL2 + NK and CD4 + T cells, triggering NK and CD4 + T-cell–mediated autoreactivity.[5] On the other hand, aberrant protein folding, if it leads to misfolding and improper aggregation, may instead trigger nonspecific inflammatory pathways against protein aggregates.[3,5]

Although the mechanism behind what triggers AS is not fully understood, what is known is that widespread inflammation is a hallmark of disease. In fact, in diagnosing AS, pain resulting from inflammatory processes allows one to differentiate between AS and mechanical chronic back pain.[1,6] Together, this extensive inflammation along with increased new bone formation leads to characteristic vertebral column remodeling. Upregulation of inflammatory processes promotes new ectopic bone formation at ligamentous insertion points throughout the axial skeleton. The enthesopathy causes ossification of the ligaments, intervertebral discs, endplates, and apophyseal structures while the ectopic bone formation results in the formation of syndesmophytes through the nucleus pulposus within each intervertebral disc.[2] In AS, syndesmophytes cause ankylosis across both zygapophysial joints and between vertebral bodies, permanently restricting the patient's capacity for movement at the spine.[6] As the inflammation progresses, the cortex and spongiosa of the vertebral bodies themselves are repeatedly destroyed and rebuilt, resulting in the formation of square vertebral bodies.[6,7] Over time, vertebral remodeling and ankylosis lead to spinal deformity in the form of the characteristic hyperkyphotic "bamboo spine."[2]

Despite the upregulation of new bone formation, AS is also associated with early osteoporosis due to the uncoupling of bone resorption and formation processes.[2,7] Increased osteoclast activity and syndesmophyte formation are linked to lower bone mineral density, weakening the spine.[6] Biomechanically, increased spinal fusion and fragility greatly increase susceptibility to vertebral column fractures. Spinal fusion prevents the spine from adequately dissipating the force of traumatic events and impairs mobility. This limited mobility when combined with the peripheral joint arthritis usually seen in AS causes gait unsteadiness which increases susceptibility to falls.[2] Thus, the rate of spinal cord injuries and fractures is greatly increased in patients with AS. While spinal deformity and trauma-related injuries are the most common conditions requiring surgical intervention in AS patients, spinal stenosis, cauda equina syndrome, and degenerative axial spine pain may also occur in a minority of patients.[6]

15.2.2 Patient Presentation

AS is most commonly diagnosed in the primary care setting. It manifests as sacroiliitis, spondylitis, and enthesitis that present as chronic and progressive inflammatory axial pain, usually during adolescence or early adulthood. Extra-axial manifestations include peripheral arthritis (25–50%), inflammatory bowel disease (26%), and psoriasis (10%).[8] The mainstays of medical treatment of AS revolve around goals of symptom relief, preservation of functionality and quality of life, and delaying or avoiding disease progression.[9] Physical therapy and nonsteroidal anti-inflammatory medications are the first and primary treatments for chronic AS. Other more aggressive disease-modifying antirheumatic medications such as sulfasalazine and methotrexate have limited roles in AS, as there are no empirical data that definitively support their use. Tumor necrosis factor and interleukin inhibitors have demonstrated efficacy in several randomized control trials, but carry a significant immunosuppressive risk profile.[10] Thus, the chronic aspects of AS are more typically managed nonsurgically with medical treatments aimed at alleviating symptoms and slowing disease progression.

Presentation for neurosurgical care most commonly occurs in the acute setting following spinal trauma.[11] The most common fractures seen are of the midcervical spine or cervicothoracic junction.[12] These fractures are highly unstable and are often displaced due to large bone lever arms created in the spine due to autofusion.[13] Unfortunately, severe neurological damage is common with these fractures, with up to 75% with neurological compromise in some series.[12,14,15] The risk of fracture progression, even with halothoracic plaster or jacket immobilization is significant given the large bone lever arms. Worsening fracture displacement can also lead to devastating neurological injury.[16] Thus, surgical stabilization is complex and warranted in most AS fractures.

15.3 Surgical Considerations

Surgical management of AS generally carries an increased risk of morbidity given the many unique challenges to performing surgery on patients with AS. Imaging studies can be difficult to obtain and interpret. The osteopenia and kyphosis make it difficult to interpret X-ray evidence.[11] Computed tomography (CT) scans and magnetic resonance imaging (MRI) are generally the recommended modality to allow for precise visualization in patients with AS.[11] Additionally, lying in the supine position is often intolerable due to pain or deformity. In these cases, the patient should either be positioned in the right decubitus position or a pillow should be used to raise the pelvis relative to the head.[11]

Intubation also becomes more challenging in patients with AS. Endotracheal intubation may be obstructed in patients where the presence of large anterior cervical osteophytes blocks the larynx or cervical flexion deformities restrict movement of the mouth or neck.[11] Imaging studies should be performed to detect the presence or absence of an obstruction prior to intubation. If endotracheal intubation fails, nasotracheal fiberoptic intubation can be used.[11,17,18] Head manipulation during intubation should be done with extreme caution. Given the brittle nature of the spine in AS, manipulation of the neck and thorax during intubation can cause iatrogenic cervicothoracic fractures.[19] Proper positioning in general is complicated by the increased risk for iatrogenic injury.[20] AS patients are at risk for complete spinal cord injury and possible death in cases where the extent of cervical kyphosis and overall sagittal alignment is inappropriately assessed.[11] To reduce the risk of injury, halo placement and increased traction prior to surgery, as well as extensive thoracic bracing have been shown to improve patient stability in cervical and thoracic fractures, respectively. Adaptations to patient beds such as the use of circle electric beds allows increases to the range of movement possible.[11] Head stabilization through a Mayfield head frame reduces inappropriate head movements.[11] When used in conjunction with a reverse Trendelenburg position, it may decrease the risk of postoperative blindness by reducing intraocular and ocular venous pressure.[11] Finally, an important adjunct for positioning AS patients with potentially unstable spines is neuromonitoring. Confirmation of pre- and postpositioning somatosensory evoked potentials and motor evoked potentials can alert the surgeon to any worsened alignment causing neurological compression during positioning, especially when moving from supine to prone position.

Aside from the challenges posed by patient positioning, patients with AS are also at an increased risk for intraoperative blood loss and epidural hematomas.[19] The spinal deformities can prevent achievement of a free-hanging abdomen.[11] The resulting increased pressure placed on the chest leads to increases in peak inspiratory pressure and ventilation issues.[11] To compensate for this, padding is sometimes used. This increased abdominal pressure can impact central venous pressure and cause distention of the epidural venous plexus.[11]

Given the patient's increased risk of both intraoperative blood loss and iatrogenic fractures, neurological monitoring is exceptionally important throughout surgery.[11,18,19] Corrective osteotomy procedures carry high risk of neurological deficits postsurgery, and local anesthesia is generally the ideal option to allow the patient to continually provide neurological feedback.[11,18] In some cases, however, such as surgeries with extensive soft-tissue exposure and prolonged periods of maintaining the prone position, awake surgeries are infeasible. In these cases, techniques like the wake-up test and continuous neurophysiological monitoring methods should be used in conjunction with general anesthesia.[18] Given the variability in sensitivity of neurophysiological monitoring strategies, it is recommended that multiple methods be used together. These methods include spinal cord evoked potentials, somatosensory cortical evoked potentials, spinal somatosensory evoked potentials, and muscle motor evoked potentials.[11,18]

15.4 Surgical Tools and Techniques

The surgical goals in treatment of AS patients with acute injury are for stabilization of fractures and correction of deformity. Standard surgical techniques aimed at improving outcomes in patients with AS include external fixation with halo immobilization and bracing, internal fixation with spinal instrumentation, and anterior release. In patients in whom only halo immobilization is utilized, the risk of delayed subluxation is greatly increased. Supplementation of halo immobilization with internal fixation significantly reduces this risk. Thus, the mainstay of AS treatment is spinal instrumentation involving lateral mass and pedicle screw and rod constructs for posterior cervical fixation, and long-segment thoracic fusion with pedicle screw and rod constructs for posterior thoracic fixation. This is supplemented with typical arthrodesis techniques using allograft or autograft and intervertebral spacing devices such as polyetheretherketone (PEEK) or titanium cages when appropriate. Optimal internal fixation in this way may obviate the need for postoperative halo immobilization entirely with cervical fractures. However, because of poor bone quality, it may be difficult to identify normal bony landmarks for screw entry points and trajectories, and thus the use of shorter-length screws and CT image guidance is recommended. Depending on the severity of fracture and deformity, different osteotomy techniques may need to be employed to achieve optimal alignment and fracture reduction. These include, but are not limited to Smith–Peterson osteotomy (SPO), pedicle subtraction osteotomy (PSO), or vertebrectomy. Other techniques to prevent acute subluxation include the use of sublaminar wires,[18] or utilization of a provisional rod threaded through posterior cervical and thoracic screws to prevent acute translation during extension.[18] These posterior fixation techniques may be combined with an anterior approach to help achieve the goals of deformity correction and improve fusion fixation with the addition of an anterior cervical discectomy and fusion (ACDF) implant. Aside from spinal instrumentation, several authors have recommend performing an initial anterior release when possible before posterior extension osteotomy and/or fusion.[21] An initial anterior release allows the surgeon to determine the level of the anterior wedge osteotomy and permits controlled correction with neck extension, reducing the risk of fracture at a random, undesired level.[18,21] That being said, given the propensity of ankylosed bone toward fracture even without excess manual force, it is not clear that an initial anterior release would provide significant clinical advantage. Additionally, in situations where performing an initial anterior release would be technically challenging such as with severe cervical kyphosis, the costs of the procedure may outweigh the benefits.[18]

With the many unique challenges of operating on a patient with AS, certain surgical tools and techniques have been developed or implemented to improve surgical outcomes in this patient population. More recently, research has focused on the use of algorithms and computational methods to guide operations. A study conducted by Kanter et al studied the impact of a clinical problem-solving algorithm designed to assist with surgical management decisions around injury and deformity.[22] The algorithm takes into account fracture site and pattern, degree of dislocation, facet pathology, cord compression, neurological deficits, deformity, and surgical urgency. Imaging with plain films, CT, and MRI are also conducted. With the use of the algorithm, 92% of patients achieved postoperative stability or improvement with a 38% complication rate.[22] Along the same lines, Pigge et al studied the effectiveness of biomechanical and mathematical preoperative planning for patients with thoracolumbar kyphotic deformity.[23] The authors utilized the ASKyphoplan computational program to perform preoperative surgical planning. The planning procedure was aimed at predicting postoperative balance and view angle.[23] The computational planning improved understanding of the biomechanical and clinical effects of lumbar spine correction osteotomy and was associated with clinical improvements in balance and view angle in all patients.[23] However, the methodology was unable to precisely predict clinical results. Achieved correction angles were between −8 and 7 degrees of the planned correction angles.[23]

While algorithms and modeling methods have shown to be useful for the preoperative stage of surgery, MIS techniques have been shown to improve outcomes in spinal surgery for fractures in patients with AS. Use of MIS is thought to reduce blood loss, physiological stress, and perioperative morbidity.[19] MIS techniques, as described by Nayak et al, involve percutaneous posterior instrumentation three levels above and three levels below the fracture.[19] Screw placement and positioning postsurgery can be guided by CT imaging. CT image guidance is recommended over intraoperative X-ray as the osteoporosis and joint fusion seen in AS complicate the interpretation of X-rays.[11,19] In patients with AS, CT image guidance can be used to bring greater accuracy to screw trajectories in order to counteract the impact of poor bone quality on the risk of screw loosening and hardware migration. To ensure a good screw–rod interface, it is recommended to pre-bend the rods to the exact contour of the screw extensions about the skin.[19]

As a standard approach to strategies for surgical stabilization of fractures and correction of significant deformity associated with AS, we maintain several specific surgical principles. First, given the highly unstable nature of AS fractures (▶ Fig. 15.1) and the difficulty in positioning AS patients, great care and consideration is taken in positioning these patients. Preservation of pre- and postpositioning neuromonitoring potentials is essential. Patient alignment must also be ideal prior to beginning the case as there is very little other laxity in the spine after surgical stabilization is completed and patient will be effectively fused in situ to that specific alignment. Next, given the fusion of the rest of the spine superior and inferior to the fracture or targeted area of correction in an AS patient, we have to consider the significant biomechanical forces to be exerted in a "lever arm" fashion around this target level. Aggressive fusion of multiple levels (often at least three levels above and below) surrounding this target level will help redistribute the tension of this "lever arm." Also, when possible, 360-degree fusion with a combined anterior–posterior approach can also strengthen the stabilization construct significantly against this "lever-arm." Finally, as

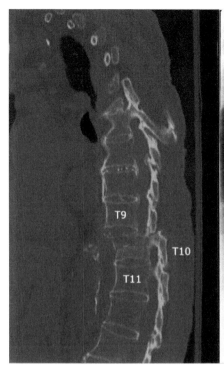
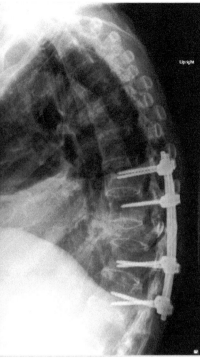

Fig. 15.1 Posterior instrumented fusion of T10 chance fracture in ankylosing spondylitis (*right*). Preoperative CT scan of a highly unstable T10 chance fracture in an ankylosing spondylitis patient following a traumatic fall. Pathological autofusion of anterior and posterior elements creates unstable lever arms similar to a long bone fracture, and distorts anatomy for more difficult screw placement (*left*). Postoperative X-ray following a T8–T12 posterior instrumented fusion for stabilization.

described above, the surface bony anatomy is often severely distorted making discerning normal entry points and determining screw trajectories challenging, even for the most experienced spine surgeons (▶ Fig. 15.1). Utilization of intraoperative CT guidance for navigation of screw placement and for delineating osteotomy boundaries has been extremely useful. Confirmation of the construct intraoperatively can also be helpful for correct suboptimal screw placements or alignment prior to closure.

15.5 Surgical Outcomes

Compared to the general population, in patients with AS, fractures from even minor trauma are known to greatly increase the risk of neurological injury and spinal deformity. Given the patient's increased vulnerability and the increased risks of operating on a patient with AS, surgical outcomes tend to be worse in this patient population compared to the general trauma population. Because of the chronic pain and inflammation associated with AS, fractures and injuries requiring surgery are often initially thought to be a part of natural disease progression, and diagnosis is delayed. Furthermore, given the progression of disease prior to surgical intervention, improvement in outcomes following surgical stabilization is often limited. A meta-analysis by Westerveld et al showed that upon admission for surgery, 67.2% of AS patients already had some neurological deficits.[24,25] Secondary neurological deterioration was frequent.[24] Even after surgery, 59.4% of patients showed no change in neurological status 3 months postoperation.[24] After surgery for spinal injury, the complication rate was 51.1% and the overall 3-month mortality was 17.7%.[24] Patients with AS were more likely to suffer from uncommon surgical complications including aortic dissection, aortic pseudoaneurysm, and tracheal rupture.[24] Rates of more common complications including

deep venous thrombosis, respiratory insufficiency, pneumonia, and postoperative wound infections were also higher in AS patients.[24]

References

[1] Khalessi AA, Oh BC, Wang MY. Medical management of ankylosing spondylitis. Neurosurg Focus. 2008; 24(1):E4

[2] Jacobs WB, Fehlings MG. Ankylosing spondylitis and spinal cord injury: origin, incidence, management, and avoidance. Neurosurg Focus. 2008; 24(1): E12

[3] Dakwar E, Reddy J, Vale FL, Uribe JS. A review of the pathogenesis of ankylosing spondylitis. Neurosurg Focus. 2008; 24(1):E2

[4] Reveille JD. Epidemiology of spondyloarthritis in North America. Am J Med Sci. 2011; 341(4):284–286

[5] Shamji MF, Bafaquh M, Tsai E. The pathogenesis of ankylosing spondylitis. Neurosurg Focus. 2008; 24(1):E3

[6] Mundwiler ML, Siddique K, Dym JM, Perri B, Johnson JP, Weisman MH. Complications of the spine in ankylosing spondylitis with a focus on deformity correction. Neurosurg Focus. 2008; 24(1):E6

[7] Cha TD, An HS. Cervical spine manifestations in patients with inflammatory arthritides. Nat Rev Rheumatol. 2013; 9(7):423–432

[8] Maxwell LJ, Zochling J, Boonen A, et al. TNF-alpha inhibitors for ankylosing spondylitis. Cochrane Database Syst Rev. 2015; 3(4):CD005468

[9] Zochling J, van der Heijde D, Burgos-Vargas R, et al. 'ASsessment in AS' International Working Group, European League Against Rheumatism. ASAS/EULAR recommendations for the management of ankylosing spondylitis. Ann Rheum Dis. 2006; 65(4):442–452

[10] Lim HJ, Moon YI, Lee MS. Effects of home-based daily exercise therapy on joint mobility, daily activity, pain, and depression in patients with ankylosing spondylitis. Rheumatol Int. 2005; 25(3):225–229

[11] Sciubba DM, Nelson C, Hsieh P, Gokaslan ZL, Ondra S, Bydon A. Perioperative challenges in the surgical management of ankylosing spondylitis. Neurosurg Focus. 2008; 24(1):E10

[12] Hunter T, Dubo H. Spinal fractures complicating ankylosing spondylitis. Ann Intern Med. 1978; 88(4):546–549

[13] Mason C, Cozen L, Adelstein L. Surgical correction of flexion deformity of the cervical spine. Calif Med. 1953; 79(3):244–246

[14] Graham B, Van Peteghem PK. Fractures of the spine in ankylosing spondylitis. Diagnosis, treatment, and complications. Spine. 1989; 14(8):803–807

[15] Graham GP, Evans PD. Spinal fractures in patients with ankylosing spondylitis. Injury. 1991; 22(5):426–427

[16] Schröder J, Liljenqvist U, Greiner C, Wassmann H. Complications of halo treatment for cervical spine injuries in patients with ankylosing spondylitis—report of three cases. Arch Orthop Trauma Surg. 2003; 123(2–3):112–114

[17] Etame AB, Than KD, Wang AC, La Marca F, Park P. Surgical management of symptomatic cervical or cervicothoracic kyphosis due to ankylosing spondylitis. Spine. 2008; 33(16):E559–E564

[18] Hoh DJ, Khoueir P, Wang MY. Management of cervical deformity in ankylosing spondylitis. Neurosurg Focus. 2008; 24(1):E9

[19] Nayak NR, Pisapia JM, Abdullah KG, Schuster JM. Minimally invasive surgery for traumatic fractures in ankylosing spinal diseases. Global Spine J. 2015; 5 (4):266–273

[20] Bron JL, de Vries MK, Snieders MN, van der Horst-Bruinsma IE, van Royen BJ. Discovertebral (Andersson) lesions of the spine in ankylosing spondylitis revisited. Clin Rheumatol. 2009; 28(8):883–892

[21] Mummaneni PV, Mummaneni VP, Haid RW, Jr, Rodts GE, Jr, Sasso RC. Cervical osteotomy for the correction of chin-on-chest deformity in ankylosing spondylitis. Technical note. Neurosurg Focus. 2003; 14(1):e9

[22] Kanter AS, Wang MY, Mummaneni PV. A treatment algorithm for the management of cervical spine fractures and deformity in patients with ankylosing spondylitis. Neurosurg Focus. 2008; 24(1):E11

[23] Pigge RR, Scheerder FJ, Smit TH, Mullender MG, van Royen BJ. Effectiveness of preoperative planning in the restoration of balance and view in ankylosing spondylitis. Neurosurg Focus. 2008; 24(1):E7

[24] Westerveld LA, Verlaan JJ, Oner FC. Spinal fractures in patients with ankylosing spinal disorders: a systematic review of the literature on treatment, neurological status and complications. Eur Spine J. 2009; 18(2):145–156

[25] Caron T, Bransford R, Nguyen Q, Agel J, Chapman J, Bellabarba C. Spine fractures in patients with ankylosing spinal disorders. Spine. 2010; 35(11):E458–E464

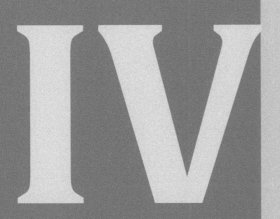

Part IV

Infection

IV

16 Epidural and Soft-Tissue Infections

Mohammed Ali Alvi, Panagiotis Kerezoudis, Sandy Goncalves, Patrick R. Maloney, Brett A. Freedman, Ahmad Nassr, Elie F. Berbari, and Mohamad Bydon

Abstract

Infections of the spinal column are uncommon. These infections have variable clinical presentation and represent a diagnostic and therapeutic challenge. Spinal column infections often originate in the disc space and are often labeled vertebral osteomyelitis, spondylitis, discitis, and spondylodiscitis. Infections can extend to adjacent paravertebral soft tissues to form epidural or other soft-tissue abscesses. Epidural abscess may be present with or without associated disc space infection. Spinal epidural abscess (SEA) and disc space infection are often the result of hematogenous seeding of a distant focus of infection or a transient bacteremia. Uncommonly, direct and iatrogenic inoculation of the fragile epidural space may also cause an SEA. Abscesses, secondary to vertebral osteomyelitis, are usually anterior to the spine. SEA is more common in the thoracic spine than in the lumbar and cervical regions. Diabetes mellitus and intravenous drug abuse are the two most common risk factors for SEAs. Common presenting symptoms include back pain, fever, or spinal tenderness. Magnetic resonance imaging can establish a radiological diagnosis. Surgical intervention may be needed in selected patients to decompress the neural elements and to establish a microbiological diagnosis.

Keywords: spine infection, epidural abscess, spine surgery, soft-tissue infection, thoracic spine, vertebral osteomyelitis, spondylodiscitis, spondylitis

Clinical Pearls

- Spinal epidural abscess (SEA) is a challenging pathology with an incidence of 0.2 to 2 cases per 10,000 hospital admissions.
- SEA may involve a hematogenous pathogenesis, that is, spread through blood vessels from other sites in the body, a nonhematogenous pathogenesis via a contaminated needle or a contiguous site including the disc space, or an iatrogenic pathogenesis, for instance from contamination during spinal surgery.
- The most important risk factors for an SEA include intravenous drug abuse and diabetes.
- The most common region affected is the thoracic region. On presentation, there is severe tenderness on palpation and percussion of the affected spinal segment, while gibbus deformity, neurological findings of dermatomal sensory and/ or motor loss, as well as bowel and bladder dysfunction are indicative of a spinal cord injury and are seen in advanced cases with extensive bony erosion.
- Magnetic resonance imaging is considered as the gold standard for establishing the diagnosis. For microbiology, depending on the situation, a biopsy may be required for culture in the absence of bloodstream infection.
- Empiric antibiotic therapy should be considered once an SEA is suspected. Prolonged antibiotic therapy is the mainstay of treatment while surgical intervention may be needed in selected patients to decompress the neural elements and to establish a microbiological diagnosis.
- Owing to modern therapeutic mechanisms, the mortality rate associated with SEA has reduced to 5 to 20%, but neurological sequelae still remain a challenge.

16.1 Introduction

Infections of the spinal column encompass a wide spectrum of pathologies including infection of the vertebral body, discitis, and epidural abscess where the epidural space, paraspinal soft tissue, or the spinal canal become infected and form a walled-off purulent mass.[1,2] Recent advances in the diagnostic imaging, including magnetic resonance imaging (MRI), has prompted a departure from the use of anatomically specific nomenclature. MRI studies have shown that most infections of the spinal column involve more than one, of the tissue planes in this area.[3] This chapter will primarily focus on spinal epidural abscesses (SEAs) while later chapters will discuss the pathogenesis and microbiological details of osteomyelitis.

Evidence of spinal infections dates back to prehistoric era circa 3400 BC as per the discovery of tuberculous spondylitis (or Pott's disease) in Egyptian mummies.[4] Recent technological advances in imaging techniques have made the diagnosis easier and timely. Modern proliferation and complexity of spine instrumentation along with increased life expectancy have led to an increase in incidence of SEA.

16.2 Epidemiology

Spine infections account for 2 to 7% of all musculoskeletal infections.[2,5,6] Reported incidence rates of vertebral osteomyelitis vary by study and have ranged between 0.2 and 6 cases per 100,000.[7,8,9] The incidence is higher in older patients and patients that are younger than 20 years of age.[10,11,12] SEA incidence rates are reported to be between 0.2 and 2 cases per 10,000 hospital admissions.[13,14,15] The increased incidence in one study of 2.7 per 10,000 admissions has been attributed to intravenous (IV) drug abuse and AIDS.[16,17] SEA predominantly affects patients aged between 30 and 70 years of age.[18] There is also a reported male preponderance with male to female ratios ranging from 2:1 to 5:1.[10,19] Other risk factors include indwelling intravascular devices, end-stage renal disease, immunosuppressive state, transplant recipients, chemotherapy, chronic indwelling catheters, splenectomy, genitourinary instrumentation, and liver cirrhosis.[20]

16.3 Pathogenesis

The details of causative organisms in osteomyelitis will be discussed in a later chapter. The origin of infection is typically classified as (1) hematogenous or (2) nonhematogenous.

Nonhematogenous infection can be the result of surgery or direct inoculation.

16.3.1 Hematogenous Spread

Hematogenous seeding is considered the most common mechanism by which the disc or epidural space often becomes infected. Pathogenic microorganisms often seed the spine via the arterial route or less commonly the vertebral venous plexus.[21] The nidus of infection forms in the metaphyseal artery, a branch of the periosteal artery. This infected thrombus leads to avascular necrosis of a portion of the metaphysis. Subsequently, the infection travels through the anastomotic arteries to reach the opposite ends of the vertebra causing vertebral body infection. The ischemia also causes aseptic necrosis of the disc space causing gradual loss of disc height and pus formation. This purulence leads to a septic thrombosis of draining veins, which serve as a conduit for infection that reach the epidural venous plexus resulting in epidural abscess.[1,2,3]

In addition to the arterial route, seeding of disc space may travel in a transvenous fashion, often involving the valveless veins of Batson's plexus.[22] This explains why infections involving the left kidney parenchyma increase the risk of spine infection given that the left kidney communicates directly with the plexus. Spine infection can also originate from other pelvic organs such as the bladder, bowel, and female genital tract.[1,2] Pathogenic microorganisms may also travel via epidural veins directly resulting in epidural abscess involving multiple segments without involvement of the bony vertebral body or disc space.[1,3]

16.3.2 Nonhematogenous Spread/Extension from an Infected Contiguous Infection

Nonhematogenous inoculation of disc or epidural space may result from the use of contaminated needles or other surgical instruments during interventional or diagnostic procedures such as discography, chemonucleolysis,[23,24] epidural anesthesia, or surgery.[3] In contrast to hematogenous spread, the infection originating in the disc space following direct inoculation spreads into the adjacent vertebral body marrow through the endplates.[2,22]

16.3.3 Iatrogenic Inoculations

Up to one-third of spinal infection cases are considered iatrogenic, resulting from contamination during spine surgery.[25,26] In spite of modern advances in surgical prophylaxis, postoperative surgical site infections have continued to jeopardize selected patient outcomes after spinal surgery.[27] The risk of postoperative spine infection is increased with extensive instrumentation.[3] Recent reports on the rate of surgical site infection after spine surgery have ranged from 0.7 to 16%.[28,29,30,31,32,33] Risk factors for postoperative infections are either nonmodifiable or modifiable. Nonmodifiable factors include patient age (> 70), the American Society of Anesthesiologists (ASA) score, diabetes mellitus (DM), cardiovascular disease, obesity, smoking, malignancy, steroid use, previous lumbar surgery, malnutrition, chronic obstructive pulmonary disease, and immunological competency.[34,35,36,37] Modifiable factors include *Staphylococcus aureus* nasal screen and decolonization, duration of surgery, blood loss, transfusions, use of instrumentation, multiple staged interventions, amount of levels fused, and prolonged hospital stay.[35,36,37,38,39,40]

16.4 Spinal Epidural Abscess

16.4.1 Risk Factors

In addition to risk factors discussed above for spondylitis, certain factors may predispose patients to develop SEA. A meta-analysis of 915 patients found that DM and IV drug abuse are among the most common risk factors and found in 15 and 8.5%, respectively.[18] Patients with DM have reduced chemotaxis, phagocytosis, and bactericidal activity of neutrophilic granulocytes which accentuate the progression to abscess. IV drug abuse is associated with an increased risk of transient bacteremia that may lead to the development of SEA as well as compromised cellular and humoral immunity.[41]

16.4.2 Source Site of Infection

Hematogenous Spread

Akin to vertebral osteomyelitis, the most mechanism of seeding of the epidural space occurs via hematogenous spread. Carbuncles, furuncles, and skin abscesses are often found to be the primary source of SEA. Cutaneous infections were found to be present in 33 to 44% cases of SEA.[18,42,43,44] Other sites include the respiratory tract (otitis media, sinusitis, or pneumonia[45]), the genitourinary tract, visceral organs, oral cavity,[46] and endocarditis.[14]

Direct Extension from a Contiguous Site

Direct extension or lymphatic spread to the epidural space from a contiguous infection, osteomyelitis, or spondylodiscitis may also occur. In one series, osteomyelitis was present in up to two-thirds of patients with SEA.[14] Inoculation of epidural space may also occur with a psoas or retropharyngeal abscess, decubitus ulcer, pharyngeal infections, mediastinitis, pyelonephritis with perinephric abscess, and dermal sinus. Traumatic injuries and spinal hematoma associated with such injuries form another important group of risk factors with frequencies of such cases ranging from 10 to 34.7%.[26,47,48]

Iatrogenic Inoculation

SEA can also be caused by iatrogenic inoculation during an invasive procedure of the spine or the surrounding vasculature.[46] Patients with evidence of any perioperative infections are at a greater risk of developing a subsequent SEA.[14] Among open procedures, lumbar discectomy has the highest risk of SEA (0.67%).[49]

Interventional, diagnostic, and therapeutic closed procedures may also be associated with an increased risk of SEA. Epidural catheterization, often employed for pain control or local anesthesia, may provide a portal of entry of skin flora such as *Staphylococcus epidermidis* or *S. aureus* in at-risk patients. The duration of catheterization is the most important risk factor. For a duration of less than 2 days, the incidence rate is 0.2 per 1,000 catheter-days[3,50,51] with longer duration of use, the rate increases to 0.77 per 1,000 catheter-days.[15,52,53,54] Overall, only 3.9% of all SEA is associated with anesthetic interventions occurring at a rate of 1 in 100,000 for epidural interventions.[18]

16.4.3 Clinical Presentation

The clinical presentation is dependent on the extent, site, and level of the SEA. A history of recent infection should be delineated. Heusner in 1948 described stages of SEA.[55] Earliest symptoms are back pain and fever often accompanied by local tenderness. The next stage is signs of spinal irritation which may be elucidated by straight leg raise (SLR) test, Kernig's (painful extension of the knee subsequent to knee and hip flexion) and Lhermitte's signs (burst of shock-like pain extending caudally from the neck), Brudzinski's reflex neck stiffness, and even extremity symptoms such as radiating pain depending on the craniocaudal level of abscess. During the third stage, patients will exhibit neurological dysfunction such as fecal or urinary incontinence, muscle weakness, and/or sensory deficits. The fourth and final stage is complete paralysis secondary to severe muscle weakness. The classic triad of back pain, fever, and neurological deficit is present in 13% of cases.[56,57,58] Atypical symptoms such as abdominal pain, headache, bowel dysfunction, and sudden paralysis have also been reported.[56,59,60] SEA leading to neurological disability is more common in cervical and thoracic spine than in the lumbar region.[3]

In one meta-analysis of 915 number of SEAs found that the thoracic region affected (50%), followed by lumbar (34%) and cervical (19%).[18] Most SEAs are located posterior to the spinal cord (80 vs. 20%).[61] However, it's worth noting that SEA originating from an adjacent osteomyelitis is often confined to the anterior portion of the spinal cord.[62] Circumferential extension of the abscess around the thecal sac is uncommon (▶ Fig. 16.1a, b).

On physical examination, patient exhibits severe tenderness on palpation and percussion of the affected spinal segment. Gibbus deformity is seen in advanced cases with extensive bony erosion. Neurological findings of dermatomal sensory and/or motor loss as well as bowel and bladder dysfunction are indicative of a spinal cord injury. Though rare, prolonged infection may cause chronic compression of the spinal cord, manifesting as long tract signs and symptoms.[3]

16.4.4 Pathogenesis of Neurological Dysfunction

Neurological signs associated with SEA are due to mechanical compression or microvascular damage.[63,64,65,66,67] In one animal model of SEA, investigators found no evidence of gross compression or histopathological thrombosis of blood vessels suggesting that mechanical compression of nerve roots is the main cause of neurological symptoms.[63] However, it is widely believed that the neurological compromise is often the result of both.[14]

16.4.5 Diagnosis

The most important step in establishing a diagnosis of SEA is having a high level of clinical suspicion based on clinical or laboratory studies.[68] It's imperative to consider SEA in the differential of back pain and irritative neurological symptoms. A combination of back pain, neurological symptoms, and elevated systemic inflammatory markers should raise the clinical suspicion of SEA. This should promptly lead providers to proceed with confirmatory radiological or microbiological testing. Any delay in establishing the diagnosis of SEA may lead to irreversible neurological sequelae including paralysis.[18] Spine MRI with and without gadolinium is considered the radiological test of choice for establishing the diagnosis of SEA.

16.4.6 Laboratory Investigation

Elevation of systemic inflammation markers such as erythrocyte sedimentation rate (ESR) and C-reactive protein (CRP) is present in a majority of the patients with SEA. Patients with recalcitrant back, signs of systemic infection, or progressive neurological symptoms should have ESR and CRP testing as part of their work-up.[69] Leukocytosis is uncommon in patients with SEA.

16.4.7 Radiological Investigation

Radiological investigations often follow clinical suspicion based on clinical presentation and laboratory testing. Spine roentgenograms are often obtained and may be able to rule out fracture, bone loss, and provide gross assessment of spinal stability.[62,70,71,72,73,74,75,76] Specific findings on radiographs in protracted SEA cases may show loss of disc height, trabecular erosion of bone, prevertebral and paravertebral soft-tissue volume, endplate destruction, vertebral collapse with loss of lordosis, and the development of gibbus or kyphotic deformity at the level of lesion.[3]

Computerized tomography (CT) of the spine offers a better sensitivity compared to radiographs and provides better visualization and extent of prevertebral and paravertebral soft-tissue inflammation as stranding and loss of normal tissue planes.[3] Distinguishing spinal cord from epidural space can sometimes be challenging on CT.[76] CT is often performed when MRI is contraindicated such as presence of implantable cardiac devices, ferromagnetic aneurysm clips, or shrapnels.[69] The advantage of CT over MRI in the evaluation of SEA is that it will be able to better delineate concomitant spondylodiscitis, with sclerotic endplate changes. CT is also performed prior to a planned spinal instrumentation in order to evaluate the quality of existing boney structures as well as the extent of bone loss (▶ Fig. 16.2b).

Myelography used to be the investigation of choice until the late 1990s.[18] It delineates the extent of epidural abscess accurately as the contrast medium can be visualized surrounding and outlining the abscess above and below it.[62,71,72,76,77,78] Myelography combined with CT may help better visualize the paraspinal space.[14,72,76] Some older publications believed the combination to be the only definitive source of diagnosis.[79]

MRI is considered the gold standard for the diagnosis of epidural abscess with greater than 90% sensitivity and specificity.[69,80] Imaging should be obtained both with and without contrast (▶ Fig. 16.3a–c). T1 image is helpful in detecting a hypointense signal in the vertebral body, specifically at the endplates signifying the loss of normal hyperintense fat signal. The

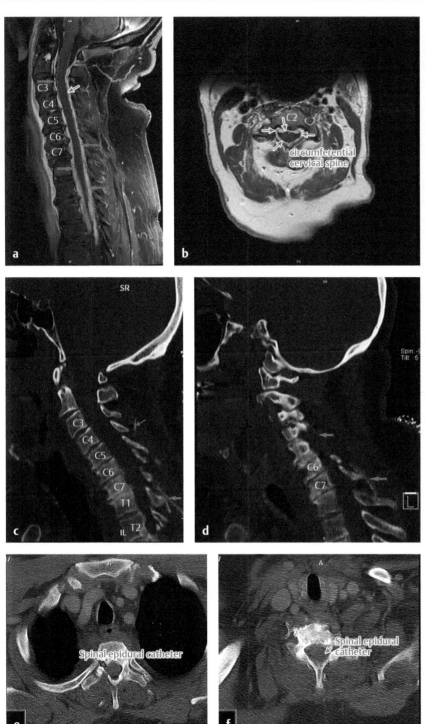

Fig. 16.1 **(a)** Preoperative sagittal T1-weighted MRI with contrast showing ventral and posterior phlegm of epidural abscess extending from C1 through T4 (*red arrows*). **(b)** Preoperative axial T1-weighted MRI with contrast showing the circumferential spread of epidural abscess at C2 level (*red arrows*). **(c–f)** Postoperative sagittal **(c,d)** and axial **(e,f)** CT scan showing the epidural catheters (*red arrows*) placed to drain the abscess. A 68-year-old man admitted with 1 to 2 weeks of intermittent thoracic back pain and fever, 3 days of right ear pain followed by right ear purulent drainage, and some shortness of breath. He was started on broad-spectrum antibiotics. CTA was negative for pulmonary embolism. Chest X-ray was unrevealing. CT of the head on revealed fluid opacification of the right mastoid and external/middle ear secondary to acute otitis media and mastoiditis. Blood cultures at the outside facility were positive for *Streptococcus pneumoniae*. MRI spine revealed findings given above **(a,b)**. His operative course consisted of multilevel decompressive hemilaminotomies and foraminotomies ("skip laminectomies") at left bottom of C3 to top of C5, right C5–6, left C7–T1, right T2–3 followed by placement of three epidural drains. "Skip laminectomies" avoid the need for instrumentation by doing the least amount of decompressive surgery as possible, needed to debride and decompress the spinal canal. Postoperatively, patient had resolution of arm and neck pain and remained neurologically intact and on appropriate microcoverage. Postoperative CT with contrast showed resolution of the long segment of epidural phlegmon previously seen on MRI and no definite enhancing lesion with mass effect is seen within the spinal canal to suggest residual/recurrent abscess.

disc height can be visualized to be markedly reduced on T1. T2 helps delineate soft-tissue edema in disc space as well as bone and paravertebral soft tissue[3] (▶ Fig. 16.4a, b). Contrast-enhanced T1 provides the best visualization of vertebral endplates, vertebral body, prevertebral and paravertebral soft tissue, and epidural space. There can also be ring-like enhancement or linear dural enhancement which is considered indications for surgery by some authors.[81,82] Some authors have recommended scanning the whole spine to exclude noncontig-uous SEA when symptoms suggestive of abscess have persisted for at least a week, when there is presence of coexisting infection outside the spinal region, and when ESR is greater than 95 mm/h.[83]

Other studies, such as indium white blood cell (WBC) scan, provide good sensitivity and specificity for detecting infections. Indium studies are better than bone scans (gallium scans), because they are specific to spine infectious as opposed to trauma or neoplastic processes.

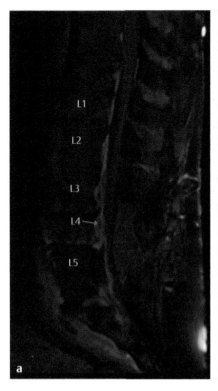

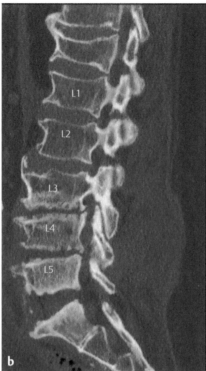

Fig. 16.2 **(a)** Sagittal T1 with contrast-enhancing imaging of the lumbar spine showing ventral SEA with osteodiscitis (*red arrow*). **(b)** Sagittal CT lumbar spine showing endplate changes consistent with sclerosis, loss of disc height, and changes consistent with osteodiscitis (*red arrow*). A 65-year-old man with history of disseminated *Streptococcus viridans* group infection, multiple previous spine surgeries, and infection of left ankle. The patient had a history of remote previous lumbar spine surgery and recent thoracic decompressive surgery. Surgical findings were consistent with granulation and inflammatory tissue without frankly purulent material and multiple intraoperative cultures negative for infection. Clinically, the patient improved significantly following surgery with resolution of the radicular bilateral leg pains.

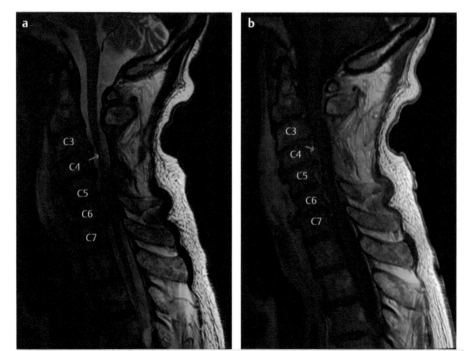

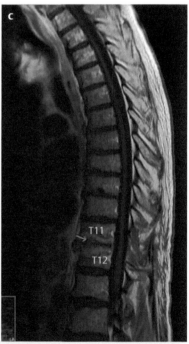

Fig. 16.3 **(a)** Sagittal T2-weighted MRI showing myelomalacia and atrophy (*red arrow*) of the spinal cord at C3-4 level. **(b)** Sagittal T1-weighted MRI with contrast showing enhancing ventral epidural abscess from C3 through C7 (*red arrow*). Also evident are degenerative changes throughout the cervical spine as well as spondylodiscitis of C3 through C5. **(c)** Sagittal T1-weighted MRI with contrast showing spondylodiscitis at T11-12 with anterior wedging and loss of disc height (*red arrow*). An 84-year-old man with history of previous posterior cervical decompression at C3-5 3 years ago and a decompression and resection of epidural cyst at T11–T12 1 year ago. Patient had a suspected immunocompromised state due to advanced age and history of lymphoma status postexploratory laparotomy, splenectomy, and lymphadenectomy 30 years ago. Presented with neck pain and B/L arm weakness and was found to have delayed spondylodiscitis and at both surgical sites secondary to sepsis. Blood cultures grew pan-sensitive septicemia by Strep G in 2/2 sets at 9 hours (7/7 bottles). CT-guided biopsy was not performed given the known source and microbiological specimen with appropriate sensitivities.

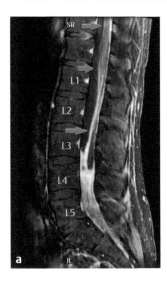 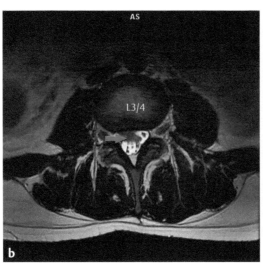

Fig. 16.4 (a) Sagittal T1-weighted MRI with contrast showing intradural enhancement extent cephalad from L4 level (*red arrows*). **(b)** Axial T2-weighted MRI showing the intradural extent of infection at L3–L4 level (*red arrow*) consistent with granulomatous disease. A 25-year-old man with history of IV drug abuse. Intraoperatively, the epidural space was found to be dry without signs of obvious infection. Subsequently, the dura was opened in the midline with a 15 blade. Upon encountering the arachnoid, no egress of CSF was noticed. A white discolored scarring of the arachnoid was seen, which was mixed in with lumbar rootlets. Scar tissue was dissected off of the rootlets and sent for microbiology. This is a classic finding for patient with history of previous meningitis which is an intradural process. This often leads to arachnoiditis and CSF loculations, scarring and obstruction of flow can occur later in life. Similar findings can occur in patient with history of subarachnoid hemorrhage (SAH) which may cause blood products to irritate the leptomeninges and cause scarring.

16.4.8 Microbiology

Establishing a microbiological diagnosis of SEA is a crucial step in confirming the diagnosis and will help guide targeted antimicrobial therapy. In patients who are neurologically stable and without hemodynamic instability or other signs of systemic sever sepsis, empiric antimicrobials should be held until establishing a microbiological diagnosis. Blood cultures should be obtained in all patients with radiologically confirmed discitis or SEA. Blood cultures are positive in 62% of the cases in patients with SEA.[57,84] In patients without a microbiologically confirmed bloodstream infection, radiologically assisted needle biopsy should be obtained from disc space or paravertebral nonepidural collections are often the next step. Specimen collection via open surgical technique may be warranted if a microbiological diagnosis has not yet been established.[61] Lumbar puncture is of low yield and should be avoided due to the risk of contaminating the central nervous system (CNS). When obtained, cerebrospinal fluid (CSF) studies reveal nonspecific elevation of protein and pleocytosis while culture is rarely positive (19%). The most common organism cultured from these sites is *S. aureus* (60–90%), with methicillin-resistant (MRSA) accounting for most of them[18,69,80,84,85,86,87] followed by gram-negative bacilli (*Escherichia coli*, etc.) (16%) and *Pseudomonas aeruginosa*, both reported frequently in the setting of IV drug abuse.[88,89] The first radiologically assisted biopsy does not establish a microbiological diagnosis in up to half of the cases.[45] In this circumstance, a repeat procedure is advocated.[90]

16.4.9 Differential Diagnosis

SEA is an uncommon cause of acute back pain but should be considered for the reasons stated above. Other important differentials for appropriate patient groups include meningitis, acute transverse myelitis, spinal cord tumors, metastatic lesion, herpes zoster, disc and degenerative bone disease, and pseudomeningocele (specially in postoperative patients).[49]

16.4.10 Management

Treatment Principles

Once the diagnosis of an epidural abscess is established, it's imperative to initiate antimicrobial therapy and evaluate the need for surgical intervention. A delay of therapy may lead to irreversible neurological damage.[91,92] A multidisciplinary approach to the diagnosis and management of SEA between an infectious diseases specialist, spine surgeon, and interventional radiologist may lead to a better outcome. Surgical decompression followed by a course of antimicrobial therapy may be appropriate.[84,93,94,95] A large meta-analysis found that 89% of patients with SEA were managed with this approach.[18] More recent data would suggest that a good proportion of patients may be managed with antimicrobial therapy alone with or without drainage performed by interventional radiology. Emergent surgical decompression should be considered in cases of progressive neurological dysfunction, evidence of impending spinal cord compression, or failure of medical or minimally invasive drainage.[14,55,93,96] For anterior SEA, anterior decompression may be an option since these cases most often arise from adjacent osteomyelitis.[18,90,94,95]

Medical Management

Empiric broad-spectrum antimicrobial therapy should be initiated in the setting of neurological compromise, hemodynamic instability, or severe signs of infections. In most other circumstances, antimicrobial therapy should be withheld until conformation of a microbiological diagnosis. Parenteral therapy at least initially is often the preferred route. Current guidelines from Infectious Diseases Society of America (IDSA) advocate the use of a total of 6 weeks of therapy in most cases of discitis. Longer therapy may be warranted for patients with extensive epidural abscess, in the absence of drainage, or with MRSA infection.

A suggested empiric antimicrobial regimen is one that combines antistaphylococcal (including MRSA) and anti–gram-negative bacilli agents, such as vancomycin,[90] combined with cefotaxime, ceftriaxone, cefepime, or ceftazidime. Cefepime or ceftazidime are preferred when *Pseudomonas aeruginosa* is likely such as intravenous drug abusers (IVDA). Some experts have vouched for adding an antistaphylococcal penicillin agent such as oxacillin or nafcillin to the regimen above to enhance antistaphylococcal activity.[97,98,99] Targeted therapy is often guided by culture results and in vitro susceptibility data. A history of type I hypersensitivity reaction to a beta-lactam should prompt the use of a fluoroquinolone such as levofloxacin or a monobactam such as aztreonam.

Surgical Management

The primary objective of surgery is to decompress the neural elements, to drain the abscess, and to establish a microbiological diagnosis.[46,90] Anteriorly, abscesses are approached by performing a decompression and, if needed, a partial or complete anterior/anterolateral corpectomy.[90] Anterior abscesses often compromise the stability of the spine. Grafting is also recommended with both autologous as well as allogenic grafts yielding optimum results.[100,101] Anterior corpectomies should be combined with posterior instrumentation to stabilize the spine, especially if there is multilevel involvement. When spinal instability is present due to destruction of vertebral body resulting in malalignment, surgery is warranted to stabilize the spine and correct the alignment to prevent further compression of neural elements.[90] Role of instrumented fusion when spinal stability is not compromised is unclear, and some experts vouch for delayed posterior fusion. This prevents graft damage which might happen if placed during the initial surgery in the presence of active infection.[102] With posterior abscesses, given their infrequent association with bone involvement, a laminectomy is often adequate to achieve optimum decompression without the need of supplemented instrumentation.[46,90] For some patients with posterior abscesses who have less severe or no neurological symptoms, percutaneous abscess drainage has also been reported. Though this decreases perioperative morbidity, the inadequate drainage of abscess is considered as a concern and hence not recommended routinely.[46]

Given the emerging trends of minimally invasive techniques aimed at decreasing perioperative morbidity, it is imperative to discuss reports of MIS surgery employed for approaching SEA. Safavi-Abbasi et al presented their experience of treating posterior epidural abscess in three patients using tubular retractor system.[103] In the presence of multiple abscesses, the authors made two separate paramedian incisions to insert two or more dilators to achieve adequate irrigation and evacuation. The dilators were entered into the center of abscesses after performing hemilaminectomies. All three patients achieved optimum resolution of symptoms and the abscess. Tan et al reported a case of anterior thoracic SEA associated with discitis and osteomyelitis, which was approached using a minimally invasive transpedicular approach. The patient had optimum outcomes and was mobilizing on postoperative day 1.[104]

16.5 Outcomes

While SEA continues to present a diagnostic and therapeutic challenge, the mortality rate has significantly reduced over the years[18] owing to early diagnosis and initiation of antibiotics which help control the spread of the pathology. The current mortality has been estimated to be from 5 to 20%.[18,69,80] The most critical factor is the dissemination of infection leading to sepsis and multiorgan failure, which is the cause of death in majority of cases.[43,105] Furthermore, permanent neurological disability as a sequel is common and is dependent on various factors. One such factor is the region of the abscess with thoracic SEA being more likely to result in adverse neurological outcomes when compared to their cervical and lumbar counterpart (36% vs. 12.5 and 7.7%, respectively[94]). Another factor is the severity of neurological symptoms at presentation, which is inversely related with outcomes. One study found a mortality rate of 21% among patients who had severe neurological disability at presentation, while 34% had permanent paraplegia.[94] Timely management is also another crucial factor that affects outcome. An older study found that a greater proportion of patients who had early intervention (< 36 hours from symptom onset) were able to regain some neurological functions, compared to those who were managed after more than 36 hours after symptom onset.[6] More recent studies have advocated for surgical decompression before 72 hours.[43] Other factors that are associated with adverse outcomes include MRSA infection, multiple coexisting medical conditions, leukocytosis, elevated CRP, increasing age (> 50 years), extent of thecal sac compression, intraoperative appearance (granulation tissue only, as opposed to pustular abscesses), sepsis, prior history of spine surgery, DM, and rheumatoid arthritis.[6,69,94,96,106,107]

16.6 Conclusion

SEA is a challenging pathology that warrants a timely and multidisciplinary approach. Timely diagnosis along prolonged antibiotic therapy is the mainstay of treatment. Surgical intervention may be needed in selected patients to decompress the neural elements and to establish a microbiological diagnosis.

References

[1] Cheung WY, Luk KDK. Pyogenic spondylitis. Int Orthop. 2012; 36(2):397–404

[2] Tyrrell PN, Cassar-Pullicino VN, McCall IW. Spinal infection. Eur Radiol. 1999; 9(6):1066–1077

[3] Vollmer DG, Tandon N. Infections of the Spine. Youmans Neurologic Surg 2011:2831–2847

[4] Taylor GM, Murphy E, Hopkins R, Rutland P, Chistov Y. First report of Mycobacterium bovis DNA in human remains from the Iron Age. Microbiology. 2007; 153(Pt 4):1243–1249

[5] Stäbler A, Reiser MF. Imaging of spinal infection. Radiol Clin North Am. 2001; 39(1):115–135

[6] Danner RL, Hartman BJ. Update on spinal epidural abscess: 35 cases and review of the literature. Rev Infect Dis. 1987; 9(2):265–274

[7] Sapico FL, Montgomerie JZ. Pyogenic vertebral osteomyelitis: report of nine cases and review of the literature. Rev Infect Dis. 1979; 1(5):754–776

[8] Kapeller P, Fazekas F, Krametter D, et al. Pyogenic infectious spondylitis: clinical, laboratory and MRI features. Eur Neurol. 1997; 38(2):94–98

[9] Hopkinson N, Stevenson J, Benjamin S. A case ascertainment study of septic discitis: clinical, microbiological and radiological features. QJM. 2001; 94(9): 465–470

[10] Grammatico L, Baron S, Rusch E, et al. Epidemiology of vertebral osteomyelitis (VO) in France: analysis of hospital-discharge data 2002–2003. Epidemiol Infect. 2008; 136(5):653–660

[11] Gahr-Traumazentrum RH. GMS Interdisciplinary Plastic and Reconstructive Surgery DGPW. Available at: http://www.egms.de/static/de/journals/iprs/2013–2/iprs000038.shtml

[12] Krogsgaard MR, Wagn P, Bengtsson J. Epidemiology of acute vertebral osteomyelitis in Denmark: 137 cases in Denmark 1978–1982, compared to cases reported to the National Patient Register 1991–1993. Acta Orthop Scand. 1998; 69(5):513–517

[13] Grewal S, Hocking G, Wildsmith JAW. Epidural abscesses. Br J Anaesth. 2006; 96(3):292–302

[14] Hlavin ML, Kaminski HJ, Ross JS, Ganz E. Spinal epidural abscess: a ten-year perspective. Neurosurgery. 1990; 27(2):177–184

[15] Kindler C, Seeberger M, Siegemund M, Schneider M. Extradural abscess complicating lumbar extradural anaesthesia and analgesia in an obstetric patient. Acta Anaesthesiol Scand. 1996; 40(7):858–861

[16] Prendergast H, Jerrard D, O'Connell J. Atypical presentations of epidural abscess in intravenous drug abusers. Am J Emerg Med. 1997; 15(2):158–160

[17] Belzunegui J, Intxausti JJ, De Dios JR, et al. Haematogenous vertebral osteomyelitis in the elderly. Clin Rheumatol. 2000; 19(5):344–347

[18] Reihsaus E, Waldbaur H, Seeling W. Spinal epidural abscess: a meta-analysis of 915 patients. Neurosurg Rev. 2000; 23(4):175–204, discussion 205

[19] Mylona E, Samarkos M, Kakalou E, Fanourgiakis P, Skoutelis A. Pyogenic vertebral osteomyelitis: a systematic review of clinical characteristics. Semin Arthritis Rheum. 2009; 39(1):10–17

[20] Berbari EF, Kanj SS, Kowalski TJ, et al. Infectious Diseases Society of America. 2015 Infectious Diseases Society of America (IDSA) Clinical Practice Guidelines for the Diagnosis and Treatment of Native Vertebral Osteomyelitis in Adults. Clin Infect Dis. 2015; 61(6):e26–e46

[21] Resnick D, Niwayama G. Osteomyelitis, septic arthritis, and soft tissue infection: organisms. In: Resnick D, ed. Diagnosis of Bone and Joint Disorders. 3rd ed. Philadelphia, PA: WB Saunders; 1995:2448–2558

[22] Tali ET. Spinal infections. Eur J Radiol. 2004; 50(2):120–133

[23] Fraser RD, Osti OL, Vernon-Roberts B. Discitis following chemonucleolysis. An experimental study. Spine. 1986; 11(7):679–687

[24] Guyer RD, Collier R, Stith WJ, et al. Discitis after discography. Spine. 1988; 13(12):1352–1354

[25] Gupta A, Kowalski TJ, Osmon DR, et al. Long-term outcome of pyogenic vertebral osteomyelitis: a cohort study of 260 patients. Open Forum Infect Dis. 2014; 1(3):ofu107

[26] Pigrau C, Rodríguez-Pardo D, Fernández-Hidalgo N, et al. Health care associated hematogenous pyogenic vertebral osteomyelitis: a severe and potentially preventable infectious disease. Medicine (Baltimore). 2015; 94(3):e365

[27] Weinstein MA, McCabe JP, Cammisa FP, Jr. Postoperative spinal wound infection: a review of 2,391 consecutive index procedures. J Spinal Disord. 2000; 13(5):422–426

[28] Veeravagu A, Patil CG, Lad SP, Boakye M. Risk factors for postoperative spinal wound infections after spinal decompression and fusion surgeries. Spine. 2009; 34(17):1869–1872

[29] Thalgott JS, Cotler HB, Sasso RC, Gardner V. Postoperative infections in spinal implants. Classification and analysis—a multicenter study. Spine. 1991; 16(8):981–984

[30] Horan TC, Culver DH, Gaynes RP. Nosocomial infections in surgical patients in the United States, January 1986–June 1992. Infect Control Urol Care. 1993. Available at: http://journals.cambridge.org/abstract_S0899823X00089923

[31] Pull ter Gunne AF, Cohen DB. Incidence, prevalence, and analysis of risk factors for surgical site infection following adult spinal surgery. Spine. 2009; 34(13):1422–1428

[32] Fang A, Hu SS, Endres N, Bradford DS. Risk factors for infection after spinal surgery. Spine. 2005; 30(12):1460–1465

[33] Smith JS, Shaffrey CI, Sansur CA, et al. Scoliosis Research Society Morbidity and Mortality Committee. Rates of infection after spine surgery based on 108,419 procedures: a report from the Scoliosis Research Society Morbidity and Mortality Committee. Spine. 2011; 36(7):556–563

[34] Olsen MA, Nepple JJ, Riew KD, et al. Risk factors for surgical site infection following orthopaedic spinal operations. J Bone Joint Surg Am. 2008; 90(1):62–69

[35] Koutsoumbelis S, Hughes AP, Girardi FP, et al. Risk factors for postoperative infection following posterior lumbar instrumented arthrodesis. J Bone Joint Surg Am. 2011; 93(17):1627–1633

[36] Christodoulou AG, Givissis P, Symeonidis PD, Karataglis D, Pournaras J. Reduction of postoperative spinal infections based on an etiologic protocol. Clin Orthop Relat Res. 2006; 444(444):107–113

[37] Cunningham ME, Girardi F, Papadopoulos EC, Cammisa FP. Spinal infections in patients with compromised immune systems. Clin Orthop Relat Res. 2006; 444(444):73–82

[38] Gelalis ID, Arnaoutoglou CM, Politis AN, Batzaleksis NA, Katonis PG, Xenakis TA. Bacterial wound contamination during simple and complex spinal procedures. A prospective clinical study. Spine J. 2011; 11(11):1042–1048

[39] Klein JD, Hey LA, Yu CS, et al. Perioperative nutrition and postoperative complications in patients undergoing spinal surgery. Spine. 1996; 21(22):2676–2682

[40] Dick J, Boachie-Adjei O, Wilson M. One-stage versus two-stage anterior and posterior spinal reconstruction in adults. Comparison of outcomes including nutritional status, complications rates, hospital costs, and other factors. Spine. 1992; 17(8) Suppl:S310–S316

[41] Brown SM, Stimmel B, Taub RN, Kochwa S, Rosenfield RE. Immunologic dysfunction in heroin addicts. Arch Intern Med. 1974; 134(6):1001–1006

[42] Redekop GJ, Del Maestro RF. Vertebral hemangioma causing spinal cord compression during pregnancy. Surg Neurol. 1992; 38(3):210–215

[43] Khanna RK, Malik GM, Rock JP, Rosenblum ML. Spinal epidural abscess: evaluation of factors influencing outcome. Neurosurgery. 1996; 39(5):958–964

[44] Maslen DR, Jones SR, Crislip MA, Bracis R, Dworkin RJ, Flemming JE. Spinal epidural abscess. Optimizing patient care. Arch Intern Med. 1993; 153(14):1713–1721

[45] Greenberg MS. Handbook of Neurosurgery. Thieme; 2010

[46] Bluman EM, Palumbo MA, Lucas PR. Spinal epidural abscess in adults. J Am Acad Orthop Surg. 2004; 12(3):155–163

[47] Hulme A, Dott NM. Spinal epidural abscess. BMJ. 1954; 1(4853):64–68

[48] Rigamonti D, Liem L, Wolf AL, et al. Epidural abscess in the cervical spine. Mt Sinai J Med. 1994; 61(4):357–362

[49] Spiegelmann R, Findler G, Faibel M, Ram Z, Shacked I, Sahar A. Postoperative spinal epidural empyema. Clinical and computed tomography features. Spine. 1991; 16(10):1146–1149

[50] Ready LB, Loper KA, Nessly M, Wild L. Postoperative epidural morphine is safe on surgical wards. Anesthesiology. 1991; 75(3):452–456

[51] Schug SA, Torrie JJ. Safety assessment of postoperative pain management by an acute pain service. Pain. 1993; 55(3):387–391

[52] Holt HM, Andersen SS, Andersen O, Gahrn-Hansen B, Siboni K. Infections following epidural catheterization. J Hosp Infect. 1995; 30(4):253–260

[53] Nyström B, Larsen SO, Dankert J, et al. The European Working Party on Control of Hospital Infections. Bacteraemia in surgical patients with intravenous devices: a European multicentre incidence study. J Hosp Infect. 1983; 4(4):338–349

[54] Phillips JMG, Stedeford JC, Hartsilver E, Roberts C. Epidural abscess complicating insertion of epidural catheters. Br J Anaesth. 2002; 89(5):778–782

[55] Heusner AP. Nontuberculous spinal epidural infections. N Engl J Med. 1948; 239(23):845–854

[56] Bremer AA, Darouiche RO. Spinal epidural abscess presenting as intra-abdominal pathology: a case report and literature review. J Emerg Med. 2004; 26(1):51–56

[57] Darouiche RO, Hamill RJ, Greenberg SB, Weathers SW, Musher DM. Bacterial spinal epidural abscess. Review of 43 cases and literature survey. Medicine (Baltimore). 1992; 71(6):369–385

[58] Davis DP, Wold RM, Patel RJ, et al. The clinical presentation and impact of diagnostic delays on emergency department patients with spinal epidural abscess. J Emerg Med. 2004; 26(3):285–291

[59] Noy ML, George S. Unusual presentation of a spinal epidural abscess. BMJ Case Rep. 2012; 2012. DOI: 10.1136/bcr-03-2012-5956

[60] Prakash A, Kubba S, Singh NP, et al. Tuberculous epidural abscess-an unusual presentation. 2004. http://imsear.li.mahidol.ac.th/handle/123456789/148243

[61] Chao D, Nanda A. Spinal epidural abscess: a diagnostic challenge. Am Fam Physician. 2002; 65(7):1341–1346

[62] Martin RJ, Yuan HA. Neurosurgical care of spinal epidural, subdural, and intramedullary abscesses and arachnoiditis. Orthop Clin North Am. 1996; 27(1):125–136

[63] Feldenzer JA, McKeever PE, Schaberg DR, Campbell JA, Hoff JT. The pathogenesis of spinal epidural abscess: microangiographic studies in an experimental model. J Neurosurg. 1988; 69(1):110–114

[64] Baker AS, Ojemann RG, Swartz MN, Richardson EP, Jr. Spinal epidural abscess. N Engl J Med. 1975; 293(10):463–468

[65] Baker CJ. Primary spinal epidural abscess. Am J Dis Child. 1971; 121(4):337–339

[66] Browder J, Meyers R. Pyogenic infections of the spinal epidural space: a consideration of the anatomic and physiologic pathology. Surgery. 1941; 10:296–308

[67] Feldenzer JA, McKeever PE, Schaberg DR, Campbell JA, Hoff JT. Experimental spinal epidural abscess: a pathophysiological model in the rabbit. Neurosurgery. 1987; 20(6):859–867

[68] Schlossberg D, Shulman JA. Spinal epidural abscess. South Med J. 1977; 70 (6):669–673

[69] Sendi P, Bregenzer T, Zimmerli W. Spinal epidural abscess in clinical practice. QJM. 2008; 101(1):1–12

[70] Goodman RR. Book Review The Practice of Neurosurgery Edited by George T. Tindall, Paul R. Cooper, and Daniel L. Barrow. 3496 pp. in three volumes, illustrated. Baltimore, Williams & Wilkins, 1996. 595. 0-683-08266-3 Neurosurgery Second edition. Edited by Robert H. Wilkins and Setti S. Rengachary. 4271 pp. in three volumes, illustrated. New York, McGraw-Hill, 1996. 550. 0-07-079991-1. N Engl J Med. 1997;336 (2):142–143

[71] Gilden DH. Clinical topics in infectious diseases. In: Schlossberg D, ed. Infections of the Nervous System. New York, NY: Springer-Verlag; 1990:396

[72] Ingham HR, Sisson PR, Mendelow AD, Kalbag RM, McAllister VL. Pyogenic neurosurgical infections. London: Edward Arnold; 1991:103–134

[73] McGahan JP, Dublin AB. Evaluation of spinal infections by plain radiographs, computed tomography, intrathecal metrizamide, and CT-guided biopsy. Diagn Imaging Clin Med. 1985; 54(1):11–20

[74] Olcott EW, Dillon WP. Plain film clues to the diagnosis of spinal epidural neoplasm and infection. Neuroradiology. 1993; 35(4):288–292

[75] Ruiz A, Post JD, Ganz WI. Inflammatory and infectious processes of the cervical spine. Neuroimaging Clin N Am. 1995; 5(3):401–425

[76] Smith AS, Blaser SI. Infectious and inflammatory processes of the spine. Radiol Clin North Am. 1991; 29(4):809–827

[77] Rengachary SS, Kennedy JD. Intracranial arachnoid and ependymal cysts. Neurosurgery. 1985; 3:2160–2172

[78] Verner EF, Musher DM. Spinal epidural abscess. Med Clin North Am. 1985; 69(2):375–384

[79] O'Sullivan R, McKenzie A, Hennessy O. Value of CT scanning in assessing location and extent of epidural and paraspinal inflammatory conditions. Australas Radiol. 1988; 32(2):203–206

[80] Nussbaum ES, Rigamonti D, Standiford H, Numaguchi Y, Wolf AL, Robinson WL. Spinal epidural abscess: a report of 40 cases and review. Surg Neurol. 1992; 38(3):225–231

[81] Tuchman A, Pham M, Hsieh PC. The indications and timing for operative management of spinal epidural abscess: literature review and treatment algorithm. Neurosurg Focus. 2014; 37(2):E8

[82] Uchida K, Nakajima H, Yayama T, et al. Epidural abscess associated with pyogenic spondylodiscitis of the lumbar spine; evaluation of a new MRI staging classification and imaging findings as indicators of surgical management: a retrospective study of 37 patients. Arch Orthop Trauma Surg. 2010; 130(1): 111–118

[83] Ju KL, Kim SD, Melikian R, Bono CM, Harris MB. Predicting patients with concurrent noncontiguous spinal epidural abscess lesions. Spine J. 2015; 15(1): 95–101

[84] Darouiche RO. Spinal epidural abscess. N Engl J Med. 2006; 355(19):2012–2020

[85] Ghobrial GM, Beygi S, Viereck MJ, et al. Timing in the surgical evacuation of spinal epidural abscesses. Neurosurg Focus. 2014; 37(2):E1

[86] Ziai WC, Lewin JJ, III. Update in the diagnosis and management of central nervous system infections. Neurol Clin. 2008; 26(2):427–468, viii

[87] Connor DE, Jr, Chittiboina P, Caldito G, Nanda A. Comparison of operative and nonoperative management of spinal epidural abscess: a retrospective review of clinical and laboratory predictors of neurological outcome. J Neurosurg Spine. 2013; 19(1):119–127

[88] Bond A, Manian FA. Spinal epidural abscess: a review with special emphasis on earlier diagnosis. BioMed Res Int. 2016; 2016:1614328

[89] Kaufman DM, Kaplan JG, Litman N. Infectious agents in spinal epidural abscesses. Neurology. 1980; 30(8):844–850

[90] Pradilla G, Nagahama Y, Spivak AM, Bydon A, Rigamonti D. Spinal epidural abscess: current diagnosis and management. Curr Infect Dis Rep. 2010; 12 (6):484–491

[91] Grieve JP, Ashwood N, O'Neill KS, Moore AJ. A retrospective study of surgical and conservative treatment for spinal extradural abscess. Eur Spine J. 2000; 9(1):67–71

[92] Karikari IO, Powers CJ, Reynolds RM, Mehta AI, Isaacs RE. Management of a spontaneous spinal epidural abscess: a single-center 10-year experience. Neurosurgery. 2009; 65(5):919–923, discussion 923–924

[93] Curry WT, Jr, Hoh BL, Amin-Hanjani S, Eskandar EN. Spinal epidural abscess: clinical presentation, management, and outcome. Surg Neurol. 2005; 63(4): 364–371, discussion 371

[94] Rigamonti D, Liem L, Sampath P, et al. Spinal epidural abscess: contemporary trends in etiology, evaluation, and management. Surg Neurol. 1999; 52(2): 189–196, discussion 197

[95] Sampath P, Rigamonti D. Spinal epidural abscess: a review of epidemiology, diagnosis, and treatment. J Spinal Disord. 1999; 12(2):89–93

[96] Soehle M, Wallenfang T. Spinal epidural abscesses: clinical manifestations, prognostic factors, and outcomes. Neurosurgery. 2002; 51(1):79–85, discussion 86–87

[97] McConeghy KW, Bleasdale SC, Rodvold KA. The empirical combination of vancomycin and a β-lactam for Staphylococcal bacteremia. Clin Infect Dis. 2013; 57(12):1760–1765

[98] Khatib R, Saeed S, Sharma M, Riederer K, Fakih MG, Johnson LB. Impact of initial antibiotic choice and delayed appropriate treatment on the outcome of Staphylococcus aureus bacteremia. Eur J Clin Microbiol Infect Dis. 2006; 25(3):181–185

[99] Lodise TP, Jr, McKinnon PS, Levine DP, Rybak MJ. Impact of empirical-therapy selection on outcomes of intravenous drug users with infective endocarditis caused by methicillin-susceptible Staphylococcus aureus. Antimicrob Agents Chemother. 2007; 51(10):3731–3733

[100] Eismont FJ, Bohlman HH, Soni PL, Goldberg VM, Freehafer AA. Pyogenic and fungal vertebral osteomyelitis with paralysis. J Bone Joint Surg Am. 1983; 65 (1):19–29

[101] Emery SE, Chan DP, Woodward HR. Treatment of hematogenous pyogenic vertebral osteomyelitis with anterior debridement and primary bone grafting. Spine. 1989; 14(3):284–291

[102] Yilmaz C, Selek HY, Gürkan I, Erdemli B, Korkusuz Z. Anterior instrumentation for the treatment of spinal tuberculosis. J Bone Joint Surg Am. 1999; 81 (9):1261–1267

[103] Safavi-Abbasi S, Maurer AJ, Rabb CH. Minimally invasive treatment of multilevel spinal epidural abscess. J Neurosurg Spine. 2013; 18(1):32–35

[104] Tan LA, Takagi I, Deutsch H. Minimally invasive transpedicular approach for evacuation of epidural abscess and debridement of disc space in a patient with discitis in the thoracic spine. Neurosurg Focus. 2013; 35(2) Suppl:Video 6

[105] Redekop GJ, Del Maestro RF. Diagnosis and management of spinal epidural abscess. Can J Neurol Sci. 1992; 19(2):180–187

[106] Pradilla G, Ardila GP, Hsu W, Rigamonti D. Epidural abscesses of the CNS. Lancet Neurol. 2009; 8(3):292–300

[107] Tompkins M, Panuncialman I, Lucas P, Palumbo M. Spinal epidural abscess. J Emerg Med. 2010; 39(3):384–390

17 Thoracic Osteomyelitis and Discitis

Venita M. Simpson, Terence Verla, and Alexander E. Ropper

Abstract

Vertebral osteomyelitis can result in severe spinal cord compression and spinal deformity. It may present nonspecifically with back pain or with paraparesis in advanced cases. Clinicians should be familiar with the epidemiology, signs, symptoms, and radiographic evidence of thoracic osteomyelitis and discitis to diagnose and treat these conditions expeditiously prior to the appearance of neurological deficits. Treatment consists of antibiotics and potentially surgery, both of which must be tailored to the individual patient and pathogen to optimize outcomes.

Keywords: osteomyelitis, discitis, bacterial infection, postinfectious deformity, sepsis

Clinical Pearls

- Pyogenic vertebral osteomyelitis (PVO) is the most common spine infection in adults. Its insidious onset sometimes delays the clinical diagnosis.
- After radiographic diagnosis by computed tomography or magnetic resonance imaging, a biopsy should be performed for tissue diagnosis to guide antibiotic therapy.
- Surgery should be considered for diagnosis, debridement of extensive bony destruction, and decompression of the thecal sac in cases of neurological compromise, instability, and deformity.
- Although previously controversial, instrumentation in the setting of active infection, such as PVO, has not been shown to have increased the risk of continued infection and may improve functional outcome in patients with instability.

17.1 Introduction

17.1.1 Epidemiology

Pyogenic vertebral osteomyelitis (PVO) is the most common spine infection in adults. It is acquired from a bacterial infection of the vertebral bodies that extends into or from adjacent intervertebral disc spaces. The annual incidence of PVO has been estimated at 0.059 episodes per 100,000 people over the past decade, with approximately 60% male predominance and a mean age of 66 years.[1] The incidence of PVO is increasing, particularly in the immunocompomised and aging populations, according to two large national studies in Japan and Denmark. An increase in pathogen resistance to antibiotics may also be a contributing factor.[2]

There are various predisposing risk factors for spondylodiscitis, which include diabetes mellitus, rheumatic diseases, immunosuppressive diseases, previous invasive treatments (pharyngeal surgery, tonsillectomy, spine surgery, etc.), and sepsis or systemic infection (pneumonia, urinary tract infection, etc.).[3] It is also increasingly recognized as a sequela of intravenous drug use, likely as a result of bacteremia.

The recent increased prevalence of the disease results from a number of factors, including improved neuroimaging capabilities, better awareness of these diseases, an increased number of elderly individuals, and a greater number of surviving immunocompromised patients, including those with cancer, human immunodeficiency virus (HIV) infection. In addition, there is a growing rate of illicit drug abuse in the United States which may contribute as well as a greater incidence of methicillin-resistant *Staphylococcus aureus* (MRSA) infections. Despite having sophisticated imaging techniques and laboratory studies, the rate of misdiagnosis at presentation for vertebral osteomyelitis and epidural abscess is still high, with an average rate of approximately 50%.[4]

Vertebral osteomyelitis is notoriously difficult to initially diagnose because of its insidious course and indolent clinical course. Typical symptoms, such as back pain, tenderness, or weight loss, may not be prominent and can be present for months before a definitive diagnosis is made. The usual radiographic sequelae of these infections such as disc space narrowing and endplate destruction may not appear for weeks after the infection. Prompt imaging is still necessary for confirmation and localization of the infection.[5]

In a systematic review by Mylona et al of 1,008 patients with PVO and excluding patients with tuberculosis and brucellosis, they found the clinical picture of PVO often was nonspecific. Back pain was by far the most common presenting symptom. Notably, fever was often absent at presentation, thus distracting the clinician from the possibility of infection and delaying the diagnosis (mean time to diagnosis, 11–59 days).[6] In these retrospective studies, the thoracic spine was affected 30% of the time, while the lumbar area was affected in 58% and cervical spine 11%. The highest rate of multifocal involvement was observed in patients with a history of intravenous drug abuse.[6]

The bacterial inoculation in PVO occurs through two main pathways: hematogenous seeding and direct inoculation. Batson et al described theories involving venous and arterial systems extensively, which describe the evolution of vertebral osteomyelitis. The Batson paravertebral plexus is a valveless venous system that allows retrograde flow of blood during times of increased intrathoracic or intra-abdominal pressure. This plexus is implicated in the spread of infection to central vertebral bodies, noncontiguous vertebral lesions, and seeding from distant sites (e.g., bacterial endocarditis).[7]

Bacteria enters areas of slower blood flow via arterial or venous conduits at the intervertebral disks or endplates, allowing extension into the vertebral column in 50% of cases.[1] Bacteria enter the bloodstream and spread hematogenously to the subchondral area adjacent to the disc. The segmental arterial supply of the spine supplies two adjacent vertebras and the disc between them, and therefore, the infection involves two vertebral endplates as well as the disc. The infection spreads in several directions, further destroying the bone, and can eventually reach the spinal cord.[5] Seeding of the spinal cord often occurs through arteries to the metaphysis of individual vertebrae, or less frequently by the Batson plexus or the deep pelvic venous system. This vascular spread of bacterial inoculation or pus can create an increase in intraosseous pressure that impedes blood flow to the vertebrae and intervertebral discs.[8] A common source that must be excluded is bacterial endocarditis. Nearly 30% of all hematogenous spinal infections are associated with concomitant bacterial endocarditis.

The bacteria *S. aureus* can cause not only a typical infection but also biomechanical instability and deformity by release of destructive enzymes such as hyaluronidase. This proteolytic enzyme can enhance the bacteria's ability to invade connective tissue such as the disc's annulus fibrosis, leading to the breakdown of its structural fibers, resulting in paraspinous disc extrusion.[8] Bone destruction, ligamentous laxity, and nerve root/spinal cord compression leading to instability, deformity, and even severe neurologic deficits or death may result from the infiltration of these pathogenic organisms.[1] Local inflammation from the response to infection may lead to thrombophlebitis or venous congestion extending to the subdural, and subarachnoid space is thought to be the mechanism of neurological injury in some cases. Surgical debridement is advocated by many as direct decompression and resection decreases possible mass effect and infectious burden, and also reduces the risk of vascular-related neurological complications.[4]

Routine invasive spinal procedures such as lumbar puncture and discography, and surgeries such as laminectomy, discectomy, and fusions can lead to direct inoculation causing bacterial colonization of the vertebral column. Direct inoculation is estimated to be causative in 15 to 40% of cases. The risk of postprocedural PVO are increased by prolonged operative time, instrumentation, posterior surgical approach, extensive soft-tissue dissection, and/or devitalization, creation of dead space, repeat surgery, surgery through previously irradiated tissue, excess blood loss, blood transfusions, and emergency surgery.[9] Less commonly, bacterial inoculation occurs through local extension from adjacent areas of infection (3% of cases), including retropharyngeal abscesses or infected aortic grafts.[1]

17.1.2 Clinical Features

Back pain is the most common symptom of osteomyelitis, accounting for the primary symptom in 67 to 100% patients from large studies (≥ 100 VO cases) and pooled data.[9] Neck or back pain with insidious onset is seen in 85% of patients, and approximately 30% of patients present with concurrent neurological deficits. Other common nonspecific findings include fever (35–60%), weight loss, nausea/vomiting, anorexia, lethargy, or confusion. Tenderness of the spine on palpation is seen in 20% of patients with pyogenic vertebral osteomyelitis.[7] Mylona et al systematically reviewed PVO clinical characteristics and reported the most common symptom is back pain (86%), with 34% of patients presenting with neurological deficits.[6] Fevers are present in 85% of culture-positive PVO versus 32% of culture-negative cases. Concomitant infections (urinary tract infection, abscesses, skin infections, pneumonia, etc.) are relatively common, and are found in 47% of culture-positive and 4% of culture-negative PVO.[1] There should be a high index of suspicion to prompt a diagnosis of PVO in the absence of fever and a non-specific insidious illness. Since the majority of PVO results from hematogenous seeding of an infection, the primary infection site, such as urinary tract or skin and soft tissue, often dominates the initial symptoms and signs.[9]

17.1.3 Workup

Standard laboratory workup may indicate an elevated white blood cell (WBC) count, erythrocyte sedimentation rate (ESR), C-reactive protein (CRP), blood culture, and urine cultures. An elevated ESR is the most reliable marker and is seen elevated in 90% of patients, while leukocytosis is seen in only 55% of VO cases, an elevated ESR is seen in 90% of patients. The CRP level, while also a nonspecific marker of inflammation, may be of more use in monitoring therapy because it has a shorter normalization time than ESR. In cases of VO, CRP level and ESR have been reported to have a sensitivity of 98 and 100%, respectively.[7]

Identification of pathogens, through either blood or tissue culture, is key to guiding antimicrobial therapy. Often a biopsy is required to identify the inciting organism and the antimicrobial sensitivities due to the low percentage of positive blood cultures in as little as 30% of cases.[7]

Mylona et al retrospectively reviewed fourteen cases of PVO, and in those cases blood cultures identified a pathogen in only 58% of the patients. When there were no positive blood cultures, when there was a failure to respond to antibiotics, or if a polymicrobial infection was suspected, a biopsy (CT- guided or open) was undertaken, providing a pathogen in 79% of the cases.[6]

Intraoperative tissue histopathology and cultures are the ideal reference tests for diagnosis of VO. However, they cannot be obtained in every patient with clinical and radiographic suspicion of VO. Therefore, the combination of multiple modalities along with clinical history and exam is reasonable for the diagnosis of VO. Image-guided percutaneous needle aspiration biopsy have a high positive predictive value for the diagnosis, but had moderate accuracy for ruling out this osteomyelitis. Image-guided percutaneous needle aspiration biopsy under computed tomography (CT) or fluoroscopic guidance has been recognized as a valuable method to obtain tissue diagnosis of vertebral disease, and the success rates of both methods are comparable. Its simplicity and cost-effectiveness led to the acceptance of this procedure as the standard tool for confirming a VO. Depending on the study, the diagnostic microbiological yields of percutaneous image-guided needle aspiration biopsy have been reported to vary from 36 to 91%.[10] The wide range of success rates depend on the organism and multiple factors, such as prior use of antimicrobial therapy, biopsy techniques, and advances in imaging studies. A retrospective study by Pupaibool et al with seven retrospective studies involving 482 patients with clinical and/or radiological suspicion of VO who underwent image-guided spinal biopsy examined the diagnostic odds ratio (DOR), likelihood ratio of a positive test (LRP), likelihood ratio of a negative test (LRN), sensitivity, and specificity of image-guided biopsy. This review found that image-guided spinal biopsy had a DOR of 45.50 (95% confidence interval [CI], 13.66–151.56), an LRP of 16.76 (95% CI, 5.51–50.95), an LRN of 0.39 (95% CI, 0.24–0.64), a sensitivity of 52.2% (95% CI, 45.8–58.5), and a specificity of 99.9% (95% CI, 94.5–100).[10] This study further confirmed the importance of image-guided biopsy for not only confirming the diagnosis but also guiding medical management with antibiotics.

17.1.4 Differential Diagnosis

The differential diagnoses of PVO stem mostly from radiographic features which encompass pathologies such as erosive osteochondrosis, extruded disc material, vertebral fracture, metastatic disease, plasmacytoma, degenerative Modic's changes, Charcot's joint, and much more. These disease processes are not typically associated with elevated ESR, CRP, and WBC count, which are markers of inflammatory response. However, in a cancer or severely osteoporotic patient, the possibility of a pathological fracture should be included in the workup. With respect to an extruded disc fragment, some radiographic features such as T2 hyperintensity of an associated disc cysts and annulus tear associated with contrast enhancement make its radiographic presentation similar to PVO.[11] This can lead to misdiagnosis as illustrated by Dunbar et al. Erosive osteochondrosis can involve the disc space, causing erosion of the vertebral body endplates and subsequent osteophytic and Modic's changes in the vertebral bodies, which can have radiographic features similar to PVO. However, there often exists extension of the T2 signal beyond the affected endplate into the disc space in PVO. In addition to baseline age-associated degenerative changes in the spinal column, the destructive arthropathy caused by Charcot's joint creates clinical and radiographic effects on the disc space and vertebral endplates with MRI features mimicking PVO.[12]

17.1.5 Radiographic Appearance

Plain radiographs have a lower sensitivity and specificity than cross-sectional imaging. However, X-rays provide important information regarding overall alignment and mechanical stability. Most suggestive findings on X-ray of osteomyelitis do not appear until later in the disease process, including osteolysis, endplate destruction, and eventual vertebral collapse.[7]

Evaluation of the entire spine should be considered in PVO, as 6% of patients demonstrate continuous lesions spanning multiple levels and 3% have noncontiguous, or skip lesions. While X-ray abnormalities for advanced cases of PVO can be found on nearly 90% of X-rays, early findings are nonspecific and difficult to identify. Early findings (2–3 weeks) may be endplate blurring, erosion of the endplate corners, disc height loss, and paraspinal soft-tissue swelling. Vertebral body destructive changes on X-ray are seen after greater than 30% bony destruction. Late PVO can demonstrate signs of bone formation, including peripheral sclerosis, osteophytosis, and osteolytic lesions.[1]

CT is the best imaging modality to evaluate instability, bony destruction, presence of gas within abscesses, and bony canal involvement. Visualization of calcifications within abscesses or identification of bone fragments can be accomplished with CT. Additionally, CT is the imaging modality used for image-guided biopsies in spinal infections. Findings of paraspinal calcifications and pedicle destruction are more common with granulomatous infections.[7] CT may demonstrate epidural granulation tissue, possibly necessitating the need for closer characterization of the epidural space with MRI.

Although CT scans can provide early information on bone integrity, they are limited when compared with MRI in identifying the extent of abscesses or spinal cord compression.[1] MRI remains the imaging modality of choice when spinal infection is suspected. MRI helps to characterize the extent and location of the infection, including associated abscesses in the epidural and paraspinal compartments. It is also the most accurate modality to characterize the presence and extent of neural compression. MRI has a reported sensitivity of 96% and specificity of 94% in the diagnosis of spinal infection.[7] Another recent series showed a sensitivity of 97.7% for detection of infection using MRI.[13]

MRI is useful in identifying some of the chronic changes that develop after development of PVO. MRI will most commonly demonstrate the contiguous involvement of two vertebrae with inflammatory change within the intervertebral disc (▶ Fig. 17.1). There is little evidence in the literature concerning the appearances of very early spinal infection on MRI and many

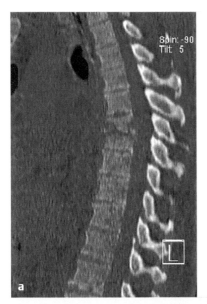
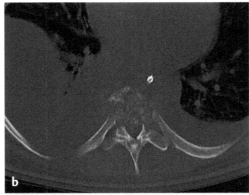
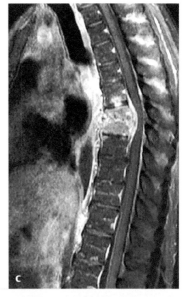

Fig. 17.1 Imaging of a 56-year-old man with thoracic osteomyelitis. **(a)** Sagittal CT scan shows a destructive osteodiscitis at T7–T8. There is collapse of the disc space and a small focal kyphotic deformity. **(b)** Axial CT image through the T7 vertebral body demonstrates a patchy, lytic appearance to the body, which is infiltrated with osteomyelitis. **(c)** Sagittal MRI T1-weighted sequence with gadolinium contrast shows diffuse enhancement in the T7–T8 vertebral bodies as well as prespinal soft-tissue enhancement. There is a large, ventral epidural abscess behind the involved bodies, which is compressing the thoracic spinal cord.

times this must be inferred based on the clinical picture and ancillary imaging.[13]

Affected discs and adjacent vertebrae may demonstrate high T2 and low T1 signal intensity early in the disease. STIR (short tau inversion recovery) sequence may demonstrate high T2 signal changes in the paraspinal soft tissues as well as inflammation and edema. Contrast is often used to display the diffuse enhancement of the subchondral bone and disc. The early MRI findings of high T2 disc signal with disc height loss and contrast uptake within the disc are highly sensitive (70–100%) for PVO diagnosis.[1] However, Carragee and Iezza reviewed 103 MRIs of patients eventually diagnosed with PVO, and found a missed diagnosis rate of 9.1% with MRIs obtained within 2 weeks of patient presentation compared with a 3.4% missed diagnosis rate for MRIs after 2 weeks.[14] An important diagnostic consideration in patients with pathological appearing vertebrae is ruling out neoplastic disease. This is usually done with laboratory tests that suggest infectious etiology, as previously discussed along with fever, and may be supported by MRI findings including disc space involvement with endplate erosion. It is common for neoplastic disease to spare the disc spaces, which sometimes can be a useful finding to distinguish these two entities. As VO progresses, further bony destruction is evident, producing a mass lesion that may cause cord compression. T1-weighted images show hypointensity in the disc and adjacent vertebral bodies, and T2-weighted images show hyperintensity in the same area. There is a loss of the margin between the involved disc and the adjacent vertebral bodies.[5] MRI with weighted postcontrast imaging may demonstrate an abscess which would appear hypointense with characteristic peripheral rim enhancement.

Dunbar et al presented several cases that confirm MRI images may be equivocal early in the course of infection. It is imperative where a history is consistent with VO, particularly if supported by positive blood cultures, that intravenous antibiotic therapy is continued and a repeat MRI performed.[13]

Some early endplate changes resemble Modic type I degenerative endplates with very subtle endplate edema associated with disc degeneration. It is important to recognize that Modic Type I changes can mimic PVO, showing a paradoxical increase in T2-weighted signal. This was demonstrated in 36% of cases of Modic Type I in a recent study. Endplate edema is also reported in association with Schmorl's nodes. It is important to recognize that these may be the very earliest signs of VO and follow up these changes with a repeat MRI when there is a clinical suspicion of spinal infection.[13]

18F-fluorodeoxyglucose positron emission tomography (18F-FDG-PET) is a three-dimensional imaging technique involving the radiopharmaceutical 18F-FDG, which has increased uptake in metabolically active tissues including in the setting of infection. A meta-analysis of 18F-FDG-PET as a diagnostic tool for VO found that from the 12 eligible studies involving a total of 224 patients, the sensitivity was 97%, specificity 88%, and with a pretest probability over 50%, the positive predictive value was 0.96 and negative predictive value 0.85.[9] A study comparing 18F-FDG-PET and MRI for VO diagnosis concluded that they showed similar accuracy, 75 versus 81%, respectively, and therefore, 18F-FDG-PET could be used when diagnostic doubt remains after MRI or if MRI is unavailable.[9]

Bone scans are nuclear medicine studies utilizing a labeled tracer, which can be 99mTc, 67Ga, or autologous radiolabeled white cells, giving two-dimensional images and are generally performed in three phases for detecting infection. Bone scans are rarely used in current practice as there are drawbacks with each of the potential tracers: autologous white cells undergo physiological uptake into active bone marrow, 67Ga is significantly taken up in the liver, bowel, bone marrow, and at post-surgical sites, and 99mTc is affected by bone remodeling. The high sensitivity of 99mTc means a negative scan effectively excludes the diagnosis.[9] Bone scintigraphy has a reported sensitivity of 86% in detecting PVO. These scans may also differentiate infectious versus metastatic lesions. Metastatic lesions tend to demonstrate multiple locations of radioactive uptake, whereas infectious processes are usually localized.[7] A combination of spine gallium/Tc99 bone scan, or computed tomography scan or a positron emission tomography scan in patients with suspected VO when MRI cannot be obtained may be useful (e.g., implantable cardiac devices, cochlear implants, claustrophobia, or unavailability).[15] Other new applications include technetium Tc-99m-ubiquicidin–derived peptides, with radioactivity as sites of infection that correlate with viable bacterial growth and radiolabeled antifungal tracers that could help distinguish fungal from bacterial spinal infections.[7]

17.2 Pathogens

Microbiological data on PVO is mostly based on blood culture, biopsy, or intraoperative cultures. *Staphylococcus aureus* stands as the most commonly isolated organism, while among gram-negative bacilli, *Escherichia coli* was the predominant etiological agent. Other organisms include *Staphylococcus epidermidis*, *Streptococcus* species, *Streptococcus pneumoniae*, *Enterococcus* and *Klebsiella* species, *Proteus mirabilis*, anaerobes, *Candida*, and *Aspergillus* species. The microbiology of PVO in drug users is an issue which remains to be clarified as both *P. aeruginosa* and *S. aureus* have been isolated from the majority of patients in various studies. PVO due to *S. epidermidis* is a frequent isolate in patients with previous spinal surgery as well as in elderly and immunocompromised patients. Therefore, one should be cautious before considering *S. epidermidis* as a contaminant in the above group of patients. Unlike *S. epidermidis*, the epidemiology of MRSA is always a nosocomial infection. Community-acquired MRSA was never isolated in a large series.[6]

Tuberculosis and brucella VO are the pathogens that most commonly present with a delayed diagnosis. Brucella VO should be considered in any patient with a history of fresh cheese consumption, animal husbandry, sweating, arthralgia, hepatomegaly, elevated alanine transaminase, and lumbar involvement on MRI. Contrarily, tuberculosis was associated more with the thoracic vertebrae.[16]

Considering the biological characteristics of *Mycobacterium tuberculosis* and *S. aureus* or *S. epidermidis*, *M. tuberculosis* rarely adheres to metal surfaces and has little or no biofilm formation; hence, the metallic implants have been successfully used in patients with spinal tuberculosis. These biological data suggest that the use of the metallic implant in an active pyogenic infection site might have a higher risk of infection persistence or reactivation than in a tuberculosis infection, even though good clinical results have been reported with spinal instrumentation in the treatment of pyogenic vertebral osteomyelitis.[17]

Polymicrobial vertebral osteomyelitis infections were associated with larger infections, higher presenting ESR value, higher mortality rate, lower clearance of infection, longer hospital stay, greater degree of vertebral instability, and greater mortality. Polymicrobial infections are associated with antibiotic resistance and lower clearance rates which can lead to a chronic or unremitting treatment course.[18] The mechanism of such has yet to be elucidated, but likely involves the additive virulence of multiple organisms and the presence of permissive conditions, such as immunosuppression, which enables bacteria to destroy healthy tissue.[18]

17.3 Treatment

17.3.1 Medical Management

Conservative management with medical therapy is a first-line option if there are no neurological deficits, if there is an identified pathogen, and if there is minimal vertebral body involvement with no or minimal instability/deformity.[5] Definitive therapy should be guided by the microbiological results of culture and susceptibility testing. In patients with normal and stable neurological examination and stable hemodynamics, one should typically hold empiric antimicrobial therapy until a microbiological diagnosis is established. However, in patients presenting with signs of sepsis, shock, or progressive decline in neurologic exam, empiric antimicrobrial therapy should be started concomitantly with establishing a microbiologic diagnosis.[15] An image-guided or intraoperative aspiration or biopsy of a disc space or vertebral endplate sample submitted for microbiological and pathological examination often establishes the microbiological or pathological diagnosis. Recent studies demonstrate a CT-guided biopsy-positive culture rate of 19 to 60% in patients with suspected PVO. Antibiotics before CT biopsy can significantly affect culture yields.[1] De Lucas et al identified a causative organism in 60% of patients not previously treated with antibiotics, compared with 23% of patients who had received antibiotics prior to biopsy.[19]

In the absence of concomitant bloodstream infection, some authors recommend obtaining a second aspiration biopsy in patients with suspected VO in whom the original image-guided aspiration biopsy specimen grew a skin contaminant (coagulase-negative staphylococci [except *Staphylococcus lugdunensis*], *Propionibacterium* species, or diphtheroids). In patients with a nondiagnostic first image-guided aspiration biopsy and suspected native vertebral osteomyelitis (NVO), further testing should be done to exclude difficult-to-grow organisms (e.g., anaerobes, fungi, *Brucella* species, or mycobacteria). In patients with suspected VO and a nondiagnostic image-guided aspiration biopsy and laboratory workup, Berbari et al suggested either repeating a second image-guided aspiration biopsy, performing percutaneous endoscopic discectomy and drainage, or proceeding with an open excisional biopsy.[15]

Conservative management with antimicrobial therapy for 6 weeks is curative in the majority of patients; however, there is limited high-quality evidence to guide the optimal time course of treatment. Some patients may need surgical debridement and/or spinal stabilization during or after a course of antimicrobial

therapy.[15] Bernard et al reviewed antibiotic treatment lengths for PVO, comparing 6- and 12-week durations of intravenous (IV) and/or oral (PO) antibiotics in an open-label, noninferiority randomized control trial, finding similar cure rates (90.9 and 90.8% cure rates, respectively) and an equal percentage of adverse events (29% each). They further noted no significant difference in treatment failure between patients receiving IV antibiotics greater than or fewer than 7 days.[20] The total duration of therapy for infections of the spine is based on many factors, including the identification of the offending organism, the extent of surgical therapy, the presence of spinal instrumentation or other hardware in the body, improvement or cessation of clinical symptoms, normalization of inflammatory markers (i.e., ESR, CRP level), and the resolution of abscesses on follow-up imaging. Several reports have recommended 6 to 8 weeks of IV therapy. In fact, less than 4 weeks of therapy is associated with a 25% incidence of recurrence.[17] Risk factors for failure of treatment were ESR greater than 55 mm/hour and CRP greater than 2.75 after 4 weeks of antibiotic treatment with an odds ratio of 5.15.[1] Rifampin has been frequently used with good eradication rates in patients with retained prosthetic devices; however, no particular antibiotic regimen has superior eradication rates.[7] In summary, antibiotic management must be tailored to the individual patient and based on sensitivity of any cultured organisms.

17.3.2 Failure of Medical Management

For those failing to eradicate the infection with medical management alone, there can be increased morbidity. Therefore, the ability to predict failure of medical management on presentation may improve the outcomes.[21]

Imaging characteristics of pretreatment MRI have been used to predict which patients are at risk of failing medical management. Hodges et al reviewed a cohort of patients with PVO who were initially managed medically and characterized their imaging, demographics, and clinic data to predict which patients would ultimately need surgical treatment. MRI T1-weighted signal changes on sagittal images of the affected segment were assessed for each group. Twenty-two patients were included in the study. Patients successfully treated medically averaged 57 ± 19% of vertebral segment involvement, whereas those failing conservative treatment averaged 89 ± 18%. Using 90% vertebral body involvement as an indication for initial surgery would have a sensitivity of 78% and specificity of 93%. Patients with thoracolumbar PVO with 90% or higher involvement of an affected motion segment should be considered for early operative management.[21]

Hodges et al found that no patient with less than 60% involvement failed with medical management. Sixty percent motion segment involvement had a sensitivity of 100% and a specificity of 57%, whereas 90% motion segment involvement had a sensitivity of 78% and a specificity of 93% in predicting failure of medical treatment and the ultimate need for surgery.[21]

Although post-infectious deformity has been well documented, there are relatively few studies focusing on risk factors associated with the development of deformity.

17.3.3 Surgical Management

Surgical intervention carries risks and financial costs; however, forgoing surgery in certain circumstance may result in permanent neurological deficit or death. VO can be a challenging condition to successfully manage surgically due to the often medically debilitated patient population, potential for regional spinal deformity, and profound local inflammatory response, which can render surgical access complicated.[22]

Indications for surgical intervention are controversial, but the consensus appears to be for obtaining cultures to aid in diagnosis, debridement of extensive bony destruction, and decompression of the thecal sac in cases of neurological compromise, stabilization, and deformity. Surgery may also be required for persistent pain; that is, continued or worsening pain despite an adequate course (6 weeks) of antibiotics.[5] However, some authors advise against surgical debridement and/or stabilization in patients who have worsening bony imaging findings at 4 to 6 weeks in the setting of improvement in clinical symptoms, physical examination, and inflammatory markers.[15] A standard laminectomy may worsen the neurologic deficit as the infectious process accelerates and may destabilize the spine, causing a flexion deformity. Kyphosis following a laminectomy in patients with PVO may require anterior column reconstruction with posterior stabilization. Therefore, a thoracic laminectomy alone is usually not recommended by most authors.

Although no definitive threshold for surgical management of PVO based on spinal instability, or kyphotic deformity exists, Dinh et al recommend using the following parameters to suggest spinal instability: vertebral body collapse greater than 50%, greater than 20 degrees of angulation, and greater than 5 degrees of vertebral translation.[20] In the setting of an infection, Bydon et al suggest the definition of spinal instability as vertebral height reduction of greater than 50%, spinal angulation exceeding 20%, sagittal displacement of a vertebra greater than 3 mm, or relative sagittal plane angulation greater than 11 degrees. Instability after laminectomy has been observed in patients with preexisting loss of lordosis or in patients undergoing multisegment decompression or greater than 30% resection of a facet joint.[23] Ultimately, surgical intervention must be tailored to the individual patient.

Surgical debridement of the infected tissue is the goal of management of spontaneous spinal infection. The patient population of PVO is usually immunocompromised, elderly, and with multiple medical comorbidities, making an aggressive surgical approach to the spine, either anteriorly or via an expanded posterior approach challenging. The reported mortality after surgical treatment is between 8 and 14%.[24]

Treatment of spinal tuberculosis led to the development of most surgical approaches to spinal infection. In the 1920s, Hibbs and Albee developed the distant operation of posterior spinal fusion for treatment of Pott's disease. In classic tuberculosis spondylodiscitis, where the disease is in the anterior column, operation through the anterior route is the rational approach for debulking, debridement and decompression, thus preserving the posterior elements of the spine.[25] Menard developed the anterolateral approach and it was expanded upon by Griffiths, Roaf, and Seddon for debridement and decompression of the cord with or without bone grafting for anterior spinal fusion.[25] The choice of surgery depends on a number of factors, including the surgeon's experience, spinal level affected, neurological deficits, and predicted spinal instability.

In cases of VO (with or without associated epidural abscess) the pathological process is ventral to the spinal cord, and an anterior, lateral, or posterolateral approach most directly addresses the compression and disease. An anterior approach affords a more complete debridement, with removal of infected tissue and devitalized vertebral bone and intervertebral disc, whereas posterior debridement affords less morbidity but risks more limited access and incomplete debridement.[1] Direct anterior approaches to the thoracic spine carries the moderate morbidity of a thoracotomy, but the advances in spinal instrumentation have allowed adequate ability to debride and reconstruct the anterior column through posterolateral approaches (e.g., transpedicular, costotransversectomy, and lateral extracavitary approaches). There are several reports of good success for treating osteomyelitis with the lateral extracavitary approach to the thoracic spine; however, other authors prefer using a transthoracic or thoracoabdominal approach. Direct visualization of the thecal sac and placement of an interbody cage simultaneously are some of the advantages to an anterior approach. The lateral extracavitary approach has the advantage of avoiding pleural or peritoneal contamination while allowing posterior fixation and fusion through the same incision. This posterior stabilization is necessary to allow early mobilization before bony fusion has taken place.[5]

However, the posterior approach may be more attractive as it is associated with earlier mobilization, more rapid rehabilitation, and, as reported in some studies, higher fusion rates. Posterior only approaches are limited by access and risk of incomplete debridement. Mohamed et al presented a series using an alternative treatment method of posterior-only decompression and stabilization without formal debridement of anterior tissue for treating spontaneous spinal infection. Of the 15 patients, 10 (66%) had a minimum 2-year follow-up and 14 patients had at least 1 year of follow-up. There were no recurrent spinal infections. There were three unplanned reoperations (one for loss of fixation, one for early superficial wound infection, and one for epidural hematoma). Nine (60%) of 15 patients were nonambulatory at presentation. At final follow-up, 8 of 15 patients were independently ambulatory, 6 required an assistive device, and 1 remained nonambulatory.[24] Long-segment fixation, without formal debridement, resulted in resolution of spinal infection in all cases and in significant neurological recovery in almost all cases.

A case report with upper thoracic (T1–T2) VO and epidural abscess utilized a transsternal approach utilizing a full median sternotomy. Pathologies involving the lower cervical and upper thoracic vertebrae can be safely and effectively accessed via this approach. Compared to other modified transsternal approaches, the full median sternotomy approach is technically simpler, provides better exposure, preserves the pectoral girdle, and allows for extension of the operative field caudally.[26]

17.3.4 Instrumentation

Beyond debridement, significant controversy exists regarding the safety of hardware implantation: one- versus two-staged procedures, anterior versus posterior instrumentation, and the use of autograft versus allograft.[1] Specific techniques and approaches to thoracic spinal instrumentation are detailed in other chapters in this book. However, special consideration should be taken when planning implantation of instrumentation in cases of osteomyelitis given the poor bone quality and the infected field. Instrumentation should be considered in the presence of pathological fractures, paravertebral or epidural abscesses, and/or spinal instability.[23] Surgical debridement with spinal instrumentation can relieve pain, correct deformity, improve neurological function, and result in early ambulation. Stabilization and correction of deformity with instrumentation presents a risk of persistent infection or recurrence with the placement of foreign material (i.e., the hardware) in the setting of infection. Thus, several authors have advised that antibiotic administration should last at least 6 to 8 weeks in patients who undergo spinal instrumentation; however, there is minimal evidence guiding this practice. Some surgeons advocate for a two-stage operation, with surgical debridement with antimicrobial therapy first followed by a delayed second stage with instrumentation to decrease the risk of residual bacteria.[27]

In the past, placing foreign material in the setting of a spinal infection was a concern for clearance of the original infection. Bydon et al retrospectively reported on 118 patients, noting similar rates of recurrent infection (8.3% for debridement and 9.8% for debridement with instrumentation) and reoperation (19.4% for debridement and 17.1% for debridement with instrumentation).[23]

Hee et al reported 21 cases that underwent posterior instrumentation or titanium cages in the surgical treatment of VO.[29] They demonstrated that posterior stabilization is important for improving sagittal alignment.[27] Liljenqvist et al also described successful outcomes in 20 patients treated with anterior surgery with titanium cage insertion and posterior instrumented fusion.[28] The other advantage is faster postoperative mobilization due to immediate stabilization with instrumentation. Korovessis et al reported that the use of an anterior titanium cage and a posterior instrumentation decreased the preoperative pain, thus allowing faster mobilization of often very sick patients.[29]

Park et al investigated a comparison of the recurrence and failure rate of patients treated surgically with noninstrumentation versus instrumentation. A total of 153 patients with PVO underwent surgical management for their infections; 94 (61.4%) underwent surgical debridement alone (noninstrumented surgery) and 59 (38.6%) underwent surgical debridement and instrumentation (instrumented surgery). The median durations of antibiotic therapy were 66 and 80 days for the noninstrumentation and instrumentation groups, respectively ($p = 0.22$). Clinical outcomes were similar between the groups, including rates of infection-related death (2.1 vs. 0%; $p = 0.52$), primary failure (1.1 vs. 5.1%; $p = 0.30$), and recurrence (4.8 vs. 6.8%; $p = 0.72$). Among the instrumentation group, there was a significant decreasing trend for recurrence according to total duration of antibiotic therapy: 22.2% (4–6 weeks), 9.1% (6–8 weeks), and 2.6% (≥ 8 weeks; $p = 0.04$).[27]

Comparing outcomes of PVO treatment consisting of either debridement with or without instrumentation, Carragee and Iezza evaluated 32 immunocompromised patients with PVO treated with a variety of anterior and posterior instrumentation techniques. Of 22 living patients who were alive without evidence of clinical recurrence at 10 years, only 1 patient had a demonstrated recurrent infection during the follow-up time period. They concluded that the use of instrumentation is considered safe in immunocompromised hosts with PVO.[14]

Despite some favorable retrospective case series, complications and treatment failures during PVO management still

occur. Arnold and colleagues reviewed 94 cases of PVO requiring surgical management with instrumentation and found a 23% (22 cases) treatment failure rate secondary to uncontrolled/recurrent infection. Ninety-one percent of these treatment failures occurred within 1 year of treatment. Nineteen of these cases underwent further debridement with an average of 2.2 repeat operations and 15 patients ultimately required hardware removal.[5]

17.3.5 Fusion Material

Anterior debridement with strut bone grafting (such as iliac crest, fibular or rib autograft) without metallic implants was previously the gold standard procedure. However, the procedure might have risks of dislodgement of the grafted bone, resulting in pseudoarthrosis with large vertebral bone defects, involvement of several vertebrae, or poor spinal alignment.[17] There are many graft choices for fusion if it is required in surgery for spinal infections. Although allograft avoids the morbidity of donor site harvesting, autograft is theorized to have superior rates of incorporation. While some concern exists with introducing allograft into infected surgical fields, several small case series suggest similar recurrent infection rates and clinical outcomes when compared with autograft.[1] Autograft is the benchmark, but large anterior defects requiring a long strut may be treated with structural allograft or titanium cages. Studies support the use of titanium cages, allograft, and recombinant human bone morphogenetic protein (rhBMP) for fusions after debridement of spinal infections.[7] The literature consists of data supporting the use of nearly all graft options including autograft, allograft, and vascularized interbodies such as pedicled rib flaps and free flaps. Despite generally favorable results, current grafting techniques have been associated with reports of pseudoarthrosis, donor site morbidity, recurrence or persistence of spinal infection, and increased mortality.[22]

Because titanium lacks porosity that can serve as a site for biofilm formation, it has been shown to have a decreased rate of infection when compared to other artificial materials such as polymethyl methacrylate, PEEK, and stainless steel. To address the concerns biofilm with implants, Demura and colleagues used spinal instrumentation with povidone–iodine–coated titanium implants. Povidone–iodine is an antiseptic agent. The antibacterial spectrum of iodine is very broad, acting not only on general bacteria but also on certain viruses, tubercle bacilli, and fungi. In addition, iodine does not cause drug resistance as induced by the administration of antibiotics. Fourteen consecutive patients with PVO underwent surgery with spinal instrumentation with iodine-containing surfaces. The infection was eradicated in all 14 patients. Both WBC and CRP levels returned to normal ranges by the final follow-up. One patient showed a lucent area around the screw and two patients showed lucencies inside the cage. However, no cage dislocations, cage migrations, or screw pullouts were noted demonstrating efficacy in the use of these iodine-coated titanium implants.[17]

The use of rhBMP-2 as the primary graft material in cases of vertebral osteomyelitis is a valuable option. The discovery of BMPs and their subsequent introduction into clinical practice has had a significant impact on modern spinal surgery. BMP functions to promote bone healing via mesenchymal stem cells producing osteoblasts via dedifferentiation of these stem cells.[22]

In fact, there is both animal and human data to suggest that BMP may be an ideal graft for cases of infection as it was shown to be associated with accelerated healing of both the fracture and the wound. rhBMP-2 improved the vascularity of the bone, ultimately led to a more rapid achievement of fracture stability, and also had a statistically significant reduced rate of infection in these studies.[22] In a retrospective study by Ondra, 20 patients with VO underwent anterior column debridement and instrumented reconstruction using rhBMP-2 and were analyzed with a mean follow-up of 40 months (range, 24–53 months). At final follow-up, all patients achieved clinical and radiographic fusion and no patient required further surgery due to either persistence or recurrence of infection.

There has also been some novel use of antibiotic- and iodine-impregnated graft materials to counter the placement of instrumentation in a patient with an active spinal infection. The antibiotic gentamicin was used with an injectable calcium sulfate/hydroxyapatite composite in combination with posterior debridement and instrumentation for spondylodiscitis. The release of the high level of gentamicin with surgical debridement resulted in improvement in pain, with CT scan confirming complete fusion after 11 months.[30]

17.4 Outcomes

In-hospital mortality has been attributed to sepsis, endocarditis, and comorbidities, while sequelae have primarily been attributed to pain and neurological defects with the diagnosis frequently delayed due to the indolent nature of the disease. Mortality ranges from 2 to 20% and there are high rates of morbidity in survivors.[13] Akiyama et al, when retrospectively examining 7,118 patients with VO, found an in-hospital mortality rate of 6%. In their study, 58.9% of the patients were men and the average age was 69.2 years.[31] There was a linear trend between higher rates of in-hospital mortality and risk factors such as older age, hemodialysis, diabetes, liver cirrhosis, malignancy, and infective endocarditis. Bhavan et al, when retrospectively examining 70 patients with VO, found an in-hospital mortality rate of 4%.[32] In their study, the mean age of the patients was 59.7 years (± 15 years) and 38 (54%) were male. Common comorbidities included diabetes (43%) and renal insufficiency (24%).[32]

Factors associated with an increased mortality include elevated CRP at admission, advanced age, and a Charlson Comorbidity index (CCI) of greater than 2.[1] The CCI is a method of predicting mortality by classifying or weighing comorbid condition. To measure disease burden, Charlson et al assigned a weighted score to each comorbid condition based on the relative risk of 1-year mortality. In a study by Marjan et al, about one-third of patients with VO were found to have a high CCI score. These patients had a significantly higher incidence of advanced changes in MRI findings and more often had complicated VO, compared with patients with low CCI score, probably due to impaired immune response caused by diabetes or chronic renal failure or because of partial modulation of immune response with medications in patients with inflammatory rheumatic diseases.[33] The altered immune system obviously had an impact on the severe disease course in these patients. High CCI scores were more frequently associated with

positive blood cultures due to bacteremia because of impaired immune system.[33]

Aagaard et al published a Danish nationwide, population-based cohort study to assess the long-term prognosis and causes of death in patients diagnosed with non-postoperative (spontaneous) pyogenic spondylodiscitis from 1994 to 2009. The authors used Kaplan–Meier survival curves and Poisson regression analyses to estimate mortality rate ratios (MRRs). This study observed increased mortality due to infections (MRR = 2.57), neoplasms (MRR = 1.40), endocrine (MRR = 3.72), cardiovascular (MRR = 1.62), respiratory (MRR = 1.71), gastrointestinal (MRR = 3.35), musculoskeletal (MRR = 5.39), and genitourinary diseases (MRR = 3.37), but also due to trauma, poisoning, and external causes (MRR = 2.78), alcohol abuse-related diseases (MRR = 5.59), and drug abuse-related diseases (6 vs. 0 deaths, MRR not calculable).[34]

Despite the surgical advances and availability of antibiotics, there is a significant mortality and relapse following PVO. Infection-related mortality and relapses appeared to be associated with S. aureus sepsis. Recurrent bacteremia, chronic draining sinuses, and paravertebral abscesses were reported to be independent risk factors for relapse.[6] A recent systematic review of 30 studies published between 1998 and 2006 by Rayes reported only 1.7% (12/689) of infection recurrence among patients who underwent instrumented surgery.[37] More recently Park et al reported a 6.8% rate of infection recurrence for the instrumented surgery group; this was comparable to the rate of 4.8% for the noninstrumented group.[27] Arnold et al reported 23.4% (22/94) treatment failure and 15.3% (13/85) infection recurrence among patients with VO who required spinal instrumentation. The recurrence rate of 15.3% was higher than the rate of 1.7% reported in a recent systematic review by Rayes and higher than Park's rate of 6.8%.[5] In the study by Arnold et al, it is noteworthy that 40.5% of the microbiologically diagnosed cases were caused by MRSA.[5] Previously MSSA was the leading cause of vertebral osteomyelitis; however, in recent years there has been a shift with MRSA becoming the predominant pathogen, along with an increased frequency of recurrences of VO.[27]

In the past, treatment of vertebral osteomyelitis was associated with a significant morbidity rate and comparatively high incidence of recurrent infection. However, in current practice there appears to be better surgical outcomes due in part to improved methods of radiological diagnosis, safer operative and anesthetic techniques, and modern segmental spinal fixation systems have led to better overall surgical outcomes.[22] Miller et al performed a retrospective review of 50 patients with VO that required surgical intervention to investigate the neurological complications, reoperation, and pain in a longitudinal manner after surgery for VO. In their study there was a statistically significant improvement in modified McCormick scale (MMS) at 12 and 24 months in the postoperative period. The statistical significance was relatively small (0.35 on MMS scale), and 54% of patients experienced no change in MMS, whereas only 34% improved. Despite these improvements, the 24-month incidence of overall adverse events was 60%. In contrast, the mean improvement in visual analog scale (VAS) was more robust and clinically significant (3.40). For VAS, a statistically significant improvement was first observed at 3 months postoperatively and continued to decrease. Moreover, 64% of patients experienced an improvement in VAS.[2] These data support the overall benefit of surgical intervention with regard to recovery of neurological function and alleviation of pain.

17.5 Conclusion

Treatment for patients with VO must be tailored to individual patients and account for the radiographic and microbiological findings. Antibiotic treatment alone is appropriate in most patients without neurological deficits, spinal deformity, or instability. Surgery may be required to treat as well as diagnose PVO in many cases. Instrumented spinal fusion can be safely performed for patients requiring immediate spinal reconstruction after debridement and decompression.

References

[1] Boody BS, Jenkins TJ, Maslak J, Hsu WK, Patel AA. Vertebral osteomyelitis and spinal epidural abscess: an evidence-based review. J Spinal Disord Tech. 2015; 28(6):E316–E327

[2] Miller JA, Achey RL, Derakhshan A, Lubelski D, Benzel EC, Mroz TE. Neurologic complications, reoperation, and clinical outcomes following surgery for vertebral osteomyelitis. Spine. 2015; 41(4):1

[3] Hahn BS, Kim KH, Kuh SU, et al. Surgical treatment in patients with cervical osteomyelitis: single institute's experiences. Korean J Spine. 2014; 11(3): 162–168

[4] Hsieh PC, Liu JC, Wang MY. Introduction: vertebral osteomyelitis and spinal epidural abscess. Neurosurg Focus. 2014; 37(2):1–2, E1

[5] Arnold PM, Baek PN, Bernardi RJ, Luck EA, Larson SJ. Surgical management of nontuberculous thoracic and lumbar vertebral osteomyelitis: report of 33 cases. Surg Neurol. 1997; 47(6):551–561

[6] Mylona E, Samarkos M, Kakalou E, Fanourgiakis P, Skoutelis A. Pyogenic vertebral osteomyelitis: a systematic review of clinical characteristics. Semin Arthritis Rheum. 2009; 39(1):10–17

[7] Cornett CA, Vincent SA, Crow J, Hewlett A. Bacterial spine infections in adults: evaluation and management. J Am Acad Orthop Surg. 2016; 24(1):11–18

[8] Srinivasan D, Terman SW, Himedan M, Dugo D, La Marca F, Park P. Risk factors for the development of deformity in patients with spinal infection. Neurosurg Focus. 2014; 37(2):E2

[9] Nickerson EK, Sinha R. Vertebral osteomyelitis in adults: an update. Br Med Bull. 2016; 117(1):121–138

[10] Pupaibool J, Vasoo S, Erwin PJ, Murad MH, Berbari EF. The utility of image-guided percutaneous needle aspiration biopsy for the diagnosis of spontaneous vertebral osteomyelitis: a systematic review and meta-analysis. Spine J. 2015; 15(1):122–131

[11] Saifuddin A, Mitchell R, Taylor BA. Extradural inflammation associated with annular tears: demonstration with gadolinium-enhanced lumbar spine MRI. Eur Spine J. 1999; 8(1):34–39

[12] Vialle R, Mary P, Tassin JL, Parker F, Guillaumat M. Charcot's disease of the spine: diagnosis and treatment. Spine. 2005; 30(11):E315–E322

[13] Dunbar JAT, Sandoe JAT, Rao AS, Crimmins DW, Baig W, Rankine JJ. The MRI appearances of early vertebral osteomyelitis and discitis. Clin Radiol. 2010; 65(12):974–981

[14] Carragee E, Iezza A. Does acute placement of instrumentation in the treatment of vertebral osteomyelitis predispose to recurrent infection: long-term follow-up in immune-suppressed patients. Spine. 2008; 33(19):2089–2093

[15] Berbari EF, Kanj SS, Kowalski TJ, et al. Infectious Diseases Society of America. 2015 Infectious Diseases Society of America (IDSA) clinical practice guidelines for the diagnosis and treatment of native vertebral osteomyelitis in adults. Clin Infect Dis. 2015; 61(6):e26–e46

[16] Eren Gök S, Kaptanoğlu E, Celikbaş A, et al. Vertebral osteomyelitis: clinical features and diagnosis. Clin Microbiol Infect. 2014; 20(10):1055–1060

[17] Demura S, Murakami H, Shirai T, et al. Surgical treatment for pyogenic vertebral osteomyelitis using iodine-supported spinal instruments: initial case series of 14 patients. Eur J Clin Microbiol Infect Dis. 2015; 34(2):261–266

[18] Issa K, Pourtaheri S, Stewart T, et al. Clinical differences between monomicrobial and polymicrobial vertebral osteomyelitis. Orthopedics. 2017; 40(2): e370–e373

[19] de Lucas EM, González Mandly A, Gutiérrez A, et al. CT-guided fine-needle aspiration in vertebral osteomyelitis: true usefulness of a common practice. Clin Rheumatol. 2009; 28(3):315–320

[20] Dinh A, Jean M, Bouchand F, et al. Impact of anti-inflammatory drugs on pyogenic vertebral osteomyelitis: a prospective cohort study. Int J Rheumatol. 2016; 2016(2):9345467

[21] Hodges FS, McAtee S, Kirkpatrick JS, Theiss SM. The ability of MRI to predict failure of nonoperative treatment of pyogenic vertebral osteomyelitis. J Spinal Disord Tech. 2006; 19(8):566–570

[22] O'Shaughnessy BA, Kuklo TR, Ondra SL. Surgical treatment of vertebral osteomyelitis with recombinant human bone morphogenetic protein-2. Spine. 2008; 33(5):E132–E139

[23] Bydon M, De la Garza-Ramos R, Macki M, et al. Spinal instrumentation in patients with primary spinal infections does not lead to greater recurrent infection rates: an analysis of 118 cases. World Neurosurg. 2014; 82(6):e807–e814

[24] Mohamed AS, Yoo J, Hart R, et al. Posterior fixation without debridement for vertebral body osteomyelitis and discitis. Neurosurg Focus. 2014; 37(2):E6

[25] Tuli SM. Historical aspects of Pott's disease (spinal tuberculosis) management. Eur Spine J. 2013; 22 Suppl 4:529–538

[26] Talia AJ, Wong ML, Lau HC, Kaye AH. Safety of instrumentation and fusion at the time of surgical debridement for spinal infection. J Clin Neurosci. 2015; 22(7):1111–1116

[27] Le HV, Wadhwa R, Mummaneni P, Theodore P. Anterior transsternal approach for treatment of upper thoracic vertebral osteomyelitis: case report and review of the literature. Cureus. 2015; 7(9):e324

[28] Park KH, Cho OH, Lee YM, et al. Therapeutic outcomes of hematogenous vertebral osteomyelitis with instrumented surgery. Clin Infect Dis. 2015; 60(9): 1330–1338

[29] Hee HT, Majd ME, Holt RT, Pienkowski D. Better treatment of vertebral osteomyelitis using posterior stabilization and titanium mesh cages. J Spinal Disord Tech. 2002; 15(2):149–156

[30] Liljenqvist U, Lerner T, Bullmann V, Hackenberg L, Halm H, Winkelmann W. Titanium cages in the surgical treatment of severe vertebral osteomyelitis. Eur Spine J. 2003; 12(6):606–612

[31] Korovessis P, Petsinis G, Koureas G. Anterior surgery with insertion of titanium mesh cage and posterior instrumented fusion performed sequentially on the same day under one anesthesia for septic spondylitis of thoracolumbar spine: is the use of titanium mesh cages safe? Spine (Phila Pa 1976). 2006; 31 (9):1014–1019

[32] Bostelmann R, Steiger HJ, Scholz AO. First report on treating spontaneous infectious spondylodiscitis of lumbar spine with posterior debridement, posterior instrumentation and an injectable calcium sulfate/hydroxyapatite composite eluting gentamicin: a case report. J Med Case Reports. 2016; 10 (1):349

[33] Akiyama T, Chikuda H, Yasunaga H, Horiguchi H, Fushimi K, Saita K. Incidence and risk factors for mortality of vertebral osteomyelitis: a retrospective analysis using the Japanese diagnosis procedure combination database. BMJ Open. 2013; 3(3):1–6

[34] Bhavan KP, Marschall J, Olsen MA, Fraser VJ, Wright NM, Warren DK. The epidemiology of hematogenous vertebral osteomyelitis: a cohort study in a tertiary care hospital. BMC Infect Dis. 2010; 10:158

[35] Marjan D, Zadravec D, Begovac J, Radiology I, Katarina S, Hospital S. Vertebral Osteomyelitis in Adult Patients. 2016; 55(1):9–15

[36] Aagaard T, Roed C, Dahl B, Obel N. Long-term prognosis and causes of death after spondylodiscitis: a Danish nationwide cohort study. Journal Infectious Diseases. 2016; 48(3):201–208

[37] Rayes M, Colen CB, Bahgat DA, Higashida T, Guthikonda M, Rengachary S, Eltahawy HA. Safety of instrumentation in patients with spinal infection. J Neurosurg Spine. 2010; 12(6):647–659

18 Fungal and Tubercular Infections of the Thoracic Spine

Kevin T. Huang, Dustin J. Donnelly, Kyle Wu, Ziev B. Moses, and John H. Chi

Abstract

Fungal and tubercular infections of the thoracic spine are uncommon occurrences in developed countries. However, because of their slow and nonspecific presentation, diagnosis is often delayed and special vigilance is necessary for timely diagnosis. One should have a particularly high suspicion in patients with immunosuppression or those from endemic areas, and individuals presenting with atypical symptoms such as fever, weight loss, and focal tenderness. Once properly recognized, the mainstays of treatment are antifungal or antitubercular chemotherapy with reversal of immunosuppression as can safely be permitted by the patient's clinical situation. Surgical debridement is often indicated in cases of fungal or tuberculous spondylitis, and in all cases where patients present with significant neurologic compression, unrelenting back pain, significant spinal instability, or deformity.

Keywords: tuberculosis of spine, fungal spondylitis, tuberculous spondylitis, Pott's disease, spinal coccidioidomycosis, spinal blastomycosis, spinal candidiasis, spinal aspergillosis

---

Clinical Pearls

- Fungal or tubercular infections of the spine should be suspected in patients who present with months of nonspecific back pain and have a history of immunosuppression or who hail from high-risk populations.
- Evaluation with magnetic resonance imaging will often reveal extensive involvement of the anterior column of the spine, but relative sparing of the intervertebral disc. Spread between vertebrae along and underneath the anterior longitudinal ligament is common.
- Treatment of tubercular infections can consist of medical therapy alone. However, most incidences of fungal infection and any case where there is significant neurologic deficit or deformity require surgical decompression and possible reconstruction.

18.1 Introduction

Fungus and tubercular infections of the thoracic spine are relatively uncommon. When they are encountered, however, they present unique challenges in both diagnosis and treatment that require special attention from clinicians due to its indolent nature. Diagnosis is often delayed due to the gradual and nonspecific nature of symptoms, factors which may be exacerbated by the complexity of immunosuppressed patients that are at particularly high risk for these infections. Treatment typically consists of prolonged antibiotic courses, but may also include neural decompression, debridement, deformity correction, and fusion of unstable elements when necessary. This chapter discusses the epidemiology, pathophysiology, presentation, diagnosis, and treatment of fungal and tubercular infections of the

thoracic spine. Information is presented both on these infections in general, and on the specifics of the most commonly encountered organisms.

18.2 Epidemiology and Pathophysiology

Systemic fungal infection is an uncommon occurrence, with an estimated incidence of approximately 306 per 1,000,000 in the United States.[1,2] This number has been increasing in recent decades, however, as the number of immunocompromised patients has increased.[1,3,4,5] Risk factors for developing invasive mycoses include stem cell or solid organ transplantation, major surgery, severe polytrauma, severe burns, human immunodeficiency virus (HIV) infection, immunosuppressive therapy, disseminated malignancy, and advanced age. Fungal infections of the spine are rarer still, with data limited to individual case series.

Fungal infections can further be subdivided into opportunistic infections, such as *Candida* species, *Aspergillus* species, *Cryptococcus neoformans*, and *Pneumocystis jirovecii*, and endemic infections such as *Coccidioides immitis/posadasii* and *Blastomyces dermatitidis*. This distinction affects presentation. Opportunistic infections require some break in the patient's normal immune barriers, and are nearly always associated with recent exposure to the health care system, including systemic use of antibiotics, corticosteroids, *tumor necrosis factor* (TNF) alpha inhibitors, chemotherapeutic agents, chronic indwelling lines, and/or recent procedures.[6] Endemic infections, on the other hand, can be acquired by simple exposure in the natural habitat and possess the inherent ability to invade deeper structures in otherwise healthy patients. Of note, *Histoplasmosis capsulatum*, though another endemic fungus that can cause invasive infection, will not be discussed as spinal involvement is exceedingly rare and typically only seen as part of a larger fungal meningitis.[7]

Systemic tuberculosis demonstrates a distinct disparity between the developed and underdeveloped populations. With an estimated prevalence of greater than 13 million worldwide, tuberculosis remains a global disease, with populations in Asia and Africa accounting for almost 90% of known cases.[8] Spinal involvement is uncommon, but it occurs in approximately 1% of affected patients and the spine is the most common site of skeletal involvement.[9,10,11] In the United States, tuberculosis remains rare, with an estimated incidence of 3 per 100,000. At-risk populations, including foreign-born residents (especially those from countries with high prevalence), immunocompromised patients, and those who are incarcerated or homeless, suffer disproportionately high rates of infection. Foreign-born residents from China (24.9 cases per 100,000), the Philippines (46.9 cases per 100,000), and Vietnam (47.8 cases per 100,000) have among the highest incidences of tuberculosis.[12]

The thoracic and thoracolumbar spines are disproportionately infected in fungal and tubercular infections as they spread through spore inhalation.[13,14] Once a nidus of infection has been established in the lungs, dissemination to the spine occurs through either hematogenous or lymphatic spread.[15,16] Venous drainage of the lungs via the bronchial veins and azygous vein or lymphatic drainage into the thoracic duct allows for an avenue of infectious spread into the paraspinal region. These, in turn, allow seeding into the cancellous bone of the spine via the external and internal venous plexuses, as well as intervertebral spread via either contiguous infection or through Batson's plexus. Arterial seeding, through gross fungemia and access through the radicular arteries and subchondral perforators of the spine, has also been hypothesized.[15]

Once there, infection causes symptoms through either structural compromise of the trabecular bone leading to instability, abscess formation and subsequent neural compression, or vascular thrombosis with resulting infarction. Because infections preferentially affect the anterior column of the spine, immediate or delayed progressive kyphotic deformity is not uncommon. This is of particular concern in pediatric patients, who are still developing their axial skeleton and whose normal anterior column growth can be hampered by the infection. Thus, many pediatric cases warrant complex reconstruction.[17] Direct intradural or intraparenchymal invasion is rare, but is associated with high morbidity.[18,19,20]

In immunosuppressed individuals, the lack of both T-cell immunity and TNF alpha activation appears to be particularly crucial factors in pathogenesis. CD4+ T cells have been shown to be critical in initial recognition of invasive fungal species of the lungs. After they encounter pathogen epitopes, these CD4+ cells are activated, and in turn activate macrophage phagocytic activity through toll-like receptor-mediated signals.[21] Similarly, TNF alpha activation is responsible for a wide range of immunoregulatory functions, including antitumor and antiviral responses. This holds true for *Mycobacterium tuberculosis* infection, where it serves a special role in stimulating recruitment of immune cells to the infected region and initiating granuloma formation. TNF alpha inhibition has been shown to interfere with granuloma formation and to cause lysis of fully formed granulomas in mice.[22] Use of TNF alpha inhibitors is associated with extrapulmonary tuberculosis, with extrapulmonary disease evident in 57% of those with TNF alpha inhibition-related tuberculosis activation.[23]

18.3 Presentation and Evaluation

As with many types of spinal infections, fungal and tubercular involvement of the spine can be difficult to diagnose due to the slow onset and nonspecific nature of symptoms. Back pain is common, but is frequently mistaken for more benign pathologies. A high index of suspicion should be maintained in patients from at-risk populations, and those who present with atypical or concerning symptoms should merit further work-up (▶ Table 18.1).

A proper history and physical is crucial for proper patient evaluations. History-taking should elucidate the time course and progression of symptoms and any associated neurologic complaints. Signs of and risk factors for infection should be identified, including a proper travel history and social history. Cancer patients should have their current treatment details explored. Patients actively undergoing chemotherapy or bone marrow transplantation present a substantially elevated risk than those with stable disease. Patients who have been infected with HIV should have the status of their infection (including

Table 18.1 Risk factors and warning signs in patients with fungal and tubercular spondylitis

At-risk populations	Warning signs on presentation

• Incarcerated
• Homeless
• Immunocompromised
  ○ Infected with human immunodeficiency virus
  ○ Ongoing chemotherapy with myelosuppression
  ○ Congenital immunodeficiency
  ○ Status post organ transplantation
  ○ Iatrogenic immunosuppression with corticosteroids or TNF alpha inhibitors
• Foreign born from endemic areas
• Concerning presentation + recent travel to endemic regions
• Previous systemic fungal or tubercular infection
• Diabetes mellitus
• Intravenous drug use
	• Fever
	• Malaise
	• Recent weight loss
	• Night sweats
	• Progressive neurologic deficit
	• Symptoms of spinal instability in young patients
	• Gross kyphotic deformity
	• Back pain resistant to standard therapy

Abbreviation: TNF, tumor necrosis factor.

CD4+ cell counts and viral loads) identified, and updated if necessary. Medication lists can also be illuminating, in particular, if a patient has been on long-term corticosteroids or TNF alpha inhibitors.

Physical examination should seek to not only identify the site of a potential lesion, but also to document the severity and extent of any neurologic deficits. Examination of the lungs can often be revealing, especially if a focal area of aeration is detected. Focal tenderness to palpation along the spine can indicate involved levels, and may indicate spread to the posterior elements or paraspinal tissues.

As in many spine cases, and especially in patients suspected of having an infectious spondylitis, the next stage in evaluation should be to pursue imaging. Both magnetic resonance imaging (MRI) and computed tomography (CT) are important to characterize the extent of bony and neural involvement, as well as the integrity of osseous structures. Standing plain radiographs can also be useful to assess the degree of any associated deformity and sagittal imbalance.

On MRI, fungal and tubercular abscesses bare similar characteristics, and can be difficult to differentiate from more commonly encountered pyogenic infections. Both tuberculous and fungal spondylitis are marked by preferential involvement of the anterior column, large paraspinal abscesses, and importantly, relative sparing of the intervertebral discs (▶ Fig. 18.1).[24,25,26] The inflammatory reaction to infectious spondylitis results in bony edema, resulting in decreased signal on T1-weighted imaging and increased signal on T2-weighted imaging in the marrow of the vertebral bodies (▶ Fig. 18.2).[27] Contrast enhancement is typical, but oftentimes can be nonspecific. The infection can often be seen spreading underneath, but contained by, the anterior longitudinal ligament. The relative sparing of the disc and ligament, particularly classic for tuberculous spondylitis, is thought

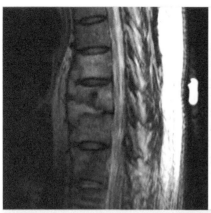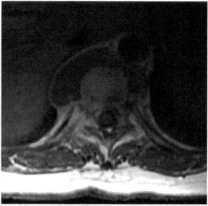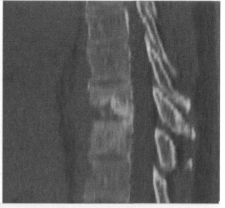

Fig. 18.1 Imaging from a 30-year-old patient who was born in China and presented with several months marked back pain. Fine-needle aspiration of the paravertebral fluid was positive for tuberculosis. (*Left*) T2-weighted sagittal MRI demonstrating involvement at the T8, T9, and T10 levels, with T9–T10 discitis, relative sparing of the T8-9 disc space, and contiguous subligamentous spread anteriorly. (*Middle*) Contrast-enhanced T1-weighted image demonstrating a characteristic large paravertebral abscess. (*Right*) Sagittal CT image demonstrating preferential lytic destruction of the anterior portion of the vertebral body.

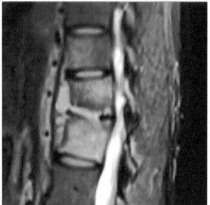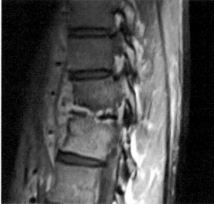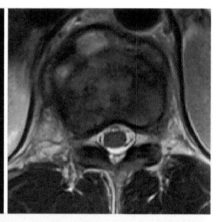

Fig. 18.2 Images from a 30-year-old man with a history of hepatitis C, intravenous drug use, and insulin-dependent diabetes mellitus. He originally presented with weeks of sharp lower thoracic back pain with radiation into his testicles. (*Left*) MRI demonstrated hyperintensity on T2-weighted imaging in the T11 and T12 vertebral bodies with associated subligamentous spread. (*Middle*) T1-weighted contrast-enhanced imaging demonstrated relative preservation of the associated disc space suggestive of fungal or tubercular disease. (*Right*) Axial image demonstrated anterior paravertebral extension of disease. Needle aspiration of the lesion leads to the eventual diagnosis of *Candida albicans* spondylitis.

to be due to the relative lack of proteases of the organism, preventing direct invasion through ligamentous structures.[28,29] Multilevel involvement is common, and can help differentiate infection from osseous tumor involvement, which can appear similarly (▶ Fig. 18.3).[30] Epidural extension can be seen, and can often be characterized by a thin, smooth, abscess wall.[31] Direct invasion of the dura with intradural abscess is an uncommon finding (▶ Fig. 18.4).

On CT imaging, extensive lytic destruction with bone sequestration is characteristic, with loss of the adjoining cortical definition.[27,32] Calcifications in adjoining paraspinal abscesses can be seen in tuberculosis cases, which is pathognomonic for the disease.[31]

In addition to the above, it is important to consider other work-up in suspected cases. A plain chest radiograph can often be the most rapid way to establish a site of primary infection. As hematogenous spread is common, blood samples to look for fungemia or systemic tuberculosis can be useful to establish a

diagnosis. Imaging of the rest of the body with CT imaging can also identify other extrapulmonary lesions and help guide systemic treatment. Systemic inflammatory markers, though nonspecific, can also help mark response to therapy going forward. Often times, however, the above work-up is either nonspecific or too slow. Thus, when necessary, image-guided needle biopsy aspiration can confirm the diagnosis and help set up a proper treatment strategy.

18.4 Organism-Specific Considerations

18.4.1 Tuberculosis

M. tuberculosis remains widely prevalent and a major cause of spinal infections in many parts of the world. Of all cases of tuberculosis, approximately 15 to 20% affect extrapulmonary locations.[33] With regard to the central nervous system, it is well known for manifesting as an indolent meningitis or spondylitis (i.e., Pott's disease), although tuberculomas may also present as focal intraparenchymal and intradural extraparenchymal lesions of the brain and spinal cord. The spine is involved in 50% of cases of skeletal spread, accounting for up to 1% of tuberculosis infections.[33,34] Pott's disease most commonly affects the thoracic spine.[9,35]

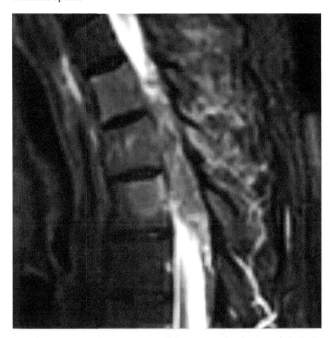

Fig. 18.3 Imaging from a 31-year-old patient with a history of alcohol and intravenous drug abuse who presented with several months of back pain. Short tau inversion recovery sagittal imaging demonstrated hyperintensity in the T2 and T3 vertebral bodies with preferential involvement of the vertebral bodies and relative disc-space sparing, as well as an epidural mass. The patient underwent laminectomy and associated mass resection, with a high clinical suspicion for tuberculosis. Final pathology demonstrated B-cell lymphoma.

The link between HIV and tuberculosis cannot be overstated, and HIV-infected patients accounted for 11% of new tuberculosis cases in 2016.[8] In the United States, there demonstrates regional variation as well, with most cases occurring in the south (40%), followed by the western region (27.4%).[35] This may underscore the population demographics of those areas.

Multidrug-resistant tuberculosis, in particular, represents a growing public health concern. Recent studies underscore the importance of diagnosing this population early on, in order to allow for appropriate treatment selection.[36,37] Similar to the general epidemiology of tuberculous spondylitis, drug-resistant tuberculosis has a predilection for the thoracic spine, occurring there 61.2% of the time.[36] Risk factors for drug-resistant tuberculosis include prior treatment, nonadherence to treatment, and short duration of treatment.

Pott's disease is associated with back pain, pathologic fractures leading to exaggerated kyphosis (including gibbus deformity), and neurologic deficits including arachnoiditis, radicular symptoms, myelopathy and frank paraplegia. Importantly, these can occur with or without pulmonary symptoms. With bony involvement, the anterior vertebral body is typically involved and endplate irregularities are present.[38] Early on in the disease course, the intervertebral disc is often spared, despite the involvement of contiguous vertebrae. While adjacent spread is the norm, noncontiguous spread is frequent.[34] While the vertebral column is typically affected, the posterior elements may be involved in 5 to 10% of cases.[39]

Intramedullary tuberculomas, though uncommon, have been previously reported. They typically appear as solid- or ring-enhancing lesions, and can be associated with cord edema and syrinx formation. Intradural extramedullary tuberculomas are typically dural-based, and, indeed, may mimic an en plaque meningioma.[40] Both extramedullary and intramedullary lesions may be associated with arachnoiditis.

Pott's disease in children presents a special case as the pediatric spine is particularly susceptible to destabilization. On average, children present with a kyphotic deformity of approximately 25 degrees due to collapse of the anterior column.[41] Even with

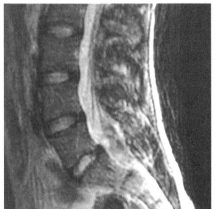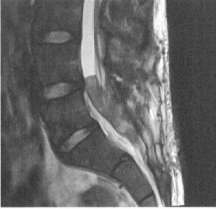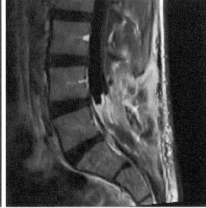

Fig. 18.4 A 22-year-old man presented with several months of episodic severe back and bilateral posterior thigh pain. (*Left*) Initial T2-weighted MRI demonstrated an intradural mass in the L5 to S1 region. The patient was taken for L4–S1 laminectomies and intradural exploration and excision of a friable mass. Though initial cultures were not able to isolate a specific organism, a presumptive diagnosis of *Candida* was made based on pathologic analysis demonstrating budding yeast and an elevated serum beta-glucan level. The patient unfortunately failed several months of antibiotic therapy due to a combination of intolerance, renal toxicity, and noncompliance. (*Middle*) Subsequent MRI demonstrated increase in the size of the intradural extension of the mass on T2-weighted imaging. (*Right*) This area demonstrated avid contrast enhancement both within the dura and in the old surgical wound, which eventually required reexploration and decompression.

successful treatment, this deformity tends to progress, with an average of 11 degrees of deformity added by the time the child is 15 years out from treatment. Thoracolumbar lesions tend to progress more severely than other locations.[41] These severe kyphotic deformities bear close monitoring, as severe deformities (those > 60 degrees) have been associated with late-onset paraplegia.[14,42] Though curves this severe are uncommon, with less than 4% of patients affected, this fact nevertheless highlights the serious long-term consequences of the disease, even after active antibiotic treatment has ended.[41]

18.4.2 Coccidioidomycosis

C. immitis and *C. posadasii* are dimorphic saprophytic fungi found in the southwestern United States and northern reaches of Mexico. They are found as mycelium in the soil of endemic regions and can remain dormant for long periods of time, before being released as spores during times of increased moisture. In humans, they are pathogenic even in immune-competent hosts, and primarily cause respiratory infections.[13]

Disseminated coccidioidomycosis is rare, occurring in only approximately 0.5% of cases. Patients with immunosuppression are at a much higher risk of extrapulmonary spread, however, with rates of extrapulmonary spread reported to be as high as 30 to 50%.[43] Of those with extrapulmonary involvement, the spine is frequently a site of infection, occurring in 10 to 60% of cases.[13,44,45] Of note, unlike in other types of fungal and tuberculous spinal infection, the intervertebral disc is frequently affected radiographically and half of patients appear to have epidural involvement.[45]

18.4.3 Blastomycosis

Similar to *C. immitis* and *C. posadasii*, *B. dermatitidis* is an invasive, dimorphic, fungal species. The organism is endemic to the eastern United States, specifically the Appalachian mountain region, Mississippi and Ohio river valleys, and parts of Ontario, Manitoba, and Quebec.[46] Similar to the *Coccidioides* species, the fungus exists in mycelium form while in the environment, but can release spores that convert to yeast form when inhaled by the human host. Blastomycosis is significantly less common than either coccidioidomycosis or histoplasmosis.[46]

An estimated 6 to 48% of blastomycosis patients have bony disease, and an estimated 25% of patients with extrapulmonary blastomycosis have evidence of osteomyelitis.[47] Because of its relative rarity, the incidence of vertebral involvement in systemic blastomycosis is difficult to determine, but previous reviews of available case series estimate that of patients with osseous spread, 26 to 37% have evidence of vertebral body involvement.[47,48,49]

In reported cases of blastomycotic spondylitis, the thoracic and thoracolumbar spines are the most commonly affected regions. Similar to other fungal infections, the anterior aspect of the vertebral body is preferentially involved, often with associated wedge-shaped compression fractures. As is classic with other organisms, large paravertebral, intramuscular abscesses are commonly reported.[47]

18.4.4 Aspergillosis

Aspergillus species are saprophytic fungi, have at least 200 known species, and have a ubiquitous presence in the environment.[50] The most commonly isolated species in humans is *Aspergillus fumigatus*.[50] Their small spores are frequently found in water, air, soil, straw, hay, and grain.[51] Humans often come in contact with *Aspergillus* by inhaling their small spores (2–4 μm) through contaminated air-handling systems.[52] However, inoculation through the gastrointestinal (GI) system by swallowing the spores or direct entry through skin wounds (e.g., surgery) are both possible. Patients may contract *Aspergillus* in the spine through direct inoculation during surgery, via hematogenous spread, or by direct extension from a pulmonary focus. As with other types of opportunistic infections, risk factors for invasive aspergillosis include chronic granulomatous disease, acquired immunodeficiency syndrome (AIDS), prolonged antibiotic use, malignancy, and intravenous drugs.[53] Vertebral osteomyelitis caused by *Aspergillus* shares many characteristics with other pyogenic causes of vertebral osteomyelitis such as a male predominance, a bimodal age distribution, and a tendency to involve the lumbar spine followed by the thoracic spine.[51]

On examination, in suspected *Aspergillus* infection, it is important to pay particular attention to the respiratory examination given the ability of this organism to initially spread from the lung. As described above, CT and MRI are helpful in examining the extent of disease and the general radiographic indicators of fungal infection apply. Diagnostic testing, with commercially available kits for galactomannan antigen can help confirm the diagnosis.[54]

18.4.5 Candidiasis

Candida species are dimorphic fungi and have a presence on the human body as commensal organisms found on the skin and GI system of healthy individuals. There are 10 pathogenic species of candida; however, it is *Candida albicans* that causes the majority of vertebral osteomyelitis cases associated with *Candida*.[55] In certain situations, *Candida* can develop into an opportunistic infection. It can seed the spine through hematogenous spread or by direct inoculation during surgery. Organisms often gain access in immunocompromised patients through intravenous lines or invasive monitoring devices, during prosthesis placement, and in the postoperative setting.[56]

Diagnostic tests can aid in earlier diagnosis of infections. However, given the widespread presence of *Candida* antibody tests lack sufficient specificity due to a prior exposure eliciting a false-positive result or the immunocompromised state preventing a true positive result.[54] Instead, testing for *Candida*-specific antigens, such as enolase or mannan can be more useful in diagnosing invasive candidiasis.

18.4.6 Cryptococcosis

C. neoformans is an encapsulated budding yeast and an opportunistic pathogen that affects immunocompromised patients. The organism is found almost universally in the soil and is found in particularly high concentrations in the stool of pigeons. Systemic infection, like the other forms of infection discussed in this chapter, is thought to stem from a primary pulmonary infection taking advantage of an immunocompromised host.[57] Systemic infection is common in patients with AIDS, with an estimated 7 to 10% of patients infected.[57] Skeletal involvement is rare, with data mostly limited to case reports and case series. Of these limited reports, however, vertebral involvement is not uncommon, with 32.5% of cases involving the vertebrae.[58]

18.5 Management and Treatment

Once recognized, treatment should be initiated as quickly as possible. The cornerstone of treatment is medical: proper antibiotics combined with reversal of the patient's immunocompromised state if possible. For cancer patients undergoing chemotherapy, this may involve temporary cessation of treatment to allow for immune reconstitution depending on the situation. For patients positive for HIV, this involves the prompt initiation, or reinitiation of antiretroviral therapy. Patients on corticosteroids and TNF alpha inhibitors should be investigated for ways that these drugs can be stopped safely.

For spinal tuberculosis, antibiotic chemotherapy consists of standard triple therapy (isoniazid, rifampin, and pyrazinamide) for at least 6 months, with kanamycin, amikacin, cycloserine, capreomycin, and ethionamide, prothionamide, and quinolones serving as second-line options.[59,60,61] Multidrug-resistant tuberculous spondylitis may require longer therapies up to possibly 24 months. For cases of systemic coccidioidomycosis, blastomycosis, and aspergillosis, limited disease in immunocompetent hosts can be considered for azole therapy alone (▶ Table 18.2).[62] However, for more serious infections, which typically encompass all cases of spinal involvement, amphotericin B is the treatment of choice, with months of subsequent chronic maintenance therapy consisting of fluconazole, itraconazole, or ketoconazole.[63,64,65] Voriconazole is used as a primary treatment for *Aspergillus* osteomyelitis, while liposomal amphotericin, caspofungin, micafungin, posaconazole, and itraconazole are available as alternative treatments.[66] Primary treatment for *Candida* osteomyelitis includes azole therapy for 6 to 12 months or liposomal amphotericin for several weeks, followed by fluconazole for 6 to 12 months.

Anidulafungin,[67] micafungin, and caspofungin or amphotericin B serve as alternates, followed by fluconazole for 6 to 12 months.[67]

For tuberculosis, historically, surgical intervention was favored in all cases as the lack of modern diagnostic technologies led to late presentation of severe disease. As increasingly good outcomes were reported with antitubercular therapy alone, however, surgery is now only recommended to attain certain clinical objectives.[68] These objectives include source control in patients failing to respond to medical therapy, decompression in those suffering from neurologic compression, and deformity correction in those with deformity greater than 30 degrees.[69,70,71,72] It should be noted that patients who present with signs of spinal instability, ankylosis and spontaneous fusion do occur.[10] Moreover, long-term progression of kyphosis can still occur.[42] As such, a surgical approach must attempt to address not only near-term symptoms but also potential long-term complications.

As part of the surgical treatment of tubercular infections, consideration must also be given to proper containment and isolation precautions. Respiratory precautions, including negative pressure isolation rooms and N95 particle filtration masks, are indicated if the patient has suspected active tuberculosis. Even if active tuberculosis is not clinically suspected, the mere presence of tubercular osteomyelitis is grounds to screen for active pulmonary infection with chest radiography and sputum cultures.[73] Intraoperatively, it is important to consider the possibility of aerosolization of infected particles during tissue manipulation. Thus, in addition to proper precautions, care should be taken to limit cauterization or vaporization of infected tissues to limit the exposure to operating room staff.

In contrast to tubercular spondylitis, for most cases of fungal spondylitis, surgical debridement is often recommended. Because of the recalcitrant nature of many fungal infections, systemic therapy is often slow to work, and recurrent cases are common. Thus, surgical debridement maximizes the chance for a successful chemotherapeutic cure, limits the amount of nearby bony destruction, and allows for neural decompression and surgical

Table 18.2 Antibiotic therapy options

Type of infection	First-line therapy	Alternative considerations
Tuberculosis	Isoniazid, rifampin, and pyrazinamide × 6 months or longer Treatment length expanded to 9–12 months for those with meningitis Isoniazid may be replaced by a later-generation quinolone in cases of intolerance of monoresistance	For multidrug-resistant tuberculosis: at least 4 of the following agents to which the organism has been proven susceptible for minimum of 20 months Alternative agents include ethambutol, later-generation quinolones, bedaquiline, delamanid, amikacin, capreomycin, kanamycin, streptomycin, linezolid, ethionamide or prothionamide, terizidone or cycloserine, amoxicillin–clavulanate, clarithromycin, clofazimine, imipenem–cilastatin, meropenem
Coccidioidomycosis	Fluconazole or itraconazole for 6–12 months	For severe infections: amphotericin B for short periods (< 3 months) followed by maintenance azole therapy for 3 years to life
Blastomycosis	Itraconazole for 12 months	For moderate-to-severe disease: amphotericin B for 1–2 weeks followed by oral itraconazole for 12 months
Aspergillosis	Voriconazole for 6–8 weeks	For moderate-to-severe disease: amphotericin for 6–8 weeks with consideration of longer-term suppressive therapy with an azole. Consideration can be given to echinocandins
Candidiasis	Fluconazole for 6–12 months or an echinocandin (caspofungin, micafungin, or anidulafungin) for 2 weeks followed by 6–12 months of azole therapy	For severe infections: amphotericin B for 2 weeks followed by 6–12 months of azole therapy

fixation in necessary cases. A notable exception occurs in spinal cryptococcosis, where medical therapy is typically sufficient and symptoms will typically resolve with antifungal therapy combined with correction of immunosuppression.

Over the last half century, technical advances in the anterior surgical approach to the thoracic spine have proven to be extremely useful in fungal and tubercular infections. As the anterior column is typically the area of key pathology in these infections, direct intervention at the site is often an effective method of debridement and fusion.[74] The anterior approach, however, does have limitations, including anatomical limitations and the need to potentially mobilize vital organs in those with preexisting medical comorbidities.[75,76] Thus, more recently others have advocated for a posterior approach, with posterolateral or transpedicular access to the anterior column to allow for debridement and reconstruction.[77,78] Combining the two approaches has also been proposed, with some investigators reporting superior kyphosis correction as a result.[59]

18.6 Conclusions

Fungal and tubercular infections of the thoracic spine are uncommon occurrences in developed countries. However, because of their slow and nonspecific presentation, diagnosis is often delayed and special vigilance in at-risk populations is necessary for timely diagnosis. Once properly recognized, the mainstays of treatment are antifungal or antitubercular chemotherapy with reversal of immunosuppression as can safely be permitted by the patient's clinical situation. Surgical debridement is important in most cases of fungal spondylitis, and in all cases where patients present with significant neurologic compression or deformity.

References

[1] Wilson LS, Reyes CM, Stolpman M, Speckman J, Allen K, Beney J. The direct cost and incidence of systemic fungal infections. Value Health. 2002; 5(1): 26–34

[2] Pfaller MA, Diekema DJ. Epidemiology of invasive mycoses in North America. Crit Rev Microbiol. 2010; 36(1):1–53

[3] Asmundsdóttir LR, Erlendsdóttir H, Gottfredsson M. Increasing incidence of candidemia: results from a 20-year nationwide study in Iceland. J Clin Microbiol. 2002; 40(9):3489–3492

[4] Marr KA, Carter RA, Crippa F, Wald A, Corey L. Epidemiology and outcome of mould infections in hematopoietic stem cell transplant recipients. Clin Infect Dis. 2002; 34(7):909–917

[5] Pfaller MA, Jones RN, Messer SA, Edmond MB, Wenzel RP. National surveillance of nosocomial blood stream infection due to Candida albicans: frequency of occurrence and antifungal susceptibility in the SCOPE Program. Diagn Microbiol Infect Dis. 1998; 31(1):327–332

[6] Smith RM, Schaefer MK, Kainer MA, et al. Multistate Fungal Infection Outbreak Response Team. Fungal infections associated with contaminated methylprednisolone injections. N Engl J Med. 2013; 369(17):1598–1609

[7] Hott JS, Horn E, Sonntag VK, Coons SW, Shetter A. Intramedullary histoplasmosis spinal cord abscess in a nonendemic region: case report and review of the literature. J Spinal Disord Tech. 2003; 16(2):212–215

[8] Global Tuberculosis Report. World Health Organization; 2016

[9] Turgut M. Spinal tuberculosis (Pott's disease): its clinical presentation, surgical management, and outcome. A survey study on 694 patients. Neurosurg Rev. 2001; 24(1):8–13

[10] Tuli SM. General principles of osteoarticular tuberculosis. Clin Orthop Relat Res. 2002(398):11–19

[11] Fuentes Ferrer M, Gutiérrez Torres L, Ayala Ramírez O, Rumayor Zarzuelo M, del Prado González N. Tuberculosis of the spine. A systematic review of case series. Int Orthop. 2012; 36(2):221–231

[12] Salinas JL, Mindra G, Haddad MB, Pratt R, Price SF, Langer AJ. Leveling of tuberculosis incidence—United States, 2013–2015. MMWR Morb Mortal Wkly Rep. 2016; 65(11):273–278

[13] Kim CW, Perry A, Currier B, Yaszemski M, Garfin SR. Fungal infections of the spine. Clin Orthop Relat Res. 2006; 444(444):92–99

[14] Jain AK, Dhammi IK. Tuberculosis of the spine: a review. Clin Orthop Relat Res. 2007; 460(460):39–49

[15] Garg RK, Somvanshi DS. Spinal tuberculosis: a review. J Spinal Cord Med. 2011; 34(5):440–454

[16] De Tavera MP, De Leon EP. Tuberculosis of the lymphatics in children; its relation to spinal tuberculosis. A clinico-radiological study. Dis Chest. 1967; 52 (4):469–477

[17] Bailey HL, Gabriel SM, Hodgson AR, Shin JS. Tuberculosis of the spine in children. 1972 [classical article]. Clin Orthop Relat Res. 2002(394):4–18

[18] Chang KH, Han MH, Choi YW, Kim IO, Han MC, Kim CW. Tuberculous arachnoiditis of the spine: findings on myelography, CT, and MR imaging. AJNR Am J Neuroradiol. 1989; 10(6):1255–1262

[19] Van Tassel P. Magnetic resonance imaging of spinal infections. Top Magn Reson Imaging. 1994; 6(1):69–81

[20] Saigal G, Donovan Post MJ, Kozic D. Thoracic intradural Aspergillus abscess formation following epidural steroid injection. AJNR Am J Neuroradiol. 2004; 25(4):642–644

[21] Rivera A, Ro G, Van Epps HL, et al. Innate immune activation and CD4 + T cell priming during respiratory fungal infection. Immunity. 2006; 25(4):665–675

[22] Winthrop KL. Risk and prevention of tuberculosis and other serious opportunistic infections associated with the inhibition of tumor necrosis factor. Nat Clin Pract Rheumatol. 2006; 2(11):602–610

[23] Keane J, Gershon S, Wise RP, et al. Tuberculosis associated with infliximab, a tumor necrosis factor alpha-neutralizing agent. N Engl J Med. 2001; 345(15): 1098–1104

[24] Pertuiset E, Beaudreuil J, Lioté F, et al. Spinal tuberculosis in adults. A study of 103 cases in a developed country, 1980–1994. Medicine (Baltimore). 1999; 78(5):309–320

[25] Whiteman ML. Neuroimaging of central nervous system tuberculosis in HIV-infected patients. Neuroimaging Clin N Am. 1997; 7(2):199–214

[26] Kwon JW, Hong SH, Choi SH, Yoon YC, Lee SH. MRI findings of Aspergillus spondylitis. AJR Am J Roentgenol. 2011; 197(5):W919–23

[27] Tali ET. Spinal infections. Eur J Radiol. 2004; 50(2):120–133

[28] Diehn FE. Imaging of spine infection. Radiol Clin North Am. 2012; 50(4):777–798

[29] Williams RL, Fukui MB, Meltzer CC, Swarnkar A, Johnson DW, Welch W. Fungal spinal osteomyelitis in the immunocompromised patient: MR findings in three cases. AJNR Am J Neuroradiol. 1999; 20(3):381–385

[30] Mahboubi S, Morris MC. Imaging of spinal infections in children. Radiol Clin North Am. 2001; 39(2):215–222

[31] Hong SH, Choi JY, Lee JW, Kim NR, Choi JA, Kang HS. MR imaging assessment of the spine: infection or an imitation? Radiographics. 2009; 29(2):599–612

[32] Sharif HS, Morgan JL, al Shahed MS, al Thagafi MY. Role of CT and MR imaging in the management of tuberculous spondylitis. Radiol Clin North Am. 1995; 33(4):787–804

[33] Trecarichi EM, Di Meco E, Mazzotta V, Fantoni M. Tuberculous spondylodiscitis: epidemiology, clinical features, treatment, and outcome. Eur Rev Med Pharmacol Sci. 2012; 16 Suppl 2:58–72

[34] Polley P, Dunn R. Noncontiguous spinal tuberculosis: incidence and management. Eur Spine J. 2009; 18(8):1096–1101

[35] De la Garza Ramos R, Goodwin CR, Abu-Bonsrah N, et al. The epidemiology of spinal tuberculosis in the United States: an analysis of 2002–2011 data. J Neurosurg Spine. 2017; 26(4):507–512

[36] Mohan K, Rawall S, Pawar UM, et al. Drug resistance patterns in 111 cases of drug-resistant tuberculosis spine. Eur Spine J. 2013; 22 Suppl 4:647–652

[37] Pawar UM, Kundnani V, Agashe V, Nene A, Nene A. Multidrug-resistant tuberculosis of the spine—is it the beginning of the end? A study of twenty-five culture proven multidrug-resistant tuberculosis spine patients. Spine. 2009; 34(22):E806–E810

[38] Jain AK, Aggarwal A, Mehrotra G. Correlation of canal encroachment with neurological deficit in tuberculosis of the spine. Int Orthop. 1999; 23(2):85–86

[39] Kumar K. A clinical study and classification of posterior spinal tuberculosis. Int Orthop. 1985; 9(3):147–152

[40] Chaudhary V, Bano S, Garga UC. Central nervous system tuberculosis: an imaging perspective. Can Assoc Radiol J. 2017; 68(2):161–170

[41] Rajasekaran S. The natural history of post-tubercular kyphosis in children. Radiological signs which predict late increase in deformity. J Bone Joint Surg Br. 2001; 83(7):954–962

[42] Tuli SM. Severe kyphotic deformity in tuberculosis of the spine. Int Orthop. 1995; 19(5):327–331

[43] Galgiani JN, Ampel NM, Blair JE, et al. Infectious Diseases Society of America. Coccidioidomycosis. Clin Infect Dis. 2005; 41(9):1217–1223

[44] Dalinka MK, Greendyke WH. The spinal manifestations of coccidioidomycosis. J Can Assoc Radiol. 1971; 22(1):93–99

[45] Wrobel CJ, Chappell ET, Taylor W. Clinical presentation, radiological findings, and treatment results of coccidioidomycosis involving the spine: report on 23 cases. J Neurosurg. 2001; 95(1) Suppl:33–39

[46] Bradsher RW, Chapman SW, Pappas PG. Blastomycosis. Infect Dis Clin North Am. 2003; 17(1):21–40, vii

[47] Saccente M, Abernathy RS, Pappas PG, Shah HR, Bradsher RW. Vertebral blastomycosis with paravertebral abscess: report of eight cases and review of the literature. Clin Infect Dis. 1998; 26(2):413–418

[48] Bassett FH, III, Tindall JP. Blastomycosis of bone. South Med J. 1972; 65(5):547–555

[49] Gehweiler JA, Capp MP, Chick EW. Observations on the roentgen patterns in blastomycosis of bone. A review of cases from the Blastomycosis Cooperative Study of the Veterans Administration and Duke University Medical Center. Am J Roentgenol Radium Ther Nucl Med. 1970; 108(3):497–510

[50] Kwon-Chung KJ, Sugui JA. Aspergillus fumigatus—what makes the species a ubiquitous human fungal pathogen? PLoS Pathog. 2013; 9(12):e1003743

[51] Vinas FC, King PK, Diaz FG. Spinal aspergillus osteomyelitis. Clin Infect Dis. 1999; 28(6):1223–1229

[52] Lutz BD, Jin J, Rinaldi MG, Wickes BL, Huycke MM. Outbreak of invasive Aspergillus infection in surgical patients, associated with a contaminated air-handling system. Clin Infect Dis. 2003; 37(6):786–793

[53] Govender S, Rajoo R, Goga IE, Charles RW. Aspergillus osteomyelitis of the spine. Spine. 1991; 16(7):746–749

[54] Yeo SF, Wong B. Current status of nonculture methods for diagnosis of invasive fungal infections. Clin Microbiol Rev. 2002; 15(3):465–484

[55] Miller DJ, Mejicano GC. Vertebral osteomyelitis due to Candida species: case report and literature review. Clin Infect Dis. 2001; 33(4):523–530

[56] Friedman BC, Simon GL. Candida vertebral osteomyelitis: report of three cases and a review of the literature. Diagn Microbiol Infect Dis. 1987; 8(1):31–36

[57] Govender S, Mutasa E, Parbhoo AH. Cryptococcal osteomyelitis of the spine. J Bone Joint Surg Br. 1999; 81(3):459–461

[58] Zhou HX, Lu L, Chu T, et al. Skeletal cryptococcosis from 1977 to 2013. Front Microbiol. 2015; 5:740

[59] Moon MS. Tuberculosis of the spine. Controversies and a new challenge. Spine. 1997; 22(15):1791–1797

[60] Kizilbash QF, Seaworth BJ. Multi-drug resistant tuberculous spondylitis: a review of the literature. Ann Thorac Med. 2016; 11(4):233–236

[61] Horsburgh CR, Jr, Barry CE, III, Lange C. Treatment of tuberculosis. N Engl J Med. 2015; 373(22):2149–2160

[62] Galgiani JN, Ampel NM, Blair JE, et al. Infectious Diseases Society of America (IDSA) clinical practice guideline for the treatment of coccidioidomycosis. Clin Infect Dis. 2016; 2016:ciw360

[63] Galgiani JN, Ampel NM, Catanzaro A, Johnson RH, Stevens DA, Williams PL, Infectious Diseases Society of America. Practice guideline for the treatment of coccidioidomycosis. Clin Infect Dis. 2000; 30(4):658–661

[64] Chapman SW, Bradsher RW, Jr, Campbell GD, Jr, Pappas PG, Kauffman CA, Infectious Diseases Society of America. Practice guidelines for the management of patients with blastomycosis. Clin Infect Dis. 2000; 30(4):679–683

[65] Chapman SW, Dismukes WE, Proia LA, et al. Infectious Diseases Society of America. Clinical practice guidelines for the management of blastomycosis: 2008 update by the Infectious Diseases Society of America. Clin Infect Dis. 2008; 46(12):1801–1812

[66] Walsh TJ, Anaissie EJ, Denning DW, et al. Infectious Diseases Society of America. Treatment of aspergillosis: clinical practice guidelines of the Infectious Diseases Society of America. Clin Infect Dis. 2008; 46(3):327–360

[67] Pappas PG, Kauffman CA, Andes DR, et al. Clinical practice guideline for the management of candidiasis: 2016 update by the Infectious Diseases Society of America. Clin Infect Dis. 2016; 62(4):e1–e50

[68] Kotil K, Alan MS, Bilge T. Medical management of Pott disease in the thoracic and lumbar spine: a prospective clinical study. J Neurosurg Spine. 2007; 6(3):222–228

[69] Parthasarathy R, Sriram K, Santha T, Prabhakar R, Somasundaram PR, Sivasubramanian S. Short-course chemotherapy for tuberculosis of the spine. A comparison between ambulant treatment and radical surgery—ten-year report. J Bone Joint Surg Br. 1999; 81(3):464–471

[70] Upadhyay SS, Sell P, Saji MJ, Sell B, Hsu LC. Surgical management of spinal tuberculosis in adults. Hong Kong operation compared with debridement surgery for short and long term outcome of deformity. Clin Orthop Relat Res. 1994(302):173–182

[71] Talu U, Gogus A, Ozturk C, Hamzaoglu A, Domanic U. The role of posterior instrumentation and fusion after anterior radical debridement and fusion in the surgical treatment of spinal tuberculosis: experience of 127 cases. J Spinal Disord Tech. 2006; 19(8):554–559

[72] Rasouli MR, Mirkoohi M, Vaccaro AR, Yarandi KK, Rahimi-Movaghar V. Spinal tuberculosis: diagnosis and management. Asian Spine J. 2012; 6(4):294–308

[73] Schirmer P, Renault CA, Holodniy M. Is spinal tuberculosis contagious? Int J Infect Dis. 2010; 14(8):e659–e666

[74] Hodgson A, Stock FE. Anterior spine fusion for the treatment of tuberculosis of the spine. J Bone Joint Surg Am. 1960; 42(2):295–310

[75] Campbell PG, Malone J, Yadla S, et al. Early complications related to approach in thoracic and lumbar spine surgery: a single center prospective study. World Neurosurg. 2010; 73(4):395–401

[76] Vidyasagar C, Murthy HK. Management of tuberculosis of the spine with neurological complications. Ann R Coll Surg Engl. 1994; 76(2):80–84

[77] Chacko AG, Moorthy RK, Chandy MJ. The transpedicular approach in the management of thoracic spine tuberculosis: a short-term follow up study. Spine. 2004; 29(17):E363–E367

[78] Zhang HQ, Lin MZ, Shen KY, et al. Surgical management for multilevel noncontiguous thoracic spinal tuberculosis by single-stage posterior transforaminal thoracic debridement, limited decompression, interbody fusion, and posterior instrumentation (modified TTIF). Arch Orthop Trauma Surg. 2012; 132(6):751–757

Part V

Tumor and Vascular

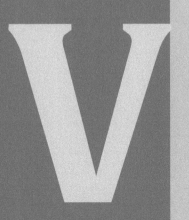

19 Primary Tumors of the Thoracic Spinal Column

Zach Pennington, C. Rory Goodwin, A. Karim Ahmed, and Daniel M. Sciubba

Abstract

Primary tumors of the thoracic spine are relatively rare pathologies with benign and malignant lesions combined affecting fewer than 10,000 Americans annually. Despite this, knowledge of the proper treatment of these lesions is essential for the complex spine surgeon, as operative intervention forms the backbone of clinical cure. Therapy comprises grading the lesions using the Enneking system to define the goals of surgery and staging using the Tomita or Weinstein–Boriani–Biagini system to assess the feasibility of that therapeutic goal. Benign lesions, for example osteoid osteomas, are usually treated surgically only after medical management has failed to relieve symptoms. By contrast, malignant lesions, e.g., chordoma and chondrosarcoma, are surgically managed in all but the most advanced cases, where adjuvant chemotherapy and radiotherapy may be indicated. Surgeries for these lesions are highly morbid and can require patients to undergo months of recovery, but said interventions improve overall survival in many patients by achieving long-term oncologic cure. Here, we describe the pathology and management of the major benign and malignant primary tumors of the thoracic spine, with specific emphasis on diagnosis and the aggressiveness of surgical intervention.

Keywords: primary spine tumor, en bloc resection, spine surgery, the Enneking grading system, multimodal therapy, tumor staging, spinal reconstruction

---

Clinical Pearls

- T2–T12 roots can be sacrificed during resection to allow for better visualization of vertebral body and minimize damage to cord.[1,2]
- Except for plasmacytomas, operable spinal malignancies should be treated per Enneking oncologic principles, which constitute en bloc resection with wide margins.
- For many tumors, local recurrence is one of the strongest predictors of survival; it can be reduced using en bloc resection.
- En bloc resection of tumors has a steep learning curve, and so patients should be referred to centers with extensive experience treating these lesions.
- Revision surgeries have a lower rate of success than index surgeries, and so it is imperative that the index surgery is conducted per the principles of oncologic surgery.

19.1 Introduction

Only 7,500 primary vertebral column tumors are seen each year,[3] constituting less than 10% of all spinal column neoplasms.[4,5] These tumors can be divided into malignant tumors, which account for 62% of all cases[6] and benign neoplasms or hamartomas, which account for the remainder. Malignant tumors are the chief concern of the spine surgeon due to their poor prognosis, but many benign lesions also require surgical intervention. This chapter discusses spine tumor staging, typing, and treatment, with a focus on tumors of the thoracic region.

19.2 Staging of Primary Tumors of the Spinal Column

Currently, there are three main staging systems for primary spinal column tumors—the Enneking system,[7,8] the Weinstein–Boriani–Biagini (WBB) system[9] (▶ Fig. 19.1), and the Tomita system[10] (▶ Fig. 19.2). They are summarized in ▶ Table 19.1 and discussed below.

19.2.1 The Enneking System

Though developed for appendicular musculoskeletal tumors,[7] the Enneking system is now widely used to classify spinal column lesions[11,12,13] based on surgical grade, local extent, and the presence of metastases. Different scales are used for benign and malignant lesions,[1,7,8,14,15,16,17] but both use clinical, histological, and radiographic evidence[8,17] and are guided by the principle that the tumor should never be entered during resection.[4]

Benign tumors are broken into three grades based on their aggressiveness and degree of circumscription.[14] Grade I (latent) lesions are generally asymptomatic, well-circumscribed, monostotic, and display contact-dependent growth inhibition.[8,14] Grade II (active) lesions possess thinner, irregular borders,[8,14] and are generally symptomatic, expansile, and histologically well-differentiated,[8] with a constant cell-to-matrix ratio throughout and an enhancing neovascular rim on computed tomography (CT).[8] Last is grade III (aggressive) lesions, which are poorly circumscribed, symptomatic, hyperplastic.[8] Unlike grade I or II lesions,[8,14] they expand extracompartmentally, and may form benign metastases.[8] Current Enneking principles allow stage I lesions to be treated with intralesional excision due to their low propensity to recur.[8] However, stage II lesions should be treated with marginal en bloc resection, unless the associated morbidity is unacceptable.[8,9] Lastly, stage III tumors require wide en bloc resection due to their tendency to recur.[8,9]

Unlike benign lesions, osseous malignancies are graded on differentiation and compromise of vertebral cortical bone—A-type lesions remain intracompartmental, whereas B-type lesions breach cortical bone.[7,8,14] Grade I (low-grade) malignancies, unlike grade III benign lesions, are necrotic, highly vascular, and hemorrhagic.[8] High-grade (grade II) malignancies are differentiated from low-grade lesions by more extensive proliferation, dedifferentiation, and nuclear atypia.[7,8,14] All malignancies with metastases are grade III, though they are generally not subdivided by degree of extracompartmental expansion.[1,7,8,14,15,16,17] Current treatment standards suggest that stage I and II lesions be treated with wide en bloc resection, despite the sacrifice of significant neurovascular structures often required in treatment of IB and IIB lesions.[8,9] It has been suggested that stage III lesions be treated with wide resection plus adjuvant radiotherapy (RT) or chemotherapy,[8] but systemic therapy and

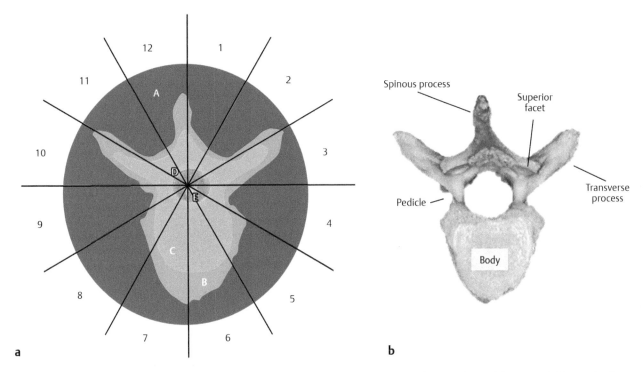

Fig. 19.1 The Weinstein–Boriani–Biagini staging system divides the vertebrae into 12 sectors and 5 tissue layers—(A) paraspinal, (B) superficial vertebral bone, (C) deep vertebral bone, (D) intradural, extramedullary space, (E) intramedullary space. **(a)** Shows the sector and **(b)** shows a labeled thoracic vertebra for reference.

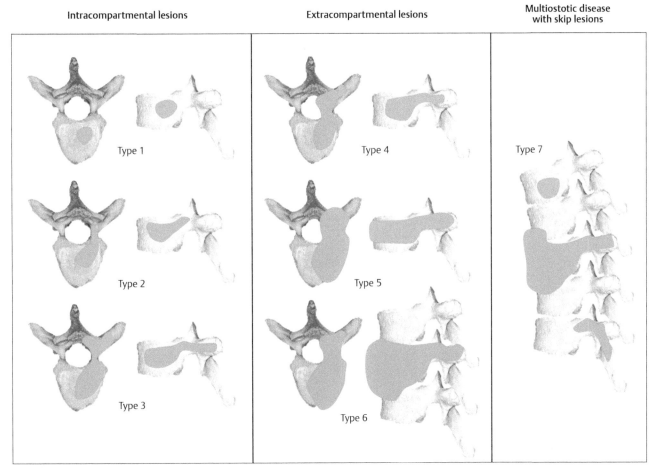

Fig. 19.2 The Tomita system assesses the feasibility of en bloc spondylectomy for a tumor based on the portions of the vertebra it involves, the extracompartmental invasion, and the presence of skip lesions. (Adapted from Tomita et al, 1994.[32])

Table 19.1 Classification systems for primary spinal tumors

System	Purpose	Classification features
Enneking	• Prescription of appropriate surgical margins	• *Benign*: Degree of expansion, definition of border, degree of hyperplasia • *Malignant*: Degree of hyperplasia, dedifferentiation, nuclear atypia, and extent beyond compartment boundary
WBB	• Prescription of optimal surgical approach	• Radial and angular position of tumor with respect to centroid of vertebral body. Described by superimposing clock face on horizontal section of vertebral body
Tomita	• Assess feasibility of en bloc resection	• Describe the number of vertebrae involved, relative positions of those vertebrae, and position of tumor within the vertebrae

Abbreviation: WBB, Weinstein–Boriani–Biagini system.

palliative care are preferable in cases where en bloc morbidity would be high.

Several studies have shown the Enneking system to have good interobserver and intraobserver reliability,[11] and have shown its use to decrease local recurrence and increase overall survival.[4]

19.2.2 The Weinstein–Boriani–Biagini System

The WBB classification differs from the Enneking staging in that it is designed to incorporate the more complex spinal anatomy[11,17,18] and seeks to describe the optimal surgical approach, not the surgical margin.[19,20,21,22] The WBB system acknowledges that true radical resection is impossible in nearly all symptomatic spinal malignancies[7,8,9] and so vertebrae are treated as the oncological compartments.

Staging begins by superimposing a clock face over a horizontal section of the vertebra so that the 12 and 1 o'clock sectors straddle the spinous process, and the 10 and 3 o'clock positions overlie the pedicles.[20] The tumor is then classified by (1) its angular position—the sectors of the clock face that it occupies, and (2) its radial position—whether it involves paraspinal musculature (A), cortical bone (B), medullary bone (C), epidural space (D), or intradural space (E).[11,20] Like the Enneking system, it has extremely high intraobserver and interobserver reliability,[11] and the two are often used together during surgical planning.[19,20,21,22]

19.2.3 The Tomita System

Like the WBB system, the Tomita system assesses spinal malignancies based on anatomical location.[10,13] However, unlike the former, its purpose is to evaluate the feasibility of resection by en bloc spondylectomy. Tumors are divided into seven numbered, increasingly inclusive classes based on location within

the spinal column: (1) the vertebral body, (2) the pedicle, (3) posterior elements, (4) the spinal canal, (5) the paravertebral area, (6) adjacent vertebrae, and (7) nonconsecutive vertebrae.[1,10,13,23,24] Tomita et al recommend wide-margin en bloc spondylectomy for type III lesions and marginal en bloc spondylectomy for type IV and V lesions.[24] They recommend against en bloc spondylectomy for type VII lesions, and leave selection of treatment type I, II, and VI lesions to the individual surgeon, as type I and II lesions do not require en bloc spondylectomy to prevent recurrence, and type VI lesions often recur, even with en bloc spondylectomy.[24]

19.3 Surgery for Thoracic Spinal Tumors

All surgical intervention begins by deciding the goal of surgery, which for most primary tumors is to attempt cure.[25] Curative treatment starts by imaging the affected region, using CT to assess bony destruction, and magnetic resonance imaging (MRI) to evaluate for spinal canal and paraspinal soft tissue invasion.[26] If imaging and clinical findings are definitive, the tumor is staged using the Enneking and WBB systems in order to determine proper margins and proper approach, respectively.[9,27] Otherwise, a biopsy should be performed to allow for definitive diagnosis prior to staging and surgical planning.[3,28,29] This definitive diagnosis allows for selection of treatment that minimizes complications, and maximizes the chance of cure. CT-guided biopsy is preferred by many,[3] as the biopsy tract can be placed in the future surgical field, which decreases recurrence.[9,30]

One of the more popular techniques for en bloc excision of thoracic tumors is the en bloc spondylectomy first described by Tomita et al.[31] The procedure involves a posterior-only approach and makes use of a specially designed T-saw, which has been shown to reduce seeding of the surgical site.[32] The procedure begins with a posterior midline incision and subperiosteal dissection encompassing three levels above and below the lesion.[10,31,33,34,35] Next, the inferior facets and spinous process of the level proximal to the specimen are osteotomized to expose the superior articular processes of the uppermost involved vertebra. Dissection continues laterally over the ribs, which are cut 3 to 4 cm lateral to the costotransverse joint. As a guideline, the dissection field must be wide enough to clear the tumor borders and allow dissection underneath the transverse processes. The pleura is then bluntly dissected from the ribs and vertebrae, and the intercostal vessels are ligated. Soft tissue around the intervertebral foramina is removed, taking care to avoid damage to the nerve roots during cervicothoracic or thoracolumbar procedures. A T-wire is then looped around the pedicle in the cephalocaudad direction using a C-shaped T-saw guide. The guide is removed and a T-saw is used to divide the pedicle. This is repeated bilaterally at each level to be resected and the posterior column is removed en bloc. The cut pedicle surfaces are sealed with bone wax to minimize bleeding and seeding of tumor cells into surgical field. Bilateral pedicle screws are placed two levels above and below the involved segments, and a temporary rod is installed on one side to maintain distraction during the corpectomy.[10] The intercostal nerves are sacrificed contralateral to the rod and blunt dissection is used to free the aorta and great vessels from anterior faces of the vertebrae.[10,31,33,34,35] Care must be taken during this step to avoid injuring the azygos system or inferior vena cava (IVC).[31] Vertebral protectors are then inserted bilaterally to create a plane between mediastinal organs and the vertebrae. The thecal sac is freed from the posterior longitudinal ligament (PLL) and vertebral body, and a cord protector is inserted in the plane between the vertebrae and thecal sac. T wires are inserted in the plane of the vertebral protectors at the levels of the vertebral discs bounding the involved segments. The anterior longitudinal ligament (ALL), discs, and PLL are then transected; the cord protector must be firmly in place during this step to avoid cord injury. Additionally, shallow grooves may be formed in the sides of the discs prior to discotomies to ensure that transection occurs in the desired plane. Following the discotomies, the specimen is rotated around the long axis of the cord and removed en bloc from the side contralateral to the rod.[10,31,33,34,35] Hemostasis is achieved and the wound may be washed with water and cisplatin to kill tumor cells that have seeded the area.[24] A bony strut or autograft-filled cage is then inserted into the anterior column defect. Permanent rods are installed, drains are inserted, and the wound is closed. The patient may also be given an orthosis to wear during the recovery period.[10,31,33,34,35]

The above procedure is modified slightly for those tumors involving the great vessels and for tumors at the cervicothoracic and thoracolumbar junctions. In these cases, a combined approach may be preferred.[24,33] For a cervicothoracic tumor, the procedure begins with a transmanubrial approach.[36,37] An osteomuscular flap containing the sternoclavicular joint, entire clavicle, and cervical musculature is formed and reflected.[36] The medial portion of the first rib, and occasionally the second and third ribs, is resected. An upper lobectomy is also performed if the lung is involved.[36] Dissection continues by freeing the esophagus, trachea, and mediastinal vasculature from the anterior surface of the vertebrae.[37] The anterior wound is then closed and the patient is rotated to the prone position, where the procedure proceeds in a fashion similar to that described for the posterior-only approach.[36,37,38] During the posterior procedure, care should be taken to dissociate the cervical and upper thoracic nerve roots from the tumor,[37] as damage to these structures is associated with significant neurological dysfunction.

For thoracolumbar tumors, a combined approach facilitates dissection of aorta branches from the vertebrae and preservation of the upper lumbar nerve roots. Whether the two approaches are performed simultaneously with posterior delivery of the tumor[39] or sequentially with delivery of the tumor through the anterior approach[40] is largely up to the individual surgeon. As with the combined approach for cervicothoracic tumors, the anterior approach is used to clear the anterior face of the spinal column—this includes taking down the diaphragm and releasing the major vessels. For posterior delivery of the specimen, the procedure is like that described for the posterior-only approach, with the exception that release of the ALL and anterior disc is done via the anterior approach.[39] However, for procedures with anterior delivery, posterior instrumentation and wound closure are performed first, followed by completion of tumor resection, tumor delivery, and reconstruction of the anterior column through the anterior approach.[40]

19.3.1 Surgical Margins

Enneking originally described four types of surgical margins[7]—intralesional, marginal, wide, and radical—but only intralesional, marginal, and wide margins are feasible in the spine due to its complex anatomy[7,8,9,27]. Intralesional resection—dissection along the tumor pseudocapsule—can be applied to the Enneking grade I benign tumors[8,41] but grade II tumors require marginal margins, or resection within the reactive tissue surrounding the tumor pseudocapsule.[8,41] Lastly, wide margins—resection of the tumor with a layer of healthy tissue—are prescribed for grade III benign lesions and all vertebral malignancies as they improve local control.[25,42,43] This improved control is the single strongest predictor of overall survival in spinal malignancies.[15,17,21,42,43,44,45]

19.3.2 Resection Technique

The last consideration in surgical planning is the resection technique. En bloc excision—removal of the entire tumor in one piece with wide margins[9,41,46]—is the only way to achieve tumor-free margins. It has the advantage of significantly improving patient's overall survival and recurrence-free survival,[4,17,23,25,41,46,47,48,49,50] and is the Enneking-appropriate approach for grade III benign lesions and all malignancies.[8] However, it has higher intraoperative mortality and morbidity, and postoperative morbidity relative to piecemeal resection.[4,10,23,41,48,51,52] This increased complication rate,[21] reported as 10 to 35% in some series,[41,46,53] and en bloc's steep learning curve led many practitioners to favor piecemeal resection. However, it is important to weigh these sequelae, the potential survival benefit,[25,41,46] and patient preference before selecting a resection technique. Current consensus holds that the risks of en bloc resection generally outweigh the benefits in benign lesions, whereas the reverse is true for localized malignancies.[17,23,30,46]

19.4 Overview of Different Lesion Types

The remainder of the chapter focuses on the main tumor types that afflict the spine, as well as the rate at which they appear in the thoracic spine. Tumor types are coarsely divided into benign lesions, which can be treated nonsurgically in some cases, and primary spinal malignancies, which are almost uniformly treated with surgery. Epidemiology and basic imaging findings are summarized in ▶ Table 19.2 and ▶ Table 19.3.

19.5 Benign Tumors and Hamartomas

19.5.1 Aneurysmal Bone Cyst

Description

Aneurysmal bone cysts are highly vascular, locally aggressive cyst-like lesions[5,54,55,56,57] characterized by significant bony destruction.[57,58,59] Two-thirds of cases are secondary to a giant cell tumor (GCT), osteoblastoma (OB), chondroblastoma, or osteosarcoma,[21,55,57,59,60,61,62,63] and nearly all affect the poste-

Table 19.2 Incidence, features, and prognosis of benign primary tumors of the spinal column

Tumor	Epidemiology and demographics	Radiological features	Adjuvant therapy	Prognosis
Aneurysmal bone cyst	• 0.14–1.4 per 100,000 • 11–30% spine; 22–43% thoracic • Women < 20	*CT*: Osteolytic *MRI*: Hypo T1; hyper T2	• Adjuvant RT contraindicated	• 10–44% recurrence • Recur within 2 y
Benign fibrous lesions	• 1–2.5% 1° bone tumor; 0.3–3.6% spine • Males; 10–20	*CT*: Osteolytic *MRI*: Iso T1; variable T2	• None	• 0% recurrence (en bloc)
Chondroblastoma	• < 1% of 1° bone tumors; 1–1.4% spine • 67% male	*CT*: Osteolytic *MRI*: Hypo rim w/ hyper core (T2)	• None	• *Recurrence*: 30%
Enostosis	• 14% of population • T1–T7 & L2–L3	*CT*: Round, osteoblastic *MRI*: Hypo T1, T2	• None	• Only 31.9% change in size w/o treatment
Eosinophilic granuloma	• 2–10 per million • 46–54% thoracic • *Age*: < 15 y; 66–75% male	*CT*: Osteolytic *MRI*: Hypo T1, hyper T2	• None	• 10-year survival: 100% • *Recurrence*: < 20%
Giant cell tumor	• 0.63 per million person-years; 22–25% thoracic • *Age*: 30–40s; 56–72% female	*CT*: Osteolytic, expansive *MRI*: Hypo T1, T2	• RT contraindicated • Denosumab	• *Recurrence*: 0% (en bloc), 46–80% (piecemeal)
Osteoid osteoma	• 9% of 1° spine tumors; 14–41.7% thoracic • *Age*: 10–20; 67–75% male	*X-ray*: Osteolytic w/ calcifications *MRI*: Hypo T1; hyper T2	• None	• *Recur*: 0% (en bloc), 4.5–10% (piecemeal) • 90% symptom relief
Osteoblastoma	• 10–25% of 1° spine tumor; 21.3–42.1% thoracic • *Age*: 10–20; 60–67% male	*CT*: Ground glass *MRI*: Hypo T1; hyper T2	• None	• *Recur*: 0% (en bloc), 10–15% (piecemeal) • > 90% pain relief
Osteochondroma	• 4–7% of 1° spine tumors; 26–27% thoracic • *Age*: early 30s; 71–75% male	*CT*: Sessile, iso *MRI*: Hypo T1, T2	• None	• *Recur*: 2–4% (piecemeal); en bloc better • 85% symptom improvement

Abbreviations: CT, computed tomography; hyper, hyperintense; hypo, hypointense; Iso, isointense; MRI, magnetic resonance imaging; recur, local recurrence rate; RT, radiotherapy.

Table 19.3 Epidemiology, features, and prognoses of malignant primary spinal tumors

Tumor	Epidemiology	Radiological features	Adjuvant therapy	Prognosis
Chordoma	• 0.08–0.5 per 100,000 PY; 10% mobile spine • *Age*: 40–50; 60–67% male	*CT*: Midline, osteolytic *MRI*: Hypo T1, hyper T2	• Adjuvant RT > 60 Gy if positive or marginal margin	• *MOS*: 84–104 mo • *Recur*: 5–17% (en bloc); > 50% (curettage)
Chondrosarcoma	• 0.24–0.5 per 100,000 • *Age*: 40–50; 67–80% male	*CT*: Osteolytic *MRI*: Hypo T1; hyper T2	• Chemotherapy and RT	• *MOS*: 72–198 mo • *Recur*: ≤ 25% (en bloc)
Ewing's sarcoma	• 1.6–3 per million • 23.3–46.7% thoracic • *Age*: < 20 y; 67% male	*CT*: Osteolytic mass *MRI*: Iso T1; hyper T2	• RT and chemotherapy (vincristine, ifosfamide or cyclophosphamide, doxorubicin, and actinomycin D)	• *MOS*: 90–98 mo • *Recur*: 12–40%
Osteosarcoma	• 0.2–0.5 per 100,000 PY; 25–45% thoracic • *Age*: 35–48 y; no gender bias	*CT*: Variable, often osteoblastic *MRI*: Low utility	• Neoadjuvant RT or chemotherapy • Post-op RT + methotrexate, cisplatin, doxorubicin, and ifosfamide	• *MOS*: 77–81 mo (en bloc) • *Recur*: 11–20% (en bloc); 44–60% (piecemeal)
Plasmacytoma	• 5–10/100,000 PY; 45.5–61.5% thoracic • *Age*: 50–60; 67% male	*CT*: Osteolytic *MRI*: Hypo T1; hyper T2 *Blood*: ↑ M protein	• Radiotherapy > 45 Gy is main treatment • Surgery is adjuvant to address symptoms	• *MOS*: 7.5–12 y

Abbreviations: CT, computed tomography; hyper, hyperintense; hypo, hypointense; Iso, isointense; MOS, median overall survival; MRI, magnetic resonance imaging; PY, person-years; recur, local recurrence rate; RT, radiotherapy.

rior elements. As much as 90% also involve the vertebral body,[26,55,57,58,61,62,64,65] creating three-column involvement and cord compression.[66] Histologically, they are characterized by a series of blood-filled channels lined with an abundant, fibrous stroma of spindle cells and osteoclast-like cells[26,57,58,59,61,62,66] occasionally showing intralesional ossification.[57]

Diagnosis

Patients often present with localized pain that worsens with activity and which has been present for 8 to 12 months.[54,55,56,58,59,60,67,68,69,70] Pain is often worse at night[26] and may present along with a palpable mass.[62,67] Neurological involvement, pathologic fracture, and spinal instability are relatively rare, but have been noted.[54,62,66,69]

On plain radiography, the lesion is expansile, well-circumscribed, and radiolucent[69] and on CT, it is expansile, eccentric, multilobulated, and osteolytic.[55,57,58,66] ABCs are often said to have a soap bubble appearance on CT,[62] with an eggshell-like capsule and visible fluid–fluid level created by previous hemorrhage.[26,62,65,69] This fluid–fluid level is best visualized on MRI, which also shows the intralesional septation.[26,55,57,59,60,62,70] Because of the abundant fluid, the lesion is generally hypointense on T1 and hyperintense on T2 MR.[69]

Treatment

ABCs generally require treatment,[55,59] though no consensus exists regarding standard of care.[71] Surgery has historically been front-line treatment, but results in the past decade have suggested that selective arterial embolization (SAE) may be equally effective in patients free of neurological dysfunction or spinal instability.[54,60,62,72,73] Additionally, SAE has lower morbidity[54,60] and reduces intraoperative blood loss in patients who crossover to surgery.[5,55,62,69,72] However, surgery, not SAE should be used in cases where the tumor shares a blood supply with the cord,[61,70] causes spinal instability, or creates rapidly progressive neurological dysfunction.

For surgical candidates, complete surgical resection is the goal, as it prevents recurrence.[5,55,60,62,63,70,72,74,75] This local control is readily achieved through en bloc resection, but many report satisfactory results with intralesional curettage of grade I or II tumors.[5,26,63,69,73,75,76] Adjuvant RT is contraindicated due to the risk of osteosarcoma induction.[54,55,56,59,60,65,70]

Prognosis

Recurrence is observed in 10 to 44% of cases and generally occurs within the first 2 years of follow-up.[56,66,68,73,75] Compared to those treated with en bloc resection, local recurrence is higher in patients treated with subtotal resection,[61,65,66] but not for those treated with SAE.[70,73]

19.5.2 Benign Fibrous Lesion

Description

Benign fibrous lesions are a class of osteolytic lesions that includes fibrous dysplasia, chondromyxoid fibroma, benign fibrous histiocytoma, and nonossifying fibroma.[14,62,77] Despite their different origins, they all feature a collagenous stroma

with cytologically normal, spindle-shaped fibroblasts arranged in fascicles or storiform patterns. The stroma may also contain woven bone, foamy macrophages, or multinucleated giant cells.[29,62,77,78,79,80,81,82,83]

Diagnosis

Benign fibrous lesions most commonly present with chronic nonspecific back pain,[29,79,80,82,83,84,85] but in rare cases may present with neurological symptoms of insidious onset.[29,77,81,85] Because of these nonspecific symptoms, diagnosis relies heavily on CT and MRI imaging.[29] CT demonstrates an expansile, blown-out lesion with ground-glass stroma and sclerotic cortex.[62,77,82]

Treatment and Prognosis

Preliminary treatment is bisphosphonates to relieve pain,[62,86] but patients with spinal instability or neurological dysfunction may require surgery.[62,87] The goal of surgery is complete resection of the tumor[29,62,77,82] as a subset of these lesions recur following subtotal resection.[29] En bloc excision is unnecessary, as piecemeal gross total resection achieves 100% local control in many cases.[29,77,78,80,82,85]

19.5.3 Chondroblastoma

Description

Chondroblastomas are extremely rare tumors derived from immature cartilage that grossly appear pink to beige, are lobulated by fibrous septa, and display multifocal calcification.[88,89,90,91,92,93,94] Histologically, they possess a high density of polygonal, chondroblast-like cells in an eosinophilic chondroid matrix with giant cells and "chicken wire" calcification.[62,88,90,91,92,94,95,96,97]

Diagnosis

The majority of patients have presented with localized pain as their chief complaint,[88,89,90,92,94,97,98,99] though a fraction also have radicular pain and/or paresis.[3,92,93,94,95,97,99,100] Furthermore, some thoracic lesions compress lung parenchyma and cause dyspnea.[93,94,97]

Chondroblastomas are aggressive, eccentric, osteolytic lesions on radiograph, with marginal sclerosis, cortical bone involvement, and occasional multifocal intralesional calcification.[88,89,90,91,92,96,97,100] The intralesional calcifications are best visualized on CT[93,97,100] and soft tissue invasion is best demonstrated as a hyperintense mass on T2-weighted MRI.[92,93,94,95,97,99,101] Because these features are nonspecific, biopsy is generally necessary for diagnosis.[3,92,97]

Treatment and Prognosis

Because of the small number of documented cases (≈30), no guidelines exist for treatment. Surgery has been the method of choice, with the goal of complete resection of the tumor,[89,90,94,98,99] as 30% of vertebral chondroblastomas have locally recurred.[94,100] Both en bloc[89,93,94,97] and curettage have been used with high success,[89,92,94,96,98,100,101] and neither is currently preferred.

19.5.4 Enostosis

Description

Enostoses, or bone islands, are hamartomas[26,102,103,104,105] less than 2 cm in diameter composed of intramedullary cortical bone.[26,104,106,107] They are histologically identical to normal lamellar bone, possess a complete haversian system,[102,104,105,108] and have an irregular or spiculated margin where they blend with surrounding cancellous bone.[102,104,105]

Diagnosis

Enostoses are generally discovered as incidental findings on imaging studies[102,104,105] and are asymptomatic in nearly 100% of cases.[105,107] Radiographically, they are identical to cortical bone and have a "cumulus cloud"[104] appearance. On CT, they are round osteoblastic lesions within normal cancellous bone characterized by an irregular or spiculated border.[102,103,104,105,106] They are hypointense on both T1- and T2-weighted MRI[26,102,103,105] and are distinguished from metastases on bone scintigraphy, as they do not show elevated levels of tracer uptake.[102,103,105,107,108]

Treatment and Prognosis

The majority of enostoses remain constant in size[103,104,105] and so do not require treatment. However, the 31.9% that do change in size can become symptomatic.[103,104,105,106,107,109] Accordingly, patients with neurological symptoms and a history of enostosis may require removal of the lesion.

19.5.5 Eosinophilic Granuloma

Description

Eosinophilic granuloma (EG) is the most benign[22,62,110] and most common[22,110,111] type of Langerhans' cell histiocytosis. It arises from the clonal expansion of Langerhans' histiocytes[62,111,112,113,114,115]—antigen-presenting cells found predominately in the skin[62,110,115]—and typically presents as a solitary bone lesion[110,111] in the vertebral body.[116,117] EG is histologically characterized by abundant Langerhans cells[69,118] with variable numbers of eosinophils, multinucleated giant cells, lymphocytes, and other leukocytes.[113,118,119]

Diagnosis

EG often shows an insidious onset with progressive osteolytic destruction leading to vertebrae plana in children and asymmetrical vertebral collapse in adults.[22,116,118] Patients commonly complain of local pain and spine stiffness, and less commonly present with spinal deformity, gait ataxia,[110,120] or other neurological impairment.[62,69,110,112,116,118,120,121,122,123,124] Said impairment may result from direct invasion of the tumor into the spinal canal or from vertebral collapse,[110,120] an event most commonly seen with thoracic and lumbar lesions.[125]

In up to 84% of thoracic lesions, EG presents as a vertebra plana with intact endplates and discs on CT or MRI.[26,62,119,122,123,125,126,127,128] Intact vertebrae contain intramedullary lytic lesions on CT, with irregular margins[69,116,124] that appear hyperintense on T2- and hypointense on T1-weighted MR.[26,62,116,121,122,125,126] Though vertebrae plana are highly characteristic of EG, they are

not pathognomic. Biopsy allows for definitive diagnosis in 70 to 100% of cases though,[22,112,113,120,124] as EG show Birbeck granules and strong CD1a staining.[62,113,115,120,121,123,129]

Treatment

General practice involves lesion biopsy and conservative management with nonsteroidal anti-inflammatory drugs (NSAIDs) and bracing,[62,69,113,116,120,121,123,127] as many pediatric cases resolve spontaneously.[124,126,127] Those patients with pain refractory to NSAIDs may get relief with methylprednisolone injection,[112,124] but for cases characterized by cord compression, deformity, or severe neurological dysfunction, surgery is preferred.[22,26,62,69,110,113,123,126] The goal of this surgery is to relieve neurological symptoms and address spinal instability, not to achieve gross total resection.[117] This is most easily accomplished via a posterior approach in thoracic regions[22,121,123] and may involve resection of the affected vertebra.[120,121]

Prognosis

Patients generally have excellent outcomes,[62,110,119,124,125] as recurrence occurs in less than 20% of solitary pediatric[112,124] and adult EG.[130] Survival rate at both five years[121,126,129] and 10 years for monostotic disease is 100%,[121] and the 5-year survival for polyostotic disease is similar.[121]

19.5.6 Giant Cell Tumor (Formerly Osteoclastoma)

Description

GCTs are highly vascularized,[5,131] expansile, osteolytic tumors[5,6,26,74] capable of producing spinal column instability[131]. They are considered to be the most aggressive benign primary spine tumor[132] and are thought to arise from osteoclasts.[74,133] Histologically, they are characterized by multinucleate giant cells with abundant eosinophilic cytoplasm, monocytes, and spindle-shaped stromal cells in a collagen-rich matrix.[3,5,14,26,62,74,134,135,136] GCTs most frequently involve the vertebral body, but may also involve the posterior elements.[5,137,138,139]

Diagnosis

Patients generally present with focal back pain that overlies the lesion persisting for 6 to 12 months.[5,14,21,69,136,137,138,139,140,141] Neurological deficits, radicular pain, and pathologic fracture are also seen in highly aggressive lesions.[5,14,136,137,139,140,142]

Radiographically, GCTs have a "moth-eaten" or "soap bubble" appearance in a blown-out vertebral body.[5,6,7,132,134,138,141] CT demonstrates a contrast-enhancing, expansive, osteolytic lesion commonly compromising the vertebral cortex.[143] MR shows a contrast-enhancing lesion with similar features, commonly accompanied by invasion of paraspinal tissue.[143] Because these features are common to many other pathologies,[6,14,132,136,141,144] definitive diagnosis requires biopsy.[6,131,132,138,145]

Treatment

As most spinal GCTs are Enneking grade II or III,[140,141,146,147] the treatment of choice is gross total resection via a wide en bloc technique. This is associated with the lowest rate of recurrence and the highest rate of long-term cure.[3,6,13,21,69,72,131,134,135,137,141,142,145,148,149,150] In cases where the tumor abuts neural elements[5,13,132,147,150] and en bloc resection is not be possible, piecemeal gross total resection may be employed.[5,69,134,140,141,145,146,150] In such cases, complete resection is essential, as it drastically reduces the rate of recurrence.[21,148,149]

Preoperative arterial embolization is highly recommended in the treatment of this highly vascular lesion,[3,5,72,74,131,132,141] as it improves visualization during resection and reduces intraoperative morbidity.[3,72,74,84,131,132,141] Despite this effectiveness as a neoadjuvant therapy, selective arterial embolization is not currently recommended as a monotherapy.[72]

The literature in support of other adjuvant therapies is insufficient to recommend their use.[6,21,134,137,140,141,146,147,149] Specifically, radiotherapy is contraindicated due to its association with iatrogenic osteosarcoma[5,14,132,134,137,139,140,146,149,150,151] and an eightfold increase in the odds of instrumentation failure.[13] The use of denosumab is similarly questionable, though several recent studies suggest that it improves the rate of surgical success[152] by preoperatively ossifying[74,135,152] or shrinking the tumor.[69,153] Lastly, the use of bisphosphonates is not supported, though some suggest they may help to prevent recurrence.[21,148]

Prognosis

GCT prognosis has improved significantly over the past two decades.[148,149] Recurrence occurs in 46 to 80% of cases treated with subtotal resection[3,6,69,133,134,141,147,149] and 25 to 50%[74,142,146,148,149] of cases treated with piecemeal gross total resection. Local control afforded by en bloc resection is superior to these two methods and approaches 100% in some series.[3,131,134,148,149] Recurrences for all interventions occur at a mean of 19 to 21 months, with 63 to 96% occurring within the first 2 years of follow-up.[14,21,134,137,142,148,149] Predictors of improved recurrence-free survival are en bloc resection, univertebral involvement, lower Enneking grade, and younger age.[21,149] Most patients show improvement of pain[74,137,146] and neurological symptoms[74,150] following surgical treatment.

19.5.7 Osteoid Osteoma

Description

Osteoid osteomas (OOs) arise from cancellous bone[3,154] and are characterized by a small, osteolytic nidus, circumscribed by a thick sclerosis of reactive bone.[26,62,154,155,156] Histologically, the nidus is highly vascularized[157] and contains osteoblasts, osteoid, and woven bone.[154,157] Nidal size traditionally distinguishes OOs (< 2 cm) from OB (> 2 cm).[3,26,69,155,157,158,159] OOs are most commonly found in the pedicles and lamina,[160,161,162] and localize to the posterior elements in 70 to 100% of cases.[26,69,155,156,159,160,163,164,165,166,167,168,169,170,171]

Diagnosis

Painful scoliosis is a near-pathognomic finding and may occur in up to 70% of cases.[154,155,156,157,160,162,164,168,172,173,174] It is most common in thoracic lesions and lesions localized to the lateral aspect of the vertebra.[174,175] It is thought to result when nidus-produced PGE_2[157,160,171,176] causes inflammation and contrac-

tion of paraspinal muscles, which flexes the spine away from the lesion.[154,155,173,174] This theory is supported by the fact that tumors usually localize to the concave aspect of the scoliotic apex[154,155,168,174] and rarely produce scoliosis when localized to the spinous process.[155] OO also classically produces focal pain that worsens at night, improves with NSAID use,[26,62,69,154,157,159,161,162,163,164,167,168,169,170,173,177] and has been present for 11 to 22 months at presentation.[62,154,166,168,170,174,177,178] It infrequently produces neurological dysfunction or radicular pain.[69,157,171]

On plain radiograph, the lesion is round and radiolucent with surrounding sclerosis[3,26,69,154,155,157,162,172] and intranidal calcification.[26,69] Small lesions may be difficult to detect on radiograph,[26,162,172,173] but are easily visualized on Tc^{99} bone scans.[62,156,160,162,179] MR also helps to visualize tumors, which are contrast-enhancing,[26,154] low-to-intermediate signal on T1, and high signal on T2.[26,69,164,170] They may also be surrounded by edema[26,154,157,166] resulting from nidal COX2 activity.[157]

Treatment

OO is a self-limiting tumor that occasionally regresses over time.[69,157,163,164,172] As such, NSAIDs are first-line therapy in most cases.[3,62,154,156,157,160,171,177] Failure of conservative therapy, development of neurological dysfunction, or onset of spinal instability recommend the patient for surgical intervention.[62,69,154,157,170,171,177] The goal of surgery is gross total resection,[3,154,157,169,179] though many groups achieve good results with only resection of the nidus.[154,160,162,173,176] En bloc resection is not required and curettage is the standard of care at many centers.[69,162,163,164,171,173,176] Though painful scoliosis resolves in 70 to 90% of cases following nidus resection[154,168,171] reconstruction is necessary in patients where the scoliosis has become structural.[69,160]

For medically refractory patients presenting with pain alone, laser or radiofrequency ablation may serve as cost-effective alternatives[172] offering quicker recovery, lower complication rates, and lower morbidity.[72,159,161,177] Their use is contraindicated in OOs directly contacting the neural elements though,[72,156,164,172] as a layer of cortical bone is necessary to act as an insulator and prevent thermal damaging to the cord or nerve roots.[160,164,169,172] This risk has led many interventional radiologists to avoid radiofrequency ablation (RFA) in all cases of spinal OO.[26,156,157,161,164,172,173,176]

Prognosis

Most patients experience good outcomes, with a 4.5 to 10% rate of recurrence in OO treated with intralesional resection and ≈ 0% rate of recurrence in those treated with wide-margin en bloc resection.[69,154,161,162,178] The higher level of recurrence in intralesional cases is thought to result from failure to completely resect the tumor nidus.[162] Symptomatic relief is also high, with greater than 90% of surgically treated patients achieving complete pain relief[154,171] and 70 to 90% of scoliotic patients showing improvement without reconstruction.[154,168,171]

19.5.8 Osteoblastoma

Description

Previously called giant OO, osteoblastoma is a potentially aggressive osteolytic tumor[5,26,62,157,180] that is grossly friable, blood-filled, and well circumscribed.[69,158,181] It most frequently affects the posterior column[5,26,138,155,158,167,168,181,182,183,184] and is histologically characterized by extensive vascularization, osteoid production, and immature woven bone.[181,183,184,185] Unlike OO, it contains large vascular spaces, giant cells,[154] and a nidus greater than 2 cm in diameter.[3,5,26,154,155,158,161]

Diagnosis

Like OO, OB commonly produces local back pain[26,154,157,158,178, 185,186] that has been present for 12 to 20 months,[62,154,158,166,168, 170,174,178,182,183,187] although fewer OB patients get relief with NSAIDs.[155,157,168,170,178,182,186] Neurological dysfunction is more common than in OO due to the larger lesion size,[154,166,170,187] but painful scoliosis is less common.[157,158,168,174]

Radiographic characteristics of lesions are similar to those of OO.[154,155,157] On CT, it has a ground-glass appearance due to multifocal mineralization within the lesion nidus.[26,69,158,182,186] And on MR, it is hypointense on T1- and hyperintense on T2-weighted images,[158,186] and may demonstrate soft tissue involvement.[5,26,157,182,185,186]

Treatment

Treatment begins with NSAID-mediated medical management of pain.[157] Those patients with neurological dysfunction or instability are treated surgically though,[170,183] as are patients who have failed conservative management.[157,161,183,188] Gross total resection of the tumor nidus is considered front-line treatment[3,161,183,188] and current recommendations suggest that this be achieved via wide en bloc excision in high-grade tumors,[3,5, 158,178,183,188,189] though lower-grade lesions can be treated with intralesional gross total resection.[5,158,182,183,185,189] As with OO, current evidence does not support adjuvant radiotherapy for local control,[5,69,185,189] and surgery is first line for treatment of recurrences[5,157,183].

Prognosis

Local control is nearly 100% in cases treated with en bloc resection,[5,185,188] but only 85 to 90% in cases treated with subtotal resection.[69,154,170,180,182,185,189] Aggressive-type lesions,[158,186,188,189] higher Enneking grade lesions, larger lesions, and cases with less extensive resection[5,166,187,188] have all been associated with higher rates of recurrence.[183,188] Both intralesional and en bloc resection create significant relief of pain in more than 90% of patients.[154,157,158,161,166,176,186,187]

19.5.9 Osteochondroma

Description

Osteochondromas, also called osteocartilaginous exostoses, are the most common type of benign bone lesion.[190,191,192,193,194] Though commonly treated as a tumor, they are actually hamartomas,[13,190,193,194,195] as they form when growth plate cartilage fragments escape the physeal plate[3,69,190,195,196,197] and produce a subperiosteal, cartilage-capped bony excrescence. This lesion then grows through endochondral ossification and creates symptoms by compressing neural elements.[192,194,195,196,197,198,199,200,201,202] Exostoses can occur secondary to radiotherapy or a genetic

condition,[3,197] and are commonly thought to cease growth at the time of epiphyseal plate closure.[62,190,192,194,200,203,204]

Histologically, exostoses are characterized by a bony stalk with a core of pathologically normal bone and cap of hyaline cartilage.[193,195,198,200,204] The cartilaginous cap resembles the physeal plate in structure[195] and is the point at which the lesion grows.[192,197,200] The majority of lesions are slow growing[69] and are found in the posterior column.[13,69,190,194,196,197,198,203,205]

Diagnosis

The vast majority (99%) of spinal lesions are asymptomatic, as they grow away from the spinal canal.[13,190,195,197,199,200,201,206,207] Symptomatic patients most commonly present with pain of gradual onset that has been present for years,[194,197,208,209] but may also present with radiculopathy or myelopathy.[3,13,192,194,197,207] Neurological symptoms are most commonly associated with thoracic lesions, which may present with neurological symptoms in as much as 85% of cases.[190] Lesions that lie in the posterior column may also present as a palpable mass.[3,190,194,195]

Radiographically, lesions present as a sessile mass iso-radio-lucent to and contiguous with the underlying vertebra.[3,13,192, 195,198,199,210] These features are considered pathognomic for exostosis,[195,200] but may be difficult to identify on plain radiograph due to the complex spinal anatomy.[3,26,69,194,195,197,200,203,208] CT is therefore the modality of choice as it allows visualization of these pathognomic radiological features.[3,13,26,190,194,195,197,198, 200,203,208] It can be complemented by MRI, which demonstrates a cartilaginous cap that is hypointense on T1 and hyperintense on T2.[26,69,195,201] MRI also differentiates osteochondroma from chondrosarcoma, which is characterized by a cap thicker than 1.5 cm in adults and 3 cm in children.[13,26,195,197,198,201,203]

Treatment

Asymptomatic exostoses are treated with observation, whereas symptomatic lesions are treated with gross total resection.[3,26, 69,192,193,197,198,205,206] Given the lesion's benign nature, piecemeal resection of the cartilaginous cap is associated with extremely high rates of local control[13,190,192,196,198] and is curative in the majority of cases.[69] Rapid progression of symptoms suggests malignant transformation[13,197] and said tumors should be treated en bloc.[3,190]

Prognosis

Osteochondromas generally have a favorable prognosis, with 85% or more of patients showing symptomatic improvement[190, 197,199,203,204,207,209] and 96 to 98% showing long-term local control.[13,193,195,203] Gross resection improves local control slightly,[190,194,197] but the difference is negligible if the cartilaginous cap is completely excised. Recurrences usually occur more than 2 years after surgery[190,197] and are rarely associated with transformation to chondrosarcoma.[197]

19.6 Malignant Tumors

Malignant tumors of the spine occur at a rate of 1 to 2 per 100,000 person-years[211] and account for less than 0.2% of all cancers.[212,213] The majority have relatively poor prognoses, though outcomes have begun to improve with the increased use of Enneking-appropriate en bloc resection.[214] Definitive diagnosis requires biopsy,[215,216,217,218] which is generally done transpedicularly to reduce recurrence.

19.6.1 Chordoma

Description

Chordoma is one of the most common primary malignancies of the spine.[3,4,19,143,212] Frequently, low grade and slow-growing,[19,215,219,220] it arises from notochordal remnants[3,26,69,143,212,217,220] and is locally aggressive, osteolytic, and often large at diagnosis.[3,16,19,26,143,217,218,220] Histologically, chordoma is characterized by cords or sheets of spindle-shaped physaliphorous cells containing hyperchromatic nuclei, mildly eosinophilic cytoplasm, and abundant mucin-filled vacuoles.[3,26,143,217,221] These cells may have indistinct borders and are surrounded by abundant myxoid matrix.[143,221] More aggressive lesions are hyperplastic,[221] possess abundant mitotic figures,[218] and demonstrate central necrosis.[143] Positive staining for the transcription factor Brachyury distinguishes chordoma from chondrosarcoma and other cartilaginous lesions.[16,143,216,218] Metastasis occurs in 5 to 30% of cases,[19,143,218,222,223,224,225] most commonly to the lungs or skeleton.[217,218]

Diagnosis

Patients present with nonspecific symptoms that have been present for months or years.[16,216,218] Pain is the most common complaint, and may be accompanied by paresthesias, weakness, or incontinence.[3,16,218,220,226] On radiograph and CT, chordomas are midline, osteolytic lesions of the vertebral body[217,218,220] with multiple septa, irregular shape, and amorphous intralesional calcification.[3,26,69,143,218,221] Chordomas generally remain extradural,[217,218] but may invade epidural space[219] and adjacent disc space.[218] MRI is the modality of choice as it allows for good delineation of soft tissue components[69,219] and identification of spinal metastases.[217,226] The appearance on MRI is similar to that of the nucleus pulposus, in that it is hyperintense on T2 MRI, hypointense on T1,[3,26,143,218] and shows moderate contrast enhancement.[217]

Treatment

Treatment of chordoma should involve a multidisciplinary team[217,226] and revolves around wide en bloc resection of the tumor.[3,16,19,69,215,217,218,219,223,225,226,227,228,229] Though associated with increased complication rates,[19,219,224] en bloc resection significantly improves overall survival and local control.[215] When en bloc resection is not possible or not accepted by the patient,[217,224] every effort should be made to achieve negative margins through piecemeal resection.[217,219,220,226,229]

Chordomas are resistant to chemotherapy and radiotherapy,[4,16,19,215,223,224,225,226,227,230] but adjuvant radiotherapy greater than 60 Gy[218,227,231] may be useful in cases where only positive or marginal margins are achieved.[217,218,227,229,232] The major disadvantage of such high-dose RT is that it can damage the spinal cord.[218,227] Recent advances in hypofractionated stereotactic radiosurgery and charged particle RT[227,229,232] have reduced this risk, as they allow higher doses of radiation to be delivered to

the tumor while maintaining extralesional doses below the safety limit of 50 Gy.[218,227] These newer radiosurgery techniques are not supported as monotherapy, except in cases of inoperable lesions, where they are the standard of care.[217,219,224,229,231,233,234,235] Unlike radiotherapy, chemotherapy is not currently supported as an adjuvant.[217,218]

Prognosis

Recurrence is incredibly common,[16,19,26,215,217,218,220,222,223,226] occurring in more than 50% of patients treated with gross total resection.[217,226] En bloc resection provides significantly better local control,[19,23,49,219,223] as high as 83 to 95% in some series.[223] The current median overall survival for isolated, surgically treated chordoma is 84 to 104 months,[16,19,23,212,213,215,220,228,229] with 5-year, 10-year, and 20-year overall survivals of 50 to 97%, 33 to 84%,[3,16,19,23,69,212,213,215,217,219,220,223,226,228,229,231,235] and 13.1%,[23,215,228] respectively. In the few series examining mobile spine lesions, local recurrence-free survival is reported to be 55 to 67.6%,[19,23,223,226] with recurrence in 25 to 48% of cases, median time to recurrence of 37 to 64 months,[19,215,219,232] and median recurrence-free survival of 37 months.[19] Positive predictors of overall survival are younger age,[226,228] smaller tumor burden,[215,225,226] use of en bloc resection,[16,19,215,219,223,225,226,229,232,235] index versus revision surgery,[16,219,220,223,225,229,235] isolated lesion,[19,212] and adjuvant radiotherapy.[3,224,227] En bloc resection with negative margins is the greatest determinant of long-term outcome though.[217,223]

19.6.2 Chondrosarcoma

Description

Chondrosarcomas are slow-growing,[21,42] low-grade[44,143,236] connective tissue sarcomas that constitute the second most common primary tumor of vertebrae.[3,4,26] They can occur as either a primary tumor or as a malignant transformation of an osteochondroma,[26,216] and are broken into four main types based on histology: conventional (classical), dedifferentiated, mesenchymal, and clear cell chondrosarcomas.[45] Conventional chondrosarcomas account for 80 to 90% of all cases and appear grossly as lobulated lesions that destroy surrounding bone.[45,71,211,237] They share radiographic features with chondromas,[45] but are distinguished by greater invasion of surrounding bone and more abundant mucoid matrix.[237] Microscopically, they are hyperplastic with pleomorphic nuclei and a matrix possessing a mixture of myxoid and hyaline features.[237] Degeneration of these conventional chondrosarcomas produces dedifferentiated chondrosarcomas, which account for 10% of all lesions.[71,238] They have the poorest prognosis, with a 5-year survival rate less than 10%,[45] and are histologically characterized by a central cartilaginous component surrounded by a peripheral sarcomatous component.[239] Mesenchymal chondrosarcomas are the next most common, accounting for 3 to 10% of all chondrosarcomas, and possess a mixture of low-grade chondrocytes and undifferentiated spindle-shaped neoplastic cells.[45,71] Clear cell chondrosarcomas account for the remaining 2% of cases.[71] They are hyperplastic, with cells featuring round, centrally placed nuclei and abundant, clear cytoplasm[45,71,238] in a matrix lacking cartilaginous features.[238]

Diagnosis

Symptoms show insidious onset and include nonfocal pain, which persists for months prior to presentation,[42,43,71,216,236,240,241] a palpable mass,[71,236,241] or neurological impairment.[43,45,240] Up to 50% of patients present with a neurological deficit.[45,236]

Radiographically, chondrosarcoma is an expansive, osteolytic lesion involving the vertebral body with or without posterior column involvement.[3,26,143,238] Low-grade tumors are circumscribed by reactive cortical bone,[143,240] but high-grade tumors usually breach the cortex.[28,236] The chondroid matrix of the tumor usually demonstrates mineralization in a "ring-and-arc" pattern on radiograph and CT.[26,45,71,242] Lesions are also generally lateralized within the vertebrae, distinguishing them from the centrally placed chordoma. On MRI, chondrosarcomas appear heterogeneously hypointense on T1, hyperintense on T2,[43,47,71] and demonstrate "rings-and-arcs" enhancement with gadolinium contrast.[26,143,238,243] MRI also allows delineation of soft tissue invasion,[3,71,143,216,238,240] and differentiation from osteochondroma.

Treatment

At present, surgery is the standard of care in treating chondrosarcoma,[212,240,242] as it is the only therapy with documented efficacy.[42,43,211,216] Resection should be executed en bloc with negative margins (▶ Fig. 19.3, ▶ Fig. 19.4), as this significantly reduces the rate of recurrence.[3,26,28,43,44,45,195,216,236,238,240,244]

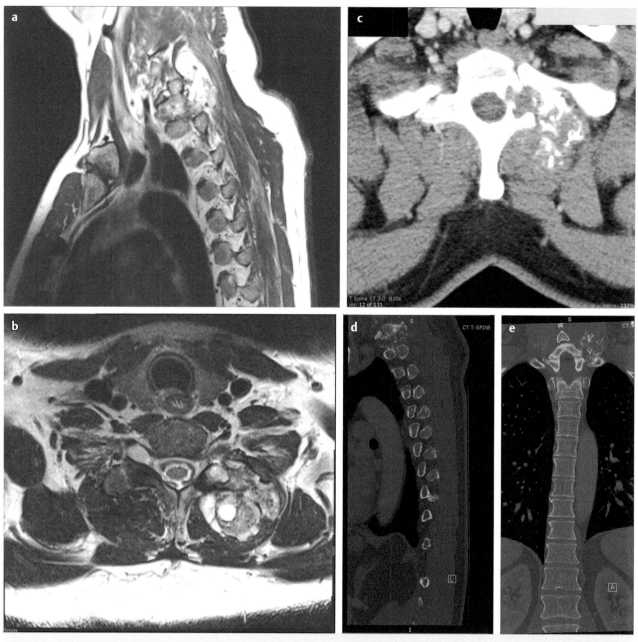

Fig. 19.3 Presentation of patient with 7-year history of left-sided neck pain and several months' history of left-sided Horner's syndrome. Patient had previously been diagnosed with benign lesion localized to left side of T1 body. Reevaluation on MRI **(a,b)** and CT **(c–e)** revealed a chondrosarcoma localized to the left side of T1 and C7 vertebrae.

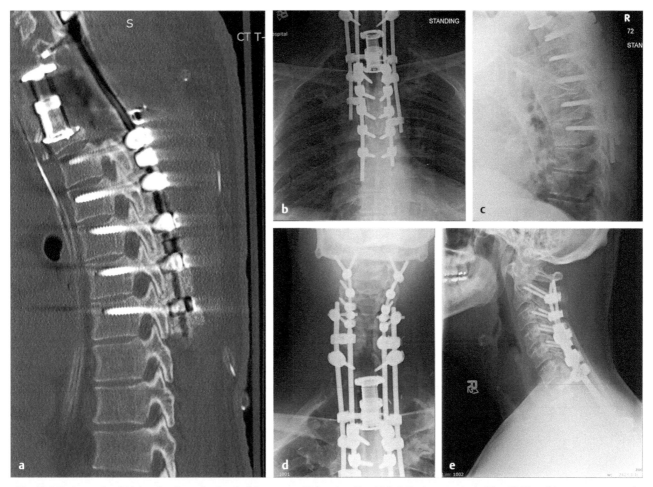

Fig. 19.4 Postoperative CT **(a)** and radiographs **(b–e)** of the same patient as in ▶ Fig. 19.3. Patient was treated with a C7–T1 en bloc corpectomy and C2–T7 fusion to address subsequent instability. Patient is free of recurrence 3 years out with full neurological function.

Piecemeal gross total resection is employed where en bloc excision is infeasible,[43,45,242] but virtually assures recurrence of the lesion.[43,45,240]

Chondrosarcomas are highly resistant to chemotherapy and traditional radiotherapy[4,15,28,42,44,45,211,216,240,241,242] though both treatments are currently used as adjuvants in cases of subtotal resection.[42,245,246] More recent studies have suggested that stereotactic radiosurgery may help to reduce recurrence when used as an adjuvant in cases of subtotal resection,[28,43,44,45,240,242,246,247] but its use as monotherapy is only indicated for inoperable lesions.[45]

Prognosis

The prognosis of chondrosarcoma is good relative to other spinal sarcomas, with overall 5- and 10-year survivals of 55 to 71% and 29 to 68%, and a median survival of 72 to 198 months in surgically treated cases.[23,42,48,212,213,228,241,246] Overall survival is highly dependent on surgical resection, with 10-year survivals of 85% for patients treated with negative margin en bloc resection, 60% for piecemeal gross total resection, and 0% for subtotal resection.[21] Recurrence in en bloc–treated patients is ≤ 25%,[21,42,43,44,45,195,240] but approaches 100% in patients treated with subtotal resection.[17,43,45,236,240,242] Negative predictors of patient

survival include tumor recurrence,[15,17,21,42,43,44,45] use of subtotal resection versus en bloc resection,[15,21,42,44,236,241,242] high tumor expression of Aurora A kinase,[248] low tumor expression of RUNX,[43] and metastases.[212,222] Of all of these factors, local recurrence is the single strongest predictor of survival.[15,17,21,42,43,44,45]

19.6.3 Ewing's Sarcoma

Description

Ewing's sarcoma (ES) is the second most common primary malignant bone tumor after osteosarcoma and is the second most common malignant primary spinal column tumor in persons under 20.[3,26,50,51,52,53,212,249,250,251] It arises from mesenchymal stem cells of bone or soft tissues and is poorly differentiated on histology.[3,51,216] Additionally, it is microscopically characterized by uniform, small, round blue cells with round nuclei and a high nucleus-to-cytoplasm ratio.[3,26,50,51,52,249,250,251,252,253,254] Cell borders are often indistinct[143] and 90% of tumors are characterized by an EWS/FLI1 translocation (t [11;22][q24;12]).[143,249,250,251,253,255,256] The majority of spinal ESs are localized to the posterior column,[69] though the anterior column is also frequently affected.[250] Metastases are common, with 25 to 35% of patients[51,69,249,251,252,255,257] having metastases at presentation, most commonly in the lungs or skeleton.[51,256,258]

Diagnosis

The majority of patients present with localized or radicular pain and 50 to 94% of patients will also present with neurological deficit.[3,26,51,69,143,250,252,255,257,259] In children these symptoms may be accompanied by weight loss, fever, and elevated serum inflammatory markers.[51,69,252]

Vertebral ES is indistinct on plain radiography, presenting as nondescript, lytic, permeative lesions.[69,254,260] It appears as an osteolytic mass on CT,[69,254,260] and on MRI it has an intermediate T1 signal,[253] an intermediate-to-high signal on T2,[26,69,143] and enhances with contrast.[143,253] MRI also shows extensive osteolysis and soft tissue invasion.[26,53]

Treatment

ES is highly sensitive to radiotherapy and chemotherapy[3,26,51,69,211,255] and so the current standard of care combines these adjuvants with wide-margin en bloc spondylectomy.[50,69,216,249,251,256] Treatment begins with four to six cycles of neoadjuvant vincristine, ifosfamide or cyclophosphamide, doxorubicin, and actinomycin D.[53,216,251,252,258,259,261,262,263] This regimen is designed to shrink the tumor[52,53] and improve the chances of achieving wide margins during resection.[53] Enneking-appropriate resection is then followed with adjuvant chemotherapy and radiotherapy to reduce recurrence.[251,252,255,264] Tumor debulking is only indicated in cases where en bloc resection is not possible, as en bloc improves the chances of long-term survival.[69,251]

Adjuvant radiotherapy has been previously shown to prolong survival[216,252,264] and reduce local recurrence in ES patients.[52,252,262] It is not currently suggested as monotherapy, though it may be used with chemotherapy alone in the case of high-grade, inoperable tumors.[52,69,253,264]

Prognosis

Most series report a 52 to 74% 5-year overall survival for spinal ES treated with modern multimodal therapy,[3,51,53,69,213,249,250,254,256,257,258,259,261,264] though this may be as high as 83.3% in cases treated with en bloc resection achieving negative margins.[51] Ten-year survival is only 34 to 47%, as median overall survival of isolated spinal lesions is 90 to 98 months.[69,212,222] Both numbers lag behind survival in nonaxial cases.[51,52,251,252,254,256,258,261] Younger age,[249,256,258] smaller tumor size,[249,258,259,265] positive response to chemotherapy,[52,249,258] absence of metastases,[52,222,249,256,258,259,262,264] long-term local control,[258,264] and en bloc resection[50,51,251,252,257] have all been associated with improved survival.[69] Recurrence occurs in 12 to 40% of cases,[50,53,250,251,255,262] though local control is better in cases with en bloc resection[51,256,257,258] and neoadjuvant chemotherapy.[52,251]

19.6.4 Osteosarcoma (Formerly Osteogenic Sarcoma)

Description

Osteochondroma is a predominately high-grade,[2,18,266] osteoid-producing tumor[267,268,269] of mesenchymal origin,[267] and is the most common malignant primary bone tumor.[52,69,211,249,267,269,270,271] It can occur as either a primary lesion, or as a sequela of Paget's disease,[1,3,26,143,236,271,272] and affects the vertebral body in more than 90% of spine cases.[69]

Osteogenic sarcomas (OGSs) are a histologically diverse group of tumors including conventional, telangiectatic, small cell, secondary, parosteal, periosteal, and high-grade and low-grade surface types of lesions.[1,211] Conventional-type OGS is by far the most common, accounting for 75 to 90% of all cases.[211,273] It is composed of highly pleomorphic tumor cells embedded in abundant collagen I–filled osteoid matrix[211,267] that is classified as osteoblastic, chondroblastic, or fibroblastic based on its properties and abundance.[267] Osteoblastic lesions are the most common subtype,[266,273] comprising 52 to 92% of OGS in some series.[236,273,274]

One feature common to nearly all osteosarcomas is the downregulation of miR-183 mRNA.[269] This leads to ezrin upregulation[275] and is integral to tumor metastasis and local invasion, as miR-183 knockdown prevents migration and local invasion in vitro.[275] miR-183 downregulation is clinically associated with higher tumor grade, poorer response to chemotherapy, local recurrence,[275] and propensity to metastasize.[275,276]

Diagnosis

Focal pain is the most common clinical finding, occurring in up to 90% of patients.[1,3,26,69,143,267,268,277,278] Neurological deficits are also common, appearing in 40 to 80% of patients,[1,2,3,69,277] as OGS has been reported to invade the spinal canal in more than 80% of patients.[26,69]

Because of the diverse histology of OGS, radiological findings vary.[166,187,266,277,279] The most common finding is an aggressive, permeative lesion that appears smooth and osteoblastic on radiograph[1,3,26,69,143,211] and may appear as an ivory body.[1,273] CT demonstrates similar findings, and is also useful in demonstrating metastases,[211] which occur in 26.7 to 32% of cases,[280,281] most commonly targeting the lungs[277,278,281] and other bones.[271,280,281] MRI is useful for demonstrating soft tissue invasion and neural element compression,[26,211,268] however, it has low utility for diagnosis, as the MRI features of OGS are nonspecific.[1,143]

Treatment

The current standard of care includes en bloc resection of the tumor with wide margins, adjuvant radiotherapy, and chemotherapy.[1,18,47,52,69,211,216,249,274,277,278] En bloc resection of thoracic tumors is most frequently accomplished via a posterior or combined approach[1,2,18] and its chance of success may be improved by preoperatively shrinking the tumor with neoadjuvant radiotherapy[1] or chemotherapy.[277] Both postoperative chemotherapy (methotrexate, cisplatin, doxorubicin, and ifosfamide)[1,211] and radiotherapy improve survival when used as adjuvants,[187,216,249] but neither should be used without surgery in the case of an operable lesion.[1,18]

Prognosis

The prognosis for osteosarcoma is quite poor[249] due to the predilection of this tumor for early and widespread metastases.[3,69]

Median overall survival is reported as 18 to 44 months for surgically treated lesions,[20,69,187,212,222,271] with 5- and 10-year overall survivals of 18 to 60%[20,212,213,222,271,277,278] and 8 to 14% for isolated spinal lesions.[212,249] However, median overall survival may be as high as 77 to 81 months for tumors treated with en bloc resection with negative margins.[18,20] Overall survival is improved by smaller tumor burden,[187,249] lower tumor grade, younger age at treatment,[249,270,277,278,281] isolated versus metastatic disease,[69,187,211,222,266,278,281] continued local control,[20,278,280] en bloc resection with negative margins,[18,187,213,249,266,274] use of adjuvant radiotherapy,[213,216,249] and good response to chemotherapy.[211,266,280,281] Local recurrence is reported in 44 to 60% of cases treated with piecemeal resection,[1,18,187,277] but only 11 to 20% of cases treated en bloc.[1,18]

19.6.5 Plasmacytomas and Multiple Myelomas

Description

Plasmacytoma—previously known as solitary myeloma[282]—and multiple myeloma are bone marrow tumors[3] that arise from abnormal proliferation of plasma cells.[3,143,283] These tumor cells release large amounts of interleukin-6 (IL-6), which causes vertebral osteolysis[3,143,283] and secondary osteoporosis.[143,283] Plasmacytoma and multiple myeloma most commonly localize to the vertebral body[143] and are histologically characterized by sheets of plasma cells.[143] These plasma cells may vary from well-differentiated cells to poorly differentiated centroblasts,[284] and are immunohistochemically characterized by Il-1β, CD56, and FGF2 expression.[283]

Diagnosis

The most common symptoms of spinal plasmacytoma are mechanical back pain (up to 100% of cases),[283,284,285,286,287] vertebral fracture (10–50% of cases),[285,286] and neurological deficits (10–24% of cases).[3,143,284,286,287,288,289] Plasmacytomas are osteolytic on radiograph[282,283,284] due to activation of osteoclasts surrounding the lesion.[3,143] CT has much higher sensitivity and shows plasmacytomas as "punched-out" lesions in the vertebra[143,284] that may be accompanied by vertebral body collapse.[284,285] Diagnosis is further aided by elevated M protein (serum) or Bence Jones protein (urine)—markers that are relatively unique to plasmacytoma and multiple myeloma.[282,283,284,285,287,290]

Treatment

All patients with tumor progression should be referred to radiation oncology for treatment[283] as plasmacytoma is highly radiation sensitive.[285,291] Radiotherapy (≥45 Gy) is the current standard of care for solitary plasmacytoma,[3,283,284,289,290,291] but may be accompanied by chemotherapy to prevent progression to multiple myeloma.[283,289,291,292] In cases of rapidly progressing neurological dysfunction or deformity secondary to vertebral collapse, patients should be offered surgery to resect the lesion and address any deformity or instability.[282,283,284,285,286,287,288,289] Unlike other sarcomas, the goal of surgery is symptom relief,[284,285] not curative resection.

Prognosis

Prognosis of plasmacytoma is quite good,[272] with a 5-year overall survival of 70 to 74%,[284,291] 10-year overall survival of 52 to 68.5%,[282,291] and median survival of 7.5 to 12 years.[283,290] The prognosis of multiple myeloma is slightly worse than this due to the systemic nature of the disease.[282,286,292] Predictors of better overall survival are decreases in serum and urine myeloma protein levels,[282,283,290,291] and treatment with chemotherapy.[287,288,289]

References

[1] Katonis P, Datsis G, Karantanas A, et al. Spinal osteosarcoma. Clin Med Insights Oncol. 2013; 7:199–208

[2] Feng D, Yang X, Liu T, et al. Osteosarcoma of the spine: surgical treatment and outcomes. World J Surg Oncol. 2013; 11(1):89

[3] Winn HR. Youmans Neurological Surgery. Vol. 3. 6th ed. Philadelphia, PA: Saunders; 2011:2979–2999, 3045–3068, 3131–3165

[4] Fisher CG, Saravanja DD, Dvorak MF, et al. Surgical management of primary bone tumors of the spine: validation of an approach to enhance cure and reduce local recurrence. Spine. 2011; 36(10):830–836

[5] Harrop JS, Schmidt MH, Boriani S, Shaffrey CI. Aggressive "benign" primary spine neoplasms: osteoblastoma, aneurysmal bone cyst, and giant cell tumor. Spine. 2009; 34(22) Suppl:S39–S47

[6] Di Lorenzo N, Spallone A, Nolletti A, Nardi P. Giant cell tumors of the spine: a clinical study of six cases, with emphasis on the radiological features, treatment, and follow-up. Neurosurgery. 1980; 6(1):29–34

[7] Enneking WF, Spanier SS, Goodman MA. A system for the surgical staging of musculoskeletal sarcoma. Clin Orthop Relat Res. 1980; 153(153):106–120

[8] Enneking WF. A system of staging musculoskeletal neoplasms. Clin Orthop Relat Res. 1986(204):9–24

[9] Boriani S, Weinstein JN, Biagini R. Primary bone tumors of the spine. Terminology and surgical staging. Spine. 1997; 22(9):1036–1044

[10] Tomita K, Kawahara N, Baba H, Tsuchiya H, Fujita T, Toribatake Y. Total en bloc spondylectomy. A new surgical technique for primary malignant vertebral tumors. Spine. 1997; 22(3):324–333

[11] Chan P, Boriani S, Fourney DR, et al. An assessment of the reliability of the Enneking and Weinstein-Boriani-Biagini classifications for staging of primary spinal tumors by the Spine Oncology Study Group. Spine (Phila Pa 1976). 2009; 34(4):384–391

[12] Jawad MU, Scully SP. In brief: classifications in brief: Enneking classification: benign and malignant tumors of the musculoskeletal system. Clin Orthop Relat Res. 2010; 468(7):2000–2002

[13] Sciubba DM, De la Garza Ramos R, Goodwin CR, et al. Total en bloc spondylectomy for locally aggressive and primary malignant tumors of the lumbar spine. Eur Spine J. 2016; 25(12):4080–4087

[14] Campanacci M, Baldini N, Boriani S, Sudanese A. Giant-cell tumor of bone. J Bone Joint Surg Am. 1987; 69(1):106–114

[15] Lee FY, Mankin HJ, Fondren G, et al. Chondrosarcoma of bone: an assessment of outcome. J Bone Joint Surg Am. 1999; 81(3):326–338

[16] Varga PP, Szövérfi Z, Fisher CG, et al. Surgical treatment of sacral chordoma: prognostic variables for local recurrence and overall survival. Eur Spine J. 2015; 24(5):1092–1101

[17] Yamazaki T, McLoughlin GS, Patel S, Rhines LD, Fourney DR. Feasibility and safety of en bloc resection for primary spine tumors: a systematic review by the Spine Oncology Study Group. Spine. 2009; 34(22) Suppl:S31–S38

[18] Dekutoski MB, Clarke MJ, Rose P, et al. AOSpine Knowledge Forum Tumor. Osteosarcoma of the spine: prognostic variables for local recurrence and overall survival, a multicenter ambispective study. J Neurosurg Spine. 2016; 25(1):59–68

[19] Meng T, Yin H, Li B, et al. Clinical features and prognostic factors of patients with chordoma in the spine: a retrospective analysis of 153 patients in a single center. Neuro-oncol. 2015; 17(5):725–732

[20] Schwab J, Gasbarrini A, Bandiera S, et al. Osteosarcoma of the mobile spine. Spine. 2012; 37(6):E381–E386

[21] Yin H, Zhou W, Meng J, et al. Prognostic factors of patients with spinal chondrosarcoma: a retrospective analysis of 98 consecutive patients in a single center. Ann Surg Oncol. 2014; 21(11):3572–3578

[22] Zhong N, Xu W, Meng T, Yang X, Yan W, Xiao J. The surgical strategy for eosinophilic granuloma of the pediatric cervical spine complicated with neurologic deficit and/or spinal instability. World J Surg Oncol. 2016; 14(1):301

[23] Cloyd JM, Acosta FL, Jr, Polley MY, Ames CP. En bloc resection for primary and metastatic tumors of the spine: a systematic review of the literature. Neurosurgery. 2010; 67(2):435–444, discussion 444–445

[24] Tomita K, Kawahara N, Murakami H, Demura S. Total en bloc spondylectomy for spinal tumors: improvement of the technique and its associated basic background. J Orthop Sci. 2006; 11(1):3–12

[25] Talac R, Yaszemski MJ, Currier BL, et al. Relationship between surgical margins and local recurrence in sarcomas of the spine. Clin Orthop Relat Res. 2002(397):127–132

[26] Orguc S, Arkun R. Primary tumors of the spine. Semin Musculoskelet Radiol. 2014; 18(3):280–299

[27] Hart RA, Boriani S, Biagini R, Currier B, Weinstein JN. A system for surgical staging and management of spine tumors. A clinical outcome study of giant cell tumors of the spine. Spine. 1997; 22(15):1773–1782, discussion 1783

[28] Hsu W, McCarthy E, Gokaslan ZL, Wolinsky JP. Clear-cell chondrosarcoma of the lumbar spine: case report and review of the literature. Neurosurgery. 2011; 68(4):E1160–E1164, discussion 1164

[29] Kuruvath S, O'Donovan DG, Aspoas AR, David KM. Benign fibrous histiocytoma of the thoracic spine: case report and review of the literature. J Neurosurg Spine. 2006; 4(3):260–264

[30] Hasegawa K, Homma T, Hirano T, et al. Margin-free spondylectomy for extended malignant spine tumors: surgical technique and outcome of 13 cases. Spine. 2007; 32(1):142–148

[31] Tomita K, Toribatake Y, Kawahara N, Ohnari H, Kose H. Total en bloc spondylectomy and circumspinal decompression for solitary spinal metastasis. Paraplegia. 1994; 32(1):36–46

[32] Abdel-Wanis Mel-S, Tsuchiya H, Kawahara N, Tomita K. Tumor growth potential after tumoral and instrumental contamination: an in-vivo comparative study of T-saw, Gigli saw, and scalpel. J Orthop Sci. 2001; 6(5):424–429

[33] Kawahara N, Tomita K, Murakami H, Demura S. Total en bloc spondylectomy for spinal tumors: surgical techniques and related basic background. Orthop Clin North Am. 2009; 40(1):47–63, vi

[34] Murakami H, Kawahara N, Abdel-Wanis ME, Tomita K. Total en bloc spondylectomy. Semin Musculoskelet Radiol. 2001; 5(2):189–194

[35] Tomita K, Kawahara N, Baba H, Tsuchiya H, Nagata S, Toribatake Y. Total en bloc spondylectomy for solitary spinal metastases. Int Orthop. 1994; 18(5):291–298

[36] Mazel C, Balabaud L, Bennis S, Hansen S. Cervical and thoracic spine tumor management: surgical indications, techniques, and outcomes. Orthop Clin North Am. 2009; 40(1):75–92, vi–vii

[37] Yoshioka K, Kawahara N, Murakami H, et al. Cervicothoracic giant cell tumor expanding into the superior mediastinum: total excision by combined anterior-posterior approach. Orthopedics. 2009; 32(7):531

[38] Oppenlander ME, Maulucci CM, Ghobrial GM, Evans NR, III, Harrop JS, Prasad SK. En bloc resection of upper thoracic chordoma via a combined simultaneous anterolateral thoracoscopic and posterior approach. Neurosurgery. 2014; 10(3) Suppl 3:380–386, discussion 386

[39] Gösling T, Pichlmaier MA, Länger F, Krettek C, Hüfner T. Two-stage multilevel en bloc spondylectomy with resection and replacement of the aorta. Eur Spine J. 2013; 22 Suppl 3:S363–S368

[40] Biagini R, Casadei R, Boriani S, et al. En bloc vertebrectomy and dural resection for chordoma: a case report. Spine. 2003; 28(18):E368–E372

[41] Bandiera S, Boriani S, Donthineni R, Amendola L, Cappuccio M, Gasbarrini A. Complications of en bloc resections in the spine. Orthop Clin North Am. 2009; 40(1):125–131, vii

[42] Fisher CG, Versteeg AL, Dea N, et al. Surgical management of spinal chondrosarcomas. Spine. 2016; 41(8):678–685

[43] Jin Z, Han YX, Han XR. Loss of RUNX3 expression may contribute to poor prognosis in patients with chondrosarcoma. J Mol Histol. 2013; 44(6):645–652

[44] Boriani S, Saravanja D, Yamada Y, Varga PP, Biagini R, Fisher CG. Challenges of local recurrence and cure in low grade malignant tumors of the spine. Spine. 2009; 34(22) Suppl:S48–S57

[45] McLoughlin GS, Sciubba DM, Wolinsky JP. Chondroma/chondrosarcoma of the spine. Neurosurg Clin N Am. 2008; 19(1):57–63

[46] Boriani S, Bandiera S, Donthineni R, et al. Morbidity of en bloc resections in the spine. Eur Spine J. 2010; 19(2):231–241

[47] Liljenqvist U, Lerner T, Halm H, Buerger H, Gosheger G, Winkelmann W. En bloc spondylectomy in malignant tumors of the spine. Eur Spine J. 2008; 17(4):600–609

[48] Rao G, Suki D, Chakrabarti I, et al. Surgical management of primary and metastatic sarcoma of the mobile spine. J Neurosurg Spine. 2008; 9(2):120–128

[49] Zou MX, Lv GH, Wang XB, Li J. Prognostic factors in spinal chordoma: an update of current systematic review and meta-analysis. J Surg Oncol. 2017; 115(4):497–500

[50] Sewell MD, Tan KA, Quraishi NA, Preda C, Varga PP, Williams R. Systematic review of en bloc resection in the management of Ewing's sarcoma of the mobile spine with respect to local control and disease-free survival. Medicine (Baltimore). 2015; 94(27):e1019

[51] Boriani S, Amendola L, Corghi A, et al. Ewing's sarcoma of the mobile spine. Eur Rev Med Pharmacol Sci. 2011; 15(7):831–839

[52] Sciubba DM, Okuno SH, Dekutoski MB, Gokaslan ZL. Ewing and osteogenic sarcoma: evidence for multidisciplinary management. Spine. 2009; 34(22) Suppl:S58–S68

[53] Vogin G, Helfre S, Glorion C, et al. Local control and sequelae in localised Ewing tumours of the spine: a French retrospective study. Eur J Cancer. 2013; 49(6):1314–1323

[54] Boriani S, De Iure F, Campanacci L, et al. Aneurysmal bone cyst of the mobile spine: report on 41 cases. Spine. 2001; 26(1):27–35

[55] Mascard E, Gomez-Brouchet A, Lambot K. Bone cysts: unicameral and aneurysmal bone cyst. Orthop Traumatol Surg Res. 2015; 101(1) Suppl:S119–S127

[56] Saccomanni B. Aneurysmal bone cyst of spine: a review of literature. Arch Orthop Trauma Surg. 2008; 128(10):1145–1147

[57] Vergel De Dios AM, Bond JR, Shives TC, McLeod RA, Unni KK. Aneurysmal bone cyst. A clinicopathologic study of 238 cases. Cancer. 1992; 69(12):2921–2931

[58] Rossi G, Rimondi E, Bartalena T, et al. Selective arterial embolization of 36 aneurysmal bone cysts of the skeleton with N-2-butyl cyanoacrylate. Skeletal Radiol. 2010; 39(2):161–167

[59] Tsagozis P, Brosjö O. Current strategies for the treatment of aneurysmal bone cysts. Orthop Rev (Pavia). 2015; 7(4):6182

[60] Amendola L, Simonetti L, Simoes CE, Bandiera S, De Iure F, Boriani S. Aneurysmal bone cyst of the mobile spine: the therapeutic role of embolization. Eur Spine J. 2013; 22(3):533–541

[61] de Kleuver M, van der Heul RO, Veraart BE. Aneurysmal bone cyst of the spine: 31 cases and the importance of the surgical approach. J Pediatr Orthop B. 1998; 7(4):286–292

[62] Ropper AE, Cahill KS, Hanna JW, McCarthy EF, Gokaslan ZL, Chi JH. Primary vertebral tumors: a review of epidemiologic, histological, and imaging findings, Part I: benign tumors. Neurosurgery. 2011; 69(6):1171–1180

[63] Zenonos G, Jamil O, Governale LS, Jernigan S, Hedequist D, Proctor MR. Surgical treatment for primary spinal aneurysmal bone cysts: experience from Children's Hospital Boston. J Neurosurg Pediatr. 2012; 9(3):305–315

[64] Capanna R, Albisinni U, Picci P, Calderoni P, Campanacci M, Springfield DS. Aneurysmal bone cyst of the spine. J Bone Joint Surg Am. 1985; 67(4):527–531

[65] Papagelopoulos PJ, Currier BL, Shaughnessy WJ, et al. Aneurysmal bone cyst of the spine. Management and outcome. Spine. 1998; 23(5):621–628

[66] Zileli M, Isik HS, Ogut FE, Is M, Cagli S, Calli C. Aneurysmal bone cysts of the spine. Eur Spine J. 2013; 22(3):593–601

[67] Ameli NO, Abbassioun K, Saleh H, Eslamdoost A. Aneurysmal bone cysts of the spine. Report of 17 cases. J Neurosurg. 1985; 63(5):685–690

[68] Hay MC, Paterson D, Taylor TK. Aneurysmal bone cysts of the spine. J Bone Joint Surg Br. 1978; 60-B(3):406–411

[69] Ravindra VM, Eli IM, Schmidt MH, Brockmeyer DL. Primary osseous tumors of the pediatric spinal column: review of pathology and surgical decision making. Neurosurg Focus. 2016; 41(2):E3

[70] Terzi S, Gasbarrini A, Fuiano M, et al. Efficacy and safety of selective arterial embolization in the treatment of aneurysmal bone cyst of the mobile spine. Spine. 2017; 42(15):1130–1138

[71] Liu G, Wu G, Ghimire P, Pang H, Zhang Z. Primary spinal chondrosarcoma: radiological manifestations with histopathological correlation in eight patients and literature review. Clin Imaging. 2013; 37(1):124–133

[72] Charest-Morin R, Boriani S, Fisher CG, et al. Benign tumors of the spine: Has new chemotherapy and interventional radiology changed the treatment paradigm? Spine. 2016; 41 Suppl 20:S178–S185

[73] Boriani S, Lo SF, Puvanesarajah V, et al. AOSpine Knowledge Forum Tumor. Aneurysmal bone cysts of the spine: treatment options and considerations. J Neurooncol. 2014; 120(1):171–178

[74] Dubory A, Missenard G, Domont J, Court C. Interest of denosumab for the treatment of giant-cells tumors and aneurysmal bone cysts of the spine. About nine cases. Spine. 2016; 41(11):E654–E660

[75] Liu JK, Brockmeyer DL, Dailey AT, Schmidt MH. Surgical management of aneurysmal bone cysts of the spine. Neurosurg Focus. 2003; 15(5):E4

[76] Mesfin A, McCarthy EF, Kebaish KM. Surgical treatment of aneurysmal bone cysts of the spine. Iowa Orthop J. 2012; 32:40–45

[77] Demiralp B, Kose O, Oguz E, Sanal T, Ozcan A, Sehirlioglu A. Benign fibrous histiocytoma of the lumbar vertebrae. Skeletal Radiol. 2009; 38(2):187–191

[78] Avanzi O, Chih LY, Meves R, Próspero JD, Brito A. Benign fibrous histiocytoma of the lumbar spine. Acta Ortop Bras. 2005; 13(2):91–92

[79] Destouet JM, Kyriakos M, Gilula LA. Fibrous histiocytoma (fibroxanthoma) of a cervical vertebra. A report with a review of the literature. Skeletal Radiol. 1980; 5(4):241–246

[80] Khor YM, Yan X. Benign fibrous histiocytoma of the thoracic spine as the cause of pyrexia of unknown origin identified by positron emission tomography/computed tomography. Spine J. 2015; 15(7):1691–1692

[81] Kim SB, Jang JS, Lee SH. Surgical treatment of benign fibrous histiocytoma as a form of intraspinal extradural tumor at lumbar spine. Asian Spine J. 2010; 4(2):132–135

[82] Skunda R, Puckett T, Martin M, Sanclement J, Peterson JE. 14-year-old boy with mild antecedent neck pain in setting of acute trauma: a rare case of benign fibrous histiocytoma of the spine. Am J Orthop. 2016; 45(3):E148–E152

[83] van Giffen NH, van Rhijn LW, van Ooij A, et al. Benign fibrous histiocytoma of the posterior arch of C1 in a 6-year-old boy: a case report. Spine. 2003; 28 (18):E359–E363

[84] Grohs JG, Nicolakis M, Kainberger F, Lang S, Kotz R. Benign fibrous histiocytoma of bone: a report of ten cases and review of literature. Wien Klin Wochenschr. 2002; 114(1–2):56–63

[85] Peicha G, Seibert FJ, Bratschitsch G, Fankhauser F, Grechenig W. Pathologic odontoid fracture and benign fibrous histiocytoma of bone. Eur Spine J. 1999; 8(2):161–163

[86] Chapurlat RD. Medical therapy in adults with fibrous dysplasia of bone. J Bone Miner Res. 2006; 21 Suppl 2:114–119

[87] Meredith CC, Kepes JJ, Johnson P, Sebastian CTS, McMahon JK, Arnold PM. Chondromyxoid fibroma of the upper thoracic spine in a 7-year-old patient. A case report and review of the literature. Pediatr Neurosurg. 2004; 40(4): 190–195

[88] Bloem JL, Mulder JD. Chondroblastoma: a clinical and radiological study of 104 cases. Skeletal Radiol. 1985; 14(1):1–9

[89] Dahlin DC, Ivins JC. Benign chondroblastoma. A study of 125 cases. Cancer. 1972; 30(2):401–413

[90] Hernández Martínez SJ, Campa Núñez H, Ornelas Cortinas G, Garza Garza R. Chondroblastoma of the fourth lumbar vertebra diagnosed by aspiration biopsy: case report and review of the literature. Acta Cytol. 2011; 55(5):473–477

[91] Jain M, Kaur M, Kapoor S, Arora DS. Cytological features of chondroblastoma: a case report with review of the literature. Diagn Cytopathol. 2000; 23 (5):348–350

[92] Kim SA, Cho KJ, Park YK, et al. Chondroblastoma of the lumbar spine: a case report and review of the literature. Korean J Pathol. 2011; 45(5):532–536

[93] Leung LYJ, Shu SJ, Chan MK, Chan CHS. Chondroblastoma of the lumbar vertebra. Skeletal Radiol. 2001; 30(12):710–713

[94] Venkatasamy A, Chenard MP, Massard G, Steib JP, Bierry G. Chondroblastoma of the thoracic spine: a rare location. Case report with radiologic-pathologic correlation. Skeletal Radiol. 2017; 46(3):367–372

[95] Ilaslan H, Sundaram M, Unni KK. Vertebral chondroblastoma. Skeletal Radiol. 2003; 32(2):66–71

[96] Masui F, Ushigome S, Kamitani K, Asanuma K, Fujii K. Chondroblastoma: a study of 11 cases. Eur J Surg Oncol. 2002; 28(8):869–874

[97] Vialle R, Feydy A, Rillardon L, et al. Chondroblastoma of the lumbar spine. Report of two cases and review of the literature. J Neurosurg Spine. 2005; 2 (5):596–600

[98] Attar A, Uğur HÇ, Çağlar YS, Erdogan A, Ozdemir N. Chondroblastoma of the thoracic vertebra. J Clin Neurosci. 2001; 8(1):59–60

[99] Chung OM, Yip SF, Ngan KC, Ng WF. Chondroblastoma of the lumbar spine with cauda equina syndrome. Spinal Cord. 2003; 41(6):359–364

[100] Kurth AA, Warzecha J, Rittmeister M, Schmitt E, Hovy L. Recurrent chondroblastoma of the upper thoracic spine. A case report and review of the literature. Arch Orthop Trauma Surg. 2000; 120(9):544–547

[101] Sohn SH, Koh SA, Kim DG, et al. A case of spine origin chondroblastoma metastasis to lung. Cancer Res Treat. 2009; 41(4):241–244

[102] Cerase A, Priolo F. Skeletal benign bone-forming lesions. Eur J Radiol. 1998; 27 Suppl 1:S91–S97

[103] Flemming DJ, Murphey MD, Carmichael BB, Bernard SA. Primary tumors of the spine. Semin Musculoskelet Radiol. 2000; 4(3):299–320

[104] Greenspan A, Steiner G, Knutzon R. Bone island (enostosis): clinical significance and radiologic and pathologic correlations. Skeletal Radiol. 1991; 20 (2):85–90

[105] Greenspan A. Bone island (enostosis): current concept—a review. Skeletal Radiol. 1995; 24(2):111–115

[106] Onitsuka H. Roentgenologic aspects of bone islands. Radiology. 1977; 123 (3):607–612

[107] Trombetti A, Noël E. Giant bone islands: a case with 31 years of follow-up. Joint Bone Spine. 2002; 69(1):81–84

[108] Hall FM, Goldberg RP, Davies JAK, Fainsinger MH. Scintigraphic assessment of bone islands. Radiology. 1980; 135(3):737–742

[109] Broderick TW, Resnick D, Goergen TG, Alazraki N. Enostosis of the spine. Spine. 1978; 3(2):167–170

[110] Garg S, Mehta S, Dormans JP. Langerhans cell histiocytosis of the spine in children. Long-term follow-up. J Bone Joint Surg Am. 2004; 86-A(8):1740–1750

[111] Islinger RB, Kuklo TR, Owens BD, et al. Langerhans' cell histiocytosis in patients older than 21 years. Clin Orthop Relat Res. 2000(379):231–235

[112] Angelini A, Mavrogenis A, Rimondi E, Rossi G, Ruggieri P. Current concepts for the diagnosis and management of eosinophilic granuloma of bone. J Orthop Traumatol. 2017; 18(2):83–90

[113] Brown CW, Jarvis JG, Letts M, Carpenter B. Treatment and outcome of vertebral Langerhans cell histiocytosis at the Children's Hospital of Eastern Ontario. Can J Surg. 2005; 48(3):230–236

[114] Willman CL, Busque L, Griffith BB, et al. Langerhans'-cell histiocytosis (histiocytosis X)—a clonal proliferative disease. N Engl J Med. 1994; 331(3):154–160

[115] Yu RC, Chu C, Buluwela L, Chu AC. Clonal proliferation of Langerhans cells in Langerhans cell histiocytosis. Lancet. 1994; 343(8900):767–768

[116] Huang W, Yang X, Cao D, et al. Eosinophilic granuloma of spine in adults: a report of 30 cases and outcome. Acta Neurochir (Wien). 2010; 152(7):1129–1137

[117] Huang WD, Yang XH, Wu ZP, et al. Langerhans cell histiocytosis of spine: a comparative study of clinical, imaging features, and diagnosis in children, adolescents, and adults. Spine J. 2013; 13(9):1108–1117

[118] Puertas EB, Milani C, Chagas JCM, et al. Surgical treatment of eosinophilic granuloma in the thoracic spine in patients with neurological lesions. J Pediatr Orthop B. 2003; 12(5):303–306

[119] Kilpatrick SE, Wenger DE, Gilchrist GS, Shives TC, Wollan PC, Unni KK. Langerhans' cell histiocytosis (histiocytosis X) of bone. A clinicopathologic analysis of 263 pediatric and adult cases. Cancer. 1995; 76(12): 2471–2484

[120] Arkader A, Glotzbecker M, Hosalkar HS, Dormans JP. Primary musculoskeletal Langerhans cell histiocytosis in children: an analysis for a 3-decade period. J Pediatr Orthop. 2009; 29(2):201–207

[121] DiCaprio MR, Roberts TT. Diagnosis and management of Langerhans cell histiocytosis. J Am Acad Orthop Surg. 2014; 22(10):643–652

[122] Hussein AA, El-Karef E, Hafez M. Reconstructive surgery in spinal tumours. Eur J Surg Oncol. 2001; 27(2):196–199

[123] Lü GH, Li J, Wang XB, Wang B, Phan K. Surgical treatment based on pedicle screw instrumentation for thoracic or lumbar spinal Langerhans cell histiocytosis complicated with neurologic deficit in children. Spine J. 2014; 14(5): 768–776

[124] Rimondi E, Mavrogenis AF, Rossi G, Ussia G, Angelini A, Ruggieri P. CT-guided corticosteroid injection for solitary eosinophilic granuloma of the spine. Skeletal Radiol. 2011; 40(6):757–764

[125] Bertram C, Madert J, Eggers C. Eosinophilic granuloma of the cervical spine. Spine. 2002; 27(13):1408–1413

[126] Lam S, Reddy GD, Mayer R, Lin Y, Jea A. Eosinophilic granuloma/Langerhans cell histiocytosis: pediatric neurosurgery update. Surg Neurol Int. 2015; 6 Suppl 17:S435–S439

[127] Mammano S, Candiotto S, Balsano M. Cast and brace treatment of eosinophilic granuloma of the spine: long-term follow-up. J Pediatr Orthop. 1997; 17(6):821–827

[128] Wei MA, Ruixue MA. Solitary spinal eosinophilic granuloma in children. J Pediatr Orthop B. 2006; 15(5):316–319

[129] Kim BE, Koh KN, Suh JK, et al. Korea Histiocytosis Working Party. Clinical features and treatment outcomes of Langerhans cell histiocytosis: a nationwide survey from Korea histiocytosis working party. J Pediatr Hematol Oncol. 2014; 36(2):125–133

[130] Lee SK, Jung TY, Jung S, Han DK, Lee JK, Baek HJ. Solitary Langerhans cell histiocytosis of skull and spine in pediatric and adult patients. Childs Nerv Syst. 2014; 30(2):271–275

[131] Elder BD, Sankey EW, Goodwin CR, et al. Surgical outcomes in patients with high spinal instability neoplasm score secondary to spinal giant cell tumors. Global Spine J. 2016; 6(1):21–28

[132] Bhojraj SY, Nene A, Mohite S, Varma R. Giant cell tumor of the spine: a review of 9 surgical interventions in 6 cases. Indian J Orthop. 2007; 41(2):146–150

[133] Thomas DM, Skubitz KM. Giant cell tumour of bone. Curr Opin Oncol. 2009; 21(4):338–344

[134] Boriani S, Bandiera S, Casadei R, et al. Giant cell tumor of the mobile spine: a review of 49 cases. Spine. 2012; 37(1):E37–E45

[135] Goldschlager T, Dea N, Boyd M, et al. Giant cell tumors of the spine: has denosumab changed the treatment paradigm? J Neurosurg Spine. 2015; 22(5):526–533

[136] Larsson SE, Lorentzon R, Boquist L. Giant-cell tumor of bone. A demographic, clinical, and histopathological study of all cases recorded in the Swedish Cancer Registry for the years 1958 through 1968. J Bone Joint Surg Am. 1975; 57(2):167–173

[137] Junming M, Cheng Y, Dong C, et al. Giant cell tumor of the cervical spine: a series of 22 cases and outcomes. Spine. 2008; 33(3):280–288

[138] Savini R, Gherlinzoni F, Morandi M, Neff JR, Picci P. Surgical treatment of giant-cell tumor of the spine. The experience at the Istituto Ortopedico Rizzoli. J Bone Joint Surg Am. 1983; 65(9):1283–1289

[139] Sanjay BKS, Frassica FJ, Frassica DA, Unni KK, McLeod RA, Sim FH. Treatment of giant-cell tumor of the pelvis. J Bone Joint Surg Am. 1993; 75(10):1466–1475

[140] Leggon RE, Zlotecki R, Reith J, Scarborough MT. Giant cell tumor of the pelvis and sacrum: 17 cases and analysis of the literature. Clin Orthop Relat Res. 2004(423):196–207

[141] Martin C, McCarthy EF. Giant cell tumor of the sacrum and spine: series of 23 cases and a review of the literature. Iowa Orthop J. 2010; 30:69–75

[142] Sung HW, Kuo DP, Shu WP, Chai YB, Liu CC, Li SM. Giant-cell tumor of bone: analysis of two hundred and eight cases in Chinese patients. J Bone Joint Surg Am. 1982; 64(5):755–761

[143] Ropper AE, Cahill KS, Hanna JW, McCarthy EF, Gokaslan ZL, Chi JH. Primary vertebral tumors: a review of epidemiologic, histological and imaging findings, part II: locally aggressive and malignant tumors. Neurosurgery. 2012; 70(1):211–219, discussion 219

[144] Sonmez E, Tezcaner T, Coven I, Terzi A. Brown tumor of the thoracic spine: first manifestation of primary hyperparathyroidism. J Korean Neurosurg Soc. 2015; 58(4):389–392

[145] Fidler MW. Surgical treatment of giant cell tumours of the thoracic and lumbar spine: report of nine patients. Eur Spine J. 2001; 10(1):69–77

[146] Hosalkar HS, Jones KJ, King JJ, Lackman RD. Serial arterial embolization for large sacral giant-cell tumors: mid- to long-term results. Spine. 2007; 32(10):1107–1115

[147] Luksanapruksa P, Buchowski JM, Singhatanadgige W, Bumpass DB. Systematic review and meta-analysis of en bloc vertebrectomy compared with intralesional resection for giant cell tumors of the mobile spine. Global Spine J. 2016; 6(8):798–803

[148] Ma Y, Li J, Pan J, et al. Treatment options and prognosis for repeatedly recurrent giant cell tumor of the spine. Eur Spine J. 2016; 25(12):4033–4042

[149] Xu W, Li X, Huang W, et al. Factors affecting prognosis of patients with giant cell tumors of the mobile spine: retrospective analysis of 102 patients in a single center. Ann Surg Oncol. 2013; 20(3):804–810

[150] Yang SC, Chen LH, Fu TS, Lai PL, Niu CC, Chen WJ. Surgical treatment for giant cell tumor of the thoracolumbar spine. Chang Gung Med J. 2006; 29(1):71–78

[151] Ma Y, Xu W, Yin H, et al. Therapeutic radiotherapy for giant cell tumor of the spine: a systemic review. Eur Spine J. 2015; 24(8):1754–1760

[152] de Carvalho Cavalcante RA, Silva Marques RA, dos Santos VG, et al. Spondylectomy for giant cell tumor after denosumab therapy. Spine. 2016; 41(3):E178–E182

[153] Thomas D, Henshaw R, Skubitz K, et al. Denosumab in patients with giant-cell tumour of bone: an open-label, phase 2 study. Lancet Oncol. 2010; 11(3):275–280

[154] Kan P, Schmidt MH. Osteoid osteoma and osteoblastoma of the spine. Neurosurg Clin N Am. 2008; 19(1):65–70

[155] Azouz EM, Kozlowski K, Marton D, Sprague P, Zerhouni A, Asselah F. Osteoid osteoma and osteoblastoma of the spine in children. Report of 22 cases with brief literature review. Pediatr Radiol. 1986; 16(1):25–31

[156] Tsoumakidou G, Thénint MA, Garnon J, Buy X, Steib JP, Gangi A. Percutaneous image-guided laser photocoagulation of spinal osteoid osteoma: a single-institution series. Radiology. 2016; 278(3):936–943

[157] Burn SC, Ansorge O, Zeller R, Drake JM. Management of osteoblastoma and osteoid osteoma of the spine in childhood. J Neurosurg Pediatr. 2009; 4(5):434–438

[158] Galgano MA, Goulart CR, Iwenofu H, Chin LS, Lavelle W, Mendel E. Osteoblastomas of the spine: a comprehensive review. Neurosurg Focus. 2016; 41(2):E4

[159] Vanderschueren GM, Obermann WR, Dijkstra SP, Taminiau AH, Bloem JL, van Erkel AR. Radiofrequency ablation of spinal osteoid osteoma: clinical outcome. Spine. 2009; 34(9):901–904

[160] Etemadifar MR, Hadi A. Clinical findings and results of surgical resection in 19 cases of spinal osteoid osteoma. Asian Spine J. 2015; 9(3):386–393

[161] Kadhim M, Binitie O, O'Toole P, Grigoriou E, De Mattos CB, Dormans JP. Surgical resection of osteoid osteoma and osteoblastoma of the spine. J Pediatr Orthop B. 2017; 26(4):362–369

[162] Quraishi NA, Boriani S, Sabou S, et al. A multicenter cohort study of spinal osteoid osteomas: results of surgical treatment and analysis of local recurrence. Spine J. 2017; 17(3):401–408

[163] Gangi A, Alizadeh H, Wong L, Buy X, Dietemann JL, Roy C. Osteoid osteoma: percutaneous laser ablation and follow-up in 114 patients. Radiology. 2007; 242(1):293–301

[164] Hadjipavlou AG, Tzermiadianos MN, Kakavelakis KN, Lander P. Percutaneous core excision and radiofrequency thermo-coagulation for the ablation of osteoid osteoma of the spine. Eur Spine J. 2009; 18(3):345–351

[165] Klass D, Marshall T, Toms A. CT-guided radiofrequency ablation of spinal osteoid osteomas with concomitant perineural and epidural irrigation for neuroprotection. Eur Radiol. 2009; 19(9):2238–2243

[166] Ozaki T, Liljenqvist U, Hillmann A, et al. Osteoid osteoma and osteoblastoma of the spine: experiences with 22 patients. Clin Orthop Relat Res. 2002(397):394–402

[167] Pettine KA, Klassen RA. Osteoid-osteoma and osteoblastoma of the spine. J Bone Joint Surg Am. 1986; 68(3):354–361

[168] Raskas DS, Graziano GP, Herzenberg JE, Heidelberger KP, Hensinger RN. Osteoid osteoma and osteoblastoma of the spine. J Spinal Disord. 1992; 5(2):204–211

[169] Rybak LD, Gangi A, Buy X, La Rocca Vieira R, Wittig J. Thermal ablation of spinal osteoid osteomas close to neural elements: technical considerations. AJR Am J Roentgenol. 2010; 195(4):W293–8

[170] Zileli M, Çagli S, Basdemir G, Ersahin Y. Osteoid osteomas and osteoblastomas of the spine. Neurosurg Focus. 2003; 15(5):E5

[171] Gasbarrini A, Cappuccio M, Bandiera S, Amendola L, van Urk P, Boriani S. Osteoid osteoma of the mobile spine: surgical outcomes in 81 patients. Spine. 2011; 36(24):2089–2093

[172] Martel J, Bueno A, Nieto-Morales ML, Ortiz EJ. Osteoid osteoma of the spine: CT-guided monopolar radiofrequency ablation. Eur J Radiol. 2009; 71(3):564–569

[173] Pourteizi HH, Tabrizi A, Bazavar M, Sales JG. Clinical findings and results of surgical resection of thoracolumbar osteoid osteoma. Asian Spine J. 2014; 8(2):150–155

[174] Saifuddin A, White J, Sherazi Z, Shaikh MI, Natali C, Ransford AO. Osteoid osteoma and osteoblastoma of the spine. Factors associated with the presence of scoliosis. Spine. 1998; 23(1):47–53

[175] Uehara M, Takahashi J, Kuraishi S, et al. Osteoid osteoma presenting as thoracic scoliosis. Spine J. 2015; 15(12):e77–e81

[176] Weber MA, Sprengel SD, Omlor GW, et al. Clinical long-term outcome, technical success, and cost analysis of radiofrequency ablation for the treatment of osteoblastomas and spinal osteoid osteomas in comparison to open surgical resection. Skeletal Radiol. 2015; 44(7):981–993

[177] Faddoul J, Faddoul Y, Kobaiter-Maarrawi S, et al. Radiofrequency ablation of spinal osteoid osteoma: a prospective study. J Neurosurg Spine. 2017; 26(3):313–318

[178] Jackson RP, Reckling FW, Mants FA. Osteoid osteoma and osteoblastoma. Similar histologic lesions with different natural histories. Clin Orthop Relat Res. 1977; 128(128):303–313

[179] Laus M, Albisinni U, Alfonso C, Zappoli FA. Osteoid osteoma of the cervical spine: surgical treatment or percutaneous radiofrequency coagulation? Eur Spine J. 2007; 16(12):2078–2082

[180] Della Rocca C, Huvos AG. Osteoblastoma: varied histological presentations with a benign clinical course. An analysis of 55 cases. Am J Surg Pathol. 1996; 20(7):841–850

[181] Lucas DR, Unni KK, McLeod RA, O'Connor MI, Sim FH. Osteoblastoma: clinicopathologic study of 306 cases. Hum Pathol. 1994; 25(2):117–134

[182] Boriani S, Capanna R, Donati D, Levine A, Picci P, Savini R. Osteoblastoma of the spine. Clin Orthop Relat Res. 1992; 278(278):37–45

[183] Elder BD, Goodwin CR, Kosztowski TA, et al. Surgical management of osteoblastoma of the spine: case series and review of the literature. Turk Neurosurg. 2016; 26(4):601–607

[184] Nemoto O, Moser RP, Jr, Van Dam BE, Aoki J, Gilkey FW. Osteoblastoma of the spine. A review of 75 cases. Spine. 1990; 15(12):1272–1280

[185] Ruggieri P, Huch K, Mavrogenis AF, Merlino B, Angelini A. Osteoblastoma of the sacrum: report of 18 cases and analysis of the literature. Spine. 2014; 39(2):E97–E103

[186] Denaro V, Denaro L, Papalia R, Marinozzi A, Di Martino A. Surgical management of cervical spine osteoblastomas. Clin Orthop Relat Res. 2007; 455(455):190–195

[187] Ozaki T, Flege S, Liljenqvist U, et al. Osteosarcoma of the spine: experience of the cooperative osteosarcoma study group. Cancer. 2002; 94(4):1069–1077

[188] Jiang L, Liu XG, Wang C, et al. Surgical treatment options for aggressive osteoblastoma in the mobile spine. Eur Spine J. 2015; 24(8):1778–1785

[189] Boriani S, Amendola L, Bandiera S, et al. Staging and treatment of osteoblastoma in the mobile spine: a review of 51 cases. Eur Spine J. 2012; 21(10):2003–2010

[190] Bess RS, Robbin MR, Bohlman HH, Thompson GH. Spinal exostoses: analysis of twelve cases and review of the literature. Spine. 2005; 30(7):774–780

[191] Samartzis D, Marco RAW. Osteochondroma of the sacrum: a case report and review of the literature. Spine. 2006; 31(13):E425–E429

[192] Tian Y, Yuan W, Chen H, Shen X. Spinal cord compression secondary to a thoracic vertebral osteochondroma. J Neurosurg Spine. 2011; 15(3):252–257

[193] Veeravagu A, Li A, Shuer LM, Desai AM. Cervical osteochondroma causing myelopathy in adults: management considerations and literature review. World Neurosurg. 2017; 97:752.e5–752.e13

[194] Zaijun L, Xinhai Y, Zhipeng W, et al. Outcome and prognosis of myelopathy and radiculopathy from osteochondroma in the mobile spine: a report on 14 patients. J Spinal Disord Tech. 2013; 26(4):194–199

[195] Murphey MD, Choi JJ, Kransdorf MJ, Flemming DJ, Gannon FH. Imaging of osteochondroma: variants and complications with radiologic-pathologic correlation. Radiographics. 2000; 20(5):1407–1434

[196] Kuraishi K, Hanakita J, Takahashi T, Watanabe M, Honda F. Symptomatic osteochondroma of lumbosacral spine: report of 5 cases. Neurol Med Chir (Tokyo). 2014; 54(5):408–412

[197] Lotfinia I, Vahedi P, Tubbs RS, Ghavame M, Meshkini A. Neurological manifestations, imaging characteristics, and surgical outcome of intraspinal osteochondroma. J Neurosurg Spine. 2010; 12(5):474–489

[198] Brastianos P, Pradilla G, McCarthy E, Gokaslan ZL. Solitary thoracic osteochondroma: case report and review of the literature. Neurosurgery. 2005; 56(6):E1379–, discussion E1379

[199] Khosla A, Martin DS, Awwad EE. The solitary intraspinal vertebral osteochondroma. An unusual cause of compressive myelopathy: features and literature review. Spine. 1999; 24(1):77–81

[200] Malat J, Virapongse C, Levine A. Solitary osteochondroma of the spine. Spine. 1986; 11(6):625–628

[201] Quirini GE, Meyer JR, Herman M, Russell EJ. Osteochondroma of the thoracic spine: an unusual cause of spinal cord compression. AJNR Am J Neuroradiol. 1996; 17(5):961–964

[202] Roblot P, Alcalay M, Cazenave-Roblot F, Levy P, Bontoux D. Osteochondroma of the thoracic spine. Report of a case and review of the literature. Spine. 1990; 15(3):240–243

[203] Gille O, Pointillart V, Vital JM. Course of spinal solitary osteochondromas. Spine. 2005; 30(1):E13–E19

[204] Giudicissi-Filho M, de Holanda CV, Borba LA, Rassi-Neto A, Ribeiro CA, de Oliveira JG. Cervical spinal cord compression due to an osteochondroma in hereditary multiple exostosis: case report and review of the literature. Surg Neurol. 2006; 66 Suppl 3:S7–S11

[205] Robbins SE, Laitt RD, Lewis T. Hereditary spinal osteochondromas in diaphyseal aclasia. Neuroradiology. 1996; 38(1):59–61

[206] Sade R, Ulusoy OL, Mutlu A, Yuce I, Kantarci M. Osteochondroma of the lumbar spine. Joint Bone Spine. 2017; 84(2):225

[207] Sakai D, Mochida J, Toh E, Nomura T. Spinal osteochondromas in middle-aged to elderly patients. Spine. 2002; 27(23):E503–E506

[208] Albrecht S, Crutchfield JS, SeGall GK. On spinal osteochondromas. J Neurosurg. 1992; 77(2):247–252

[209] Sharma MC, Arora R, Deol PS, Mahapatra AK, Mehta VS, Sarkar C. Osteochondroma of the spine: an enigmatic tumor of the spinal cord. A series of 10 cases. J Neurosurg Sci. 2002; 46(2):66–70, discussion 70

[210] Schellinger KA, Propp JM, Villano JL, McCarthy BJ. Descriptive epidemiology of primary spinal cord tumors. J Neurooncol. 2008; 87(2):173–179

[211] Rozeman LB, Cleton-Jansen AM, Hogendoorn PCW. Pathology of primary malignant bone and cartilage tumours. Int Orthop. 2006; 30(6):437–444

[212] Mukherjee D, Chaichana KL, Gokaslan ZL, Aaronson O, Cheng JS, McGirt MJ. Survival of patients with malignant primary osseous spinal neoplasms: results from the Surveillance, Epidemiology, and End Results (SEER) database from 1973 to 2003. J Neurosurg Spine. 2011; 14(2):143–150

[213] Mukherjee D, Chaichana KL, Parker SL, Gokaslan ZL, McGirt MJ. Association of surgical resection and survival in patients with malignant primary osseous spinal neoplasms from the Surveillance, Epidemiology, and End Results (SEER) database. Eur Spine J. 2013; 22(6):1375–1382

[214] Groves ML, Zadnik PL, Kaloostian P, et al. Epidemiologic, functional, and oncologic outcome analysis of spinal sarcomas treated surgically at a single institution over 10 years. Spine J. 2015; 15(1):110–114

[215] Gokaslan ZL, Zadnik PL, Sciubba DM, et al. Mobile spine chordoma: results of 166 patients from the AOSpine Knowledge Forum Tumor database. J Neurosurg Spine. 2016; 24(4):644–651

[216] Ozturk AK, Gokaslan ZL, Wolinsky JP. Surgical treatment of sarcomas of the spine. Curr Treat Options Oncol. 2014; 15(3):482–492

[217] Stacchiotti S, Sommer J, Chordoma Global Consensus Group. Building a global consensus approach to chordoma: a position paper from the medical and patient community. Lancet Oncol. 2015; 16(2):e71–e83

[218] Williams BJ, Raper DMS, Godbout E, et al. Diagnosis and treatment of chordoma. J Natl Compr Canc Netw. 2013; 11(6):726–731

[219] Boriani S, Bandiera S, Biagini R, et al. Chordoma of the mobile spine: fifty years of experience. Spine. 2006; 31(4):493–503

[220] Choi D, Melcher R, Harms J, Crockard A. Outcome of 132 operations in 97 patients with chordomas of the craniocervical junction and upper cervical spine. Neurosurgery. 2010; 66(1):59–65, discussion 65

[221] Crapanzano JP, Ali SZ, Ginsberg MS, Zakowski MF. Chordoma: a cytologic study with histologic and radiologic correlation. Cancer. 2001; 93(1):40–51

[222] Mukherjee D, Chaichana KL, Adogwa O, et al. Association of extent of local tumor invasion and survival in patients with malignant primary osseous spinal neoplasms from the surveillance, epidemiology, and end results (SEER) database. World Neurosurg. 2011; 76(6):580–585

[223] Ruggieri P, Angelini A, Ussia G, Montalti M, Mercuri M. Surgical margins and local control in resection of sacral chordomas. Clin Orthop Relat Res. 2010; 468(11):2939–2947

[224] Yamada Y, Laufer I, Cox BW, et al. Preliminary results of high-dose single-fraction radiotherapy for the management of chordomas of the spine and sacrum. Neurosurgery. 2013; 73(4):673–680, discussion 680

[225] Zou MX, Huang W, Wang XB, Li J, Lv GH, Deng YW. Prognostic factors in spinal chordoma: a systematic review. Clin Neurol Neurosurg. 2015; 139:110–118

[226] Stacchiotti S, Gronchi A, Fossati P, et al. Best practices for the management of local-regional recurrent chordoma: a position paper by the Chordoma Global Consensus Group. Ann Oncol. 2017; 28(6):1230–1242

[227] Holliday EB, Mitra HS, Somerson JS, et al. Postoperative proton therapy for chordomas and chondrosarcomas of the spine: adjuvant versus salvage radiation therapy. Spine. 2015; 40(8):544–549

[228] McMaster ML, Goldstein AM, Bromley CM, Ishibe N, Parry DM. Chordoma: incidence and survival patterns in the United States, 1973–1995. Cancer Causes Control. 2001; 12(1):1–11

[229] Park L, Delaney TF, Liebsch NJ, et al. Sacral chordomas: impact of high-dose proton/photon-beam radiation therapy combined with or without surgery for primary versus recurrent tumor. Int J Radiat Oncol Biol Phys. 2006; 65(5):1514–1521

[230] Stacchiotti S, Longhi A, Ferraresi V, et al. Phase II study of imatinib in advanced chordoma. J Clin Oncol. 2012; 30(9):914–920

[231] Chen YL, Liebsch N, Kobayashi W, et al. Definitive high-dose photon/proton radiotherapy for unresected mobile spine and sacral chordomas. Spine. 2013; 38(15):E930–E936

[232] DeLaney TF, Liebsch NJ, Pedlow FX, et al. Long-term results of Phase II study of high dose photon/proton radiotherapy in the management of spine chordomas, chondrosarcomas, and other sarcomas. J Surg Oncol. 2014; 110(2):115–122

[233] Imai R, Kamada T, Tsuji H, et al. Working Group for Bone, Soft Tissue Sarcomas. Carbon ion radiotherapy for unresectable sacral chordomas. Clin Cancer Res. 2004; 10(17):5741–5746

[234] Imai R, Kamada T, Sugahara S, Tsuji H, Tsujii H. Carbon ion radiotherapy for sacral chordoma. Br J Radiol. 2011; 84(Spec No 1):S48–S54

[235] Rotondo RL, Folkert W, Liebsch NJ, et al. High-dose proton-based radiation therapy in the management of spine chordomas: outcomes and clinicopathological prognostic factors. J Neurosurg Spine. 2015; 23(6):788–797

[236] Shives TC, McLeod RA, Unni KK, Schray MF. Chondrosarcoma of the spine. J Bone Joint Surg Am. 1989; 71(8):1158–1165

[237] Rosenberg AE, Nielsen GP, Keel SB, et al. Chondrosarcoma of the base of the skull: a clinicopathologic study of 200 cases with emphasis on its distinction from chordoma. Am J Surg Pathol. 1999; 23(11):1370–1378

[238] Collins MS, Koyama T, Swee RG, Inwards CY. Clear cell chondrosarcoma: radiographic, computed tomographic, and magnetic resonance findings in 34 patients with pathologic correlation. Skeletal Radiol. 2003; 32(12):687–694

[239] Dahlin DC, Beabout JW. Dedifferentiation of low-grade chondrosarcomas. Cancer. 1971; 28(2):461–466

[240] Boriani S, De Iure F, Bandiera S, et al. Chondrosarcoma of the mobile spine: report on 22 cases. Spine. 2000; 25(7):804–812

[241] York JE, Berk RH, Fuller GN, et al. Chondrosarcoma of the spine: 1954 to 1997. J Neurosurg. 1999; 90(1) Suppl:73–78

[242] Strike SA, McCarthy EF. Chondrosarcoma of the spine: a series of 16 cases and a review of the literature. Iowa Orthop J. 2011; 31:154–159

[243] Aoki J, Sone S, Fujioka F, et al. MR of enchondroma and chondrosarcoma: rings and arcs of Gd-DTPA enhancement. J Comput Assist Tomogr. 1991; 15(6):1011–1016

[244] Mesfin A, Ghermandi R, Castiello E, Donati DM, Boriani S. Secondary chondrosarcoma of the lumbar spine in hereditary multiple exostoses. Spine J. 2013; 13(9):1158–1159

[245] Foweraker KL, Burton KE, Maynard SE, et al. High-dose radiotherapy in the management of chordoma and chondrosarcoma of the skull base and cervical spine: part 1—Clinical outcomes. Clin Oncol (R Coll Radiol). 2007; 19(7):509–516

[246] Jiang B, Veeravagu A, Feroze AH, et al. CyberKnife radiosurgery for the management of skull base and spinal chondrosarcomas. J Neurooncol. 2013; 114(2):209–218

[247] Gwak HS, Yoo HJ, Youn SM, et al. Hypofractionated stereotactic radiation therapy for skull base and upper cervical chordoma and chondrosarcoma: preliminary results. Stereotact Funct Neurosurg. 2005; 83(5–6):233–243

[248] Liang X, Wang D, Wang Y, Zhou Z, Zhang J, Li J. Expression of aurora kinase A and B in chondrosarcoma and its relationship with the prognosis. Diagn Pathol. 2012; 7(84):84

[249] Arshi A, Sharim J, Park DY, et al. Prognostic determinants and treatment outcomes analysis of osteosarcoma and Ewing sarcoma of the spine. Spine J. 2017; 17(5):645–655

[250] Marco RAW, Gentry JB, Rhines LD, et al. Ewing's sarcoma of the mobile spine. Spine. 2005; 30(7):769–773

[251] Wan W, Lou Y, Hu Z, et al. Factors affecting survival outcomes of patients with non-metastatic Ewing's sarcoma family tumors in the spine: a retrospective analysis of 63 patients in a single center. J Neurooncol. 2017; 131(2):313–320

[252] Biswas B, Rastogi S, Khan SA, et al. Developing a prognostic model for localized Ewing sarcoma family of tumors: a single institutional experience of 224 cases treated with uniform chemotherapy protocol. J Surg Oncol. 2015; 111(6):683–689

[253] Huang WY, Tan WL, Geng DY, et al. Imaging findings of the spinal peripheral Ewing's sarcoma family of tumours. Clin Radiol. 2014; 69(2):179–185

[254] Ilaslan H, Sundaram M, Unni KK, Dekutoski MB. Primary Ewing's sarcoma of the vertebral column. Skeletal Radiol. 2004; 33(9):506–513

[255] Mirzaei L, Kaal SE, Schreuder HW, Bartels RH. The neurological compromised spine due to Ewing sarcoma. what first: surgery or chemotherapy? Therapy, survival, and neurological outcome of 15 cases with primary Ewing sarcoma of the vertebral column. Neurosurgery. 2015; 77(5):718–724, discussion 724–725

[256] Serlo J, Helenius I, Vettenranta K, et al. Surgically treated patients with axial and peripheral Ewing's sarcoma family of tumours: A population based study in Finland during 1990–2009. Eur J Surg Oncol. 2015; 41(7):893–898

[257] Indelicato DJ, Keole SR, Shahlaee AH, et al. Spinal and paraspinal Ewing tumors. Int J Radiat Oncol Biol Phys. 2010; 76(5):1463–1471

[258] Bacci G, Forni C, Longhi A, et al. Long-term outcome for patients with non-metastatic Ewing's sarcoma treated with adjuvant and neoadjuvant chemotherapies. 402 patients treated at Rizzoli between 1972 and 1992. Eur J Cancer. 2004; 40(1):73–83

[259] Venkateswaran L, Rodriguez-Galindo C, Merchant TE, Poquette CA, Rao BN, Pappo AS. Primary Ewing tumor of the vertebrae: clinical characteristics, prognostic factors, and outcome. Med Pediatr Oncol. 2001; 37(1):30–35

[260] Grubb MR, Currier BL, Pritchard DJ, Ebersold MJ. Primary Ewing's sarcoma of the spine. Spine. 1994; 19(3):309–313

[261] Bacci G, Boriani S, Balladelli A, et al. Treatment of nonmetastatic Ewing's sarcoma family tumors of the spine and sacrum: the experience from a single institution. Eur Spine J. 2009; 18(8):1091–1095

[262] Schuck A, Ahrens S, von Schorlemer I, et al. Radiotherapy in Ewing tumors of the vertebrae: treatment results and local relapse analysis of the CESS 81/86 and EICESS 92 trials. Int J Radiat Oncol Biol Phys. 2005; 63(5):1562–1567

[263] Womer RB, West DC, Krailo MD, et al. Randomized controlled trial of interval-compressed chemotherapy for the treatment of localized Ewing sarcoma: a report from the Children's Oncology Group. J Clin Oncol. 2012; 30(33):4148–4154

[264] Akagunduz OO, Kamer SA, Kececi B, et al. The role of radiotherapy in local control of nonextremity Ewing sarcomas. Tumori. 2016; 102(2):162–167

[265] Barr SJ, Schuette AM, Emans JB. Lumbar pedicle screws versus hooks. Results in double major curves in adolescent idiopathic scoliosis. Spine. 1997; 22(12):1369–1379

[266] Joo MW, Shin SH, Kang YK, et al. Osteosarcoma in Asian populations over the age of 40 years: a multicenter study. Ann Surg Oncol. 2015; 22(11):3557–3564

[267] Klein MJ, Siegal GP. Osteosarcoma: anatomic and histologic variants. Am J Clin Pathol. 2006; 125(4):555–581

[268] Lefebvre G, Renaud A, Rocourt N, Cortet B, Ceugnart L, Cotten A. Primary vertebral osteosarcoma: five cases. Joint Bone Spine. 2013; 80(5):534–537

[269] Mu Y, Zhang H, Che L, Li K. Clinical significance of microRNA-183/Ezrin axis in judging the prognosis of patients with osteosarcoma. Med Oncol. 2014; 31(2):821

[270] Ottaviani G, Jaffe N. The epidemiology of osteosarcomas. In: Jaffe N, Bruland ØS, Bielack S, eds. Pediatric and Adolescent Osteosarcoma. Vol. 152. 1st ed. New York, NY: 2009:3–13. Available at: https://link.springer.com/chapter/10.1007%2F978-1-4419-0284-9_1. Accessed October 3, 2018

[271] Schoenfeld AJ, Hornicek FJ, Pedlow FX, et al. Osteosarcoma of the spine: experience in 26 patients treated at the Massachusetts General Hospital. Spine J. 2010; 10(8):708–714

[272] Kelley SP, Ashford RU, Rao AS, Dickson RA. Primary bone tumours of the spine: a 42-year survey from the Leeds Regional Bone Tumour Registry. Eur Spine J. 2007; 16(3):405–409

[273] Ilaslan H, Sundaram M, Unni KK, Shives TC. Primary vertebral osteosarcoma: imaging findings. Radiology. 2004; 230(3):697–702

[274] Bhatia R, Beckles V, Fox Z, Tirabosco R, Rezajooi K, Casey ATH. Osteosarcoma of the spine: dismal past, any hope for the future? Br J Neurosurg. 2014; 28(4):495–502

[275] Zhu J, Feng Y, Ke Z, et al. Down-regulation of miR-183 promotes migration and invasion of osteosarcoma by targeting Ezrin. Am J Pathol. 2012; 180(6):2440–2451

[276] Zhao H, Guo M, Zhao G, et al. miR-183 inhibits the metastasis of osteosarcoma via downregulation of the expression of Ezrin in F5M2 cells. Int J Mol Med. 2012; 30(5):1013–1020

[277] Lim JBT, Sharma H, MacDuff E, Reece AT. Primary osteosarcoma of the spine: a review of 10 cases. Acta Orthop Belg. 2013; 79(4):457–462

[278] Zils K, Bielack S, Wilhelm M, et al. Osteosarcoma of the mobile spine. Ann Oncol. 2013; 24(8):2190–2195

[279] Sundaresan N, Rosen G, Huvos AG, Krol G. Combined treatment of osteosarcoma of the spine. Neurosurgery. 1988; 23(6):714–719

[280] Bacci G, Picci P, Ferrari S, et al. Primary chemotherapy and delayed surgery for nonmetastatic osteosarcoma of the extremities. Results in 164 patients preoperatively treated with high doses of methotrexate followed by cisplatin and doxorubicin. Cancer. 1993; 72(11):3227–3238

[281] Bielack SS, Kempf-Bielack B, Delling G, et al. Prognostic factors in high-grade osteosarcoma of the extremities or trunk: an analysis of 1,702 patients treated on neoadjuvant cooperative osteosarcoma study group protocols. J Clin Oncol. 2002; 20(3):776–790

[282] Bataille R, Sany J. Solitary myeloma: clinical and prognostic features of a review of 114 cases. Cancer. 1981; 48(3):845–851

[283] Dimopoulos MA, Moulopoulos LA, Maniatis A, Alexanian R. Solitary plasmacytoma of bone and asymptomatic multiple myeloma. Blood. 2000; 96(6):2037–2044

[284] Huang W, Cao D, Ma J, et al. Solitary plasmacytoma of cervical spine: treatment and prognosis in patients with neurological lesions and spinal instability. Spine. 2010; 35(8):E278–E284

[285] Qian Y, Jing J, Tian D, Yang H. Partial tumor resection combined with chemotherapy for multiple myeloma spinal cord compression. Ann Surg Oncol. 2014; 21(11):3661–3667

[286] Rehak S, Maisnar V, Malek V, et al. Diagnosis and surgical therapy of plasma cell neoplasia of the spine. Neoplasma. 2009; 56(1):84–87

[287] Zhang J, Zhong Y. Clinical analysis of 36 multiple myeloma patients with extramedullary plasmacytoma invasion of the spinal canal. Hematol Oncol. 2015; 33(2):75–79

[288] Amelot A, Moles A, Cristini J, et al. Predictors of survival in patients with surgical spine multiple myeloma metastases. Surg Oncol. 2016; 25 (3):178–183

[289] Zadnik PL, Goodwin CR, Karami KJ, et al. Outcomes following surgical intervention for impending and gross instability caused by multiple myeloma in the spinal column. J Neurosurg Spine. 2015; 22(3):301–309

[290] Wilder RB, Ha CS, Cox JD, Weber D, Delasalle K, Alexanian R. Persistence of myeloma protein for more than one year after radiotherapy is an adverse prognostic factor in solitary plasmacytoma of bone. Cancer. 2002; 94(5): 1532–1537

[291] Ozsahin M, Tsang RW, Poortmans P, et al. Outcomes and patterns of failure in solitary plasmacytoma: a multicenter Rare Cancer Network study of 258 patients. Int J Radiat Oncol Biol Phys. 2006; 64(1):210–217

[292] Avilés A, Huerta-Guzmán J, Delgado S, Fernández A, Díaz-Maqueo JC. Improved outcome in solitary bone plasmacytomata with combined therapy. Hematol Oncol. 1996; 14(3):111–117

20 Metastatic Disease of the Thoracic Spinal Column

Ori Barzilai, Mark H. Bilsky, and Ilya Laufer

Abstract

Therapy for metastatic tumor treatment serves a palliative function and must be directed toward improvement of the patient's quality of life. The goals of spinal metastatic tumor treatment include restoration or preservation of neurological function and spinal column stability, pain relief, and local tumor control. NOMS provides an evidence-based decision framework for treatment plan development in patients with spinal metastases and consists of neurological, oncological, mechanical, and systemic considerations. Data demonstrating the ability of SRS to safely deliver ablative radiation doses and achieve durable local control has revolutionized the type and extent of surgical procedures currently utilized. Extensive, often morbid, surgeries aiming for complete tumor removal or cytoreduction are being replaced with less invasive surgical options such as separation surgery or minimally invasive procedures. Separation surgery is a posterolateral approach to circumferential spinal cord decompression and stabilization. Minimally invasive surgeries (MISs) are currently used often as they entail limited perioperative morbidity, allow for quick recovery, and have shown to lead to less blood loss, low transfusion rates, and short hospitalizations. Spinal instability neoplastic score facilitates diagnosis of spinal mechanical instability, with patients with instability requiring cement or instrumented stabilization. Familiarity with the surgical, radiation, and systemic therapy options allows tailoring of optimal treatment strategy.

Keywords: spine, tumor, MESCC, NOMS, separation surgery, radiosurgery, SRS

Clinical Pearls

- Back pain in cancer patients should trigger magnetic resonance imaging in order to determine the presence of spinal metastases.
- NOMS provides evidence-based decision framework for treatment plan development in patients with spinal metastases and consists of neurological, oncological, mechanical, and systemic considerations.
- Primary tumor histology determines the optimal radiotherapy selection, with radiosensitive tumors responding to conventionally fractionated radiotherapy and radioresistant tumors requiring stereotactic radiosurgery for durable control.
- Patients with spinal cord compression due to solid tumor metastases require surgical decompression and stabilization followed by radiotherapy.
- Spinal instability neoplastic score facilitates diagnosis of spinal mechanical instability, with patients with instability requiring cement- or instrumented stabilization.

20.1 Introduction

The number of people requiring treatment for spinal metastatic tumors continues to increase due to increasing elderly population and improved survival of cancer patients. The goals of spinal metastatic tumor treatment include restoration or preservation of neurological function and spinal column stability, pain relief, and local tumor control. Therapy for metastatic tumor treatment serves a palliative function and must be directed toward improvement of the patient's quality of life. Familiarity with the surgical-, radio-, and systemic therapy options allows selection of optimal treatment strategy. The current chapter focuses on the presentation, diagnosis and decision-making, and surgery for spinal metastases.

20.2 Diagnostic Evaluation

20.2.1 Back Pain

Metastatic tumors frequently present with pain. Biological and mechanical pain represent the two primary pain patterns. Biological pain generally increases in severity during the night or early morning, without a clear exacerbation by movement. While the etiology of this pain pattern required further research, the pain is likely due to tumor-associated inflammation and the diurnal variation of endogenous steroid production playing a likely role and lower steroid production during the night contributing to increased pain. This hypothesis is supported by the pain relief, generally achieved by administration of glucocorticoids. Pain relief after glucocorticoid administration generally serves as a good predictor of pain relief after radiotherapy. On the other hand, mechanical pain becomes more severe with movement and does not respond to steroid administration. Mechanical pain is generally attributable to vertebral fractures and requires surgical stabilization. In the thoracic spine, mechanical back pain is often elicited with recumbency or position change. Pain attributable to fractures in the thoracolumbar junction generally radiates to the lumbar spine. Gathering of back pain history may facilitate differentiation of biological and mechanical pain patters. During the physical examination patients should be observed while supine, sitting, standing, and ambulating and during position changes in order to make note of pain during movement that would be consistent with symptoms of mechanical instability.

20.2.2 Neurological Symptoms

Neurological symptoms generally develop after the prodrome of back pain and may consist of radiculopathy due to nerve root compression or myelopathy due to compression of the spinal cord. Pain radiating into the arm, leg, or band-like thoracic pain may be indicative of nerve root compression caused by tumor.

The development of neurological deficits attributable to compression of the spinal cord may have a variable time course and severity. Patients may experience ataxia or loss of proprioception, diminished sensation, paresthesia, weakness, and disturbances in bowel or bladder function. Radicular thoracic pain generally presents as unilateral or bilateral band-like pain radiating around the thorax and radiculopathy due to T1 tumors may radiate to the axilla or hand. Signs and symptoms of thoracic spinal cord compression may include diminished or altered sensation below the level of the tumor, ataxia and leg weakness, and bowel and bladder dysfunction. Neurological examination consists of proprioception, light touch and pin-prick sensation, muscle strength assessment, ambulation and testing for clonus, hyperreflexia, and Babinski's sign.

20.2.3 Imaging

Back pain or neurological symptoms or radiculopathy or myelopathy in cancer patients should trigger urgent magnetic resonance (MR) imaging of the spine. While X-rays may serve as an initial screen for fractures, they lack the soft tissue definition required for diagnosis of spinal tumors. Imaging of the full spinal axis is generally recommended since patients frequently present with multifocal spinal metastases. MR imaging has excellent sensitivity and specificity for osseous metastases, epidural and paraspinal tumor extension, and evaluation of the degree of spinal cord compression. Computed tomography (CT) imaging provides additional information about the osseous structure and may be useful in evaluation of fractures. CT imaging of the chest, abdomen, and pelvis or whole-body positron emission tomography imaging are required to assess the systemic tumor burden, and play an important role in therapeutic decision making.

20.3 Treatment Strategies

20.3.1 NOMS

Treatment goals for patients with spine metastases are palliative and include preservation or restoration of neurological function, maintenance of spinal stability, palliation of pain, and durable local tumor control. There are several treatment options including surgery, systemic therapy, radiation therapy, or combinations of these modalities. Selecting the optimal treatment in this complicated population is challenging and recent technological advancement, particularly in the field of radiosurgery along with advancement in systemic therapy owed to new biological treatments, complicates decision-making. The NOMS framework, consisting of **n**eurological, **o**ncological, **m**echanical, and **s**ystemic considerations, facilitates clear patient description and treatment decisions. This framework incorporates evidence-based treatment recommendations and can also be adopted to incorporate new technology and therapies. The neurological and oncological considerations are used in concert in order to determine the optimal radiotherapy and to determine whether the patient requires surgical decompression. The mechanical consideration serves as an independent indication for intervention, since spinal instability represents a mechanical problem requiring mechanical repair, such as

cement or instrumented stabilization. The systemic consideration looks at the patient's survival prognosis, extent of metastatic tumor burden, and medical comorbidities in order to determine whether they can tolerate the proposed treatment plan.

Neurological

The neurological evaluation combines a clinical examination and radiological evaluation. Clinically, patients are assessed for myelopathy or functional radiculopathy. The radiological evaluation focuses on the degree of epidural spinal cord compression (ESCC). Generally, it is not expected to find myelopathy on physical examination without radiographic evidence of epidural cord compression. Thus, although myelopathy on physical examination is an important factor, most of the weight of decision making relies on the degree of ESCC.

The degree of ESCC is evaluated using a three-point scale originally developed by Bilsky et al and validated by the Spine Oncology Study Group (SOSG).[1] The ESCC scale consists of six grades of compression: grade 0, grade 1A, grade 1B, grade 1C, grade 2, and grade 3. Grade 0 signifies bone-only disease; 1A, epidural impingement, without deformation of the thecal sac; 1B, deformation of the thecal sac, without spinal cord abutment; 1C, deformation of the thecal sac with spinal cord abutment, but without cord compression; 2, spinal cord compression, but with cerebrospinal fluid (CSF) visible around the cord; and 3, spinal cord compression, no CSF visible around the cord (▶ Fig. 20.1).

Oncological

The oncological evaluation accounts for the tumor histological type and responsiveness to available therapies. Modern anti-cancer treatments are revolutionizing cancer care and to date, these therapies include conformal external beam radio therapy (cEBRT), stereotactic radiosurgery (SRS), chemotherapy, hormones, immunotherapy, or biologics. Albeit the major advancements in cancer care, the mainstay of treatment for spinal metastasis remains radiation treatment. Historically, cERBT was adopted as the standard of care for patients with spinal metastases of all histologies.[2] With surgical advancement and improved instrumentation, stronger evidence in support of combination surgical decompression combined with cEBRT became available.[3,4,5] cEBRT delivers radiation through one to two beams to a treatment field that includes, but is not confined to, the tumor area. As there are organs at risk (OAR), particularly the spinal cord, within the radiation field, the dose of radiation is limited.[6] Tumors are considered either radioresistant or radiosensitive depending on the response to cEBRT.[7,8,9] Clinically, this results in the lower median response duration after cEBRT, repeatedly seen in radioresistant histologies in the literature.[10,11,12] Lymphoma, seminoma, and myeloma are considered radiosensitive histologies along with solid tumors such as breast, prostate, ovarian, and neuroendocrine.[10,13] Renal, thyroid, hepatocellular, colon, and non-small cell lung carcinomas, sarcoma, and melanoma represent radioresistant tumors.[8,9,10,13] It is important to realize that regardless of the degree of ESCC, patients with radiosensitive tumors can be treated effectively with cEBRT.[7,9]

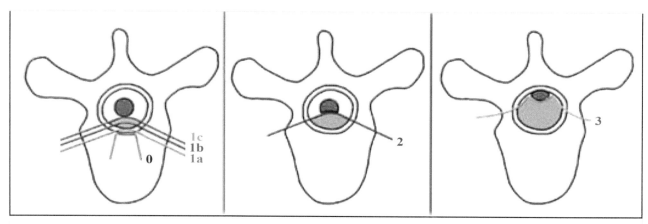

Schematic representation of the 6-point ESCC grading scale.

Grade 0	Bone-only disease
Grade 1a	Epidural impingment, without deformation of thecal sac
Grade 1b	Deformation of thecal sac, without spinal cord abutment
Grade 1c	Deformation of thecal sac, with spinal cord abutment, without cord compression
Grade 2	Spinal cord compression, with cerebral spinal fluid (CSF) visible around the cord
Grade 3	Spinal cord compression, no CSF visible around the cord

Fig. 20.1 Epidural spinal cord compression (ESCC) score. (Adapted with permission from Bilsky MH, Laufer I, Fourney DR, Groff M, Schmidt MH, Varga PP, Vrionis FD, Yamada Y, Gerszten PC, Kuklo TR. Reliability analysis of the epidural spinal cord compression scale. J Neurosurg Spine. 2010 Sep;13 (3):324-8.)

In contrast, radiosurgery can provide conformal high-dose per fraction radiation optimizing the dosimetry while minimizing injury to OARs. The safe and effective implementation of SRS is a result of technological advancements in noninvasive patient immobilization; intensity-modulated image-guided radiation therapy (IGRT) delivery systems, and sophisticated planning software.[14,15] Accordingly, SRS yields a clinical benefit regardless of histology, providing a more durable symptomatic response and higher local control rate.[5,12,16,17,18] To unify treatment planning, the International Spine Radiosurgery Consortium updated contouring and planning guidelines for spinal radiosurgery planning[19,20] and recent consensus guidelines have also been created for postoperative target contouring.[21]

Mechanical

Mechanical instability serves as an indication for surgery regardless of the degree of ESCC or the radiosensitivity of the tumor as radiotherapy and systemic therapy do not restore mechanical stability of the spine. Evaluation of spinal stability is an important consideration independent from both the cancer and neurological assessments. Pathological fracture from tumor and traumatic fracture represent different pathologies and thus have distinct biomechanical implications. In order to ease the assessment of mechanical stability and to unify reporting the SOSG developed a scoring system; the spinal instability neoplastic score (SINS) (▶ Table 20.1). SINS accounts for six parameters: location, pain, alignment, lesion character (i.e., lytic vs. blastic), vertebral body collapse, and posterior element involvement. High SINSs[3,11,22,23,24,25] are considered unstable and require surgical stabilization, low SINSs (0–6) are considered stable, and intermediate SINSs (7–12) are considered potentially unstable. The intermediate lesions are evaluated and treated on case-to-case basis at the discretion of the spine surgeon.[22]

Table 20.1 Spinal instability neoplastic score[22]

SINS component		Score
Location	Junctional (occiput-C2, C7-T2, T11-L1, L5-S1)	3
	Mobile spine (C3-C6, L2-L4)	2
	Semi-rigid (T3-T10)	1
	Rigid (S2-S5)	0
Pain	Yes	3
	Occasional pain but not mechanical	1
	Pain-free lesion	0
Bone lesion	Lytic	2
	Mixed (lytic/blastic)	1
	Blastic	0
Radiographic spinal alignment	Subluxation/translation present	4
	De novo deformity (kyphosis/scoliosis)	2
	Normal alignment	0
Vertebral body collapse	>50% collapse	3
	<50% collapse	2
	No collapse with >50% body involved	1
	None of the above	0
Posterolateral involvement of spinal elements	Bilateral	3
	Unilateral	1
	None of the above	0
Total	Stable	0-6
	Indeterminate	7-12
	Unstable	13-18

Systemic

The systemic evaluation of NOMS relates to the patients' comorbidities, overall disease burden, and ability to withstand the proposed treatment. As treatment for metastatic spine disease is of palliative nature, estimation of the expected survival and overall risk–benefit ratio are of great importance. Treatment goals are focused on whether the patients are likely to adequately recover from the indicated procedure and continue systemic therapy. Patients most often undergo an MR imaging of the entire spinal axis and histology-specific staging. Medical workup should be directed toward known patient comorbidities, but often includes pulmonary function tests, Dopplers, and echocardiogram.

The prevention, diagnosis, treatment, and general management of cancer have recently been influenced by major scientific advances. Modern technologies allow for the assessment of genomic and proteomic alterations and epigenetic and posttranslational modifications at the molecular level.[23] The understanding

of how these influence tumors of the spine is ongoing. Albeit focus has been directed largely to nonspinal tumors, interest in understanding the effect on spine cancer is growing.[24,25]

20.3.2 Surgical Techniques

The spine surgeon's armamentarium for treatment of metastatic ESCC has significantly grown in recent years owing to technological and engineering advancements. Extensive, often morbid, surgeries aiming for complete tumor removal or cytoreduction are being replaced with less invasive surgical options such as separation surgery or minimally invasive procedures. Data demonstrating the ability of SRS to safely deliver ablative radiation doses and achieve durable local control have brought forth separation surgery. Separation surgery employs a posterolateral approach to circumferential spinal cord decompression and stabilization. No attempt for cytoreduction is made and the bulk of the tumor is often left in situ (▶ Fig. 20.2). The rationale

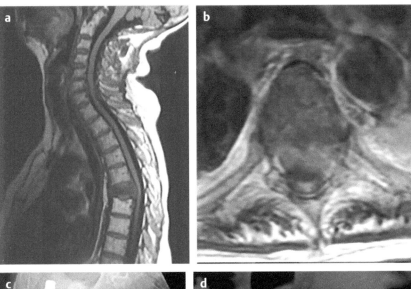
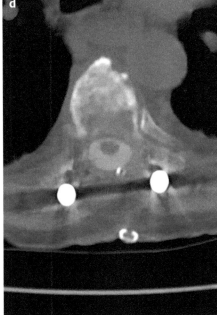

Fig. 20.2 A 61-year-old woman with history of non-small cell lung carcinoma developed interscapular pain was diagnosed with T6 metastasis. (a) Sagittal and (b) axial MR images showing a T6 pathological compression fracture with high-grade epidural tumor extension and spinal cord compression. Patient underwent separation surgery with T4-8 posterolateral instrumented stabilization (c) and T5-7 laminectomy with transpedicular circumferential spinal cord decompression (d).

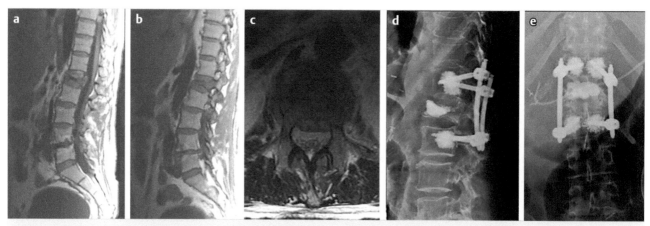

Fig. 20.3 A 78-year-old man with history of metastatic colon adenocarcinoma developed severe lower back pain exacerbated by movement. Sagittal **(a,b)** MR images showing L1 pathological burst fracture with extension into posterior elements, without high-grade epidural tumor extension on axial imaging **(c)**. Patient underwent percutaneous T12-L2 instrumented stabilization with screw cement augmentation and L1 balloon kyphoplasty **(d,e)**.

for this surgery arises from data demonstrating that SRS treatment failures occur when less than 15 Gy is delivered to a portion of the clinical treatment volume[6] and this dose cannot be delivered to the entire tumor margin without risking spinal cord injury unless a safe distance between the tumor and the spinal cord is created.[3] Therefore, separating the tumor from the spinal cord, creating a 1 to 2 mm distance, allows for optimal SRS planning with adequate dosimetry and low morbidity. This method of separation surgery with concomitant radiosurgery has been shown to be safe and effective in achieving durable local tumor control in several patient series.[4,11,26] More extensive open surgical approaches including corpectomies and combined anterior–posterior approaches[12,16] are sometimes necessary, particularly in the setting of deformity; however, these are becoming less frequent due to enhanced collaboration between oncologists and surgeons allowing for earlier referral and integration of SRS to the treatment plan. In centers and regions without SRS, more aggressive surgeries are still warranted, especially in metastases with known resistance to cEBRT and some centers and literature still support more aggressive surgeries including en bloc resections,[17] particularly in the setting of solitary renal cell and thyroid spine metastases.

Minimally invasive surgeries (MISs) are currently used often as they entail limited perioperative morbidity, allow for quick recovery, and have shown to lead to less blood loss, low transfusion rates, and short hospitalizations.[18,27,28,29] Rapid recovery and return to systemic treatment is an important goal in patients with spinal tumors. Unlike open surgeries where the risk of wound complications frequently delays radiation therapy, with MIS, radiation can sometimes be started within a week surgery.[2,30] Current MIS techniques for the treatment of spinal metastases include percutaneous instrumentation, mini-open approaches for decompression,[5] and tumor removal with or without tubular/expandable retractors and thoracoscopy/endoscopy (▶ Fig. 20.3).

Often, the indication for intervention is based on mechanical instability alone, without a need to decompress the spinal cord. Several options are available for stabilization in the setting of a pathological fracture. Traditionally, stabilization was achieved

via open surgery with low complication rates.[31] Recent advances in MIS techniques, in particular, intraoperative navigation systems and improved pedicle screw and rod systems, have led percutaneous stabilization to be used extensively. Percutaneous approaches spare the paraspinal musculature and posterior elements.[32] To overcome poor bone quality in cancer patients (due to the osteolytic tumors, chemotherapy, radiation, and other comorbidities), new systems have been developed including fenestrated pedicle screws (for injection of polymethylmethacrylate bone cement through the screw) and expandable screws, both methods aim to reduce pullout rates.[33,34,35] Another widely accepted stabilizing method is percutaneous cement augmentation. Evidence strongly supports kyphoplasty and vertebroplasty for symptomatic compression fractures due to metastatic disease.[36,37,38,39] Prospective randomized data have showed significant pain reduction and improvement in disability indexes that persist for up to 6 months when kyphoplasty was performed compared to a noninterventional control arm in patients with tumorous compression fractures.[38] This has been demonstrated in other data supporting kyphoplasty for symptomatic osteolytic tumors to control pain, provided that no overt instability or myelopathy is present.[36,37] Likewise, pain reduction has been shown after vertebroplasty in patients with spinal metastases.[40]

References

[1] Bilsky MH, Laufer I, Fourney DR, et al. Reliability analysis of the epidural spinal cord compression scale. J Neurosurg Spine. 2010; 13(3):324–328

[2] Yang Z, Yang Y, Zhang Y, et al. Minimal access versus open spinal surgery in treating painful spine metastasis: a systematic review. World J Surg Oncol. 2015; 13:68

[3] Yamada Y, Bilsky MH, Lovelock DM, et al. High-dose, single-fraction image-guided intensity-modulated radiotherapy for metastatic spinal lesions. Int J Radiat Oncol Biol Phys. 2008; 71(2):484–490

[4] Moulding HD, Elder JB, Lis E, et al. Local disease control after decompressive surgery and adjuvant high-dose single-fraction radiosurgery for spine metastases. J Neurosurg Spine. 2010; 13(1):87–93

[5] Donnelly DJ, Abd-El-Barr MM, Lu Y. Minimally invasive muscle sparing posterior-only approach for lumbar circumferential decompression and stabilization to treat spine metastasis—technical report. World Neurosurg. 2015; 84 (5):1484–1490

[6] Lovelock DM, Zhang Z, Jackson A, et al. Correlation of local failure with measures of dose insufficiency in the high-dose single-fraction treatment of bony metastases. Int J Radiat Oncol Biol Phys. 2010; 77(4):1282–1287

[7] Gerszten PC, Mendel E, Yamada Y. Radiotherapy and radiosurgery for metastatic spine disease: what are the options, indications, and outcomes? Spine. 2009; 34(22) Suppl:S78–S92

[8] Mizumoto M, Harada H, Asakura H, et al. Radiotherapy for patients with metastases to the spinal column: a review of 603 patients at Shizuoka Cancer Center Hospital. Int J Radiat Oncol Biol Phys. 2011; 79(1):208–213

[9] Maranzano E, Latini P. Effectiveness of radiation therapy without surgery in metastatic spinal cord compression: final results from a prospective trial. Int J Radiat Oncol Biol Phys. 1995; 32(4):959–967

[10] Rades D, Fehlauer F, Stalpers LJ, et al. A prospective evaluation of two radiotherapy schedules with 10 versus 20 fractions for the treatment of metastatic spinal cord compression: final results of a multicenter study. Cancer. 2004; 101(11):2687–2692

[11] Laufer I, Iorgulescu JB, Chapman T, et al. Local disease control for spinal metastases following "separation surgery" and adjuvant hypofractionated or high-dose single-fraction stereotactic radiosurgery: outcome analysis in 186 patients. J Neurosurg Spine. 2013; 18(3):207–214

[12] Fang T, Dong J, Zhou X, McGuire RA, Jr, Li X. Comparison of mini-open anterior corpectomy and posterior total en bloc spondylectomy for solitary metastases of the thoracolumbar spine. J Neurosurg Spine. 2012; 17(4):271–279

[13] Rades D, Fehlauer F, Schulte R, et al. Prognostic factors for local control and survival after radiotherapy of metastatic spinal cord compression. J Clin Oncol. 2006; 24(21):3388–3393

[14] Alongi F, Arcangeli S, Filippi AR, Ricardi U, Scorsetti M. Review and uses of stereotactic body radiation therapy for oligometastases. Oncologist. 2012; 17 (8):1100–1107

[15] Chang BK, Timmerman RD. Stereotactic body radiation therapy: a comprehensive review. Am J Clin Oncol. 2007; 30(6):637–644

[16] Molina C, Goodwin CR, Abu-Bonsrah N, Elder BD, De la Garza Ramos R, Sciubba DM. Posterior approaches for symptomatic metastatic spinal cord compression. Neurosurg Focus. 2016; 41(2):E11

[17] Cloyd JM, Acosta FL, Jr, Polley MY, Ames CP. En bloc resection for primary and metastatic tumors of the spine: a systematic review of the literature. Neurosurgery. 2010; 67(2):435–444, discussion 444–445

[18] Hansen-Algenstaedt N, Kwan MK, Algenstaedt P, et al. Comparison between minimally invasive surgery and conventional open surgery for patients with spinal metastasis: a prospective propensity score-matched study. Spine. 2017; 42(10):789–797

[19] Cox BW, Spratt DE, Lovelock M, et al. International Spine Radiosurgery Consortium consensus guidelines for target volume definition in spinal stereotactic radiosurgery. Int J Radiat Oncol Biol Phys. 2012; 83(5):e597–e605

[20] Potters L, Kavanagh B, Galvin JM, et al. American Society for Therapeutic Radiology and Oncology, American College of Radiology. American Society for Therapeutic Radiology and Oncology (ASTRO) and American College of Radiology (ACR) practice guideline for the performance of stereotactic body radiation therapy. Int J Radiat Oncol Biol Phys. 2010; 76(2):326–332

[21] Redmond KJ, Lo SS, Soltys SG, et al. Consensus guidelines for postoperative stereotactic body radiation therapy for spinal metastases: results of an international survey. J Neurosurg Spine. 2017; 26(3):299–230

[22] Fourney DR, Frangou EM, Ryken TC, et al. Spinal instability neoplastic score: an analysis of reliability and validity from the spine oncology study group. J Clin Oncol. 2011; 29(22):3072–3077

[23] Goodwin CR, Abu-Bonsrah N, Bilsky MH, et al. Clinical decision making: integrating advances in the molecular understanding of spine tumors. Spine. 2016; 41 Suppl 20:S171–S177

[24] Caruso JP, Cohen-Inbar O, Bilsky MH, Gerszten PC, Sheehan JP. Stereotactic radiosurgery and immunotherapy for metastatic spinal melanoma. Neurosurg Focus. 2015; 38(3):E6

[25] Shankar GM, Choi BD, Grannan BL, Oh K, Shin JH. Effect of immunotherapy status on outcomes in patients with metastatic melanoma to the spine. Spine. 2017; 42(12):E721–E725

[26] Rock JP, Ryu S, Shukairy MS, et al. Postoperative radiosurgery for malignant spinal tumors. Neurosurgery. 2006; 58(5):891–898, discussion 891–898

[27] Hikata T, Isogai N, Shiono Y, et al. A retrospective cohort study comparing the safety and efficacy of minimally invasive versus open surgical techniques in the treatment of spinal metastases. Clin Spine Surg. 2017; 30(8):E1082–E1087

[28] Rao PJ, Thayaparan GK, Fairhall JM, Mobbs RJ. Minimally invasive percutaneous fixation techniques for metastatic spinal disease. Orthop Surg. 2014; 6 (3):187–195

[29] Kumar N, Malhotra R, Maharajan K, et al. Metastatic spine tumor surgery: a comparative study of minimally invasive approach using percutaneous pedicle screws fixation versus open approach. Clin Spine Surg. 2017; 30(8): E1015–E1021

[30] Disa JJ, Smith AW, Bilsky MH. Management of radiated reoperative wounds of the cervicothoracic spine: the role of the trapezius turnover flap. Ann Plast Surg. 2001; 47(4):394–397

[31] Amankulor NM, Xu R, Iorgulescu JB, et al. The incidence and patterns of hardware failure after separation surgery in patients with spinal metastatic tumors. Spine J. 2014; 14(9):1850–1859

[32] Kim CH, Chung CK, Sohn S, Lee S, Park SB. Less invasive palliative surgery for spinal metastases. J Surg Oncol. 2013; 108(7):499–503

[33] Frankel BM, Jones T, Wang C. Segmental polymethylmethacrylate-augmented pedicle screw fixation in patients with bone softening caused by osteoporosis and metastatic tumor involvement: a clinical evaluation. Neurosurgery. 2007; 61(3):531–537, discussion 537–538

[34] Elder BD, Lo SF, Holmes C, et al. The biomechanics of pedicle screw augmentation with cement. Spine J. 2015; 15(6):1432–1445

[35] Gazzeri R, Roperto R, Fiore C. Surgical treatment of degenerative and traumatic spinal diseases with expandable screws in patients with osteoporosis: 2-year follow-up clinical study. J Neurosurg Spine. 2016; 25(5):610–619

[36] Mendel E, Bourekas E, Gerszten P, Golan JD. Percutaneous techniques in the treatment of spine tumors: what are the diagnostic and therapeutic indications and outcomes? Spine. 2009; 34(22) Suppl:S93–S100

[37] Papanastassiou ID, Filis AK, Gerochristou MA, Vrionis FD. Controversial issues in kyphoplasty and vertebroplasty in malignant vertebral fractures. Cancer Contr. 2014; 21(2):151–157

[38] Berenson J, Pflugmacher R, Jarzem P, et al. Cancer Patient Fracture Evaluation (CAFE) Investigators. Balloon kyphoplasty versus non-surgical fracture management for treatment of painful vertebral body compression fractures in patients with cancer: a multicentre, randomised controlled trial. Lancet Oncol. 2011; 12(3):225–235

[39] Fourney DR, Schomer DF, Nader R, et al. Percutaneous vertebroplasty and kyphoplasty for painful vertebral body fractures in cancer patients. J Neurosurg. 2003; 98(1) Suppl:21–30

[40] Xie P, Zhao Y, Li G. Efficacy of percutaneous vertebroplasty in patients with painful vertebral metastases: a retrospective study in 47 cases. Clin Neurol Neurosurg. 2015; 138:157–161

21 Intradural Extramedullary Tumors

Ibrahim Hussain and Ali A. Baaj

Abstract

Intradural extramedullary tumors of the thoracic spine are predominantly meningiomas, schwannomas, and neurofibromas. Other lesions, like lymphoma or metastases, can occur but are far less likely. While most of these lesions are benign and rarely progress to malignant forms, surgical resection is indicated for tumors that cause spinal cord compression or become symptomatic. Even for ventrally situated tumors, a posterior or posterolateral approach can result in adequate decompression in most cases. Instrumented fusion in association with tumor resection should be considered for lesions that require laminectomies at three or more levels, junctional levels, or when bilateral facetectomies are required. All patients should have neurophysiologic monitoring during the procedure to prevent catastrophic spinal cord injury by reversible causes. Gross total resection is curative in most cases; however, adjuvant radiation has shown benefit for recurrent tumors.

Keywords: intradural extramedullary, spinal cord, tumor, schwannoma, meningioma, neurofibroma

---

Clinical Pearls

- Surgical resection is the gold standard for the treatment of symptomatic intradural extramedullary (IDEM) thoracic tumors or those with radiographic evidence of spinal cord compression.
- Radiosurgery has shown benefit as a primary treatment modality or as adjuvant treatment for recurrent tumors; however, this is an area of current research.
- Most thoracic IDEM tumors can be resected safely from a posterolateral approach, precluding high-risk lateral and anterior approaches.
- Instrumented fusion should be considered for tumors that require three or more laminectomies for dural exposure, or for those at transitional levels.
- Intraoperative neurophysiologic monitoring (somatosensory evoked potentials and motor evoked potentials) should be used on all surgeries to prevent spinal cord injury from reversible causes, including spinal cord rotation maneuvers and low mean arterial pressures leading to spinal cord hypoperfusion.

21.1 Introduction

Intradural extramedullary (IDEM) tumors occur in the thoracic spine in 26 to 29% of cases[1,2] and can cause significant morbidity by spinal cord compression or involvement of thoracic nerve roots. While these tumors can present in individuals of all ages, in the pediatric population they are most often associated with leptomeningeal metastases from intracranial tumors.[3] In the adult population, there are broadly three tumor subtypes which predominate, which are meningiomas, schwannomas, and neurofibromas (the latter two are often grouped together as nerve sheath tumors). Presenting symptoms include localized thoracic back pain, radicular pain, dermatomal paresthesias, and myelopathy. Optimal management is based on a number of factors, including age at presentation, symptomatology, radiographic degree of spinal cord compression, rate of growth, and location within the thecal sac. The focus of this chapter will be on these three tumor types; however, a subset of rarer tumors can also be seen in the thoracic IDEM compartment, including metastases, paragangliomas, epidermoid, hemangiomas, and lymphoma.[4,5]

21.2 Tumor Subtypes

21.2.1 Meningioma

Meningiomas of the spinal canal account for 25 to 45% of all IDEM spinal tumors.[6] While histologically similar to those seen intracranially, spinal meningiomas account for only 2% of all central nervous system meningiomas.[7] These tumors have a nearly 4:1 predilection for the female sex in adults, for reasons that remain to be elucidated, and are most commonly diagnosed in the fifth and sixth decades of life. Histopathologically, the vast majority are World Health Organization grade I, and rarely progress to higher grades. In this regard, invasion of the spinal cord is typically not seen; however, long-standing tumors can be scarred to the spinal cord making a distinct plane difficult to distinguish. These tumors are over three times as likely to form in the thoracic spine compared with the cervical spine and are exceedingly rare in the lumbar spine.[7]

There is a strong association of these tumors forming in the context of neurofibromatosis type 2 (NF2). This inherited cancer predisposition syndrome is caused by mutation in the *NF2* gene on chromosome 22. A diagnosis of multiple intradural meningiomas should prompt investigation into this genetic syndrome, which are characterized by café au lait spots and the development of intracranial schwannomas (most commonly vestibular schwannomas).

21.2.2 Nerve Sheath Tumors

IDEM nerve sheath tumors can be divided into two primary subtypes, schwannomas and neurofibromas. These tumors are usually indistinguishable on imaging and require histopathology to obtain a definitive diagnosis. Schwannomas are the most common IDEM tumors of the spine in general; however, these are less commonly seen in the thoracic spine compared with meningiomas. These tumors are benign and arise from the Schwann cells of nerve roots. Pathologic evaluation of schwannomas demonstrates spindled (Antoni A) areas and microcystic (Antoni B) areas comprised of macrophages and collagen, and tumors express S100 protein on immunohistochemistry.[8] Neurofibromas not only arise from Schwann cells, but also incorporate nonneoplastic nerve components, including axons, perineural cells, and fibroblasts.[8] As with IDEM meningiomas, multiple IDEM schwannomas should raise the suspicious of NF2. Moreover, in a similar regard, both schwannomas and neurofibromas have the ability to transform into malignant peripheral nerve sheath tumors which are aggressive tumors that carry poor prognosis and most commonly observed in patients with a history of NF1.[9]

21.3 Imaging Characteristics

Gadolinium contrast-enhanced magnetic resonance imaging is the primary imaging modality used for diagnosis of thoracic IDEM tumors. Meningiomas homogenously contrast enhance and are well circumscribed. A broad-based dural attachment and/or a dural tail indicating the initial growth point of the tumor are commonly seen (▶ Fig. 21.1 and ▶ Fig. 21.2). T1- and T2-weighted hypointensities can indicate calcifications as seen with their intracranial counterparts. Computed tomography (CT) imaging should be considered for patients that will require instrumented fusion following resection to assess for bony anatomy and quality. CT imaging may also more clearly demonstrate calcifications in the region of the tumor or dural margin (most commonly with meningiomas) and posterior vertebral body scalloping due to long-standing mass effect (most commonly with schwannomas). Unlike intracranial meningiomas, hyperostosis of surround bony structures is typically not seen when confined to the intradural compartment.

Schwannomas can demonstrate solid and cystic regions that heterogeneously contrast enhance due to internal hemorrhage or intracystic fluid signal intensity. These tumors are also more likely to present with intradural and extradural components (▶ Fig. 21.3 and ▶ Fig. 21.4), sometimes forming a characteristic dumbbell shape, as the tumor expands on the medial and lateral side of the foramen that it exits. CT imaging may demonstrate bony remodeling from these slow-growing tumors, including expanded foramen, thinned pedicles, and/or posterior vertebral bodies scalloping.

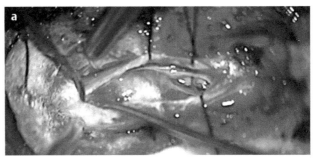
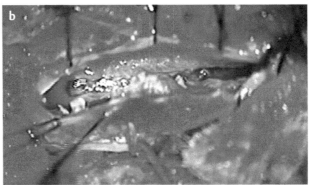
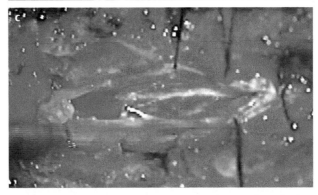

Fig. 21.2 Intraoperative photographs of a dorsally located intradural extramedullary meningioma. **(a)** The tumor is apparent immediately after dural opening. Dural edges are tacked up with 4–0 nylon sutures to aid in visualization and to prevent blood from entering the subarachnoid space. **(b)** After partial debulking, note the broad based dural attachment of the tumor. **(c)** Following complete resection of the tumor, the dorsal surface of the spinal cord is visualized and decompressed.

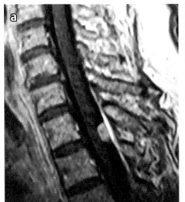
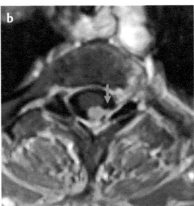
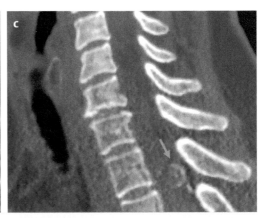

Fig. 21.1 **(a)** Sagittal and **(b)** axial T1 postcontrast MRI of a high thoracic intradural extramedullary (IDEM) meningioma. Note the broad dural attachment and dural tail (*arrow*). **(c)** Sagittal CT image of the same IDEM meningioma with characteristic calcifications (*arrow*), as commonly seen with intracranial meningiomas.

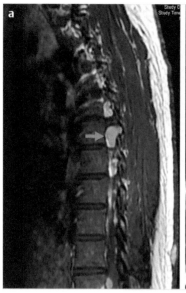
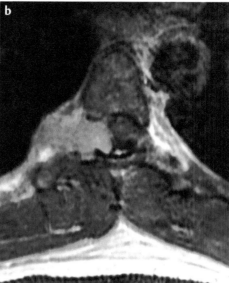

Fig. 21.3 (a) Sagittal and (b) axial T1 postcontrast MRI of a high thoracic intradural extramedullary schwannoma. Note extension of the tumor along the exiting nerve root through the foramen (*arrow*). On sagittal images, also note expansion of the foramen caused by longstanding bony remodeling.

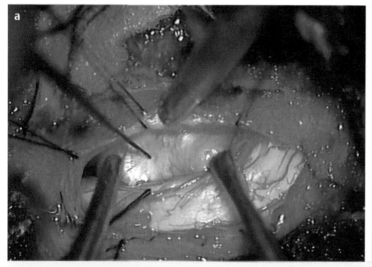
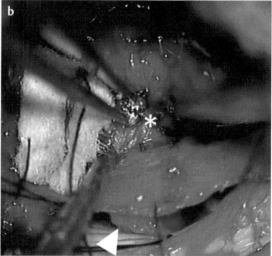

Fig. 21.4 Intraoperative photographs of a dorsally located intradural extramedullary schwannoma. (a) Intradural component of the tumor causing severe spinal cord compression. Note the characteristic white, glistening appearance of the tumor. (b) Following debulking of the intradural component of the tumor (*white arrowhead*), attention is turned to the extradural component which has extended through the exiting foramen (*).

21.4 Nonoperative and Operative Management

Thoracic IDEM tumors including meningioms and nerve sheath tumors are typically slow growing and rarely transform to more malignant forms. Small tumors with no significant mass effect or overt symptoms can be observed with serial imaging every 6 to 12 months. If symptoms progress, there is rapid growth, or if spinal cord compression is present, then surgical resection is considered the gold standard for treatment. There are currently no approved medications for the treatment of these tumors. It is important to note that as with other IDEM tumors, the natural history is for these lesions to grow, thus surgical excision is more likely to yield gross total resection with preservation of neurologic function with smaller tumors that have not had time

to scar to the underlying spinal cord pia or reach larger sizes that require concordant larger laminectomies and dural openings. Stereotactic radiosurgery as a primary treatment modality and for recurrence after open resection has been described. Studies have shown little to no tumor growth during 26 month follow-up periods with no subacute or long-term spinal cord toxicity following treatment.[1,2,10] However, further investigations are ongoing to discern the role of radiosurgery as an alternative versus as an adjunct to open surgical resection.

21.4.1 Surgical Techniques and Considerations

The majority of thoracic IDEM tumors can be resected safely from a posterolateral approach. Fusion of the thoracic spine can be considered for all tumors that require laminectomies at junctional levels (T1 and T12) and when laminectomies at three or more levels are necessary. For nerve sheath tumors that extend out of the foramen or large ventrally situated tumors, unilateral or bilateral facetectomies may be required which introduce further instability where instrumented fusion should be strongly considered to prevent postoperative kyphotic deformity.

Following wide laminectomies, the initial durotomy incision is based on the location of the tumor within the spinal canal. A midline durotomy is used for most dorsally located tumors, though this durotomy can be made just off midline for eccentrically located tumors. For ventrally located tumors, a side approach can be determined prior to opening the dura, which can then influence the laterality off midline of dural opening. Also for ventrally located tumors, dentate ligament transection is often required. Once cut, a suture can be placed through the dentate ligament, which then allows the surgeon to roll the spinal cord in order to better visualize and access the tumor. If intraoperative neurophysiologic monitoring changes occur during the maneuver, it should be immediately aborted and the spinal cord returned to its original orientation.

Once the tumor is visualized, exploration for nerve involvement should be performed. For schwannomas and neurofibromas, the afferent and efferent nerves should be identified prior to debulking. With the exception of T1, thoracic nerve roots can be sacrificed with minor neurologic deficits, which predominantly involve dermatomal paresthesias. Bipolar cautery followed by microscissor transection frees the tumors from the nerve, with the same technique performed at the caudal end. Depending on the tumor size and consistency, two general approaches for tumor resection can be taken. A plane should be identified on the ventral, dorsal, and lateral margins. Then following transection of the afferent and efferent nerve, the tumor should be extracted en bloc. For larger tumors that are densely adherent to dura or spinal cord pia, piecemeal resection can be performed. Cautery and sharp excision, suction, or ultrasonic aspiration can be used. Care should be taken to prevent thermal injury and current spread to the spinal cord when using cautery.

For meningiomas, attention should be focused on resecting as much of the dural attachment as possible, including the dural tail. In some situations, gross total resection can be achieved without sacrificing native dura. However, when this is not possible, leaving residual tumor is advised, considering the technical difficulties in sewing in a patch and higher probability of cerebrospinal fluid (CSF) leak. Dura should be closed with running sutures in a watertight fashion. Closure can be augmented with fibrin sealant gel as needed. A Valsalva maneuver at the end of the closure should confirm adequate watertight dural closure.

21.4.2 Surgical Adjuncts

Intraoperative neurophysiologic monitoring (somatosensory evoked potentials and motor evoked potentials) should be used on all surgeries for thoracic IDEM tumors. For tumors involving or extending to the upper thoracic spine into the low cervical spine, continuous electromyographic monitoring of the T1-innervated muscles can be performed. Sphincter monitoring should also be performed for tumors located in the low thoracic spine extending into the lumbar spine near the level of the conus. During resection, loss or decreasing amplitudes of signal should prompt the following maneuvers. First, technical errors should be explored (disconnected needle, wiring, computer/software processing issues). Once technical issues have been excluded, mean arterial pressure should be assessed. Hypoperfusion of the spinal cord during manipulation can lead to drops in amplitude, which should be immediately corrected by raising mean arterial pressure to 90 mm Hg or above. An experienced anesthesiologist should keep in constant communication during this portion of the case. Once technical and blood pressure issues have been excluded, then reversal of preceding surgical manipulation steps should performed until signals rebound.

Another useful adjunct to have available is ultrasonography. After laminectomies are performed, ultrasound can be used to visualize the tumor, which will usually appear hyperechoic to the adjacent spinal cord. This will give an indication as to whether the laminectomies need to be extended either cranially or caudally. During closure, a subfascial drain can be left to low or gravity suction. High or thin, clear output should raise concern for CSF leak. If this occurs, the drain should be removed and the exit site stitched close to prevent a cutaneous–dural fistula, which can lead to meningitis.

21.5 Postoperative Care and Complication Management

Postoperatively attention should be focused on pain control and preventing CSF leak. Depending on the location with thoracic spine, patients should be positioned with the head of the bed up to at least 30 degrees for T5 and above versus flat in bed (T7–T12). Tumors requiring durotomy at T5-7 are positioned based on surgeon preference, as there is no strong evidence to position one way or another. A strict bowel regimen should be in place to prevent straining with bowel movements that could exacerbate a small CSF leak and also to prevent opioid-induced constipation while taking pain medications. In situations where a watertight dural closure cannot be achieved, or for CSF leak postoperatively, lumbar drainage should be aggressively considered. Physical therapy should be pursued once patients mobilize. Mobilization should be encouraged on postoperative day one if there is low concern for CSF leak and deep vein thrombosis chemoprophylaxis should also be initiated. Postoperative imaging to assess for residual tumor can be obtained prior to discharge versus at 3 months follow-up if the patient is clinically stable. Most stable patients can be discharged within 2 to 5 days postoperatively.

References

[1] Gerszten PC, Chen S, Quader M, Xu Y, Novotny J, Jr, Flickinger JC. Radiosurgery for benign tumors of the spine using the Synergy S with cone-beam computed tomography image guidance. J Neurosurg. 2012; 117 Suppl:197–202

[2] Gerszten PC, Quader M, Novotny J, Jr, Flickinger JC. Radiosurgery for benign tumors of the spine: clinical experience and current trends. Technol Cancer Res Treat. 2012; 11(2):133–139

[3] Huisman TA. Pediatric tumors of the spine. Cancer Imaging. 2009; 9 Spec No A:S45–S48

[4] Barbagallo GMV, Maione M, Raudino G, Certo F. Thoracic intradural-extramedullary epidermoid tumor: the relevance for resection of classic subarachnoid space microsurgical anatomy in modern spinal surgery. Technical note and review of the literature. World Neurosurg. 2017; 108:54–61

[5] Lee JH, Jeon I, Kim SW. Intradural extramedullary capillary hemangioma in the upper thoracic spine with simultaneous extensive arachnoiditis. Korean J Spine. 2017; 14(2):57–60

[6] Postalci L, Tugcu B, Gungor A, Guclu G. Spinal meningiomas: recurrence in ventrally located individuals on long-term follow-up; a review of 46 operated cases. Turk Neurosurg. 2011; 21(4):449–453

[7] Maiti TK, Bir SC, Patra DP, Kalakoti P, Guthikonda B, Nanda A. Spinal meningiomas: clinicoradiological factors predicting recurrence and functional outcome. Neurosurg Focus. 2016; 41(2):E6

[8] Rodriguez FJ, Folpe AL, Giannini C, Perry A. Pathology of peripheral nerve sheath tumors: diagnostic overview and update on selected diagnostic problems. Acta Neuropathol. 2012; 123(3):295–319

[9] Carroll SL, Ratner N. How does the Schwann cell lineage form tumors in NF1? Glia. 2008; 56(14):1590–1605

[10] Gerszten PC, Burton SA, Ozhasoglu C, McCue KJ, Quinn AE. Radiosurgery for benign intradural spinal tumors. Neurosurgery. 2008; 62(4):887–895, discussion 895–896

22 Intramedullary Spinal Cord Tumors

Rohit Mauria, Jakub Godzik, and Steven W. Chang

Abstract

Intramedullary spinal cord tumors are the least common type of spinal cord tumor, comprising about 4 to 10% of primary central nervous system tumors. Among intramedullary spinal cord tumors, the most common are astrocytomas, followed by ependymomas and hemangioblastomas. Although these tumors are often benign and slow growing, patients may experience severe pain, dysfunction, and deformity leading to poor quality of life. Magnetic resonance imaging (MRI) is critical in the diagnosis of these tumors and in clinical decision-making for patients. Open microsurgical resection is the first-line definitive step in the management of these patients. Although gross total resection is associated with better survival and long-term neurologic function, it can be challenging to accomplish safely, with surgery carrying a risk of clinically significant neurologic deficit and negative impact on patients' quality of life. Given the proximity of vital neurologic structures to these tumors, proper surgical planning and technique are essential to successful neurologic outcomes. The optimal trajectory for the resection of intramedullary spinal cord tumors is dictated by the location of the lesion and is constrained by the vascular and spinal cord anatomy. The three basic approaches that are used are the posterior midline, dorsal root entry zone, and lateral. When surgical resection is contraindicated, adjuvant radiotherapy is preferable, although it has potentially severe adverse effects. When both of these treatment modalities are contraindicated, chemotherapy can be considered.

Keywords: astrocytoma, ependymoma, hemangioblastoma, intramedullary, spinal cord tumor

Clinical Pearls

- Intramedullary spinal cord tumors are the least common spinal cord tumor. The most common types are astrocytomas, ependymomas, and hemangioblastomas.
- Although magnetic resonance imaging is critical in the diagnosis of these tumors and in clinical decision-making for patients, open surgical biopsy remains the first definitive step in management.
- Given the proximity of vital neurologic structures to these tumors, proper surgical planning and technique are key to successful neurologic outcomes.
- The optimal trajectory for the resection of intramedullary spinal cord tumors is dictated by the location of the lesion and constrained by vascular and spinal cord anatomy. The three basic approaches are the posterior midline, dorsal root entry zone, and lateral.

22.1 Introduction

Intramedullary spinal cord tumors comprise about 4 to 10% of primary central nervous system tumors.[1] These rare neoplasms can cause severe pain, dysfunction, and deformity, all of which further contribute to poor quality of life for patients.[2,3,4] About 35% of all spinal tumors in children are classified as intramedullary tumors, in contrast to 10% in adults.[5] Ependymomas are the most common subtype, comprising 60% of all spinal cord tumors, followed by astrocytomas at 30% and hemangioblastomas at 2 to 15%.[5,6,7]

Intramedullary spinal cord tumors are often benign and slow growing.[8] In most patients, back pain is the predominant presenting symptom, followed by motor or sensory disturbances and urinary incontinence.[2,4] Some studies show an association between intramedullary tumors with syringomyelia and even scoliosis in advanced cases.[3,4] Magnetic resonance imaging (MRI) has become the recommended imaging modality for identification and evaluation of intramedullary tumors.[2] The presence of spinal cord edema and high signal intensity on T2-weighted MRIs is common to all intramedullary tumors.[9] Despite studies elucidating the differentiating characteristics among the most common subtypes, the diagnosis nonetheless remains an area of focused research.[9]

The recommended initial treatment modality for intramedullary spinal cord tumors is microsurgical resection, followed by adjuvant therapy in certain cases. Although gross total resection is associated with better survival and better long-term neurologic function,[8,10,11] it can be challenging to accomplish safely, with surgery carrying a risk of clinically significant neurologic deficit and a potentially negative impact on the patient's quality of life.[8,11,12] Several variables influence outcome, with preoperative functional status and neurologic status as well as tumor histology being the best predictors.[4,12,13] Given the proximity of vital neurologic structures to these tumors, proper surgical planning and technique are key to successful neurologic outcomes.[12]

22.2 Incidence and Epidemiology

Extradural, intradural extramedullary, and intradural intramedullary tumors make up the three main groups of spinal cord tumors. The vast majority of spinal cord neoplasms are classified as extradural, with intramedullary tumors being the least common at approximately 10% of all spinal tumors.[5,6,7,14,15] The intracranial counterparts are more common than those in the spinal cord, occurring at about a 4:1 ratio. Although intramedullary tumors are infrequent, the incidence is greater in children than in adults, accounting for 35% and 10% of spinal cord tumors, respectively.[5] Interestingly, neuroepithelial types are the primary type of intramedullary tumor.[4,15] Syringomyelia occurs in about 25 to 58% of people with intramedullary spinal tumors, most commonly in the lower cervical region.[16,17]

The main subtypes of spinal cord tumors are astrocytomas, ependymomas, and hemangioblastomas.[18,19] Ependymomas are the most common intramedullary spinal cord tumor in adults and are often found in the cervical or thoracic region.[2,6] Myxopapillary ependymomas are World Health Organization grade I and commonly originate from the filum terminale.[20] Making up about 60% of spinal cord tumors, ependymomas typically carry a good prognosis[2,7] and are frequently associated with the presence of syringomyelia as well as neurofibromatosis type 2 (NF2).[17,21] In most cases, these tumors are considered benign, and they occur equally in both sexes.[16]

Astrocytomas are the second most common intramedullary spinal cord neoplasm, comprising about 30% of spinal cord tumors.[5,6] Most of these tumors are low grade, with a 5-year survival rate of more than 70%, although the higher-grade ependymomas carry a much lower survival rate.[6] These tumors have an established association with neurofibromatosis type 1 due to a germline mutation in chromosome 17q11, which codes for the tumor suppressor neurofibromin.[17,21,22,23,24] Similar to ependymomas, astrocytomas most commonly affect the cervical level and are strongly associated with syrinx formation.[2] In terms of age disparity, adults usually present with high-grade tumors, whereas children typically present with low-grade tumors.[25]

Hemangioblastomas are the third most common intramedullary spinal tumor, making up about 2 to 10% of all intramedullary neoplasms.[16,26,27,28] They are considered benign mesenchymal tumors most likely originating from vascular endothelial growth factor-secreting cells.[2,5,16] Commonly found in the cervical spine, these tumors carry an excellent prognosis.[2] Hemangioblastomas often occur as a solitary tumor, mainly in the posterior portion of the spinal cord, and most occur in patients younger than 40 years of age.[5,16] As many as one-fourth of these patients have signs of von Hippel–Lindau syndrome, an inherited cancer syndrome affecting many systems with visceral and central nervous system manifestations.[15,29] This syndrome, caused by a deletion in chromosome 3q, is also associated with retinal hemangiomas, renal and pancreatic cysts, and renal cell carcinoma.[29]

Cancer metastasis to the intramedullary spinal cord is relatively rare, affecting only about 1 to 3% of patients with intramedullary neoplasms; however, with improving survival of patients with metastatic disease, this disease entity is more frequently encountered.[30,31] Lung cancer is responsible for approximately one-half of the primary tumor metastases to the spinal cord, which is particularly significant because lung cancer is associated with the highest mortality rate of any cancer type.[30,32] Unfortunately, the prognosis of patients with this diagnosis is dismal, and the median survival time is about 4 months.[2]

Lipomas comprise about 1% of intraspinal tumors and usually occur in the extramedullary region, although they are also found in the intramedullary location. These neoplasms are associated with spinal dysraphism and are associated with an excellent long-term prognosis with gross total resection.[5,16] Various other types of intramedullary spinal neoplasms can be found as well, but because the incidence is low, the literature on these pathologies is scarce. Gangliogliomas are slow growing and rare in the adult population.[6] Dermoid and epidermoid tumors, as well as teratomas (▶ Fig. 22.1), are other neoplasms that can present in this location; sacrococcygeal teratomas are the most commonly diagnosed tumors among newborns, with an incidence of approximately 1 case per 14,000 live births.[33]

22.3 Clinical Features

Intramedullary spinal cord tumors can manifest in various ways, but because of their location, many cause common symptoms that can make differentiation of tumor type difficult. Most of their clinical features are related to tumor growth rate, location, and degree of invasion. The most common symptom is pain—either back pain, radicular pain, or central pain.[29] This pain is often caused by dural distention and is exacerbated in the recumbent position.[16] The next most common symptoms include motor symptoms, which are often bilateral with corresponding upper motor signs such as spasticity.[16,29,34] Sphincter disturbances, such as urinary incontinence, are common, with an incidence as high as 45%,[4] whereas hydrocephalus occurs about 8% of the time.[4,35] Paresthesias often occur later and at first more distally.[34] Interestingly, rapidly progressive scoliosis in an adult can be a sign of an intramedullary tumor, highlighting the importance of a wide differential diagnosis in the evaluation of de novo scoliosis or a rapidly progressive deformity.[16]

In addition to the common symptoms, clinical features unique to certain types of tumor can, in certain situations, help elucidate the pathology. More specifically, motor and sensory symptoms initially occur most often in patients with ependymomas and astrocytomas[6]; syringomyelia is also common in patients with these two neoplasms. Children with low-grade ependymomas often present with an inability to meet normal developmental milestones, whereas those with astrocytomas often have marked pain at night, specifically abdominal pain.[2] Sensory symptoms can occur initially in persons with hemangioblastomas because of the predisposition of the tumor to arise in the dorsal spinal cord, which in rare cases can result in subarachnoid hemorrhage or intramedullary hemorrhage.[6] Patients with gangliogliomas commonly present with paraparesis and radicular pain, and about 40% present with obvious scoliosis.[2,6,36] Finally, when considering all the patient's symptoms, it is important to note the factors that contribute to symptom development and severity, such as age, degenerative changes, spinal canal size, and comorbidities.

22.4 Magnetic Resonance Imaging

MRI is the preferred imaging modality for diagnosing and characterizing intramedullary spinal cord tumors. Discerning among spinal ependymomas, astrocytomas, and hemangioblastomas on MRI can be challenging, but several radiologic characteristics allow these tumors to be identified with relatively high accuracy.[9] Ependymomas appear as a local enlargement with symmetric growth in the central region of the spinal cord. They appear hyperintense on T2-weighted MRIs and hypointense or isointense on T1-weighted MRIs, with enhanced margins on T1-weighted contrast images (▶ Fig. 22.2).[6,12]

Astrocytomas can be challenging to differentiate. They appear as fusiform expansions of the spinal cord with poorly defined margins and asymmetrical growth.[2] They show hypointensity or isointensity on T1-weighted MRIs and hyperintensity on T2-weighted MRIs.[6] Both ependymomas and astrocytomas have heterogeneous enhancement with contrast, so differentiation on the basis of MRIs alone can be difficult.[2]

Hemangioblastomas are extremely vascularized tumors with homogenous enhancement, unlike ependymomas and astrocytomas.[6,37] They appear isointense on T1-weighed MRIs and hyperintense on T2-weighted MRIs, and they are associated with cysts and syringomyelia. Angiography is a useful modality to visualize feeding vessels.[6]

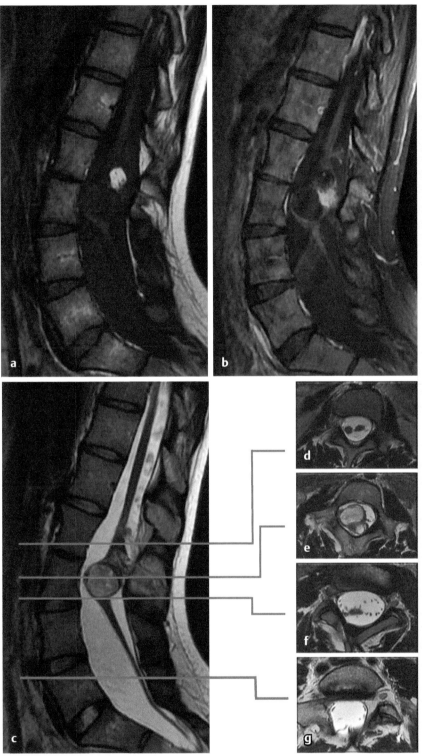

Fig. 22.1 A 20-year-old woman presented with lower back pain after prolonged standing with no abnormalities on physical examination. Imaging demonstrates an intradural, intramedullary heterogeneously enhancing mass at the conus medullaris with associated dysraphism (spina bifida, tethered spinal cord, and vertebral body changes). Sagittal **(a)** T1-weighted noncontrast, **(b)** T1-weighted postcontrast, **(c)** T2-weighted magnetic resonance images (MRIs). Red lines on **(c)** indicate axial T2-weighted MRIs **(d-g)** through the lesion. The final pathology findings were consistent with teratoma. (Used with permission from Barrow Neurological Institute, Phoenix, Arizona.)

Gangliogliomas have hypointense characteristics on T1-weighted magnetic resonance images (MRIs) and are hyperintense on T2-weighted MRIs with patchy contrast enhancement.[6,36] Signs of scoliosis and tumor cysts may also be visible. Lymphoma shows homogenous contrast enhancement on T1-weighted MRIs and hyperintensity on diffusion-weighted and T2-weighted MRIs.[2]

Metastatic intramedullary tumors are often single, encapsulated, and eccentrically located lesions. They have characteristic "rim" and "flame" signs that aid in distinguishing between a metastasis and primary spinal cord neoplasms.[38] The rim sign is a complete or partial region of gadolinium enhancement, whereas the flame sign is a poorly defined gadolinium-enhancing region.[38] These lesions are isointense on T1-weighted MRIs

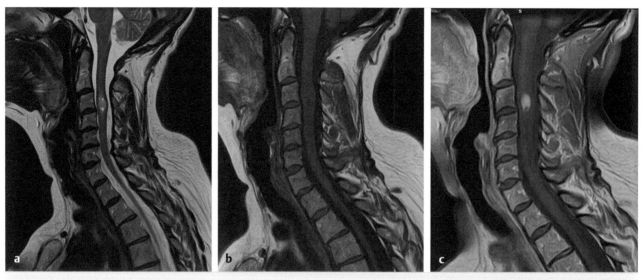

Fig. 22.2 A 54-year-old woman presented with paresthesias and neck soreness at C3-4. A C3–C4 laminoplasty was performed for resection of an ependymoma. Pathology was consistent with a World Health Organization grade II tumor. Sagittal **(a)** T2-weighted, **(b)** T1-weighted noncontrast, and **(c)** T1-weighted contrast-enhanced magnetic resonance images. (Used with permission from Barrow Neurological Institute, Phoenix, Arizona.)

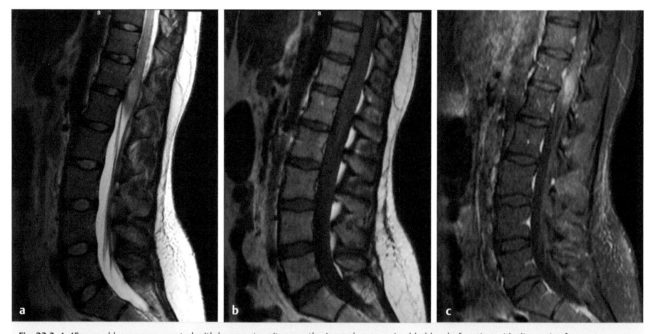

Fig. 22.3 A 45-year-old woman presented with lower extremity paresthesias and progressive bladder dysfunction with diagnosis of conus glioblastoma multiforme. Sagittal **(a)** T2-weighted sequence, **(b)** T1-weighted noncontrast, and **(c)** T1-weighted contrast-enhanced magnetic resonance images. (Used with permission from Barrow Neurological Institute, Phoenix, Arizona.)

and hyperintense on T2-weighted MRIs. Although it is a rare entity, a first-time presenting intramedullary glioblastoma has been described in the literature (▶ Fig. 22.3).[39,40]

22.5 Differential Diagnosis

Many other pathologies share characteristics with intramedullary spinal tumors. Various vascular and inflammatory lesions that share symptoms or imaging patterns with these tumors include spinal cord infarctions, multiple sclerosis, transverse

myelitis, and spinal vascular lesions (e.g., dural arteriovenous fistulas, spinal cord abscesses, and cavernous malformations). An extensive diagnostic workup is critical to properly diagnose and treat the condition when one of these disease processes is suspected.

Spinal cord infarctions occur with a bimodal age distribution. The main etiologies in children are trauma and cardiac malformations, whereas atherosclerosis is the most common cause among adults.[41] Symptoms appear acutely, with back pain, urinary incontinence, and bowel incontinence being the most common symptoms. Sensory deficits are seen early and frequently. MRI is the gold standard for imaging spinal cord ischemia. Hyperintensity is usually present inside the spinal cord on T2-weighted and diffusion-weighted imaging.[42,43]

Multiple sclerosis is considered an autoimmune acquired chronic relapsing demyelinating disease of the central nervous system. This disease should always be part of the differential diagnosis because of its high prevalence, especially among young adult women. The relapsing-remitting type of multiple sclerosis is the most common, in which patients present with episodic symptoms, then recover between episodes.[44] Paresthesia, dysesthesias, ataxia, vertigo, and urinary incontinence are often present, with a wide variety of neurologic deficits also possible.[44] MRI is used to confirm diagnosis, showing isointensity to hypointensity on T1-weighted images and hyperintensity on T2-weighted images.[45,46] These lesions are separated in time and space and are frequently located peripherally in the spinal cord, with poor margins.

Transverse myelitis is another severe inflammatory disease of the spinal cord with destructive sequelae. This disease can present at any age with ascending paresthesias, weakness that affects the flexor muscles of the legs and extensors of the arms, bowel and bladder dysfunction, and autonomic irregularities.[47] Unlike the other previously discussed lesions, about 40% of transverse myelitis cases do not have findings on MRI.[48] In patients with MRI findings, T1-weighted images are isointense or hypointense, and T2-weighted images show a poorly defined hyperintense signal.[49]

Dural arteriovenous fistulas or vascular malformations can manifest within the spinal cord and as a different entity than primary intramedullary tumors. Patients are often older at presentation and have progressive symptoms of weakness and urinary and bowel incontinence.[50,51] On MRI, hyperintensity on T2-weighted images is commonly seen secondary to edema; a mass lesion with flow voids can also be appreciated.[50,51] The primary diagnostic imaging modality in these cases is dedicated spinal angiography.

Spinal cord abscesses occur most commonly in the thoracic spine. Symptoms include typical signs of infection, such as fever, chills, and back pain, as well as weakness, paresthesia, and bowel or bladder incontinence. Unlike with a fracture, percussion tenderness is rarely observed. MRI will demonstrate rim enhancement and restricted diffusion on diffusion-weighted images, hypointensity on T1-weighted images, and hyperintensity on T2-weighted images.

Cavernous malformations are rare vascular malformations composed of a cluster of dilated thin-walled capillaries. These lesions may occur within the spinal cord, making up about 5% of intramedullary lesions.[52] Pain, paresthesia, and weakness are the most common symptoms, with patterns of clinical features ranging from several discernible episodes of neurologic decline, to slow progressive decline, to acute onset. For diagnosis, MRI is the gold standard imaging modality. Heterogeneous signal intensity on T1- and T2-weighted images is characteristic and signifies the presence of hemosiderin.[52] The often-described "popcorn appearance" signifies products of different ages, and low signal intensity on T2-weighted images indicates hemosiderin.

It is evident that several debilitating diseases should be considered when an intramedullary spinal cord tumor is suspected. Almost all patients present very similarly clinically, with some important differences found on imaging. Therefore, knowledge of a wide scope of neurologic disorders is required to make an accurate assessment.

22.6 Treatment Considerations

The standard of care for most patients with an intramedullary spinal tumor is open biopsy and microsurgical resection.[2] A clear plane of dissection is critical in successful microsurgical treatment, and is therefore critical in selecting the optimal treatment. A poor plane of dissection leads to a decreased likelihood of gross total resection and a higher likelihood of postoperative morbidity and mortality.[1,4] In general, if surgical resection is contraindicated, adjuvant radiotherapy is preferable[12]; however, radiotherapy carries the potential for severe adverse effects, such as radiation necrosis and myelopathy, which must be considered in the counseling of patients.[29,53] Radiotherapy is typically used sporadically on the basis of tumor histology and recurrence.[54] When surgical resection and radiotherapy are not indicated, chemotherapy is chosen as the treatment modality.[29,30] While it may not be the mainstay for treatment of intramedullary spinal tumors, it is considered as an adjuvant therapy for various patients.[54] However, chemotherapy often leads to a high incidence of chemotherapy-related toxicity,[53] such as renal impairment.

Most ependymomas have a clear plane of dissection between the tumor and parenchyma in the spine. Thus, gross total resection is the primary goal of treatment because the extent of resection is a predictor of overall survival.[29,55] Subtotal resection with adjuvant radiotherapy is required if the plane of dissection is not clear and if it is evident that surgery will cause decreased neurologic function. Reports in the surgical literature document a 5-year survival rate of approximately 70% for these patients.[30] There is scarce literature regarding the use of chemotherapy in spinal cord ependymomas. However, promising results have been demonstrated for the use of etoposide on recurrent spinal cord ependymomas.[54,56] Similarly, adjuvant radiotherapy for spinal ependymomas has resulted in improvements in progression-free survival and overall survival[57]; radiation doses ranging from 4,000 cGy to 5,400 cGy are associated with a survival rate as high as 100%.[14,54]

Typically, astrocytomas do not have a good plane of dissection, making subtotal resection more common.[2] Their invasive nature leads to a higher neurologic morbidity associated with surgery and lower survival.[58] Recurrence rates of almost 50% have been found, for which radiotherapy is then used as the next stage of treatment.[13,29] However, because of controversy regarding the use of radiotherapy in children (the primary demographic group associated with astrocytomas), chemotherapy is considered a valid adjuvant treatment to surgery.[2] A study by Chamberlain[59] showed a median survival of 23 months among 22 patients who underwent temozolomide treatment. The *BRAF-KIAA1549* fusion gene and the *NF1* gene are prevalent among patients found to have spinal pilocytic astrocytomas, for whom surgical resection is favorable if done before severe neurologic decline.[21] Mutation of *TP53*, an important tumor-suppressor gene involved in the cell cycle, and of *H3F3A*, a gene involved in gene expression, has been observed in various cases of spinal glioblastoma.[21] Unfortunately, patients with spinal glioblastomas have had poor results with various treatment modalities, with vascular endothelial growth factor inhibition being the only targeted therapy approved by the U.S. Food and Drug Administration.[21,60]

Postoperative radiotherapy has been associated with improved survival for patients with high-grade infiltrative spinal astrocytomas but not for patients with pilocytic tumors.[61] Radiotherapy is also recommended for recurring tumors. More specifically, low-grade astrocytomas should have a total dose of 5,040 cGy in 180-cGy fractions over 28 days, with high-grade astrocytomas having a total dose of 5,400 cGy in the same fractions.[29,62]

In contrast, chemotherapy treatments are traditionally administered only after surgical and radiotherapy treatments have been attempted. In a 2008 study, two different doses of temozolomide were used to treat 22 patients with low-grade spinal gliomas.[59] Twelve of the 22 patients had stabilized after two treatment cycles, the median overall survival rate was almost 2 years, and progression-free survival was 27% at 2 years. Interestingly, Gwak et al[63] reported in 2014 that bevacizumab in combination with temozolomide can inhibit the growth of intramedullary gliomas better than temozolomide alone. The combination therapy also led to greater cell apoptosis, most likely due to the inhibition of autophagy.

Hemangioblastomas are primarily removed via surgical resection.[2,26] Gross total resection is often possible because of the clear dissection plane, but a low possibility of intraoperative bleeding always exists. Preoperative embolization has been shown to reduce this risk.[64] Sterotactic radiosurgery is reserved for patients with recurrent hemangioblastomas or hemangioblastomas that cannot be resected.[6] Antiangiogenic therapy is used for patients with concurrent von Hippel–Lindau disease.[65]

Surgical resection is also the treatment of choice for patients with gangliogliomas. Because gross total resection is possible, with favorable long-term outcomes, radiotherapy postoperatively or as adjunctive treatment is not normally recommended.[6] The 5-year progression-free survival rate is approximately 67%.[66]

Methotrexate is the standard treatment for patients with primary central nervous system lymphomas, but it has been combined with the alkylating agent temozolomide, with favorable results, because of the high prevalence of tumor recurrence.[67,68] Maximal safe resection remains the treatment of choice for patients with dermoid and epidermoid tumors, lipomas, and hamartomas.[2,29]

22.7 Operative Considerations and Surgical Pearls

In all cases, the surgical strategy must be tailored to match the individual patient by balancing safety and function preservation against the benefits of tumor debulking and decompression. Before surgical resection of any tumor, proper evaluation of imaging must be done to ensure the safest approach to maximize a good outcome. Basic tenets of surgical resection include exposure, dural opening, biopsy, and debulking or resection. We also recommend diligent use of multimodal intraoperative neuromonitoring to help facilitate safe resection.[8]

Surgical exposure of the dura mater can be attained via soft tissue dissection, with bone removal either through a laminoplasty or laminectomy to provide sufficient access to the solid part of the tumor (▶ Fig. 22.4). If additional lateral exposure is necessary, a costrotransversectomy or facetectomy may be performed. Laminoplasty has been noted to lead to decreased hospitalization times, postoperative pain, and cerebrospinal fluid (CSF) leaks. The long-term impact on preventing spinal deformity remains controversial.[69] Once adequate dural exposure is achieved (▶ Fig. 22.5a), placement of a CSF suction device is recommended (▶ Fig. 22.5b); the dura is opened in a linear fashion with placement of arachnoid dural tack-up sutures directly to adjacent muscle for maximum exposure (▶ Fig. 22.5c). If additional anterolateral visualization is needed, dentate ligaments may be transected to gently rotate the spinal cord (▶ Fig. 22.6).

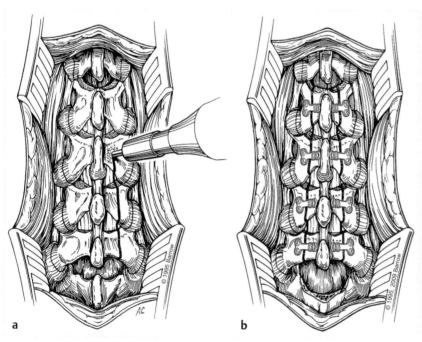

a   b

Fig. 22.4 Illustrations demonstrating laminoplasty technique **(a)** using a footplate drill and **(b)** showing the spine after instrumentation with laminoplasty plates. Care must be taken to reapproximate the bone edges closely to avoid iatrogenic injury or prominence. (Used with permission from Barrow Neurological Institute, Phoenix, Arizona.)

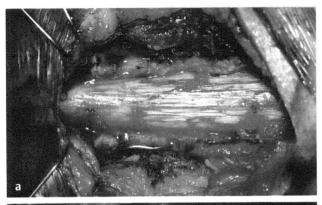
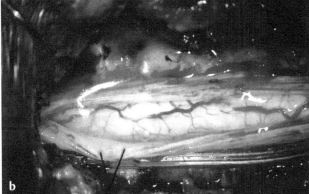
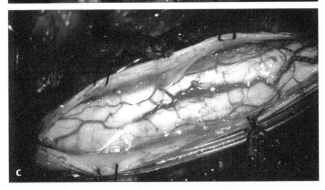

Fig. 22.5 Intraoperative photographs demonstrate the surgical exposure for resection of a cervical midline intramedullary spinal cord tumor. **(a)** Visualization of dura mater after laminoplasty, with fishhooks in place. **(b)** Linear opening of dura with single tack-up suture placed to secure the cerebrospinal fluid suction device. **(c)** Multiple tack-up sutures are placed and attached to adjacent muscles to aid visualization. (Used with permission from Barrow Neurological Institute, Phoenix, Arizona.)

Safe entry zones have been elucidated for certain tumors and should be considered to minimize iatrogenic injury (▶ Fig. 22.7). These zones are based in part on intrinsic spinal cord vascular anatomy, which supplies the cord in a centripetal fashion from pial perforators and sulcocommissural arteries based off the posterior spinal artery and anterior spinal artery, respectively (▶ Fig. 22.8). It is important to note that many intramedullary tumors receive vascular supply from the anterior spinal artery traveling within the anterior median raphe. The posterior median sulcus approach is performed through the posterior median septum for centrally located tumors, such as astrocytomas and ependymomas, whereas a direct transpial approach is more favorable for hemangioblastomas and cavernous malformations.[70] For more laterally situated tumors, a more posterolateral trajectory through the dorsal root entry zone and substantia gelatinosa may be beneficial. An additional option involves a lateral trajectory between the dorsal and ventral spinocerebellar tracts.

The first surgical step involves a myelotomy with a linear pial opening to expose the entire dorsal extent of the tumor mass for biopsy and histopathologic diagnosis (▶ Fig. 22.9a, b). Next, a cleavage plane is identified to facilitate tumor removal. In large part, the ability to achieve maximal resection is dictated by the degree of infiltration by the tumor and maintenance of the surgical plane. In certain less aggressive tumor types, such as ependymomas, there is less tissue infiltration, which allows for the development of a surgical plane that facilitates complete resection. Ependymomas typically have a well-demarcated margin and are dark red or gray in appearance; these tumors are typically resectable en bloc, with a well-defined cleavage border that can be developed using a blunt instrument. Hemangioblastomas have a characteristic sunset yellow appearance. In contrast, higher-grade tumors that are necrotic tend to be different in appearance from normal tissue and can be easily suctioned or bluntly dissected (▶ Fig. 22.9c).[71] In other situations, low-grade tumors may resemble normal parenchyma, making positive identification of margins more challenging. Astrocytomas, for example, typically have a less well-demarcated margin with the spinal cord, and they are pale yellow and glassy in appearance. A worthwhile surgical strategy involves inside to outside intratumoral resection to preserve injury to traversing spinal tracts. A critical consideration in such high-grade tumors or tumors with poorly defined borders is the balancing of surgical goals with surgical morbidity and patient safety; particularly in high-grade tumors, such as glioblastoma, we recommend tumor debulking or expansile duraplasty with subsequent adjuvant systemic therapy.

Finally, multimodal intraoperative neuromonitoring, such as somatosensory evoked potentials and motor evoked potentials, can provide critical information regarding the status of anatomical tracts. Evidence suggests that, in certain circumstances, multimodal monitoring may help guide the determination of surgical margins and thus lead to alterations in operative strategies to improve neurologic functioning and outcomes.[8,72,73]

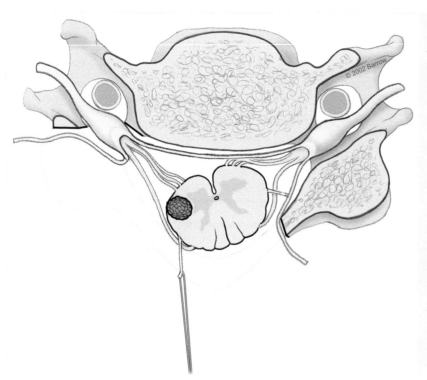

Fig. 22.6 Illustration demonstrates gentle spinal cord rotation to allow access to lateral entry zone, which is facilitated by retraction of dentate ligaments. (Used with permission from Barrow Neurological Institute, Phoenix, Arizona.)

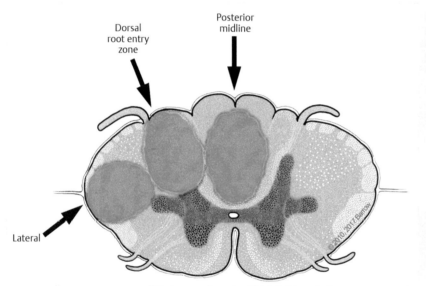

Fig. 22.7 Illustration demonstrates three zones of entry for a myelotomy: lateral, dorsal root entry zone, and posterior midline. (Used with permission from Barrow Neurological Institute, Phoenix, Arizona.)

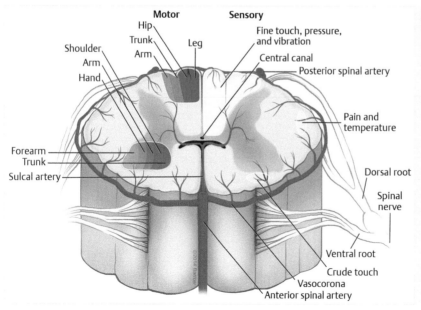

Fig. 22.8 Illustration demonstrates that the vascular supply to the spinal cord is primarily via the anterior spinal artery and posterior spinal artery. This cross-section of the spinal cord demonstrates sensory and motor nerve pathways. (Used with permission from Barrow Neurological Institute, Phoenix, Arizona.)

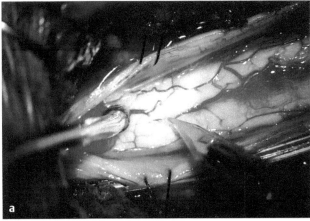

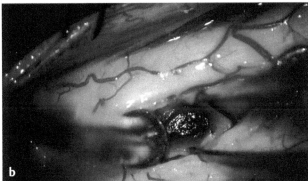

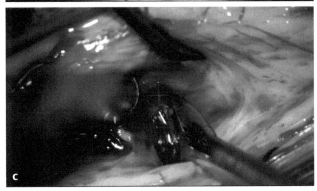

Fig. 22.9 Intraoperative photographs demonstrate the surgical technique for a myelotomy. **(a)** A central midline incision over the dorsal medial sulcus is made with a sharp cutting instrument. **(b)** Exposure of the tumor is performed with gentle retraction on the medial structure. **(c)** A well-demarcated margin is observed and the tumor is debulked. (Used with permission from Barrow Neurological Institute, Phoenix, Arizona.)

References

[1] Boström A, Kanther NC, Grote A, Boström J. Management and outcome in adult intramedullary spinal cord tumours: a 20-year single institution experience. BMC Res Notes. 2014; 7:908

[2] Tobin MK, Geraghty JR, Engelhard HH, Linninger AA, Mehta AI. Intramedullary spinal cord tumors: a review of current and future treatment strategies. Neurosurg Focus. 2015; 39(2):E14

[3] Papagelopoulos PJ, Peterson HA, Ebersold MJ, Emmanuel PR, Choudhury SN, Quast LM. Spinal column deformity and instability after lumbar or thoracolumbar laminectomy for intraspinal tumors in children and young adults. Spine. 1997; 22(4):442–451

[4] Bansal S, Ailawadhi P, Suri A, et al. Ten years' experience in the management of spinal intramedullary tumors in a single institution. J Clin Neurosci. 2013; 20(2):292–298

[5] Mechtler LL, Nandigam K. Spinal cord tumors: new views and future directions. Neurol Clin. 2013; 31(1):241–268

[6] Grimm S, Chamberlain MC. Adult primary spinal cord tumors. Expert Rev Neurother. 2009; 9(10):1487–1495

[7] Duong LM, McCarthy BJ, McLendon RE, et al. Descriptive epidemiology of malignant and nonmalignant primary spinal cord, spinal meninges, and cauda equina tumors, United States, 2004–2007. Cancer. 2012; 118(17):4220–4227

[8] Verla T, Fridley JS, Khan AB, Mayer RR, Omeis I. Neuromonitoring for intramedullary spinal cord tumor surgery. World Neurosurg. 2016; 95:108–116

[9] Arima H, Hasegawa T, Togawa D, et al. Feasibility of a novel diagnostic chart of intramedullary spinal cord tumors in magnetic resonance imaging. Spinal Cord. 2014; 52(10):769–773

[10] Epstein FJ, Farmer JP, Freed D. Adult intramedullary spinal cord ependymomas: the result of surgery in 38 patients. J Neurosurg. 1993; 79(2):204–209

[11] Yang S, Yang X, Hong G. Surgical treatment of one hundred seventy-four intramedullary spinal cord tumors. Spine. 2009; 34(24):2705–2710

[12] Samartzis D, Gillis CC, Shih P, O'Toole JE, Fessler RG. Intramedullary spinal cord tumors: part II—management options and outcomes. Global Spine J. 2016; 6(2):176–185

[13] Karikari IO, Nimjee SM, Hodges TR, et al. Impact of tumor histology on resectability and neurological outcome in primary intramedullary spinal cord tumors: a single-center experience with 102 patients. Neurosurgery. 2011; 68(1):188–197, discussion 197

[14] Harrop JS, Ganju A, Groff M, Bilsky M. Primary intramedullary tumors of the spinal cord. Spine. 2009; 34(22 Suppl):S69–S77

[15] Tihan T, Chi JH, McCormick PC, Ames CP, Parsa AT. Pathologic and epidemiologic findings of intramedullary spinal cord tumors. Neurosurg Clin N Am. 2006; 17(1):7–11

[16] Samartzis D, Gillis CC, Shih P, O'Toole JE, Fessler RG. Intramedullary spinal cord tumors: part I—epidemiology, pathophysiology, and diagnosis. Global Spine J. 2015; 5(5):425–435

[17] Samii M, Klekamp J. Surgical results of 100 intramedullary tumors in relation to accompanying syringomyelia. Neurosurgery. 1994; 35(5):865–873, discussion 873

[18] Kucia EJ, Bambakidis NC, Chang SW, Spetzler RF. Surgical technique and outcomes in the treatment of spinal cord ependymomas, part 1: intramedullary ependymomas. Neurosurgery. 2011; 68(1 Suppl Operative):57–63, discussion 63

[19] Kucia EJ, Maughan PH, Kakarla UK, Bambakidis NC, Spetzler RF. Surgical technique and outcomes in the treatment of spinal cord ependymomas: part II: myxopapillary ependymoma. Neurosurgery. 2011; 68(1 Suppl Operative): 90–94, discussion 94

[20] Bydon M, Mathios D, Aguayo-Alvarez JJ, Ho C, Gokaslan ZL, Bydon A. Multiple primary intramedullary ependymomas: a case report and review of the literature. Spine J. 2013; 13(10):1379–1386

[21] Zadnik PL, Gokaslan ZL, Burger PC, Bettegowda C. Spinal cord tumours: advances in genetics and their implications for treatment. Nat Rev Neurol. 2013; 9(5):257–266

[22] Minehan KJ, Shaw EG, Scheithauer BW, Davis DL, Onofrio BM. Spinal cord astrocytoma: pathological and treatment considerations. J Neurosurg. 1995; 83(4):590–595

[23] Rosenbaum T, Wimmer K. Neurofibromatosis type 1 (NF1) and associated tumors. Klin Padiatr. 2014; 226(6/7):309–315

[24] Hirbe AC, Gutmann DH. Neurofibromatosis type 1: a multidisciplinary approach to care. Lancet Neurol. 2014; 13(8):834–843

[25] Houten JK, Cooper PR. Spinal cord astrocytomas: presentation, management and outcome. J Neurooncol. 2000; 47(3):219–224

[26] Gonzalez LF, Spetzler RF. Treatment of spinal vascular malformations: an integrated approach. Clin Neurosurg. 2005; 52:192–201

[27] Snyder LA, Spetzler RF. Resection of sporadic spinal hemangioblastomas. World Neurosurg. 2014; 82(5):629–631

[28] Oppenlander ME, Spetzler RF. Advances in spinal hemangioblastoma surgery. World Neurosurg. 2010; 74(1):116–117

[29] Chamberlain MC, Tredway TL. Adult primary intradural spinal cord tumors: a review. Curr Neurol Neurosci Rep. 2011; 11(3):320–328

[30] Balmaceda C. Chemotherapy for intramedullary spinal cord tumors. J Neurooncol. 2000; 47(3):293–307

[31] Wilson DA, Fusco DJ, Uschold TD, Spetzler RF, Chang SW. Survival and functional outcome after surgical resection of intramedullary spinal cord metastases. World Neurosurg. 2012; 77(2):370–374

[32] Howlader N, Noone AM, Krapcho M, et al. SEER Cancer Statistics Review. 2014. Available at: https://seer.cancer.gov/csr/1975_2014/

[33] Hambraeus M, Arnbjörnsson E, Börjesson A, Salvesen K, Hagander L. Sacro-coccygeal teratoma: a population-based study of incidence and prenatal prognostic factors. J Pediatr Surg. 2016; 51(3):481–485

[34] Abul-Kasim K, Thurnher MM, McKeever P, Sundgren PC. Intradural spinal tumors: current classification and MRI features. Neuroradiology. 2008; 50(4): 301–314

[35] Mirone G, Cinalli G, Spennato P, Ruggiero C, Aliberti F. Hydrocephalus and spinal cord tumors: a review. Childs Nerv Syst. 2011; 27(10):1741–1749

[36] Yang C, Li G, Fang J, et al. Intramedullary gangliogliomas: clinical features, surgical outcomes, and neuropathic scoliosis. J Neurooncol. 2014; 116(1): 135–143

[37] Colombo N, Kucharczyk W, Brant-Zawadzki M, Norman D, Scotti G, Newton TH. Magnetic resonance imaging of spinal cord hemangioblastoma. Acta Radiol Suppl. 1986; 369:734–737

[38] Rykken JB, Diehn FE, Hunt CH, et al. Intramedullary spinal cord metastases: MRI and relevant clinical features from a 13-year institutional case series. AJNR Am J Neuroradiol. 2013; 34(10):2043–2049

[39] Tai P, Dubey A, Salim M, Vu K, Koul R. Diagnosis and management of spinal metastasis of glioblastoma. Can J Neurol Sci. 2015; 42(6):410–413

[40] Maslehaty H, Cordovi S, Hefti M. Symptomatic spinal metastases of intracranial glioblastoma: clinical characteristics and pathomechanism relating to GFAP expression. J Neurooncol. 2011; 101(2):329–333

[41] Vargas MI, Gariani J, Sztajzel R, et al. Spinal cord ischemia: practical imaging tips, pearls, and pitfalls. AJNR Am J Neuroradiol. 2015; 36(5):825–830

[42] Thurnher MM, Bammer R. Diffusion-weighted MR imaging (DWI) in spinal cord ischemia. Neuroradiology. 2006; 48(11):795–801

[43] Masson C, Pruvo JP, Meder JF, et al. Study Group on Spinal Cord Infarction of the French Neurovascular Society. Spinal cord infarction: clinical and magnetic resonance imaging findings and short term outcome. J Neurol Neurosurg Psychiatry. 2004; 75(10):1431–1435

[44] Goldenberg MM. Multiple sclerosis review. P&T. 2012; 37(3):175–184

[45] Janardhan V, Suri S, Bakshi R. Multiple sclerosis: hyperintense lesions in the brain on nonenhanced T1-weighted MR images evidenced as areas of T1 shortening. Radiology. 2007; 244(3):823–831

[46] Okuda DT, Mowry EM, Beheshtian A, et al. Incidental MRI anomalies suggestive of multiple sclerosis: the radiologically isolated syndrome. Neurology. 2009; 72(9):800–805

[47] West TW. Transverse myelitis—a review of the presentation, diagnosis, and initial management. Discov Med. 2013; 16(88):167–177

[48] Scotti G, Gerevini S. Diagnosis and differential diagnosis of acute transverse myelitis. The role of neuroradiological investigations and review of the literature. Neurol Sci. 2001; 22 Suppl 2:S69–S73

[49] DeSanto J, Ross JS. Spine infection/inflammation. Radiol Clin North Am. 2011; 49(1):105 127

[50] Marcus J, Schwarz J, Singh IP, et al. Spinal dural arteriovenous fistulas: a review. Curr Atheroscler Rep. 2013; 15(7):335

[51] Willinsky R, Goyal M, terBrugge K, Montanera W. Tortuous, engorged pial veins in intracranial dural arteriovenous fistulas: correlations with presentation, location, and MR findings in 122 patients. AJNR Am J Neuroradiol. 1999; 20(6):1031–1036

[52] Kharkar S, Shuck J, Conway J, Rigamonti D. The natural history of conservatively managed symptomatic intramedullary spinal cord cavernomas. Neurosurgery. 2007; 60(5):865–872, discussion 865–872

[53] Allen JC, Aviner S, Yates AJ, et al. Children's Cancer Group. Treatment of high-grade spinal cord astrocytoma of childhood with "8-in-1" chemotherapy and radiotherapy: a pilot study of CCG-945. J Neurosurg. 1998; 88(2):215–220

[54] Juthani RG, Bilsky MH, Vogelbaum MA. Current management and treatment modalities for intramedullary spinal cord tumors. Curr Treat Options Oncol. 2015; 16(8):39

[55] Guidetti B, Mercuri S, Vagnozzi R. Long-term results of the surgical treatment of 129 intramedullary spinal gliomas. J Neurosurg. 1981; 54(3):323–330

[56] Chamberlain MC. Etoposide for recurrent spinal cord ependymoma. Neurology. 2002; 58(8):1310–1311

[57] Chen P, Sui M, Ye J, Wan Z, Chen F, Luo C. An integrative analysis of treatment, outcomes and prognostic factors for primary spinal anaplastic ependymomas. J Clin Neurosci. 2015; 22(6):976–980

[58] Babu R, Karikari IO, Owens TR, Bagley CA. Spinal cord astrocytomas: a modern 20-year experience at a single institution. Spine. 2014; 39(7):533–540

[59] Chamberlain MC. Temozolomide for recurrent low-grade spinal cord gliomas in adults. Cancer. 2008; 113(5):1019–1024

[60] Karsy M, Guan J, Sivakumar W, Neil JA, Schmidt MH, Mahan MA. The genetic basis of intradural spinal tumors and its impact on clinical treatment. Neurosurg Focus. 2015; 39(2):E3

[61] Minehan KJ, Brown PD, Scheithauer BW, Krauss WE, Wright MP. Prognosis and treatment of spinal cord astrocytoma. Int J Radiat Oncol Biol Phys. 2009; 73(3):727–733

[62] Isaacson SR. Radiation therapy and the management of intramedullary spinal cord tumors. J Neurooncol. 2000; 47(3):231–238

[63] Gwak SJ, An SS, Yang MS, et al. Effect of combined bevacizumab and temozolomide treatment on intramedullary spinal cord tumor. Spine. 2014; 39(2): E65–E73

[64] Lee DK, Choe WJ, Chung CK, Kim HJ. Spinal cord hemangioblastoma: surgical strategy and clinical outcome. J Neurooncol. 2003; 61(1):27–34

[65] Madhusudan S, Deplanque G, Braybrooke JP, et al. Antiangiogenic therapy for von Hippel–Lindau disease. JAMA. 2004; 291(8):943–944

[66] Jallo GI, Freed D, Epstein F. Intramedullary spinal cord tumors in children. Childs Nerv Syst. 2003; 19(9):641–649

[67] Flanagan EP, O'Neill BP, Porter AB, Lanzino G, Haberman TM, Keegan BM. Primary intramedullary spinal cord lymphoma. Neurology. 2011; 77(8):784–791

[68] Kasenda B, Ferreri AJ, Marturano E, et al. First-line treatment and outcome of elderly patients with primary central nervous system lymphoma (PCNSL)—a systematic review and individual patient data meta-analysis. Ann Oncol. 2015; 26(7):1305–1313

[69] McGirt MJ, Garcés-Ambrossi GL, Parker SL, et al. Short-term progressive spinal deformity following laminoplasty versus laminectomy for resection of intradural spinal tumors: analysis of 238 patients. Neurosurgery. 2010; 66(5): 1005–1012

[70] Takami T, Naito K, Yamagata T, Ohata K. Surgical management of spinal intramedullary tumors: radical and safe strategy for benign tumors. Neurol Med Chir (Tokyo). 2015; 55(4):317–327

[71] Brotchi J, Fischer G. Spinal cord ependymomas. Neurosurg Focus. 1998; 4(5):e2

[72] Barzilai O, Lidar Z, Constantini S, Salame K, Bitan-Talmor Y, Korn A. Continuous mapping of the corticospinal tracts in intramedullary spinal cord tumor surgery using an electrified ultrasonic aspirator. J Neurosurg Spine. 2017; 27 (2):161–168

[73] Scibilia A, Terranova C, Rizzo V, et al. Intraoperative neurophysiological mapping and monitoring in spinal tumor surgery: sirens or indispensable tools? Neurosurg Focus. 2016; 41(2):E18

23 Surgical Management of Thoracic Spinal Arteriovenous Malformations

Benjamin I. Rapoport and Jared Knopman

Abstract

Vascular malformations of the spinal cord are rare, but carry significant risk of spinal cord compromise, particularly in the thoracic watershed region, which is the spinal cord segment most vulnerable to ischemic injury. In this chapter we focus on arteriovenous malformations (AVMs) and arteriovenous fistulas (AVFs) of the thoracic spinal cord. We review the relevant spinal vascular anatomy, the pathologic mechanisms by which spinal vascular malformations (SVMs) can cause acute or progressive neurological deficits, and the natural history of these lesions. Selective spinal angiography is the gold standard for diagnosing and characterizing SVMs, whose highly variable and dynamic angioarchitecture, together with adjacent normal spinal vascular anatomy, must be well understood in order to plan safe, effective, individualized treatment. Finally, we discuss endovascular and microsurgical approaches to treating AVMs and dural and pial AVFs of the thoracic spinal cord.

Keywords: spinal vascular malformation (SVM), spinal arteriovenous malformation (AVM), spinal arteriovenous fistula (AVF), spinal dural AVF, spinal pial AVF

Clinical Pearls

- Vascular malformations of the spinal cord carry significant risk of spinal cord compromise, particularly in the thoracic watershed region, which is the spinal cord segment most vulnerable to ischemic injury.
- The natural history of most spinal cord vascular malformations is progressive neurological decline over a period of several years. Therefore, treatment should be aimed at safely obliterating these lesions soon after diagnosis, in order to stabilize or reverse initial neurological deficits, and to prevent future spinal cord compromise.
- Selective, catheter-based spinal angiography is the gold standard for diagnosing and characterizing spinal vascular malformations (SVMs), and their highly variable and dynamic angioarchitecture, together with the surrounding normal spinal vascular anatomy, must be well understood in order to plan safe, effective, and individualized treatment.
- The most appropriate treatment strategy for spinal arteriovenous malformations (AVMs) may be endovascular, microsurgical, or hybrid, depending on lesion angioarchitecture.
- Spinal dural arteriovenous fistulas (AVFs) are the most common SVMs, comprising 60 to 80% of all SVMs. They are often amenable to straightforward microsurgical ligation, due to the location of the fistula in the portion of the segmental radiculomeningeal branch within the dura associated with the segmental sensory nerve root. The exposure typically requires only a one- or two-level thoracic laminectomy and small dural incision. The sensory nerve root provides a clear intradural landmark.

- Spinal pial AVFs are highly variable in their angioarchitecture. Giant pial AVFs are best treated endovascularly when possible, while small and large pial AVFs are more safely managed by microsurgery, in order to protect small branches to normal spinal cord from direct catheterization.
- Spinal AVMs are typically approached endovascularly when possible, and though safe and complete obliteration may not always be possible, it may not be needed in order to favorably alter the natural history of the lesion.

23.1 Introduction, Definitions, and Classifications

In this chapter we review the classification, diagnosis, evaluation, and surgical and endovascular management of arteriovenous malformations (AVMs) and arteriovenous fistulas (AVFs) of the thoracic spine. The general approach to spinal vascular malformations (SVMs) at our institution has been published elsewhere, and we adhere to that framework in the present discussion.[1]

Many classification systems for SVMs have been described. Here, for simplicity, we classify these lesions on the basis of their angioarchitectural features. Vascular lesions that contain an arteriovenous shunt, AVMs and AVFs, are amenable to surgical and endovascular treatment. The vascular lesions that do not contain an arteriovenous shunt, capillary telangiectasias, and cavernous hemangiomas, in the rare cases in which procedural intervention is indicated, are amenable to surgical management alone, as they are anatomically inaccessible via transcatheter routes. The fundamental distinction between AVFs and AVMs is that an AVF contains a direct connection between an artery and a vein, whereas an AVM contains a network of abnormal vessels, referred to as a "nidus," separating the arterial and venous sides of the lesion. (Some lesions may contain both nidal and direct fistulous components, making them difficult to classify.)

AVMs can be further classified based on the location of the nidus, which may lie either within or at the surface of the spinal cord. The nidal location has important endovascular and open surgical treatment implications. We use a straightforward system based on the location of the nidus or fistulous connection, outlined in ▶ Table 23.1.

23.2 Vascular Anatomy of the Thoracic Spine

In order to understand SVMs and their surgical and endovascular management, it is important to establish a background understanding of normal spinal arterial and venous anatomy. This subject has been comprehensively reviewed by several authors.[2] Here we briefly survey the elements of spinal vascular anatomy most relevant to the subject of this chapter. The reader is referred to ▸ Fig. 23.1 and ▸ Fig. 23.2, which illustrate the segmental arterial supply to the spine and spinal cord, respectively, and to ▸ Fig. 23.3, which illustrates the venous anatomy of the spinal cord.

The arterial supply to the spinal cord is provided by one anterior spinal artery (ASA) and two posterior spinal arteries (PSAs).

The ASA is formed from small left and right ASAs, each of which arises from the corresponding vertebral artery. The ASA is located in the anterior median sulcus, and supplies approximately the anterior two thirds of the spinal cord, including the anterior horns, ventral and lateral corticospinal tracts, and the

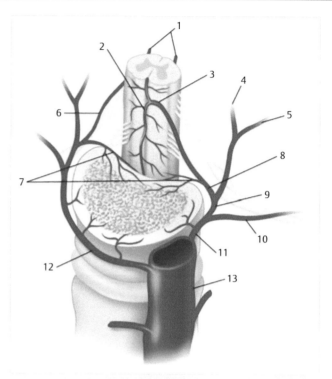

Fig. 23.1 Segmental arterial anatomy of the spine. (1) Posterior spinal arteries, (2) anterior spinal artery, (3) great anterior radiculomedullary artery (artery of Adamkiewicz), (4) medial musculocutaneous branch, (5) lateral musculocutaneous branch, (6) posterior radiculomedullary artery, (7) retrocorporeal arteries, (8) spinal branch, (9) posterior (dorsal) branch, (10) anterior (ventral) branch, (11) left segmental artery (posterior intercostal artery), (12) right segmental artery (posterior intercostal artery), and (13) aorta. (Reproduced with permission from Santillan A, Nacarino V, Greenberg E, et al. Vascular anatomy of the spinal cord. J Neurointerv Surg 2012;4:67–74.)

Table 23.1 Topographic classification of spinal AVM

Type	Location of nidus or fistula	Alternative names
AVM	Intramedullary	Type II, "glomus AVM"
	Pial	
	Epidural	
	Intramedullary and extramedullary	Type III, "juvenile AVM," "metameric AVM"
AVF	Pial	Type IV, "spinal cord AVF," "perimedullary AVF"
	Dural	Type I, "dural AVF," "dorsal intradural AVF"
	Epidural	

Abbreviation: AVF, arteriovenous fistula; AVM, arteriovenous malformation.

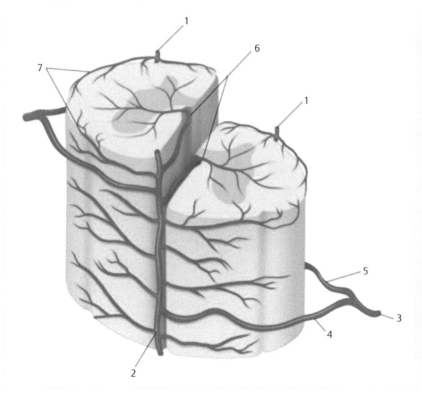

Fig. 23.2 Segmental arterial anatomy of the spinal cord. (1) Posterior spinal arteries, (2) anterior spinal artery, (3) spinal branch, (4) anterior radiculomedullary artery, (5) posterior radiculomedullary artery, (6) central (sulcal) arteries, and (7) vasocorona. (Reproduced with permission from Santillan A, Nacarino V, Greenberg E, et al. Vascular anatomy of the spinal cord. J Neurointerv Surg 2012;4:67–74.)

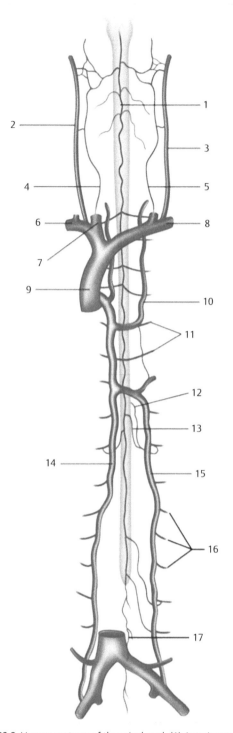

Fig. 23.3 Venous anatomy of the spinal cord. (1) Anterior median vein, (2) right deep cervical vein, (3) left deep cervical vein, (4) right vertebral vein, (5) left vertebral vein, (6) subclavian vein, (7) internal jugular vein, (8) left brachiocephalic vein, (9) superior vena cava, (10) accessory hemiazygous vein, (11) intercostal veins, (12) posterior radiculomedullary vein, (13) anterior radiculomedullary vein, (14) azygous vein, (15) hemiazygous vein, (16) lumbar veins, and (17) vein of the filum terminale. (Reproduced with permission from Santillan A, Nacarino V, Greenberg E, et al. Vascular anatomy of the spinal cord J Neurointerv Surg 2012;4:67–74.)

spinothalamic tracts. At thoracic levels, the aorta gives rise to segmental radiculomedullary feeding arteries that provide collateral supply to the territory of the ASA. (Each segmental artery also gives rise to radiculomeningeal branches that supply the dura at segmental levels; these branches become especially relevant in the setting of spinal dural AVFs.) The most significant of these is the great anterior segmental medullary artery (the artery of Adamkiewicz), which typically arises on the left, between the levels of T8 and L2. In part as a result of this configuration, the spinal cord watershed is located in the upper thoracic region, so compromise of the ASA carries a high risk of paralysis.

The PSAs also arise from the vertebral arteries, but descend along the spinal cord posterolaterally, supplying the posterior columns. At thoracic levels, the PSAs anastomose with segmental radiculomedullary branches from the intercostal arteries.

Venous drainage from the spinal cord occurs through an intradural system and an extradural system. The intradural venous system comprises the intramedullary veins and the pial veins, while the extradural system involves the veins of the spine and the epidural venous plexus (Batson's plexus). The ventral spinal cord is drained by a longitudinal midline anterior spinal vein, as well as by anterolateral veins, which receive drainage from segmental sulcal veins. Venous drainage from the posterior columns and dorsal horns is into the longitudinal posteromedian and posterolateral veins.

23.3 Epidemiology

SVMs are overall rare, and account for approximately one-tenth of central nervous system vascular malformations. The detection rate of new cases has been estimated at less than 15 per million per year in the general population. Of these, spinal dural AVFs are the most common, constituting 60 to 80% of all SVMs.[3]

23.4 Presentation and Clinical Features

Patients with SVMs may present clinically with signs of myelopathy (sensory or motor deficits, bladder or bowel dysfunction, proprioceptive deficits, hyperreflexia), or with pain or a neurological deficit in a radicular distribution. They may also present with back pain or progressive spinal column deformity. The dominant pathophysiologic mechanism is determined by the hemodynamics of the lesion; the principal mechanisms are hemorrhage, ischemia due to venous hypertension or arterial steal, and mass effect.

Pain or neurological deficit that is acute in onset may signify a hemorrhage. Rupture of a spinal AVM can cause acute spinal injury due to spinal subarachnoid hemorrhage or hematomyelia (spinal intraparenchymal hemorrhage). The clinical presentation of a ruptured spinal AVM varies depending on the level and site of the injury within the spinal cord, but typically includes lower extremity motor and sensory deficits, with or without proprioceptive deficits and bowel or bladder dysfunction. Hemorrhage also typically produces a sudden onset of severe upper back or interscapular pain without nuchal rigidity. The likelihood of hemorrhage is increased in the presence of intranidal or flow-related aneurysms, particularly aneurysms of the ASA.

AVMs with drainage into the perimedullary venous system are prone to cause venous hypertension. The classic lesions of this type are the spinal dural or pial AVF. In lesions containing an arteriovenous shunt into the valveless perimedullary veins, arterial pressure is transmitted directly into the perimedullary venous system. These veins become "arterialized," developing tortuous courses and thickened walls. As the pressure in the venous system approaches arterial pressure, the arteriovenous pressure gradient falls, and the rate of tissue perfusion declines proportionally, resulting in hypoxia of the spinal cord. Additionally, the intrinsic veins of the spinal cord are also exposed to elevated pressures, resulting in disruption of the blood–spinal cord barrier and cord edema. Venous pressure in the draining veins is a function of arterial pressure, and therefore increases, with concomitant exacerbation of symptoms, during exercise.

Conus medullaris syndrome is common in the setting of certain spinal AVMs. The reason for this is that because the spinal venous system is valveless, the degree of venous hypertension increases in the more gravity-dependent regions of the spine. As the conus medullaris is the most dependent segment of the spinal cord when posture is upright, venous hypertension is most pronounced there. Venous hypertension can be verified angiographically, by demonstrating of a prolonged venous phase on angiogram of the artery of Adamkiewicz.

Arterial steal phenomena may also arise in lesions containing high-flow arteriovenous shunts, as such shunts can divert flow from normal, adjacent spinal cord tissue. Lesions fed by the ASA are especially prone to cause arterial steal, as the ASA is poorly collateralized.

Mass effect is an uncommon mechanism for myelopathy in SVMs, but large intranidal or flow-related aneurysms or dilated venous varices may cause cord or nerve root compression.

23.5 Arteriovenous Malformations

Spinal cord AVMs typically come to attention in childhood or young adulthood, in the setting of acute spinal cord compromise due to spinal intraparenchymal hemorrhage or compression myelopathy. Most patients recover partially from an initial hemorrhage, but the probability of second and subsequent hemorrhages is high, and the tendency is for patients to experience progressive deterioration of spinal cord function.

23.6 Pial Arteriovenous Fistula

Large and giant spinal cord pial AVFs often come to attention in childhood and adolescence, while small pial AVFs typically present later in life. Large and giant lesions can present with acute spinal cord compromise in the setting of spinal subarachnoid hemorrhage (usually due to venous rupture), progressive sensorimotor deficits due to vascular steal or venous hypertension, or mass effect on the spinal cord or nerve roots from dilated veins. Small lesions rarely rupture, and typically cause slowly progressive neurological deficits due to venous hypertension.

23.7 Dural Arteriovenous Fistula

Spinal dural AVFs typically cause progressive myelopathy through venous hypertension and hypoperfusion of the spinal cord. Back or leg pain is common, and symptoms are typically exacerbated by actions that increase intraabdominal pressure, such as straining, or bending at the waist. Patients typically present in adulthood, and by the time of diagnosis many patients already experience bladder or bowel dysfunction or sexual dysfunction.

23.8 Intramedullary–Extramedullary Arteriovenous Malformation and Angiomatosis

Intramedullary–extramedullary AVMs and angiomatosis typically present in childhood and young adulthood, sometimes in the setting of an identifiable syndrome such as Osler–Weber–Rendu or Cobb syndrome. Children present with pain and progressive myelopathy due to mass effect, arterial steal, or hemorrhage.

23.9 Pathophysiology

AVMs and fistulas are believed to form as a result of structural deficits in the embryologic arteriolar–capillary network that normally separates the intracranial arterial and venous circulations. Development of these capillary beds takes place in the period between 40 and 80 mm embryonic length, corresponding to gestational age between 11 and 14 weeks. Most AVMs appear to develop prior to the end of this period, but further details as to the formation of these lesions are not well understood.[4]

An AVM is a vascular malformation in which arterial circulation flows directly into the venous drainage system without an intervening capillary bed. The center of such a lesion, where there is a transition from the arterial to the venous system, is known as the nidus, and contains no neural parenchyma. The fundamental danger of these lesions arises from the feeding of the high-flow, high-pressure arterial system into the low-pressure venous system; these configurations establish the potential for a pressure-flow mismatch that overcomes the strength of the vascular wall, resulting in vascular rupture and hemorrhage.

Because AVMs lack a high-resistance capillary bed separating the arterial from the venous side of the circulation, they tend to have low resistance and consequently high blood flow, with an associated tendency to undergo active remodeling (mediated, in part, by vascular endothelial growth factor) and to increase in size and tortuosity over time.

23.10 Spinal Cord Arteriovenous Malformation

Spinal cord AVMs account for 20 to 30% of SVMs. They are high-flow lesions, and are supplied by at least one branch of the ASA or PSA. The spinal AVM comprises a network of arteriovenous shunts that drain into the spinal veins. Aneurysms associated with the feeding arteries and within the nidus are common.

Spinal cord AVMs show no preference for spinal cord level. They may arise within the parenchyma (intramedullary), at the spinal cord surface (pial), or within the epidural space (epidural). They may also cross tissue boundaries, exhibiting both intramedullary and extramedullary components.

23.11 Pial Arteriovenous Fistula

A pial AVF comprises one or more direct, intradural arteriovenous shunts, without intervening nidus, located on the pial surface of the spinal cord. The arterial supply arises from one or more branches of the ASA or PSA, and the venous shunt drains into dilated spinal cord veins. Pial AVFs can be classified further according to size and flow rate of the direct arteriovenous shunt.

The type I (small) pial AVF is a single, slow-flow shunt between a normal caliber ASA and a slightly dilated spinal vein. Type I lesions are typically located on the anterior surface of the conus medullaris or filum terminale.

The type II (large) pial AVF comprises one or more shunts in parallel, resulting in greater total flow than is observed in a small AVF, and compensatory "ampullary" (proximal) dilation of the draining vein. Large pial AVFs are most commonly located in the posterolateral aspect of the conus medullaris, in which case they are supplied by one or more slightly dilated branches of a PSA.

The type III (giant) pial AVFs contain one or more high-flow shunts, also supplied by dilated arterial branches of the ASA, PSA, or both. In the case of a giant pial AVF, however, the arterial feeders converge to a single shunt, which drains into a collection of grossly dilated, arterialized draining veins. While giant pial AVFs are most common in the conus medullaris, they are also found at cervical and thoracic levels.

23.12 Dural Arteriovenous Fistula

Spinal dural AVFs are the most common type of spinal AVF. Several synonymous terms are used to refer to these lesions: type I malformations, spinal dural AVFs, intradural dorsal AVFs, dorsal extramedullary AVFs, and angioma venosum racemosum.

Spinal dural AVFs derive their arterial supply from radiculomeningeal branches of segmental spinal arteries (anterior or posterior radicular arteries). Their venous drainage is centripetal into the spinal cord and medullary veins. A critical anatomic feature of these lesions is that the shunt itself is typically located in the dura around the sensory ganglion of the proximal nerve root.

These lesions become symptomatic due to flow reversal in the perimedullary spinal cord veins, resulting in spinal cord venous hypertension, cord ischemia, and in extreme cases, necrotizing myelopathy.

Some authors have proposed that spinal cord autoregulation is accomplished, in part, by a glomerulus-like vascular structure located within the two dural leaflets. The function of this structure is to maintain constant intraspinal venous pressure in the setting of frequent changes in intraabdominal and intrathoracic pressures. The structure comprises the terminal portion of the radiculomedullary vein, which becomes tortuous and narrow in the arachnoid and dura, preventing venous blood from flowing intradurally from the epidural plexus. The wall of the radiculomedullary vein transitions to form a meningeal cuff, which

is thought to connect spinal arteries with the perimedullary veins. This model of the spinal arteriovenous anatomy is the basis for the recommendation that both endovascular and microsurgical treatment should aim to obliterate the origin of the proximal draining vein in order to permanently obliterate a spinal dural AVF.[5,6]

23.13 Epidural Arteriovenous Fistula

An epidural AVF represents an arterial shunt into the epidural venous plexus. This lesion carries high morbidity, though it is extremely rare, appearing in several case reports and small series. Epidural AVFs most commonly arise in the cervical spine, though they have also been described in the lumbar region, sacrum, and pelvis. We include them for completeness in describing the anatomic classification of SVMs, but will not discuss them further here, as they are hardly relevant to surgery of the thoracic spine.

23.14 Intramedullary–Extramedullary Arteriovenous Malformation and Angiomatosis

Intramedullary–extramedullary (also referred to as intradural–extradural) AVMs represent metameric vascular lesions that may involve any or all tissue compartments within one or more adjacent spinal levels, including spinal cord, dura, vertebral bodies, paravertebral soft tissues, and skin. They commonly involve multiple feeding arteries over adjacent spinal levels. Many cases of intramedullary–extramedullary spinal AVMs are associated with developmental syndromes. Cobb syndrome, in particular, is associated with complete AVM involvement of affected somite levels.

23.15 Genetics and Associated Syndromes

AVMs are not congenital; as discussed in the previous section, they are the result of developmental errors that arise during embryogenesis. However, several syndromes have known associations with SVMs, including some with both cutaneous and vascular manifestations: Osler–Weber–Rendu, Klippel–Trénaunay–Weber, Parkes Weber, and Cobb syndromes, as well as neurofibromatosis type I. Ventral intradural AVFs have particular associations with these syndromes. Cobb syndrome involves the skin, vertebrae, and spinal cord of the affected metameres, and AVMs are found in a metameric distribution.[6]

23.16 Diagnosis and Evaluation
23.16.1 Noninvasive Imaging

Magnetic resonance imaging (MRI) has nearly 100% sensitivity for detecting spinal cord AVMs, and is the imaging modality of choice for initial evaluation and follow-up of these lesions. On

MRI, spinal AVMs appear as signal voids within or on the surface of the spinal cord, corresponding to dilated arteries or veins. Other features of these lesions are also detected on MRI, including hematomyelia and spinal cord edema.

Decisions with regard to treatment and the feasibility of surgical or endovascular intervention are almost always based on spinal angiography, which is considered the definitive imaging modality for evaluating spinal cord vascular malformations.

23.16.2 Spinal Angiography

Even in the era of high-quality MRI and noninvasive vascular imaging, conventional catheter spinal angiography remains the definitive imaging modality for diagnosis and classification of SVMs. Catheter angiography still provides maximal spatial resolution, and, most importantly, an ability to isolate segments of the vascular system, and to visualize and study the dynamic flow patterns through lesions of interest.

Spinal angiography under general anesthesia can provide higher quality images of the thoracic region, as longer periods of apnea can be maintained during angiography, to reduce motion artifact, without causing discomfort to the patient.

We routinely perform spinal angiography through a 5 French sheath in the femoral artery, using a 5 French diagnostic catheter. In the thoracic spine, the catheters we most commonly use for catheterization of segmental arteries are the Cobra 2 or Simmons 2 (Terumo Medical, Somerset, NJ) and the Mikaelson and Modified Hook (Merit Medical, South Jordan, UT).

A nonselective angiogram from the aorta can be obtained by power injection through a pigtail, high-flow catheter positioned in the descending aorta at a midthoracic level (injecting at 10 mL/s for a total volume of 35 mL). Similarly, a retrograde bilateral femoral angiogram can be used to study the lumbar and lower thoracic levels nonselectively. In this technique, using bilateral 5 French femoral sheaths, 40 mL of contrast is injected at 20 mL/s into each femoral artery, resulting in opacification of the dorsal aorta at abdominal and lower thoracic levels up to the level of T10. This technique fills the lower thoracic and lumbar segmental arteries without filling the visceral arteries.

Individual segmental arteries must be selectively catheterized and evaluated in almost every case of a SVM. It is important to note that even though a vascular lesion may localize to the thoracic spine, its arterial supply may arise from lumbar or cervical levels, so catheter angiography must take this into account.

In the setting of a spinal AVM, spinal angiography should also be used to evaluate spinal cord venous drainage. This can be accomplished by selective angiography of the artery of Adamkiewicz. When thoracolumbar myelopathy is due to severe venous hypertension, venous drainage after injection of the artery of Adamkiewicz is prolonged or absent. Improvement in venous drainage after treatment of the lesion is a good prognostic factor.[6]

23.17 Natural History and Implications for Treatment

The natural history of untreated SVMs varies according to lesion type and location. The thoracic spinal cord is particularly

vulnerable to ischemia, as it is less well collateralized than the cervical and lumbar segments, so special care must be taken when considering treatment of thoracic SVMs.

23.18 Spinal Cord Arteriovenous Malformation

The natural history of untreated spinal cord AVMs is toward progressive neurological deterioration following an initial event, with a prognosis that varies according to specific lesion type. Extramedullary AVMs tend to present later in life, with 85% of patients asymptomatic until age 40. After an initial event, however, there is a tendency toward steady, progressive decline in neurological function, with major neurological impairment by 4 to 6 years from the initial event. Intramedullary AVMs, by contrast, present prior to age 40 in more than 85% of cases. For intramedullary AVMs of the thoracic spine, 40% of patients are no longer independent 5 years from presentation, and at 15 years 60% are no longer independent.[7]

As these lesions are often curable, and almost always at least partially treatable in ways that favorably alter the natural history, there is a general agreement that treatment soon after diagnosis is advisable. Microsurgical, endovascular, and combined approaches are possible, and will be discussed in the sections that follow.

23.19 Dural and Pial Arteriovenous Fistula

The natural history of dural and pial AVFs of the spinal cord is incompletely understood, as no cohort has been observed longitudinally without intervention. The best data are derived from observational studies performed in the 1970s, which suggest that within 3 years of initial presentation, 50% of patients with untreated SVMs develop severe neurological disability, as defined by requiring crutches to walk, or being wheelchair bound and unable to stand independently.[8]

Treatment considerations for dural and pial AVFs are therefore similar to those for spinal cord AVMs with respect to the timing and indications. The choices of modality are also similar, and will be discussed in the sections that follow.

23.20 Intramedullary–Extramedullary Arteriovenous Malformation and Angiomatosis

Intramedullary–extramedullary AVMs and angiomatoses are the most complex SVMs, and they are consequently the most difficult to treat. No optimal treatment strategy has been described. Curative treatment via microsurgical, endovascular, or combined approaches is extremely difficult, and carries high likelihood of procedural morbidity, as the lesions are entangled within normal spinal cord parenchyma. Treatment of these lesions is typically palliative, directed toward relief of symptoms caused by hematoma, arterial steal, venous hypertension, or mass effect.

23.21 Preoperative Assessment and Planning

In the present era, treatment of thoracic SVMs is almost always multimodal. Some lesions can be treated through endovascular techniques alone, some can be treated through open surgical techniques alone, and some require combined endovascular and open surgical approaches. In almost all cases, however, the treatment begins with selective spinal angiography, and partial or complete embolization is considered prior to open surgery.

The primary considerations when planning treatment of a SVM are the location of the lesion in the axial and longitudinal planes, the hemodynamics and angioarchitecture of the lesion, and the neurological status of the patient. Posttreatment status is highly correlated with preoperative neurological function, so early treatment, prior to neurological deterioration, is recommended. Nevertheless, stabilization or partial improvement in neurological function is sometimes achievable when a lesion is treated even after it has severely compromised spinal cord function.

Some lesions require surgical management. Superselective angiography through a microcatheter must be performed prior to embolization of a SVM, in order to rule out the presence of a branch to an anterior or PSA originating from a vascular pedicle common to the lesion. In particular, spinal dural AVFs that have arterial feeders arising from a pedicle common to an anterior or PSA branch should be treated with open surgery rather than endovascular embolization. In such cases, open microsurgical occlusion of the pathologic branch can be performed with greater selective precision, avoiding the potential complication of occluding arterial supply to a spinal cord artery.

As comprehensive management of SVMs requires collaboration between open microsurgical and endovascular surgical teams, it is important for each to understand the capabilities and limitations of the other. We therefore discuss both treatment modalities here.

23.22 Endovascular Treatment

In approaching a spinal cord vascular malformation, several general anatomic considerations must be addressed: anterior or PSA supply, collateral supply to or from adjacent spinal levels, collateral supply via pial collateral vessels, venous drainage, and the optimal point at which to occlude the arteriovenous shunt or shunts. It is particularly important to realize that spinal vascular lesions are dynamic, and their flow patterns and architecture may change during treatment.

The angioarchitecture and hemodynamics of a SVM must be precisely defined prior to any treatment, and they must be understood in the context of the surrounding normal vascular anatomy of the spinal cord. The ASA supplies the anterior two-thirds of the spinal cord, including the majority of the spinal cord grey matter and the corticospinal and spinothalamic tracts. The PSAs supply the dorsal one-third of the spinal cord, and have more anastomoses than the anterior system. As a result, there may be sufficient collateral circulation for the spinal cord to tolerate occlusion of a posterior radiculomedullary branch supplying a PSA, or at least for such an occlusion to result in at most a posterior column syndrome. However,

occlusion of an anterior radiculomedullary branch to the ASA carries high risk for causing a spinal cord stroke and anterior cord syndrome.

Vascular anastomoses at levels adjacent to a SVM must be characterized prior to embolization. Anastomoses to the ASA from adjacent levels must be understood and protected during embolization. Such anastomoses are not always apparent prior to treatment, as high-flow malformations may "steal" from small anastomoses. Hemodynamic changes must therefore be anticipated during treatment. In particular, when a high-flow lesion is occluded, collateral anastomoses from which the lesion had been stealing flow may reopen. If one of these anastomoses with a spinal artery, inadvertent embolization of the newly patent artery must be avoided.

Pial anastomoses must also be understood. The pial perimedullary network connects the anterior and PSAs, so embolization of a posterior radiculomedullary artery can result in inadvertent embolization of the ASA.

The optimal occlusion point of an arteriovenous shunt must be determined prior to occlusion. The venous drainage of arteriovenous shunts must be preserved. In an AVM, occlusion of the venous drainage can cause increased pressure in the nidus, resulting in hemorrhage. In an AVF, occlusion of the venous drainage can lead to venous hypertension and cord ischemia. On the other hand, proximal occlusion of an arterial feeder to an arteriovenous shunt can be worse than ineffective, for two reasons. First, collateral arterial anastomoses supplying normal cord can be recruited to supply the shunt, and when this happens the shunt steals flow from normal cord, resulting in steal-induced cord ischemia. Second, proximal occlusion precludes further access for subsequent embolization.

23.23 Spinal Cord Arteriovenous Malformation

The goal in treating spinal cord intramedullary AVMs is to favorably alter the natural history, intervening at an early stage to stabilize or reverse neurlogic deficits and reduce future risk of hemorrhage. Curative treatment without compromising normal spinal cord is not always possible through endovascular, microsurgical, or even combined approaches; however, even partial embolization can preserve neurological function and improve overall prognosis.

Endovascular embolization is an important, first-line treatment strategy for intramedullary spinal cord AVMs, either in isolation or as an adjunct to microsurgical resection.

The angioarchitecture of an intramedullary spinal cord AVM does not always favor definitive cure. As a result, repeated, partial embolization may be an acceptable approach to treatment, favorably altering the natural history by slowing or arresting progressive cord compromise, without obliterating the lesion. Successive particle embolization can be used in this manner. Particle embolization permits slow, stepwise embolization, in a carefully controlled manner, with an ability to observe dynamic changes in the lesion and surrounding normal arterial anatomy during embolization. Particle embolization tends to permit recanalization over time, so periodic (usually annual) retreatment is necessary. In a series of thoracic AVMs treated with periodic particle embolization, 57% of patients improved neurologically after the initial embolization, and 63% improved neurologically after the final embolization. Repeated treatments were required because the recanalization rate was 80%, but there was a clear clinical benefit, with favorable alteration of the natural history, with persistence of clinical improvement after treatment even in the setting of AVM recanalization. It is hypothesized that successive embolization preserves some neurological function by protecting the spinal cord from prolonged exposure to the AVM.[9]

When the configuration of the AVM permits, liquid embolic agents such as n-butyl cyanoacrylate (n-BCA) and Onyx (ev3, Irvine, CA) should be used to embolize the lesion from within or as close to the AVM nidus as possible. These agents provide essentially permanent occlusion, with very low rates of recanalization. A hazard of these agents is the speed with which they act, resulting in a risk to small perforating arteries supplying normal spinal cord, which may only reappear angiographically as the steal from high-flow components is reduced during embolization.

Several series confirm that it is possible to embolize more than half of the target lesion in more than 80% of patients, with good clinical outcome in more than 80% of patients, and fixed neurological deficit in fewer than 15% of patients (severe deficits in fewer than 5%). The completeness of the embolization is not clearly correlated with clinical outcome.[10,11]

Most procedural morbidity in the setting of spinal AVM embolization is associated with catheterization of the ASA. We recommend use of a flow-guided catheter for this purpose, when possible. The catheter should be positioned within or as close to the nidus as possible, ideally in a sulcal branch that has turned off the longitudinal axis of the ASA, so as to minimize inadvertent embolization of a small, normal branch.

23.24 Pial Arteriovenous Fistula

The guiding principle behind treatment of pial AVFs is to obliterate the fistula at the point of arteriovenous connection, and to intervene early at an early stage, soon after presentation, to prevent spinal cord compromise and neurological deterioration. Endovascular embolization may also be used as an adjunct to microsurgical treatment, but any treatment approach must achieve complete and permanent occlusion of the point of arteriovenous connection in order to achieve cure and prevent long-term recurrence.

Liquid embolic materials, alone or in conjunction with detachable coils as a scaffold, are ideal for endovascular treatment of pial AVFs, as their degree of penetration into the nidus, to the point of arteriovenous connection, can be controlled. Particle embolization should be used only when endovascular therapy is used as an adjunct to microsurgical treatment, as particle-based occlusions are prone to recanalization. Furthermore, particles may pass through the shunt into the venous circulation, resulting in venous thrombi or pulmonary embolism.

As discussed in a previous section, pial AVFs vary greatly in their angioarchitecture. As a result, endovascular treatment must be individualized to each specific lesion.

Endovascular embolization is typically the treatment modality of choice for giant (type III) pial AVFs. These lesions are amenable to safe microcatheterization of the feeding arteries, which are dilated in response to high flow. Giant pial AVFs can be treated by deploying coils into the fistula as a scaffold for a liquid embolic agent such as n-BCA glue or Onyx (ev3, Irvine, CA). The objective of this approach is to prevent migration of the embolic agent through to the venous side of the high-flow shunt. Embolization must be performed at the fistulous connection and proximal draining vein, but not more proximally on the arterial side, so as to prevent subsequent recruitment of inaccessible collateral feeding arteries and recanalization of the fistula.

Embolization of large (type II) pial AVFs can be challenging, as these lesions typically contain at least one transmedullary or perimedullary feeding artery that is unsafe to catheterize. Small (type I) pial AVFs can be difficult to treat endovascularly, as superselective catheterization and microcatheter placement within the fistula may be dangerous when the feeding artery is a small, distal branch of the ASA. When the angioarchitecture of an AVF poses these technical challenges, microsurgical treatment may be preferable, particularly when the lesion is located on the dorsal or dorsolateral surface of the spinal cord.

23.25 Dural Arteriovenous Fistula

Endovascular management of spinal dural AVFs is similar to that of spinal AVMs, with several logical differences. Catheterization of dural AVFs typically requires microwire-assisted navigation, as these lesions are usually slower-flow lesions than AVMs, which may be catheterized using flow-guided microcatheters. Prior to embolization, superselective angiography should be performed through the microcatheter to ensure that no small branch to the ASA was missed on an initial angiogram from the segmental artery.

Importantly, spinal dural AVFs that receive arterial branches from the same pedicle as either the ASA or a PSA should be treated by microsurgical ligation, rather than by endovascular embolization.

23.26 Surgical Management

23.26.1 Spinal Cord Arteriovenous Malformation

Microsurgical obliteration of intramedullary spinal cord AVMs has been described in small case series, but is rarely achieved in practice.[12,13] Nevertheless, a microsurgical approach must be considered when safe angiographic access to the AVM cannot be achieved, as in cases in which the feeding spinal artery branches are long and tortuous. In these cases, microsurgical resection may be appropriate. In the cervical spine and in the filum terminale, both dorsal and ventral lesions can be approached safely for resection. In the thoracic spine, however, dorsal intramedullary AVMs are considerably safer and more straightforward to approach microsurgically than ventral lesions. In all cases, a superficial location makes the AVM more amenable to safe resection.

The microsurgical approach to intramedullary spinal cord AVMs is similar to that of cranial AVMs. Bipolar coagulation and ligation of the arterial feeders must be performed first, while preserving the venous drainage, in order to avoid intraoperative

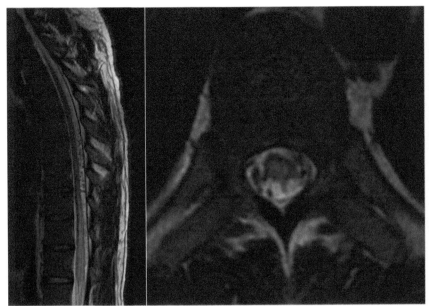

Fig. 23.4 Dural arteriovenous fistula of the thoracic spine (MRI). Sagittal (left) and axial (right) T2-weighted MRI sequences demonstrate an intradural extramedullary vascular nidus along the posterior aspect of the thoracic spinal cord, spanning the T6-9 levels, compatible with a type I spinal dural arteriovenous fistula. There is diffuse high T2 signal and an expansile appearance of the distal spinal cord and conus medullaris, compatible with venous hypertension.

rupture of the lesion. Associated aneurysms may be remodeled with bipolar cauterization, or they may be resected.

23.26.2 Pial Arteriovenous Fistula

The goal of microsurgical treatment of a pial AVF is to obliterate the fistulous connection between the arterial and venous system, while preserving all spinal artery branches.

Small (type I) and large (type II) pial AVFs are often best treated microsurgically, for reasons discussed in an earlier section. When the angioarchitecture of a pial AVF precludes definitive endovascular treatment, curative microsurgical ligation may nevertheless be possible, particularly when the fistula is located on the dorsal or dorsolateral aspect of the spinal cord and therefore accessible via standard thoracic laminectomy. The limitations of endovascular approaches in the face of multiple transmedullary or perimedullary feeding arteries, or a small feeding branch arising from a spinal artery, do not apply to the open microsurgical approach, in which arachnoid dissection and direct exposure of the feeding arteries facilitate precise ligation, without the attendant risks of catheterizing and occluding small arteries supplying normal spinal cord. Giant (type III) pial AVFs, on the other hand, which have massively dilated draining veins, are associated with increased risk of intraoperative hemorrhage and may be more easily treated by endovascular embolization.

23.26.3 Dural Arteriovenous Fistula

The spinal dural AVF represents one vascular lesion in contemporary vascular neurosurgery in which the microsurgical approach very often offers distinct advantages relative to endovascular treatment. The reason for this preference pertains to the typical anatomic configuration of a dural AVF in the thoracic spine, whose arterial supply is typically derived, as discussed in an earlier section, from a single radiculomeningeal branch of a segmental artery, with the shunt itself located in the dura around the sensory nerve root. When this configuration is

present, the fistula can be cured via ligation at a single point, which can be accessed in straightforward fashion via thoracic laminectomy. Moreover, test occlusion can be performed prior to ligation, with continuous neurophysiologic monitoring of the long spinal cord tracts, to ensure that no spinal artery branches will be compromised by permanent ligation at the targeted site.

▸ Fig. 23.4, ▸ Fig. 23.5, ▸ Fig. 23.6, ▸ Fig. 23.7, ▸ Fig. 23.8, ▸ Fig. 23.9, and ▸ Fig. 23.10 illustrate the approach to microsurgical treatment of spinal dural AVFs at our institution. The patient presented with progressive difficulty walking and myelopathy localizing to the midthoracic spine. MRI of the thoracic spine demonstrated an intradural extramedullary vascular nidus along the posterior aspect of the thoracic spinal cord, spanning the T6-9 levels, compatible with a type I spinal dural AVF; there was high T2 signal and an expansile appearance of the distal spinal cord and conus medullaris, compatible with venous hypertension. In the illustrated case, as demonstrated in the selective catheter angiogram shown in ▸ Fig. 23.5, the fistula is supplied by the radiculomeningeal branch of the left T7 segmental artery. A decision was made to treat the lesion surgically, and a coil was placed (▸ Fig. 23.6) to assist in localizing the level of the feeding artery intraoperatively, prior to laminectomy. Following a thoracic laminectomy at the targeted level, the appropriate nerve root is identified, and the dura is incised and retracted. A system of dilated perimedullary veins is readily identified (▸ Fig. 23.7). Arachnoid dissection at the sensory nerve root permits precise identification of the arteriovenous connection (▸ Fig. 23.8). We place a temporary aneurysm clip at this point for several minutes, and assess the resulting change in hemodynamics in three ways. First, direct observation under the operating microscope typically reveals an immediate color change in the previously arterialized venous complex (▸ Fig. 23.9). When normal blood flow is restored after the fistula is disconnected, the venous complex deepens in color, reflecting the return of venous (purple hue) blood to the venous circulation, which had previously been arterialized (red hue) by the fistula. Second, continuous neurophysiologic monitoring of motor and somatosensory evoked potentials is performed, to ensure

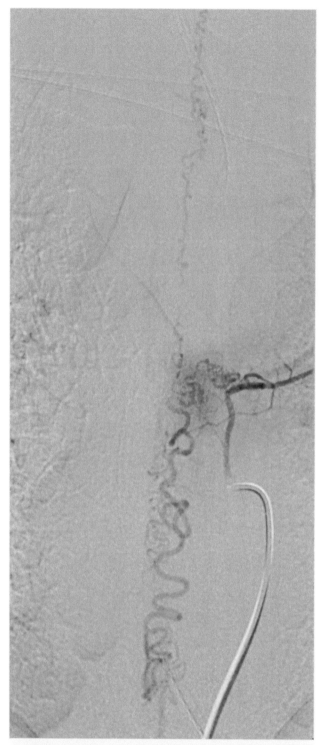

Fig. 23.5 Dural arteriovenous fistula of the thoracic spine (angiogram). Diagnostic spinal angiogram obtained by selective catheterization of the left T7 segmental artery demonstrates an arteriovenous fistula with the primary arterial feeder originating form left T7 segmental intercostal artery. There is evidence of severe venous congestion with delayed venous outflow into a perimedullary venous system. The artery of Adamkiewicz was found to originate from the left T9 segmental artery.

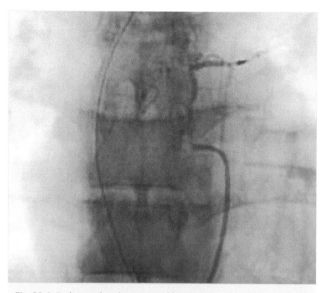

Fig. 23.6 Endovascular placement of localization coil. A nylon coil was deployed in the left T7 segmental artery, distal to the fistula, to assist in localizing the lesion for microsurgical ligation.

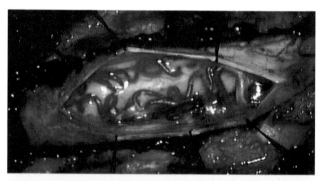

Fig. 23.7 Dilated intradural venous plexus. Intraoperative view of the dorsal surface of the spinal cord through the operating microscope after thoracic laminectomy and dural opening, demonstrating a plexus of dilated, arterialized perimedullary veins in the subarachnoid space.

that the temporary occlusion has not caused cord ischemia by compromising a spinal artery branch. Finally, we perform an indocyanine green injection as a form of intraoperative angiography to confirm obliteration of the arteriovenous shunt. After taking these precautions, we remove the temporary clip and ligate the radiculomeningeal branch at the location of the clip, using bipolar cautery (▸ Fig. 23.10).

23.27 Postoperative Care

Postoperative care following microsurgical or endovascular treatment of spinal AVMs is for the most part routine. One exception pertains to the postoperative management of AVMs and AVFs following endovascular embolization. Treatment of

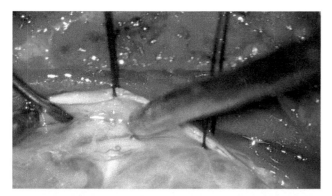

Fig. 23.8 Radiculomeningeal feeding artery. Intraoperative view of the left T7 radiculomeningeal artery, after arachnoid dissection, coursing parallel to the left T7 sensory nerve root. The adjacent, dilated, dorsal perimedullary veins are clearly arterialized, having the same reddish hue as the feeding artery itself.

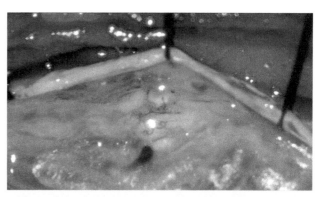

Fig. 23.10 Obliteration of the dural arteriovenous fistula. The temporary clip has been removed, and the fistulous connection has been ligated using microsurgical bipolar cautery. The color change in the previously arterialized veins, noted after placement of the temporary clip, is seen to persist, confirming closure of the fistula and restoration of the normal separation between the arterial and venous circulations.

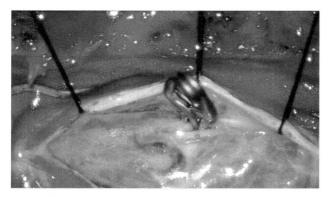

Fig. 23.9 Test occlusion by placement of a temporary clip. Temporary occlusion of the fistula at the point of arteriovenous connection is achieved intraoperatively, using a temporary vascular clip. The purpose of this maneuver is to ensure adequacy of ligation at the chosen point, which is confirmed in part by the color change in the surface veins from red to purple, consistent with restoration of the normal separation between the arterial and venous circulations. Additionally, motor and sensory evoked potentials are tested during this test occlusion to ensure that permanent ligation of the feeding artery will not cause a spinal cord stroke.

these lesions may result in progressive, retrograde thrombosis of the veins draining a fistula, or thrombosis of normal spinal arteries in the case of an AVM, with associated exacerbation of symptoms. These situations can be avoided by intensive care unit monitoring and treatment with intravenous heparin drip for 24 to 48 hours following embolization, with target partial thromboplastin time of 50 to 60 seconds.[14]

References

[1] Patsalides A, Knopman J, Santillan A, Tsiouris AJ, Riina H, Gobin YP. Endovascular treatment of spinal arteriovenous lesions: beyond the dural fistula. AJNR Am J Neuroradiol. 2011; 32(5):798–808

[2] Santillan A, Nacarino V, Greenberg E, Riina HA, Gobin YP, Patsalides A. Vascular anatomy of the spinal cord. J Neurointerv Surg. 2012; 4(1):67–74

[3] Özkan N, Kreitschmann-Andermahr I, Goerike SL, et al. Single center experience with treatment of spinal dural arteriovenous fistulas. Neurosurg Rev. 2015; 38(4):683–692

[4] Albright LA, ed. Principles and Practice of Pediatric Neurosurgery. 3rd ed. New York, NY: Thieme; 2014

[5] Manelfe C, Lazorthes G, Roulleau J. Artères de la dure-mère rachidienne chez l'homme [Arteries of the human spinal dura mater]. Acta Radiol Diagn (Stockh). 1972; 13(0):829–841

[6] Merland JJ, Riche MC, Chiras J. Intraspinal extramedullary arteriovenous fistulae draining into the medullary veins. J Neuroradiol. 1980; 7(4):271–320

[7] Hurth M, Houdart R, Djindjian R, Rey A, Djindjian M. Arteriovenous malformations of the spinal cord: clinical, anatomical and therapeutic consideration: a series of 150 cases. Prog Neurol Surg. 1978; 9:238–266

[8] Aminoff MJ, Logue V. The prognosis of patients with spinal vascular malformations. Brain. 1974; 97(1):211–218

[9] Biondi A, Merland JJ, Reizine D, et al. Embolization with particles in thoracic intramedullary arteriovenous malformations: long-term angiographic and clinical results. Radiology. 1990; 177(3):651–658

[10] Rodesch G, Hurth M, Alvarez H, David P, Tadie M, Lasjaunias P. Embolization of spinal cord arteriovenous shunts: morphological and clinical follow-up and results—review of 69 consecutive cases. Neurosurgery. 2003; 53(1):40–49, discussion 49–50

[11] Corkill RA, Mitsos AP, Molyneux AJ. Embolization of spinal intramedullary arteriovenous malformations using the liquid embolic agent, Onyx: a single-center experience in a series of 17 patients. J Neurosurg Spine. 2007; 7(5):478–485

[12] Boström A, Krings T, Hans FJ, Schramm J, Thron AK, Gilsbach JM. Spinal glomus-type arteriovenous malformations: microsurgical treatment in 20 cases. J Neurosurg Spine. 2009; 10(5):423–429

[13] Zozulya YP, Slin'ko EI, Al-Qashqish II. Spinal arteriovenous malformations: new classification and surgical treatment. Neurosurg Focus. 2006; 20(5):E7

[14] Knopman J, Zink W, Patsalides A, Riina HA, Gobin YP. Secondary clinical deterioration after successful embolization of a spinal dural arteriovenous fistula: a plea for prophylactic anticoagulation. Interv Neuroradiol. 2010; 16(2):199–203

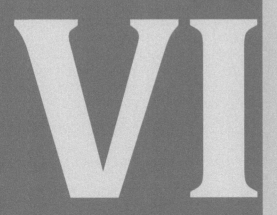

VI

24 Classifications of Thoracic Spinal Fractures

Hai Le and Christopher M. Bono

Abstract

The thoracolumbar junction (T10–L2) is a unique transition zone between the relatively rigid thoracic spine (T1–T10) and the more mobile lower lumbar spine (L3–L5). At this junction, the spine is subject to great biomechanical stress and, consequently, the thoracolumbar spine is the most common site of failure from blunt trauma. To the authors' knowledge, there are no classification systems specific to the thoracic spine. Thus, thoracic and lumbar injuries are most often considered together in classification systems. The earliest classification of thoracolumbar fractures dates back to Boehler's sentinel work in 1929, when he first categorized fractures based on the mechanism of injury and fracture morphology. Denis' three-column spine model marked an important point in history, as this classification offered insight into the stability of the spine and attempted to guide treatment. Since these publications, additional classifications have been developed, each of which has advanced our understanding in characterizing and managing thoracolumbar trauma. This chapter reviews the common classification schemes for thoracic injuries, specifically detailing their historical context as well as highlighting their advantages and disadvantages.

Keywords: thoracic spine, thoracolumbar spine, thoracolumbar fracture, classification, spine trauma, thoracolumbar trauma

Clinical Pearls

- The thoracolumbar junction (T10–L2) is the most common site of spinal failure from blunt trauma.
- Both thoracic and lumbar injuries are considered together in classification systems.
- Boehler published the first classification in 1929, organizing injuries into five categories on the basis of the mechanism of injury and fracture morphology.
- Watson-Jones simplified injuries into three categories and emphasized the importance of the posterior ligamentous complex (PLC) to the stability of the spinal column.
- Nicoll classified injuries into four groups on an anatomical basis and offered treatment guidelines based on the neurological status and spinal stability.
- Holdsworth introduced the two-column concept and upheld that the posterior column, and thus the integrity of the PLC, was the determining factor of stability.
- Under his three-column principle, Denis proposed that the middle column was integral to spinal stability. The extent of thoracolumbar trauma could be measured by three degrees of instability.
- McAfee et al grouped thoracolumbar trauma into six patterns of injuries determined solely by sagittal computed tomography imaging.
- According to their mechanistic classification, Ferguson and Allen categorized injuries into six groups depending on the

mode on failure of the anterior and posterior spinal elements.
- The Gaines load sharing classification was the first to incorporate a point system to quantify injury severity and guide surgical treatment.
- The Magerl/AO classification was the most comprehensive system and subcategorized thoracolumbar trauma into 53 distinct injuries.
- The thoracolumbar injury classification and severity score (TLICS) assigned a comprehensive injury severity score to every thoracolumbar trauma based on the injury morphology, integrity of the PLC, and neurological status. The TLICS score helped guide clinical decision-making.
- The AOSpine classification assigned a thoracolumbar AOSpine injury score (TL AOSIS) score to every thoracolumbar trauma based on the fracture morphology, neurological status, and patient-specific modifiers. Operative versus nonoperative treatment was recommended depending on the TL AOSIS score.

24.1 Introduction

The thoracic spine is a complex three-dimensional structure made up of bones, soft tissues (intervertebral discs and ligaments), and the neural elements (spinal cord and nerve roots). It can fail under supraphysiological forces in flexion, compression, extension, distraction, lateral bending, axial rotation, translation, shear, or any combination thereof. The same directional forces can produce different fracture patterns and severity of injury depending on the position of the spine at the instantaneous moment of injury. Injuries can be broadly considered to be mechanically stable or unstable. Either may be associated with a neurological deficit. In distinction from the more mobile and flexible lumbar spine, the thoracic spine is additionally stabilized from the interaction with the ribs. Thus, more energy is required to lead to injury of this more rigid spinal region.

Adding to these complexities is the diversity of treatment options for thoracic injuries which can vary widely between institutions and surgeons. In following, there is currently no universally accepted classification that can perfectly characterize these injuries, predict treatment outcomes, or unanimously guide clinical decision-making.

Starting with Boehler's original work and Holdsworth's two-column concept and progressing to more modern systems such as the thoracolumbar injury classification and severity score (TLICS) and the thoracolumbar AOSpine injury score (TL AOSIS), it is this chapter's goal to review the milestones along this 90-year journey of thoracic spine fracture classification. Much has been learned about the natural history and behavior of specific injuries with certain types of management. Below, we detail the development of various fracture classifications in chronological order and underscore how each has added to our understanding of injury care (▶ Table 24.1).

Table 24.1 Summary of classifications of thoracolumbar fractures

Classification	Boehler	Watson-Jones	Nicoll	Holdsworth	Denis	McAfee	Ferguson & Allen	McCormack	Magerl/AO	TLICS	AOSpine TLICS
Basis of classification	Mechanism of injury, fracture morphology	Mechanism of injury, fracture morphology (specifically of vertebral body)	Mechanism of injury, fracture morphology	Mechanism of injury to two spinal columns, fracture morphology	Mechanism of injury to three spinal columns	Three modes of failure of middle column	Mechanism of injury to anterior and posterior elements	Vertebral body comminution, fragment apposition, kyphosis correction	Failure of spinal column by three main forces (compression, distraction, or rotation)	Injury morphology, neurological status, integrity of PLC	Fracture morphology, neurological status, patient-specific modifiers
Major categories	5	3	4	5	4	6	6	3	3	3	3
	Compression Flexion distraction Extension Shear Rotational	Simple wedge Comminuted Fracture dislocation	Anterior wedge Lateral wedge Fracture dislocation Isolated fracture of neural arch	Simple wedge Rotational fracture dislocation Extension dislocation Vertical compression Shear	Compression Burst Seat-belt type (flexion distraction) Fracture dislocation	Wedge compression Stable burst Unstable burst Chance Flexion distraction Translational	Compressive flexion Distractive flexion Lateral flexion Torsional flexion Translation Vertical compression Distractive flexion	Three major variables, each is graded between one to three degrees of severity 3 points minimum, 9 points maximum	Vertebral body compression Anterior and posterior element injury with distraction Anterior and posterior element injury with rotation	Three major variables 1 point minimum, 10 points maximum	Three major variables 0 point minimum, 13 points maximum
Subcategories	–	–	–	–	21 types and subtypes	–	–	Many combinations of injuries	53 groups and subgroups with specifications	Many combinations of injuries	Many combinations of injuries
Significance	First TL trauma classification	Emphasis of PLC on stability Provided methods of reduction, prognosis of neurological deficits and treatment outcomes	Differentiated stable versus unstable TL fractures Provided treatment guidelines depending on neurological status and spinal stability	Introduced two-column concept with emphasis on posterior column for spinal stability Described burst fractures	Introduced three-column concept with emphasis on middle column for spinal stability Described extent of TL trauma based on three degrees of instability	Classified injuries on basis of sagittal CT Provided surgical treatment guidelines Differentiated stable versus unstable burst fractures, bony versus ligamentous flexion–distraction injuries	Introduced concept of anterior and posterior elements	First-point system Treatment guidelines based on total severity score	The most comprehensive classification	Introduced neurological status as major factor in TL classification Treatment guidelines based on total severity score	Newest classification Introduced patient-specific modifiers to TL classification

Abbreviations: PLC, posterior ligamentous complex; TL, thoracolumbar.

Note: This table summarizes the different classifications of thoracolumbar trauma with an emphasis on the basis of each classification and its contribution to our understanding of thoracolumbar classification and management.

24.2 Boehler: 1929

The first published classification of thoracolumbar injuries was reported by Boehler in 1929. In his seminal work, Boehler reviewed the plain radiographs of patients with spinal injury during World War I and developed his classification scheme based on the mechanism of injury and fracture morphology. He grouped thoracolumbar trauma into five categories: compression, flexion distraction, extension, shear, and rotational injuries.[1]

24.3 Watson-Jones: 1938

In 1938, Watson-Jones was credited as the first to emphasize the importance of the posterior ligamentous complex (PLC) to the stability of the thoracolumbar spinal column.[2] The PLC is the capsuloligamentous structures supporting the vertebral arch comprising the facet joint capsule, ligamentum flavum, interspinous ligament, and supraspinous ligament (▶ Fig. 24.1). Like Boehler, Watson-Jones' classification scheme was based on the mode of injury and fracture pattern, specifically of the vertebral body. He simplified thoracolumbar trauma into three categories: simple wedge fractures, comminuted fractures, and fracture dislocations.

Simple wedge fractures were the most common that he observed. He felt these were caused by axial loading. With this fracture pattern, Watson-Jones observed that the intervertebral disc was generally preserved and therefore ankylosis of the fractured segment to an adjacent segment over time was rare. He additionally postulated that the wedging through an intact

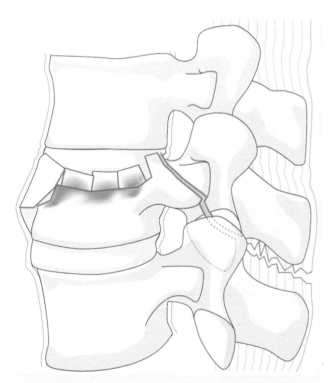

Fig. 24.1 Posterior ligamentous complex (PLC). Illustrative example of an injury to the PLC, which comprises four capsuloligamentous structures: facet capsule, ligamentum flavum, interspinous ligament, and supraspinous ligament. (Copyright AO Foundation, Switzerland. Reproduced with permission.)

disc increased the strain on the facet joints which could lead to persistent pain. In contrast, the disc in comminuted fractures was felt to be more generally disrupted, and thus ankylosis was found to occur more commonly. Interestingly, despite being what we would consider to be higher energy injuries, these fractures tend to be less painful because of the "autofusion" that would occur anteriorly. Finally, fracture dislocations were a distinct group that was found to have a higher risk for spinal cord injury (SCI). Such injuries carried a particularly poor prognosis in the high thoracic spine. According to his writings, Watson-Jones insisted on obtaining "perfect reduction" to achieve the best clinical outcomes, similar to burgeoning appendicular (long-bone) fracture recommendations.

24.4 Nicoll: 1949

Nicoll further advanced the work of Watson-Jones and in 1949 published his thoracolumbar classification system organized on an anatomical basis into four main categories: anterior wedge fractures, lateral wedge fractures, fracture dislocations, and isolated fractures of the neural arch.[3] Nicoll also acknowledged the importance of the PLC, most importantly the interspinous ligament, in predicting stability. Like Watson-Jones, he observed that in anterior wedge fractures, the fulcrum of angular deformity lies at the nucleus pulposus, and therefore compromise of the interspinous ligament must take place to produce instability. Radiographically, disruption of the interspinous ligament was implied if there was separation of the spinous processes.

Nicoll divided wedge fractures into anterior and lateral types. He believed lateral wedge fractures occurred when the axial skeleton was forced forward and to one side (i.e., a flexion-rotation mechanism). This force would lead to fractures of the transverse processes on the concave side and of the intervertebral joints on the convex side of the spinal column. Nicoll reported that this fracture pattern had a poorer prognosis than its anterior counterpart. Neural arch fractures were thought to be caused by rotational injuries. Nicoll observed that bilateral arch fractures anywhere in the thoracic spine were stable. Like Watson-Jones, he called for perfect reduction, stating that "a good anatomical result is indispensable to a good functional result."

Nicoll offered treatment guidelines based on the neurological status of the patient and spinal stability. In patients with a normal neurological examination, the first step was to establish whether the fracture was stable or unstable. Wedge fractures with intact interspinous ligament and neural arch fractures were considered stable. Stable fractures would undergo so-called "functional treatment," which does not require reduction or immobilization. Wedge fractures with rupture of the interspinous ligament were considered unstable, being treated with reduction and immobilization to minimize the risk of deformity and disability. Understand that all treatment at this time was closed as there were no internal fixation options for the spine at the time.

24.5 Holdsworth: 1963

Holdsworth introduced the two-column concept of spinal stability in 1963.[4,5] The anterior column comprises the anterior

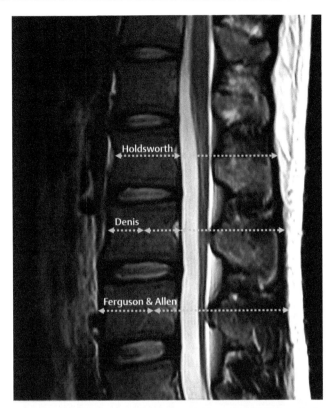

Fig. 24.2 Spinal columns and elements. Holdsworth divided the spinal column into the anterior (from ALL to PLL) and posterior column (comprising the neural arches, facets, and PLC). Denis divided the spine into the anterior (from ALL to anterior half of body/disc), middle (from posterior half of body/disc to PLL), and posterior column (comprising the posterior bony elements and ligamentous complex). Ferguson and Allen divided the spinal column into the anterior (from ALL to anterior two-thirds of body/disc) and posterior element (from posterior one-third of body/disc to PLC).

Table 24.2 Denis' thoracolumbar classification

Fracture type	Spinal column		
	Anterior	Middle	Posterior
Compression	Compression	–	–
Burst	Compression	Compression	–
Seat-belt type (flexion distraction)	± Compression	Distraction	Distraction
Fracture dislocation	Compression, rotation, shear	Distraction, rotation, shear	Distraction, rotation, shear

Source: Data from Denis.[6]
Note: Denis classified thoracolumbar trauma into four major groups, depending on the mode of failure of one, two, or all three spinal columns. Each column can fail under forces in compression, distraction, rotation, shear, or any combination thereof.

24.6 Denis: 1983

In 1983, Denis advanced the two-column concept by dividing Holdsworth's anterior column into separate anterior and middle columns.[6,7] His three-column principle changed the way surgeons considered stability and managed thoracolumbar trauma. The three columns consist of the anterior (ALL to anterior half of the vertebral body and disc), middle (posterior half of the vertebral body and disc to the PLL), and posterior column (posterior bony elements and ligamentous complex) (▶ Fig. 24.2). In contrast to Watson-Jones, Nicoll, and Holdsworth, Denis maintained that disruption of the PLC (or posterior column) alone is insufficient to results in spinal instability. Instead, his definition of instability required two adjacent columns to be compromised. Accordingly, spinal instability develops when the middle column fails either with the anterior or posterior columns (or both).[1,6,7,8]

In short, Denis denoted that the middle column was the key to predicting neurological injury and stability. Compression of the middle column (or vertical collapse) can cause narrowing of the neuroforaminae and injury to the exiting nerve roots. More importantly, posterior displacement of the vertebral body fragmens (or retropulsion) can lead to compression of the spinal cord (▶ Fig. 24.3).

Denis divided thoracolumbar trauma into minor and major injuries. Minor injuries included fractures of the transverse processes, articular processes, pars, and spinous processes. Major injuries were classified into four groups from most to least stable: compression, burst, seat-belt type (flexion distraction), and fracture dislocation. These four fracture patterns are due to failure of one, two, or all three columns (▶ Table 24.2).[1,8] Compression fractures occur from axial force causing isolated failure of the anterior column. In minor compression fractures, only the anterior column fails in compression. In severe compression fractures, the middle column serves as a hinge, so the posterior column may fail in tension. Like Nicoll, Denis distinguished two types of compression fractures, anterior and lateral. Burst fractures occur when the anterior and middle columns fail in compression. Denis described five different types of burst fractures. Seat-belt type fractures involve the middle and posterior columns, which fail in tension. The axis lies at the anterior column, which may fail in compression. Fracture dislocations are complex and arise when all three columns

longitudinal ligament (ALL), vertebral body, disc, and posterior longitudinal ligament (PLL). The posterior column comprises the osseoligamentous structures posterior to the PLL, which include the neural arches, facets, and PLC (▶ Fig. 24.2). The major contribution that this system made, which still stands today, is that the posterior column, and thus the integrity of the PLC, was deemed the determining factor of stability.

Morphologically, Holdsworth classified thoracolumbar trauma based on clinical and radiographic findings into five categories: simple wedge fractures, rotational fracture dislocations, extension dislocations, vertical compression fractures, and shear fractures. Wedge fractures are caused by pure flexion and are inherently stable. Flexion rotation results in fracture dislocations with disruption of the PLC, which pose high risk of neurological injury. Extension causes failure of the anterior column, specifically rupture of the intervertebral disc and avulsion injury of the ALL. Extension dislocations are stable in flexion, so immobilization in this position was recommended. Holdsworth was the first to introduce the concept of a burst fracture. Of note, he felt that these injuries were generally stable because the ligaments remained intact. Finally, shear force across the posterior column can produce instability and spondylolisthesis and therefore neurological injury was common.

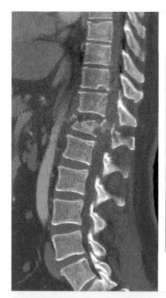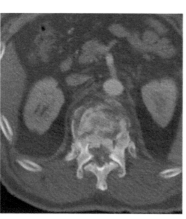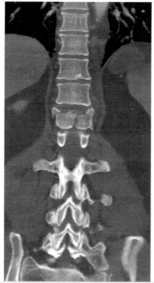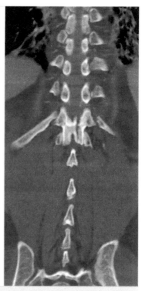

Fig. 24.3 Burst fracture. Sagittal, axial, and coronal CT images demonstrating a burst fracture at T12 with retropulsion of the fractured fragments into the spinal canal. (Copyright AO Foundation, Switzerland. Reproduced with permission.)

fail from a combination of flexion rotation, shear, and flexion distraction forces (▶ Fig. 24.4). The main drawback of Denis' classification is it quickly branches from 4 major fracture patterns into 21 different types and subtypes.

Denis was one of the first to describe the extent of thoracolumbar trauma based on the degree of instability.[6] First degree instability is purely mechanical with risk of progressive kyphotic deformity. It describes the severe compression and seat-belt type fractures. Second degree instability is purely neurological. This includes the stable burst fractures. Third degree instability combines mechanical and neurological instability and accounts for the unstable burst fractures and fracture dislocations.

24.7 McAfee: 1983

McAfee et al developed a simple thoracolumbar fracture classification in 1983 based on computed tomography (CT) imaging.[9] Like Denis, the authors maintained that the integrity of the middle column is essential to spinal stability. They observed three modes of failure of the middle column as determined on the sagittal CT reconstruction: axial compression, axial distraction, and translation. Based on these modes of failure, six patterns of thoracolumbar trauma were established: wedge compression, stable burst, unstable burst, Chance fracture, flexion distraction, and translational.

One advantage of the McAfee system over Denis' classification is the simplification of thoracolumbar fractures into six types with no subtypes. McAfee et al were among the first to provide surgical treatment guidelines based on how the middle column fails. Interestingly, these guidelines were based on hook constructs, which was the only widely available form of internal fixation of the spine at the time. Compression injuries were treated with distraction instrumentation, distraction injuries by compression instrumentation, and translation by segmental spinal instrumentation (created by so-called claw constructs of sections of hooks above and below the injury).

This group has been credited for subcategorizing burst fractures as stable or unstable, based on involvement of the posterior column, an important distinction from Denis' system in which all burst fractures were by definition unstable. This classification also distinguished between bony flexion–distraction injuries (so-called Chance fractures) versus ligamentous flexion–distraction injuries (▶ Fig. 24.5). The latter group was usually unstable and therefore felt to require surgical intervention.[1] Of note, this classification scheme was developed on the basis of CT imaging, a relatively new technology at the time that was not yet widely available at all centers.

24.8 Ferguson and Allen: 1984

In 1984, Ferguson and Allen presented their "mechanistic classification," which catalogued thoracolumbar injuries based on the mechanism of failure of the anterior and posterior spinal elements,[10] similar to their more widely adopted classification of cervical spine injuries. The authors divided the spine into elements rather than columns. The junction between the anterior two-thirds and posterior one-third of the vertebral body marks the division into the anterior and posterior elements (▶ Fig. 24.2). Ferguson and Allen observed that the spine can fail in six ways: compressive flexion, distractive flexion, lateral flexion, torsional flexion, translation vertical compression, and distractive flexion. Like McAfee et al, they maintained that the mechanism of injury can help guide the instrumentation of choice for surgical stabilization.[10]

24.9 McCormack: 1994

McCormack et al were the first to assign a point system in a classification of thoracolumbar trauma in 1994, known as the Gaines load sharing classification.[11] This classification is based on three variables and attempt to predict the behavior of the injury with a posterior short-segment pedicle screw construct

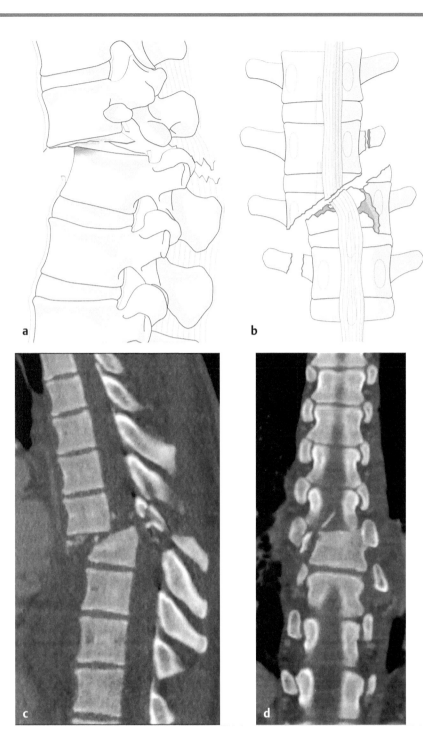

Fig. 24.4 Fracture dislocation. Sagittal (**a**) and coronal (**b**) illustration and sagittal (**c**) and coronal (**d**) CT reconstruction demonstrating a fracture dislocation of the thoracic spine with complete dissociation between the cephalad and caudal segments at the level of injury. (Copyright AO Foundation, Switzerland. Reproduced with permission.)

(i.e., screws at the level above and below the injury only). The first variable is vertebral body comminution, or how damaged the vertebral body is; the second is fragment apposition, or how spread out the fragments are; and the third is kyphosis correction, or how much surgical correction of kyphosis is required (▶ Table 24.3). Each variable is then assigned a degree of severity (1 point for mild, 2 points for moderate, and 3 points for severe). The sum of all three variables (minimum of 3 and maximum of 9) gives the total severity score.

Treatment guidelines are recommended based on the total severity score. For injuries with a total severity score of less than or equal to 6, short-segment posterior instrumentation is recommended. A total severity score of greater than or equal to 7 predicts failure of short-segment posterior instrumentation as determined by screw breakage. Therefore, these injuries require some form of anterior column support. Specifically, if there is no fracture dislocation, anterior instrumentation with strut graft fusion is sufficient. If there is fracture dislocation, combined staged posterior followed by anterior instrumented fusion was recommended.

This point system makes it possible to quantify the severity of thoracolumbar trauma. However, the authors

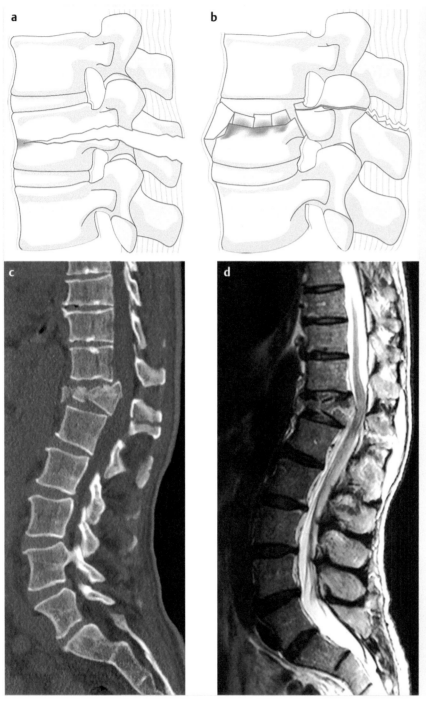

Fig. 24.5 Flexion–distraction injury. **(a)** illustrates a purely osseous flexion–distraction injury (i.e., Chance fracture). Compare that to **(b)**, which shows a flexion–distraction injury with disruption of both osseous and ligamentous structures. Sagittal CT **(c)** and MRI **(d)** showing a flexion–distraction injury at T12. (Copyright AO Foundation, Switzerland. Reproduced with permission.)

noted that this classification does not take into account the integrity of the PLC or the mechanism of injury. Because ligamentous injury and neurological status are not addressed, they concluded that this classification "cannot be used to make decisions on surgical indications." Furthermore, this classification was established from a retrospective study of patients who had undergone surgical stabilization; therefore, it cannot be applied to patients who have not undergone surgery (i.e., the degree of kyphosis correction cannot be determined).

24.10 Magerl/AO: 1994

The most comprehensive classification to date was proposed by Magerl et al in 1994 based on the AO principles and 3-3-3 classification scheme applied to extremity fractures. This study was the largest at the time, having considered the mechanism of injury and pathomorphological characteristics of 1,445 consecutive cases (▶ Table 24.4). The authors observed that the spinal column failed by three principal forces, each of which leads to a type of fracture. Compression force produces type A injuries,

Table 24.3 Gaines load sharing classification

Degree of severity (points)	Comminution/ involvement[a]	Fragment apposition[b]	Deformity correction[c]
Mild (1)	Little (< 30%)	Minimal	Little (≤ 3°)
Moderate (2)	More (30–60%)	Spread (≥ 2 mm displacement of < 50% of body)	More (4–9°)
Severe (3)	Gross (> 60%)	Wide (≥ 2 mm displacement of > 50% of body)	Most (≥ 10°)

[a]Based on sagittal CT
[b]Based on axial CT
[c]Based on lateral plain radiograph
Source: Data from McCormack et al.[11]
Note: The load sharing classification was based on three variables: fracture comminution, fragment apposition, and kyphosis correction. Each variable is assigned a degree of severity. Their sum yields the total severity score. Short-segment posterior instrumentation is recommended for injuries with a total severity score of ≤ 6. Anterior column support is recommended for injuries with a total severity score of > 7.

which comprise the vertebral body compression fractures (▶ Table 24.4). Type A injuries generally involve the anterior column while leaving the PLC intact. Of note, the authors used the term column as defined by Holdsworth. Distraction force produces type B injuries, which comprise anterior and posterior element injuries with distraction. Type B injuries are due to transverse disruption of one or both spinal columns. Axial torque (or rotation) produces type C injuries, which comprise anterior and posterior element injuries with rotation. In type C injuries, both columns are injured with potential for rotational and translational displacement.

Each type of fracture is further characterized into groups and subgroups with specifications, leading to an overwhelming 53 distinct thoracolumbar injuries. The severity of injury, and thus neurological deficit and spinal instability, progresses from type A through C and within groups and subgroups. This descriptive classification is all-encompassing and accounts for nearly all possible fracture patterns. Given its complexity, this classification may be useful for research endeavors but impractical for clinical practice. Its complexity also leads to poor inter- and intraobserver reliability.[12]

24.11 TLISS/TLICS: 2005

The TLICS, and its short-lived predecessor thoracolumbar injury severity score (TLISS), was introduced by the Spine Trauma Study Group in 2005.[13,14] The TLISS was based on injury mecha-

Table 24.4 Magerl/AO classification

Type	Group	Subgroup	Specification
A: vertebral body compression	A1: impaction	A1.1: endplate impaction	
		A1.2: wedge impaction	A1.2.1: superior A1.2.2: lateral A1.2.3: inferior
		A1.3: vertebral body collapse	
	A2: split	A2.1: sagittal split	
		A2.2: coronal split	
		A2.3: pincer	
	A3: burst	A3.1: incomplete burst	A3.1.1: superior A3.1.2: lateral A3.1.3: inferior
		A3.2: burst split	A3.2.1: superior A3.2.2: lateral A3.2.3: inferior
		A3.3: complete burst	A3.3.1: pincer A3.3.2: flexion A3.3.3: axial
B: anterior and posterior element injury with distraction	B1: posterior disruption predominantly ligamentous (flexion distraction)	B1.1: with transverse disruption of disc	B1.1.1: flexion subluxation B1.1.2: anterior dislocation B1.1.3: flexion subluxation/anterior dislocation with fracture of articular processes
		B1.2: with type A fracture of vertebral body	B1.2.1: flexion subluxation B1.2.2: anterior dislocation B1.2.3: flexion subluxation/anterior dislocation with fracture of articular processes
	B2: posterior disruption predominantly osseous (flexion distraction)	B2.1: transverse bicolumn fracture	
		B2.2: with transverse disruption of disc	B2.2.1: disruption through pedicle and disc B2.2.2: disruption through pars and disc (flexion spondylolysis)
		B2.3: with type A fracture of vertebral body	B2.3.1: fracture through pedicle B2.3.2: fracture through pars (flexion spondylolysis)

Table 24.4 continued

Type	Group	Subgroup	Specification
	B3: anterior disruption through disc (hyperextension shear)	B3.1: hyperextension subluxation	B3.1.1: without injury of posterior column B3.1.2: with injury of posterior column
		B3.2: hyperextension spondylolysis	
		B3.3: posterior dislocation	
C: anterior and posterior element injury with rotation	C1: type A injury with rotation	C1.1: rotational wedge	
		C1.2: rotational split	C1.2.1: sagittal split C1.2.2: coronal split C1.2.3: pincer C1.2.4: vertebral body separation
		C1.3: rotational burst	C1.3.1: incomplete C1.3.2: burst split C1.3.3: complete
	C2: type B injury with rotation	C2.1: B1 injury with rotation (flexion distraction with rotation)	C2.1.1: rotational flexion subluxation C2.1.2: rotational flexion subluxation with unilateral articular process fracture C2.1.3: unilateral dislocation C2.1.4: rotational anterior dislocation without/with fracture of articular processes C2.1.5: rotational flexion subluxation without/with unilateral articular process fracture + type A fracture C2.1.6: unilateral dislocation + type A fracture C2.1.7: rotational anterior dislocation without/with fracture of articular processes + type A fracture
		C2.2: B2 injury with rotation (flexion distraction with rotation)	C2.2.1: rotational transverse bicolumn fracture C2.2.2: unilateral flexion spondylolysis with disruption of disc C2.2.3: unilateral flexion spondylolysis + type A fracture
		C2.3: B3 injury with rotation (hyperextension-shear with rotation)	C2.3.1: rotational hyperextension-subluxation without/with fracture of posterior vertebral elements C2.3.2: unilateral hyperextension-spondylolysis C2.3.3: posterior dislocation with rotation
	C3: rotational-shear injury	C3.1: slice fracture	
		C3.2: oblique fracture	

Source: Data from Magerl F, Aebi M, Gertzbein SD, Harms J, Nazarian S. A comprehensive classification of thoracic and lumbar injuries. Eur Spine J 1994;3(4):184–201.

Note: The Magerl/AO classification is the most comprehensive thoracolumbar fracture classification. It grouped injuries based on how the spinal column failed under compression (type A fractures), distraction (type B) or rotation (type C) force. Each type of fracture is further characterized into groups and subgroups with specifications, leading to 53 distinct thoracolumbar injuries.

nism alone, while the TLICS also considered fracture morphology. Vaccaro et al established the TLICS based on three characteristics: injury morphology, integrity of the PLC, and neurological status. The injury morphology and integrity of the PLC were determined from plain radiography, CT imaging, and magnetic resonance imaging (MRI). The neurological status was graded by the American Spinal Injury Association (ASIA) system, with A designating complete SCI and ASIA B, C and D designating varying grades of incomplete injuries. The subgroups in each major variable are assigned points depending on the extent of involvement or severity (▶ Table 24.5). The points from the three variables are summed to give a comprehensive injury severity score (combined score of 1 minimum to 10 maximum), which is used to guide clinical decision-making. Specifically, nonoperative treatment is recommended for injuries with a combined score of less than or equal to 3, while operative treatment is recommended for injuries with a combined score

of greater than or equal to 5. A score of 4 can be managed either operatively or nonoperatively.

In addition to providing a guideline of when to consider surgery for a particular thoracolumbar injury, the TLICS goes further by suggesting which surgical approach might be carried out based on two general principles. First, an incomplete SCI generally requires anterior decompression. Second, disruption of the PLC generally requires posterior stabilization. Depending on the integrity of the PLC and the neurological status, either an anterior, posterior, or combined approach is recommended (▶ Table 24.6). Despite their logic, there is considerable variability in surgeon decision-making making it difficult to hold these treatment recommendations as a standard of care.

The TLICS is the first classification of thoracolumbar injuries that incorporates neurological status. It has been demonstrated to be both reliable and reproducible.[15,16,17] However, there are two minor drawbacks of the TLICS. First, although the integrity

Table 24.5 Thoracolumbar injury classification and severity score (TLICS)

Variable	Qualifiers	Points
Injury morphology		
• Compression	Burst	1
		2
• Translational/ rotational		3
• Distraction		4
Neurological status		
• Intact		0
• Nerve root		2
• Cord, conus medullaris	Complete	2
	Incomplete	3
• Cauda equina		3
Integrity of PLC		
• Intact		0
• Suspected/ indeterminate		2
• Injured		3

Abbreviation: PLC, posterior ligamentous complex.
Source: Data from Vaccaro et al.[14]
Note: Under the TLICS classification, different points are allotted for the injury morphology, neurological status, and PLC integrity. Their summation yields a combined injury severity score for a particular thoracolumbar injury. Nonoperative treatment is recommended for injuries with a combined score of ≤ 3, while operative treatment is recommended for injuries with a combined score of ≥ 5. A score of 4 can be managed either operatively or nonoperatively.

Table 24.6 TLICS recommended surgical approach

	PLC	
Neurological status	Intact	Disrupted
Intact	Posterior	Posterior
Root injury	Posterior	Posterior
Incomplete SCI or cauda equina	Anterior	Combined
Complete SCI or cauda equina	Anterior or posterior	Posterior or combined

Abbreviations: PLC, posterior ligamentous complex; SCI, spinal cord injury; TLICS, thoracolumbar injury classification and severity score.
Source: Data from Vaccaro et al.[14]
Note: The TLICS guides the recommended surgical approach (anterior, posterior, or combined) based on the last two components of the classification scheme, specifically the patient's neurological status and the integrity of the PLC.

of the PLC can be inferred from plain radiography and CT imaging (by widening of the interspinous space, facet diastasis, or facet subluxation/dislocation), it may still be difficult for inexperienced practitioners to determine the integrity of the PLC without MRI. This is problematic in polytrauma patients who may be unfit for MRI. Therefore, this "suspected/indeterminate" subgroup can cause confusion and affect clinical decision-making. Second, since determination of the neurological status from the ASIA classification necessitates that patients are not in spinal shock, the TLICS classification is difficult to interpret in the first 24 to 48 hours from injury.[1]

24.12 AOSpine TLICS and TL AOSIS: 2013

In a concerted effort to establish a comprehensive yet practical classification, an international team of spine trauma experts convened at the AOSpine Spinal Cord Injury and Trauma Knowledge Forum and introduced the AOSpine thoracolumbar injury classification system (AOSpine TLICS) in 2013.[18] This system considered three factors in classifying thoracolumbar trauma: fracture morphology, neurological status, and patient-specific modifiers.

Classification of the fracture morphology is based on three main injury patterns: type A (compression), type B (tension band disruption), and type C (displacement/translation) (▶ Fig. 24.6). Type A fractures are compression injuries due to

failure of the anterior structures under axial loading. These injuries are further divided into five subtypes (A0–A4). A0 subtypes consist of minor, nonstructural fractures such as those involving the spinous or transverse processes. These fractures are stable. A1 subtypes consist of wedge-compression fractures affecting a single endplate without involvement of the posterior wall of the vertebral body. A2 subtypes consist of split/pincer fractures in which both endplates are involved; like A1 subtypes, the posterior wall remains intact. A3 subtypes consist of incomplete burst fractures affecting a single endplate with involvement of the posterior wall. Finally, A4 subtypes are complete burst fractures with involvement of both endplates as well as the posterior wall. With incomplete or complete burst fractures, a vertical fracture of the lamina is usually present. Type B fractures are distraction injuries due to failure of the anterior or posterior tension band. These injuries are further divided into three subtypes (B1–B3). B1 subtypes result from transosseous tension band disruption, also known as bony Chance fractures. These injuries are a pure failure of the posterior tension band through one motion segment. B2 subtypes result from osseous and/or ligamentous failure of the posterior tension band combined with a type A (compression) fracture. B3 subtypes result from a hypertension injury through the disc or vertebral body. The ALL is commonly disrupted. Finally, type C fractures are displacement/translation injuries due to failure of all elements leading to dissociation between the cephalad and caudal segments at the level of injury. These injuries are not divided into subtypes and can occur concurrently with type A or B fractures.

Under the AOSpine TLICS, the neurological status at the time of presentation is graded as follows: N0 (no neurological deficit), N1 (transient deficit), N2 (radicular symptoms), N3 (incomplete SCI or any degree of cauda equina injury), N4 (complete SCI), and Nx (unknown neurological status secondary to altered mental status).

The third factor of the AOSpine TLICS is descriptive and provides details on two patient-specific modifiers. An M1 modifier is designated when injury to the posterior tension band is indeterminate, and an M2 modifier is designated when a patient has a comorbidity that argues either for or against surgery.

The AOSpine classification has demonstrated good interobserver and intraobserver reliability among spine surgeons.[19,20] Recently, Kepler et al established a spine injury score for the

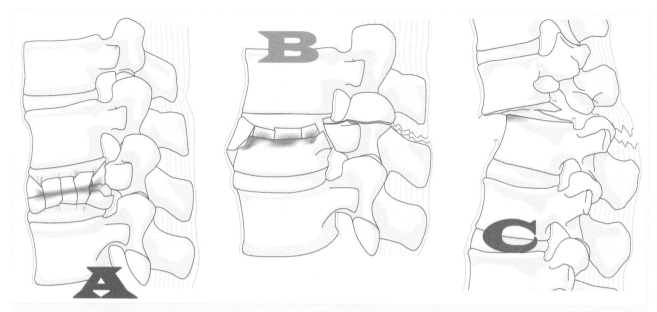

Fig. 24.6 AOSpine TLICS. Type A fractures are compression fractures resulting from excessive axial force. Type B fractures are distraction injuries resulting from disruption of the anterior or posterior tension band. Type C fractures are injuries resulting from complete fracture dislocation of the spinal column. (Copyright AO Foundation, Switzerland. Reproduced with permission.)

AOSpine TLICS called the TL AOSISbased on a survey of 100 spine surgeons worldwide (▶ Table 24.7).[21] Different points are allocated for the three major variables of the AOSpine TLICS (i.e., fracture morphology, neurological status, and patient-specific modifiers). Their summation represents the TL AOSIS for a specific thoracolumbar injury. Nonoperative treatment is recommended for a TL AOSIS of less than or equal to 3 while operative treatment is recommended for a TL AOSIS of greater than or equal to 5. A score of 4 can be managed either operatively or nonoperatively.[22] The AOSpine TLICS and TL AOSIS are relatively new and therefore their practicality is yet to be determined.

24.13 Acknowledgment

We would like to acknowledge the AOSpine for granting us permission to reuse their illustrations. "AOSpine is a clinical division of the AO Foundation—an independent medically guided nonprofit organization. The AOSpine Knowledge Forums are pathology focused working groups acting on behalf of AOSpine in their domain of scientific expertise. Each forum consists of a steering committee of up to 10 international spine experts who meet on a regular basis to discuss research, assess the best evidence for current practices, and formulate clinical trials to advance spine care worldwide. Study support is provided directly through AOSpine's Research department and AO's Clinical Investigation and Documentation unit."

Table 24.7 Thoracolumbar AOSpine injury score (TL AOSIS)

Variable	Points
Fracture morphology	
Type A: compression fractures	
• A0	0
• A1	1
• A2	2
• A3	3
• A4	5
Type B: tension band injuries	
• B1	5
• B2	6
• B3	7
Type C: translational injuries	8
Neurological status	
• N0	0
• N1	1
• N2	2
• N3	4
• N4	4
• Nx	3
Patient-specific modifiers	
• M1	1
• M2	0

Source: Data from Kepler et al.[21]

Note: Under the thoracolumbar AOSpine injury score (TL AOSIS), different points are allotted for the fracture morphology, neurological status, and patient-specific modifiers. Their summation yields a combined TL AOSIS score. Nonoperative treatment is recommended for thoracolumbar injuries with a TL AOSIS score of ≤ 3, while operative treatment is recommended for injuries with a TL AOSIS score of ≥ 5. A score of 4 can be managed either operatively or nonoperatively.

References

[1] Azam MQ, Sadat-Ali M. The concept of evolution of thoracolumbar fracture classifications helps in surgical decisions. Asian Spine J. 2015; 9(6):984–994

[2] Watson-Jones R. The results of postural reduction of fractures of the spine. J Bone Joint Surg. 1938; 20(3):567–586

[3] Nicoll EA. Fractures of the dorso-lumbar spine. J Bone Joint Surg Br. 1949; 31B(3):376–394

[4] Holdsworth FW. Fractures, dislocations, and fracture-dislocations of the spine. J Bone Joint Surg. 1963; 45B(1):6–20

[5] Holdsworth F. Fractures, dislocations, and fracture-dislocations of the spine. J Bone Joint Surg Am. 1970; 52(8):1534–1551

[6] Denis F. The three column spine and its significance in the classification of acute thoracolumbar spinal injuries. Spine. 1983; 8(8):817–831

[7] Denis F. Spinal instability as defined by the three-column spine concept in acute spinal trauma. Clin Orthop Relat Res. 1984(189):65–76

[8] Bernstein MP, Baxter AB, Harris JH. Imaging thoracolumbar spine trauma. In: Pope TL, Harris JH, eds. Harris & Harris' Radiology of Emergency Medicine. Philadelphia, PA: Lippincott Williams & Wilkins; 2013:265–306

[9] McAfee PC, Yuan HA, Fredrickson BE, Lubicky JP. The value of computed tomography in thoracolumbar fractures. An analysis of one hundred consecutive cases and a new classification. J Bone Joint Surg Am. 1983; 65(4):461–473

[10] Ferguson RL, Allen BL, Jr. A mechanistic classification of thoracolumbar spine fractures. Clin Orthop Relat Res. 1984(189):77–88

[11] McCormack T, Karaikovic E, Gaines RW. The load sharing classification of spine fractures. Spine. 1994; 19(15):1741–1744

[12] Blauth M, Bastian L, Knop C, Lange U, Tusch G. Interobserverreliabilität bei der Klassifikation von thorakolumbalen Wirbelsäulenverletzungen[Inter-observer reliability in the classification of thoraco-lumbar spinal injuries]. Orthopade. 1999; 28(8):662–681

[13] Vaccaro AR, Zeiller SC, Hulbert RJ, et al. The thoracolumbar injury severity score: a proposed treatment algorithm. J Spinal Disord Tech. 2005; 18(3):209–215

[14] Vaccaro AR, Lehman RA, Jr, Hurlbert RJ, et al. A new classification of thoracolumbar injuries: the importance of injury morphology, the integrity of the posterior ligamentous complex, and neurologic status. Spine. 2005; 30(20):2325–2333

[15] Bono CM, Vaccaro AR, Hurlbert RJ, et al. Validating a newly proposed classification system for thoracolumbar spine trauma: looking to the future of the thoracolumbar injury classification and severity score. J Orthop Trauma. 2006; 20(8):567–572

[16] Lenarz CJ, Place HM, Lenke LG, Alander DH, Oliver D. Comparative reliability of 3 thoracolumbar fracture classification systems. J Spinal Disord Tech. 2009; 22(6):422–427

[17] Lewkonia P, Paolucci EO, Thomas K. Reliability of the thoracolumbar injury classification and severity score and comparison with the Denis classification for injury to the thoracic and lumbar spine. Spine. 2012; 37(26):2161–2167

[18] Vaccaro AR, Oner C, Kepler CK, et al. AOSpine Spinal Cord Injury & Trauma Knowledge Forum. AOSpine thoracolumbar spine injury classification system: fracture description, neurological status, and key modifiers. Spine. 2013; 38(23):2028–2037

[19] Azimi P, Mohammadi HR, Azhari S, Alizadeh P, Montazeri A. The AOSpine thoracolumbar spine injury classification system: a reliability and agreement study. Asian J Neurosurg. 2015; 10(4):282–285

[20] Kepler CK, Vaccaro AR, Koerner JD, et al. Reliability analysis of the AOSpine thoracolumbar spine injury classification system by a worldwide group of naïve spinal surgeons. Eur Spine J. 2016; 25(4):1082–1086

[21] Kepler CK, Vaccaro AR, Schroeder GD, et al. The Thoracolumbar AOSpine Injury Score. Global Spine J. 2016; 6(4):329–334

[22] Vaccaro AR, Schroeder GD, Kepler CK, et al. The surgical algorithm for the AOSpine thoracolumbar spine injury classification system. Eur Spine J. 2016; 25(4):1087–1094

25 Complete and Incomplete Thoracic Spinal Cord Injuries

Vijay Yanamadala and John H. Shin

Abstract

Thoracic spinal injuries include complete and incomplete injuries, and are a major cause of morbidity and mortality resulting from either destabilization of the bony spine or neurological injury to the spinal cord or spinal nerves. Prompt medical and surgical treatment is essential to minimizing chronic functional disability. Major nonoperative issues are immobilization and management of hypoxia and hypotension to reduce secondary neurological damage to the spinal cord. Accurate diagnosis of the injury requires careful neurological examination and imaging. Optimal surgical decisions depend on the need for decompression, reduction of any induced deformity, and maintenance and/or restoration of spinal stability. This report reviews the commonly used criteria, guidelines, and approaches for operative management of thoracic spinal cord injury.

Keywords: spinal injury, spinal cord damage, vertebral fractures, spinal fusion, spinal stability

Clinical Pearls

- The goals of surgery in thoracic spinal cord injury include decompression of the spinal cord, correction of deformity, reduction of fractures, and the restoration of stability.
- Patients with incomplete thoracic spinal cord injuries often present with deficits that localize to specific areas of spinal cord injury, such as Brown–Sequard syndrome.
- Patients with Brown–Sequard syndrome have the best prognosis among patients with spinal cord injury. Most patients recover enough motor function to maintain ambulatory status.
- The thoracolumbar injury classification and severity score (TLICS) is based on morphology of the injury, integrity of the posterior ligamentous complex, and neurological status of the patient to provide prognosis and treatment guidelines.

25.1 Introduction

About 12,000 Americans sustain an acute spinal cord injury (SCI) every year, and in 2013 there existed a nationwide population of 273,000 who were living with the chronic consequences of SCI.[1] Patient with SCI comprise only 10 to 20% of all patients with spinal fractures.[2] For each patient with SCI many more suffer from bony or ligamentous injury. Common causes of SCI include motor vehicle accidents (MVA, 37%), falls (29%), violence (14%), and sports (9%).[1]

SCIs are often life changing for the patient and his or her family. They can cause great anxiety in the acute phase and substantial disability in the long term. Despite many refinements in the medical management and technological innovations in the surgical treatment, more than 99% of hospitalized patients with SCI are left with residual neurological dysfunction. The nature of residual neurological disability ranges complete

tetraplegia (12%), incomplete tetraplegia (41%), complete paraplegia (18%), and incomplete paraplegia (19%).[1,3] Spinal injuries without SCI have more favorable outcomes but correct diagnosis and treatment is necessary to limit chronic disability.

25.2 Pathophysiology of Spinal Cord Injury

The immediate effect of the injury is direct disruption of the neurological tissue by pressure or laceration from the spinal bones or foreign bodies. Simultaneous disruptions of blood vessels may cause bleeding in the spinal cord and result in a hematoma with potential to cause further pressure damage. Starting immediately and evolving over weeks, a number of vascular, eurohumoral, and cellular mechanisms are activated that cause secondary neurological injury. Vascular effects include hypotension from hemorrhagic or neurogenic shock leading to vasoconstriction and ischemic-reperfusion injury. Cellular effects include tissue hypoxia, free radical activation, cytokine release, lipid peroxidation, and apoptosis.[4,5] About 3 to 25% of damage to the spinal cord is estimated to occur after the initial injury. Hence, it is important to optimize care and minimize further loss of neurological function after the primary injury.[5]

25.3 Spinal Stability

In addition to consideration of spinal cord injury, the decision between operative and nonoperative management of spinal trauma depends on whether the spine is considered stable or unstable. Multiple theoretic models have been developed to assess spinal stability. The most commonly used model is the three-column model of Denis[6] consisting of an anterior column (anterior longitudinal ligament, the anterior two-thirds of the vertebral body, and the anterior annulus fibrosis), a middle column (posterior one-third of the vertebral body, the posterior longitudinal ligament, and posterior annulus fibrosis), and a posterior column (the posterior ligamentous complex connecting the neural arches and consisting of facet capsules, ligamentum flavum, and the interspinous and supraspinous ligaments). Failure of two or more columns results in spinal instability. More recent criteria for stability will also be discussed in this chapter.

25.4 Emergency Room and Intensive Care Management

25.4.1 Neurological Assessment

For 48 to 72 hours after SCI, the patient may be in spinal shock, a transient state of neurological unresponsiveness below the level of injury due to injury-induced hyperpolarization of spinal cord neurons. This stage is recognized by the loss of the bulbocavernosus reflex (contraction of anal sphincter in response to

Table 25.1 International standards for neurological classification of spinal cord injury by the American Spinal Injury Association (ASIA): ASIA Impairment Scale (AIS), 2011[7]

A = Complete	No sensory or motor function is preserved in the sacral segments S4–S5
B = Sensory incomplete	Sensory but not motor function is preserved below the neurological level and includes the sacral segments S4–S5, and no motor function is preserved more than three levels below the motor level on either side of the body
C = Motor incomplete	Motor function is preserved below the neurological level,[a] and more than half of key muscle functions below the single neurological level of injury have a muscle grade < 3 (grades 0–2)
D = Motor incomplete	Motor function is preserved below the neurological level,[a] and at least half (half or more) of key muscle functions below the neurological level of injury have a muscle grade > 3
E = Normal	If sensation and motor function as tested with the International Standards for Neurological Classification of Spinal Cord Injury are graded as normal in all segments, and the patient had prior deficits, then the AIS grade is E. Someone without a spinal cord injury does not receive an AIS grade

[a]For an individual to receive a grade of C or D, that is, motor incomplete status, he or she must have either (1) voluntary anal sphincter contraction or (2) sacral sensory sparing with sparing of motor function more than three levels below the motor level for that side of the body. The International Standards at this time allows even non-key muscle function more than three levels below the motor level to be used in determining motor incomplete status (AIS B vs. C).
Note: When assessing the extent of motor sparing below the level for distinguishing between AIS B and C, the motor level on each side is used; whereas to differentiate between AIS C and D (based on proportion of key muscle functions with strength grade 3 or greater), the neurological level of injury is used.

Table 25.2 Spinal Cord Independence Measure[8]

Self-care (subscore 0–20)	Feeding: 0–5
	Bathing: 0–5
	Dressing: 0–5
	Grooming: 0–5
Respiration and sphincter management (subscore 0–40)	Respiration: 0–10
	Sphincter management—bladder: 0–15
	Sphincter management—bowel: 0–10
	Use of toilet: 0–5
Mobility (subscore 0–40)	Mobility in bed and action to prevent pressure sores: 0–6
	Transfers: bed–wheelchair: 0–2
	Transfers: wheelchair–toilet–tub: 0–2
	Mobility indoors (short distances): 0–8
	Mobility for moderate distances: 0–8
	Mobility outdoors: 0–8
	Stair management: 0–4
	Transfers: wheelchair–car: 0–2
	Mobility in bed and action to prevent pressure sores: 0–6
	Transfers: bed–wheelchair: 0–2
	Transfers: wheelchair–toilet–tub: 0–2

squeezing of the glans penis or tugging on the urinary catheter). Prognostication about permanent neurological loss should be postponed till the resolution of spinal shock.

Neurological examination should include an inspection of face, head, and spine for lacerations, ecchymosis, and angular or rotational deformities. Patient should be log-rolled to palpate the entire spine. Absence of posterior, midline, and spinal tenderness in an awake and alert patient makes cervical SCI unlikely.

The American Spinal Injury Association (ASIA) recommended International Standards for Neurological Classification of Spinal Cord Injury in 1997 and last revised them in 2011 (▶ Table 25.1).[7] These have become the current standard of care in assessment of patients with SCI. Several other scales have also been proposed. Of these, the Spinal Cord Independence Measure (SCIM, ▶ Table 25.2) that incorporates measures of self-care, respiration, and sphincter management and mobility is particularly useful for following patients during the recovery phase of SCI.[4,8]

25.4.2 Radiological Assessment

Common radiological imaging tests for spine trauma include plain film radiographs, computed tomography (CT), and magnetic resonance imaging (MRI). CT scan is more sensitive than radiography but incurs more radiation exposure. MRI with short T1 inversion recovery (STIR) sequences is more sensitive in revealing soft tissue injuries such as disc herniation, ligamentous tears, and spinal cord contusion but may also produce more false positives. MR or CT angiography is useful to evaluate injury to the blood vessels such as the vertebral arteries.

25.4.3 Hypotension

Blood pressure may be low due to hemorrhagic or neurological shock. Hypotensive shock is usually due to associated injuries in large blood vessels or abdominal viscera. Neurological shock results from loss of sympathetic tone due to injured autonomic tracts in the spinal cord.

Vasopressor agents should be given to maintain a goal mean arterial pressure (MAP) of above 85 mm Hg.[9]

25.4.4 Hypoxia

Hypoxia should be avoided to prevent further injury to neurological tissues. Patients need to be intubated carefully without spinal movement.

25.4.5 Steroids

High-dose intravenous methylprednisolone is no longer recommended by either the American Association of Neurological Surgeons (AANS) or the Congress of Neurological surgeons (CNS) because the marginal benefit observed in the second and third National Acute Spinal Cord Injury Study trials (NASCIS II and III) did not outweigh potential adverse effects.[10,11,12]

25.5 Assessment of Thoracic Spine Injuries

Injuries to the thoracic spine often result in paraplegia and loss of sensory function below the level of the lesion. Function of the upper extremities is preserved. Higher lesions (T1–T8) result in more neurological deficits than lower thoracic lesion (T9–T12) especially with motor function of abdominal muscles and truncal stability.

A variety of autonomic functions may be impaired with lesions of the thoracic spinal cord. **Autonomic dysreflexia** may occur due to overreaction to sensory stimuli in the absence of inhibitory controls from the brain resulting in episodic hypertension and associated symptoms such as headache, flushing, vomiting, nasal congestion, and blurred vision. Other syndromes include abnormalities of thermal regulation with lesion above T8 and neurogenic shock (mentioned above) with lesions above T6.

Thoracic spinal cord injuries may be classified as **complete** or **incomplete** as assessed using the ASIA scale (▶ Table 25.1).

Complete spinal cord injury may occur with or without physical transection of the spinal cord, and may be known as segmental syndrome. It is characterized by complete absence of sensory and motor function in the most distal dermatomal segments of the spinal cord, S4 and S5. Variable degree of function may be preserved above this level depending on the spinal level of injury. Patients generally have urinary and fecal incontinence. Males may have priapism.

Incomplete spinal cord injury is characterized by some preservation of the sensory or motor function in the areas of innervation by S4–S5 dermatomal segments of the spinal cord, such as voluntary anal contraction and preserved perianal sensation, a feature referred to as "sacral sparing." In compressive injuries, the sacral pathways may be spared because they are located most medially in the laminated arrangement of neural pathways.

Anterior cord syndrome is caused by damage to the anterior part of the thoracic cord either by direct compression or by interruption of blood flow in the anterior spinal artery. In particular, anterior cord syndrome is typically observed in patients with underlying disease of the aorta, such as atherosclerosis, aortic aneurysm, or aortic dissection. Damage to the lateral corticospinal tract causes loss of motor function, and damage to the lateral spinothalamic tracts causes loss of pain and temperature sensation, both below the level of the injury. The posterior columns are spared resulting in preservation of proprioception and vibration sense. The prognosis is worst of any incomplete SCI with only 10 to 15% chance of recovery.[13,14]

Posterior cord syndrome is a rare condition caused by damage to posterior part of the spinal cord injuring the dorsal columns resulting in loss of proprioception and vibration sense below the level of injury. The lateral corticospinal and spinothalamic tracts are spared resulting in preservation of motor function and of pain and temperature sense. This syndrome is caused more often by medical than surgical conditions such as syphilis (tabes dorsalis) and vitamin B_{12} deficiency. Interruption of blood flow in the posterior spinal artery can also cause posterior cord syndrome.

Brown–Sequard syndrome is caused by injury localized mostly to one-half of the spinal cord such as in knife injuries, gunshot wounds, or vertebral fractures. There is loss of motor function and proprioception and vibration sense on the ipsilateral side and loss of pain and temperature on the contralateral side, below the level of the injury.[15] The lateral spinothalamic tracts cross over to the other side at two levels above the origin. Patients with Brown–Sequard syndrome have the best prognosis among patients with SCI with most people recovering enough motor function to maintain ambulatory status. Retention of dominant hand motor function is particularly impactful on prognosis.[16]

Central cord syndrome is the most common form of incomplete SCI overall but is almost always due to injury to the cervical spinal cord and is rare with isolated injuries to the thoracic cord. The mechanism of injury is most commonly hyperextension of the spine, particularly in the elderly. It is characterized by greater loss of motor function on the upper than lower extremities.[17] There are often significant improvements in gross sensorimotor function, though fine motor function may not improve. Factors predictive of improvement in function may include younger age, absence of spasticity, and a higher level of education.[18,19]

25.5.1 Prognostic Factors

Prognosis following thoracic spinal cord injury is largely related to severity of the injury as assessed by the ASIA grading scale. An ASIA grade of A has been shown to predict an 8.3% chance of ambulatory ability within 1 year, while a grade of D has a 97.3% chance.[20] Conversion from complete injury (ASIA grade A) to incomplete is uncommon but may occur. A predictive tool has been reported that uses five factors to successfully differentiate between nonwalkers, dependent walkers, and independent walkers.[21] These factors include age greater than 65 years, motor function in the L3 myotome, motor function in the S1 myotome, light touch score in the L3 dermatome, and light touch score in the S1 dermatome. Further studies are still needed to identify additional prognostic factors of functional status after spinal cord injury.

25.6 Operative Management

Goals of surgery: These include decompression of injured neurological tissues, correction of deformity, reduction of fractures, and restoration of stability by fixation using instruments and fusion using bone grafts.[22]

Timing of surgery: While some older studies reported lack of benefit and even deterioration with early surgery, most recent studies suggest benefit of early intervention including a prospective trial—the Surgical Timing in Acute Spinal Cord Injury Study (STASCIS).[23]

The thoracolumbar spine may be surgically approached anteriorly, posteriorly, laterally, or by using a combination of these approaches. The posterior approach with a transpedicular corpectomy generally requires fusion at more levels than the lateral approach.

The thoracolumbar injury classification and severity score (TLICS) is based on morphology of the injury, integrity of the posterior ligamentous complex, and neurological status of the patient to provide prognosis and treatment guidelines (▶ Table 25.3 and ▶ Table 25.4).[24]

Table 25.3 Thoracolumbar injury classification and severity score[24]

Morphology	Points
Compression fracture	1
Burst fracture	2
Translational/rotational	3
Distraction	4
Neurological involvement	
Intact	0
Nerve root	2
Cord, conus medullaris	
• Incomplete	3
• Complete	2
Cauda equina	3
Posterior ligamentous complex	
Intact	0
Injury suspected/indeterminate	2
Injured	3

Table 25.4 Management per thoracolumbar injury classification and severity score[24]

Management	Total score
Nonoperative	0–3
Nonoperative or operative	4
Operative	≥ 5

25.6.1 Major Thoracolumbar Injuries

Compression Fracture

Compression fractures account for 50% of thoracolumbar fractures.[25] They are weight-induced fractures of fragile, commonly osteoporotic, bone. Axial compression may be combined with flexion forces to cause injury, and the middle and posterior columns are often preserved. It is a common fracture, occurring in 0.5 to 1.5 million people in the United States annually.[26,27] Patients are typically over age 65, and present with localized pain, sometimes with dermatomal distribution. Neurological deficits are rare. Radiographs of the entire spine should be obtained. Neither CT nor MRI imaging is necessary unless plain films are inconclusive.[28] The American Academy of Orthopedic Surgeons recommends that most patients should be managed conservatively with calcitonin, bisphosphonates, and observation.[29] Nonoperative management can include an orthosis if kyphosis is less than 30 degrees.[22] Otherwise, operative options include kyphoplasty for severe pain persisting for more than 6 weeks, and surgical decompression and stabilization in rare cases of instability with progressive neurological deficit. Spinal fusion can be performed, and a posterior approach is typically preferred.[25]

Burst Fracture

A burst fracture is a vertebral fracture that compromises both the anterior and middle columns of the Denis three-column system (see earlier section on "Spinal Stability"). These fractures are commonly unstable. The mechanism of injury involves axial loading with flexion, particularly at the thoracolumbar junction, and the posterior column is frequently compromised.[25] Patients commonly present with neurological deficit secondary to canal compromise from retropulsion of bone. Neurological deterioration is uncommon as retropulsed fragments resorb with time. Plain films will commonly show the extent of the disease, and CT scans are indicated if fracture is observed on plain film, or if the plain film is inadequate. MRI is

most useful for assessing compromise of the spinal canal. Patients without neurological deficit may be treated with an orthosis if the kyphosis is less than 30 degrees, canal compromise is less than 50%, and there is less than 50% loss of anterior body height. Operative management of burst fracture includes anterior decompression and spinal stabilization using a posterior approach, sometimes with additional anterior decompression and stabilization.[12]

Three-Column Injury: Chance Fracture

Chance fractures are bony injuries that involve the entire spinal column, and are commonly caused by flexion–distraction.[30] The classic mechanism of injury is a tight seatbelt, and gastrointestinal injuries are commonly associated. Plain radiographs and CT imaging to assess degree of bony injury, and MRI to assess injury to posterior elements are recommended. Immobilization with a cast or orthosis may be appropriate for patients who are neurologically intact with stable injuries. Operative management for patients with neurological deficit and/or unstable injury includes decompression and stabilization. Fusion with posterior instrumentation is advised, though posterior instrumentation without fusion has recently been successful.[25]

25.7 Prognosis and Conclusion

Thoracic spinal injuries are commonly associated with damage to the spinal cord resulting in complete or partial paraplegia. The prognosis for neurological recovery remains poor after complete SCI but is fair for incomplete SCI.

References

[1] Spinal cord injury facts and figures at a glance. J Spinal Cord Med. 2014; 37 (4):479–480

[2] Kanwar R, Delasobera BE, Hudson K, Frohna W. Emergency department evaluation and treatment of cervical spine injuries. Emerg Med Clin North Am. 2015; 33(2):241–282

[3] The 2014 annual statistical report for the spinal cord injury model systems. National Spinal Cord Injury Statistical Center, Birmingham, Alabama. https://www.nscisc.uab.edu/reports.aspx. Accessed on June 27, 2015

[4] Ropper AE, Neal MT, Theodore N. Acute management of traumatic cervical spinal cord injury. Pract Neurol. 2015; 15(4):266–272

[5] Schwartz G, Fehlings MG. Secondary injury mechanisms of spinal cord trauma: a novel therapeutic approach for the management of secondary pathophysiology with the sodium channel blocker riluzole. Prog Brain Res. 2002; 137:177–190

[6] Denis F. The three column spine and its significance in the classification of acute thoracolumbar spinal injuries. Spine. 1983; 8(8):817–831

[7] Kirshblum SC, Burns SP, Biering-Sorensen F, et al. International standards for neurological classification of spinal cord injury (revised 2011). J Spinal Cord Med. 2011; 34(6):535–546

[8] Catz A, Itzkovich M, Agranov E, Ring H, Tamir A. SCIM—Spinal Cord Independence Measure: a new disability scale for patients with spinal cord lesions. Spinal Cord. 1997; 35(12):850–856

[9] Vale FL, Burns J, Jackson AB, Hadley MN. Combined medical and surgical treatment after acute spinal cord injury: results of a prospective pilot study to assess the merits of aggressive medical resuscitation and blood pressure management. J Neurosurg. 1997; 87(2):239–246

[10] Walters BC, Hadley MN, Hurlbert RJ, et al. American Association of Neurological Surgeons, Congress of Neurological Surgeons. Guidelines for the management of acute cervical spine and spinal cord injuries: 2013 update. Neurosurgery. 2013; 60 Suppl 1:82–91

[11] Bracken MB, Shepard MJ, Collins WF, et al. A randomized, controlled trial of methylprednisolone or naloxone in the treatment of acute spinal-cord injury. Results of the Second National Acute Spinal Cord Injury Study. N Engl J Med. 1990; 322(20):1405–1411

[12] Bracken MB, Shepard MJ, Holford TR, et al. Administration of methylprednisolone for 24 or 48 hours or tirilazad mesylate for 48 hours in the treatment of acute spinal cord injury. Results of the Third National Acute Spinal Cord Injury Randomized Controlled Trial. National Acute Spinal Cord Injury Study. JAMA. 1997; 277(20):1597–1604

[13] Field-Fote E. Spinal cord injury: an overview. In: Field-Fote E, ed. Spinal Cord Injury Rehabilitation. F.A. Davis; 2009

[14] Pollard ME, Apple DF. Factors associated with improved neurologic outcomes in patients with incomplete tetraplegia. Spine. 2003; 28(1):33–39

[15] Brown-Séquard C-É. De la transmission croisée des impressions sensitives par la moelle épinière. Comptes rendus de la Société de biologie. 1851; 2:33–44– (1850)

[16] Kirshblum SC, O'Connor KC. Predicting neurologic recovery in traumatic cervical spinal cord injury. Arch Phys Med Rehabil. 1998; 79(11):1456–1466

[17] Morse SD. Acute central cervical spinal cord syndrome. Ann Emerg Med. 1982; 11(8):436–439

[18] Dvorak MF, Fisher CG, Hoekema J, et al. Factors predicting motor recovery and functional outcome after traumatic central cord syndrome: a long-term follow-up. Spine. 2005; 30(20):2303–2311

[19] Roth EJ, Lawler MH, Yarkony GM. Traumatic central cord syndrome: clinical features and functional outcomes. Arch Phys Med Rehabil. 1990; 71(1):18–23

[20] van Middendorp JJ, Hosman AJ, Pouw MH, Van de Meent H, EM-SCI Study Group. Is determination between complete and incomplete traumatic spinal cord injury clinically relevant? Validation of the ASIA sacral sparing criteria in a prospective cohort of 432 patients. Spinal Cord. 2009; 47(11):809–816

[21] van Middendorp JJ, Hosman AJ, Donders AR, et al. EM-SCI Study Group. A clinical prediction rule for ambulation outcomes after traumatic spinal cord injury: a longitudinal cohort study. Lancet. 2011; 377(9770):1004–1010

[22] Weiss DB, Milewski MD, Thompson SR, Stannard JP. Trauma. In: Miller M, Thompson S, Hart J, eds. Review of Orthopedics. 6th ed. Saunders; 2012:773–779

[23] Fehlings MG, Vaccaro A, Wilson JR, et al. Early versus delayed decompression for traumatic cervical spinal cord injury: results of the Surgical Timing in Acute Spinal Cord Injury Study (STASCIS). PLoS One. 2012; 7(2):e32037

[24] Lee JY, Vaccaro AR, Lim MR, et al. Thoracolumbar injury classification and severity score: a new paradigm for the treatment of thoracolumbar spine trauma. J Orthop Sci. 2005; 10(6):671–675

[25] Kim BG, Dan JM, Shin DE. Treatment of thoracolumbar fracture. Asian Spine J. 2015; 9(1):133–146

[26] Kondo KL. Osteoporotic vertebral compression fractures and vertebral augmentation. Semin Intervent Radiol. 2008; 25(4):413–424

[27] Alexandru D, So W. Evaluation and management of vertebral compression fractures. Perm J. 2012; 16(4):46–51

[28] Lenchik L, Rogers LF, Delmas PD, Genant HK. Diagnosis of osteoporotic vertebral fractures: importance of recognition and description by radiologists. AJR Am J Roentgenol. 2004; 183(4):949–958

[29] Esses SI, McGuire R, Jenkins J, et al. The treatment of symptomatic osteoporotic spinal compression fractures. J Am Acad Orthop Surg. 2011; 19(3):176–182

[30] Davis JM, Beall DP, Lastine C, Sweet C, Wolff J, Wu D. Chance fracture of the upper thoracic spine. AJR Am J Roentgenol. 2004; 183(5):1475–1478

26 Posterior Approaches for Thoracic Spine Fractures

Michael J. Nanaszko and U. Kumar Kakarla

Abstract

The thoracic region is one of the most common anatomic sites for vertebral fractures, including compression type, burst, chance, and translation–rotation injuries. Associated spinal cord injury can also be found in these patients, and the treatment remains controversial despite many decades of widely accepted surgical treatment. Treatment indications include the need for stabilization, the need for decompression of neural elements, and persistent pain despite conservative management. Fundamental to the formulation of an appropriate treatment plan are a detailed patient history and a thorough physical examination, in combination with imaging (e.g., plain radiographs, computed tomograms, and magnetic resonance imaging [MRI]) of the region of interest. MRI of the spinal region of interest is used to evaluate the soft-tissue injury, the integrity of intervertebral discs and the posterior ligamentous complex, and spinal hematomas. The two main surgical approaches that allow posterior stabilization of the thoracic spine are open and percutaneous pedicle screw fixation, both of which can facilitate the goals of surgery: reduction of the fracture, stabilization with decompression of the neural elements, and reconstruction of the normal spinal alignment. Early stabilization of the spine is generally recommended to optimize patient outcomes. An alternative posterior treatment approach in select patients is kyphoplasty, a minimally invasive, percutaneous technique that uses a fast-setting polymer to help reconstruct the pathologic vertebral body. Posterior segmental fixation, whether through an open or a percutaneous approach, and kyphoplasty can lead to both fracture stabilization and good long-term pain and neurologic outcomes, but thoughtful patient selection and meticulous surgical technique are paramount to achieving these results.

Keywords: kyphoplasty, minimally invasive technique, pedicle screw fixation, thoracic spine fracture

Clinical Pearls

- An open posterior approach is robust and versatile in treatment of any type of thoracic spinal fractures.
- Somatosensory evoked potentials and motor evoked potentials are mandatory along with post positional X-rays to confirm alignment with thoracic fractures.
- Placement of pedicle screws and temporary fixation on one side is recommended before decompression and further destabilization in unstable spinal fractures.
- Costovertebral/transpedicular approach can be used in ventral spinal cord decompression and anterior column reconstruction.
- Pedicle screw fixation via open or percutaneous minimally invasive surgical techniques renders fixation of all three columns of the thoracic spine.
- Fixed angle pedicle screws render best rigid fixation of spine along with restoration of alignment in fracture dislocations.

26.1 Introduction

Traumatic or pathologic fractures of the thoracic spine may lead to neurologic injury, may compromise spinal alignment, may cause instability of the vertebral column, and may serve as the source of acute or chronic pain. In contrast to fractures involving the lumbar spine, fractures of the thoracic spine put the spinal cord at increased risk. Posterior reduction and instrumentation are recommended for most uncomplicated thoracic spine fractures when there is injury to the posterior ligamentous complex, gross instability, or worsening neurologic function in a patient with spinal canal compromise. A posterior approach can be used to treat fractures that involve the anterior, middle, or posterior columns, with a relatively simple and better complication profile, and with results that are at least comparable to those of an anterior or lateral approach. Individual patient factors, such as osteoporosis or concurrent injuries, should be considered when deciding whether to perform an anterior, a lateral, or a posterior approach.

Two main approaches, open and percutaneous, allow posterior stabilization of the thoracic spine. Since each technique has numerous advantages and disadvantages, the decision underlying the optimal approach depends both on the pathology of the fracture and on the surgeon's experience and preference.

Before 1950, thoracic spine fractures were treated either by an external orthosis or by placement of sublaminar hooks or wire[1] (▶ Fig. 26.1). Originally described by Michele and Krueger[1] in 1949, pedicle screw fixation is now the most widely selected method of posterior fixation. Unlike sublaminar hooks or wires, pedicle screw fixation does not require the posterior elements to be intact. Since traumatic disruption of the thoracic spine typically disrupts the posterior elements, pedicle screw fixation is the preferred method. Furthermore, the sublaminar hook and wire systems require entry into the spinal canal, which poses a risk of spinal cord compression or compromise. In contrast, pedicle screw fixation obviates this risk by allowing tangential entry around the spinal canal, and it results in an increased rate of arthrodesis.[2,3] However, pedicle screw instrumentation does have disadvantages, primarily the higher cost associated with the use of these expensive systems. Nonetheless, they are preferable, and numerous clinical and biomechanical studies have demonstrated that pedicle screw constructs, when placed correctly, are superior to hook constructs in terms of rigid fixation, correction of spinal malalignment (coronal or sagittal), and prevention of future loss of correction.[3]

Successful fixation of a thoracic spine fracture requires extensive knowledge of the anatomy of the spine. Furthermore, optimization of the length and diameter of the pedicle screws allows for maximization of posterior fixation, but it must be weighed against possible caudal or medial penetration resulting in adverse risk to the dura mater and neural structures. Numerous reports in the surgical literature describe the ideal entry points and trajectory[2,4] and discuss the advantages of anatomic versus straightforward placement of the pedicle screws. In our practice, we generally favor the straightforward

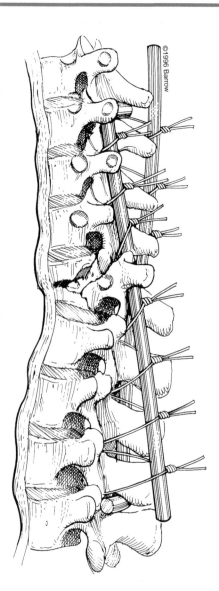
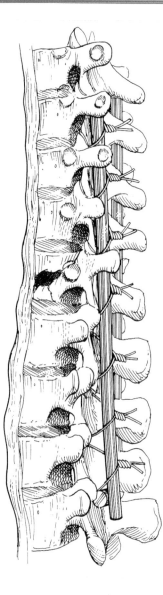

Fig. 26.1 Illustration of segmental fixation of a thoracic fracture with the use of sublaminar wires, one method of nonpedicle screw fixation employed before 1950. Unlike pedicle screw fixation, sublaminar wires require the posterior elements to be intact. (Used with permission from Barrow Neurological Institute, Phoenix, AZ.)

trajectory for placement of pedicle screws (parallel to the superior end plate), and we use the anatomy of the patient to identify the optimal thoracic entry point.

Unlike spinal fixation, kyphoplasty is a relatively simple and safe procedure that facilitates relief of pain from and healing of simple compression fractures of the thoracic spine. Properly selected patients who have no significant comorbidities, no bleeding diathesis, and no canal compromise may benefit from vertebral augmentation with polymethyl methacrylate (PMMA) cement.

26.2 Open Posterior Approach

26.2.1 Indications

Careful patient selection is important in determining whether to perform an open reduction, that is, an internal fixation of a thoracic spine fracture from a posterior approach. Patients with multiple medical comorbidities, especially those involving the cardiopulmonary system, must be thoroughly evaluated and

cleared medically for surgery. As always, conservative management, including bracing, should be attempted first in patients without neurologic deficits and gross instability on supine or upright radiographs.

Surgical fixation of a thoracic spine fracture is indicated in the presence of a progressive neurologic deficit, retropulsed bone fragments or hematoma requiring decompression of the spinal cord, malalignment of the spine, or gross instability. Other indications for surgical fixation include the failure of conservative management, including persistent pain despite adequate nonoperative treatment and delayed fracture healing or nonhealing. Most pathologic conditions (dorsal, lateral, or ventral) can be addressed by using an open posterior approach.

26.2.2 Surgical Technique

General endotracheal intubation is preferable, with the patient positioned prone on a Jackson table or a radiolucent operating room table to allow for an unobstructed view during surgery, if necessary. Care is taken to ensure that all pressure points and bony prominences are padded properly, thereby avoiding pressure ulcers and skin tears. The anterior chest wall should also have enough space to allow for adequate ventilation throughout the operation.

Neuromonitoring is critical, and we recommend the use of somatosensory evoked potentials (SSEPs) of both the upper and lower extremities, as well as motor evoked potentials (MEPs). After the patient is positioned, anteroposterior (AP) or lateral fluoroscopy can be used in conjunction with MEPs to verify spinal alignment and rule out compression of the spinal cord, especially in patients with gross spinal instability or retropulsed fragments that could migrate after positioning or during the operation.

In patients whose MEPs of the lower extremities diminish or disappear after positioning, one should first eliminate technical error before increasing the mean arterial pressure to greater than 85 mm Hg to allow for increased spinal cord perfusion. One should also consider AP or lateral fluoroscopy to determine whether cord compression has been caused by a change in spinal alignment. Irrespective of whether this is the case, the goal should be to decompress the spinal cord as quickly as possible when there is a change in MEPs indicating potential neural compromise.

Localization is easiest with AP fluoroscopy, given the presence of the thoracic ribs and the lack of proximity to the L5-S1 disc space or C2 vertebral body. When localizing the vertebral level, one should verify that the vertebral body end plates are aligned; the fractured level is often apparent on imaging. Lateral fluoroscopy can be difficult to use for localization, particularly in the upper thoracic spine, because of thoracic kyphosis and the angle of the ribs. Lateral fluoroscopy can also be difficult to use in obese patients, osteoporotic patients, and patients with severe spinal deformities.

After the skin is infiltrated with the surgeon's choice of analgesic, a standard midline posterior approach is performed, followed by opening of the fascia and subperiosteal dissection of the paraspinal muscles to identify the relevant anatomy, including the spinous process, lamina, and bony anatomy, spanning medially from the facet to the lateral tip of the transverse process. We attempt to limit soft-tissue exposure to only the planned fixation levels and, most importantly, to avoid disruption of the facet capsules located above and below those levels. As a general rule, thoracic spine fractures are treated by instrumenting a minimum of one level above and one level below the index level of disruption. When adequate fixation is unlikely, such as because of poor bone quality, the instrumentation can usually be increased to two or three levels above and below the disrupted level. The disc space above the apex of the construct must be intact to decrease the risk of proximal junctional kyphosis or failure.

The biomechanics of pedicle screws have been proven to be superior to those of hooks,[5] with pullout strength directly correlated with the outer diameter of the screw. Thus, an increase in the diameter of the screw leads to increased pullout strength, especially with bicortical purchase. However, as screws that are too large can lead to pedicle breakage, it is important to select the screw size that will optimize bony purchase without placing the pedicle at risk of fracture. Screw length can be measured on preoperative imaging, or it can be measured in situ by using a ball-tipped probe. However, the length of screw that is generally recommended approximates 70 to 80% of the vertebral

body, which translates to 40 to 45 mm in the lower thoracic spine, 35 to 40 mm in the middle thoracic spine, and 30 to 35 mm in the upper thoracic spine. There is limited benefit in oversizing screw length, as it does not add to pullout strength or improve the rate of arthrodesis, and it also places structures in the thoracic cavity at risk for penetration. Lateral perforation poses risk to both the pleural cavity and the aorta.

Pedicle diameter varies greatly in the thoracic spine, with the T4-6 pedicles generally regarded as the smallest and the T12 pedicle regarded as the largest (▶ Fig. 26.2). On average, the width of the T1-4 pedicles is 5.6 to 7.9 mm, the width of the T4-9 pedicles is 4.7 to 6.1 mm, and the width of the T10 to T12 pedicles is 6.3 to 7.8 mm.[6] In general, we recommend placing screws at the fractured level, if such placement is feasible, which often results in the use of shorter screws at the index level.

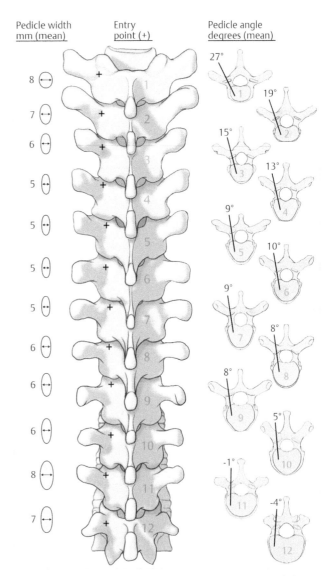

Fig. 26.2 Thoracic spinal anatomy can be quite variable in medial–lateral angulation, pedicle height, and pedicle diameter. In general, T4-6 have a small pedicle diameter and T12 has the largest pedicle diameter. (Reproduced with permission from Hartl R, Theodore N, Dickman CA, Sonntag VKH. Technique of thoracic pedicle screw fixation for trauma. Oper Tech Neurosurg 2004;7(1):22–30.)

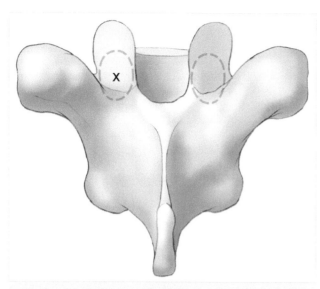

Fig. 26.3 The pedicle screw insertion site in the thoracic spine is located at the junction of the midpoint of the superior facet (an inferior facetectomy at the level above can aid in its identification) and the proximal one-third of the transverse process. (Reproduced with permission from Hartl R, Theodore N, Dickman CA, Sonntag VKH. Technique of thoracic pedicle screw fixation for trauma. Oper Tech Neurosurg 2004;7(1):22–30.)

26.2.3 Pedicle Screw Insertion Technique

Thoracic pedicle screw insertion can be performed through a variety of different approaches, including freehand, with use of laminotomy, and with fluoroscopy or computed tomography (CT) image guidance. Verification of the optimal placement of screws can be demonstrated by using a ball-tipped probe or palpation, postinsertion C-arm fluoroscopy, or intraoperative (O-arm fluoroscopy) or postoperative CT images.

The proper entry point for thoracic pedicle screws requires knowledge of pertinent thoracic anatomy, which can be distorted in trauma patients. However, in general, the insertion site can be found at the junction of the midpoint of the superior facet (performing an inferior facetectomy at the level above can aid in its identification) and the proximal one-third of the transverse process (▶ Fig. 26.3). The bisected transverse process helps to identify T1-4 and T10-12, whereas the starting point for T5-9 is generally more cephalad on the pedicle. In addition, entry points that are more cephalad in the thoracic spine tend to be more lateral. We recommend using a 7- to 9-mm drill bit to identify the entry point, to decorticate the transverse process, and to prevent medialization of the screw head and lateralization of the screw tip. The pedicle probe finder, or gearshift, can then be used to cannulate the pedicle, using anatomic landmarks to allow for the appropriate amount of cranial or caudal trajectory and to allow for sufficient medialization. The gearshift should gently fall into the pedicle with steady and minimal resistance. The gearshift is initially inserted more laterally, to avoid medial wall (and thus spinal canal) violation, before being inserted to a depth of 20 mm. The ball-tipped probe can then be used to assess for any breaches of the pedicle or of the four surrounding walls (superior, inferior, medial, and lateral). Lateral breakouts are more common given the thinner lateral wall of the pedicle. If a breakout occurs, the gearshift can be reinserted with the curve aimed more medially into the vertebral body once past the 20-mm depth to finish cannulation of the level, followed again by use of the ball-tipped probe to evaluate for any breach.

Tapping the tract can also be performed before screw placement, and we recommend undertapping using a tap diameter 1 mm smaller than the planned screw diameter. If the tract is small or there is any concern about possible deviation of the screw, then the tract can be tapped using a cannulated tap over a Kirschner wire. After the level is tapped, the ball-tipped probe is used once again to check for any breaches. The depth of the tract can be assessed by using the ball-tipped probe to feel for cortical bone at its tip and by using a hemostat to measure the length, then comparing the length with any available preoperative images. In addition, when bone quality is not an issue, we recommend placement of fixed-angle screws to facilitate reduction of malalignment just before rod placement. Otherwise, polyaxial screws can be used. Placing screws using C-arm or O-arm fluoroscopy is much more time consuming, but it may result in more accurate screw placement. When pedicle location is uncertain, a small laminotomy can aid in medial, superior, and inferior localization of the pedicle. Screw placement can again be verified by AP or lateral fluoroscopy, CTs, or even triggered electromyography from the intercostal and abdominal muscles.

The salvage technique for pedicle breaches or misplaced screws involves attempting to place a new tract along a different trajectory, although limited pedicle diameters in the thoracic spine often limit this approach. Reentry into the previous tract may be avoided by using Kirschner wires and cannulated taps. Otherwise, extrapedicular screws can be placed by attempting a more lateral entry point and an "in-out-in" technique that travels through the transverse process, then back into the vertebral body[4] (▶ Fig. 26.4). However, in general, when the ideal placement of a screw is doubtful, it is best to simply leave it out. Pedicle screws can also be augmented by injection of PMMA, hydroxyapatite, calcium phosphate, or carbonated apatite. Augmentation is generally recommended for patients who are at increased risk of screw pullout, such as osteoporotic patients.

26.2.4 Fracture Reduction

After placement and verification of the screws, the next step is usually decompression of the neural elements, reduction of the fractured elements, or attempted restoration of normal coronal or sagittal alignment. Spinal stenosis at the fractured level necessitates a laminectomy to decompress the spinal cord and evacuation of any associated spinal epidural hematoma. Further decompression and more ventral access can be achieved through either a transpedicular approach or a costotransversectomy, as described later.

Transpedicular decompression allows access to ventral pathology that may otherwise be challenging to access or that risks injury to the spinal cord by retraction. Cancellous bone can cause significant bleeding during these approaches, which can be controlled with Floseal hemostatic matrix (Baxter Healthcare Corp.) or thrombin-soaked Gelfoam absorbable gelatin

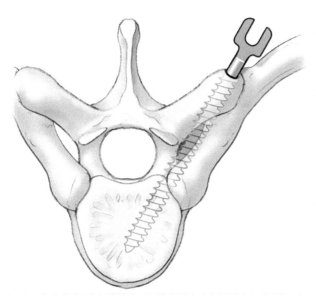

Fig. 26.4 One salvage technique for pedicle breaches or misplaced screws involves extrapedicular placement by attempting a more lateral entry point and an "in-out-in" technique that travels through the transverse process, then back into the vertebral body. (Reproduced with permission from Hartl R, Theodore N, Dickman CA, Sonntag VKH. Technique of thoracic pedicle screw fixation for trauma. Oper Tech Neurosurg 2004;7(1):22–30.)

powder (Pfizer, Inc.). In addition, placing a contralateral temporary rod before decompression allows for relative stability of the spine before progressive destabilization and removal of bone. A complete laminectomy should be performed at the index levels, which identifies the dura mater and exiting nerve roots. With the use of either a high-speed bur or Leksell or Kerrison rongeurs, the facet complex can then be removed, which facilitates exposure of the thoracic pedicle. The pedicle can then be drilled down, which allows for safe passage of a reverse-angled curette anterior to the thecal sac and the removal of any retained fractured fragments.

If a more midline or contralateral exposure is necessary, we recommend extending the approach to include a costotransversectomy. During this approach, the length and number of ribs resected depends on the amount of access desired. In general, a 5-cm-long proximal rib resection is sufficient for safe access to the vertebral level. Contralateral visualization, if necessary, can be improved with the use of angled mirrors or an endoscope. The rib below the index level must be exposed (e.g., sixth rib for access to T5–T6 level) with meticulous care, including by careful subperiosteal dissection, to preserve the neurovascular bundle located below the rib. Although sacrifice of a thoracic nerve root is often necessary, it is important to try to preserve the arterial supply, especially in the lower thoracic spine given the variable location of the artery of Adamkiewicz (most commonly, left-sided at T10–T12). The key steps in this approach include removal of the transverse process, division of the costotransverse ligaments using a Cobb elevator (Sklar Surgical Instruments, West Chester, PA), removal of the rib head using rib cutters or Kerrison rongeurs, and complete disarticulation anteriorly using periosteal elevators, with care taken to avoid disrupting the ventral pleura. After these steps, one should have

an unobstructed view of the anterior vertebral body, disc space, neural foramen, and spinal canal and should be able to achieve thorough decompression of the ventral spinal cord.

After complete decompression of the neural elements has been achieved, the focus shifts to restoration of spinal alignment. Ligamentotaxis can be used to achieve the desired fracture reduction and realignment. One method for restoring normal alignment involves gentle distraction using an interlaminar distractor, which can alternatively be placed in between screw heads. Before attempting these maneuvers, however, one should ensure that no ventral compression remains, and the patient should be monitored for any changes in SSEPs or MEPs pre- and postreduction. If fixed-angle screws were placed, it is generally easier to achieve the desired correction after placing the rods. After rod placement, a 7-mm or 9-mm bur can be used to decorticate and then place locally harvested autograft or allograft. We generally place a 7F fully fluted Jackson–Pratt drain in the cavity to help minimize dead space and allow for prevention of postoperative hematomas and seromas. In addition, copious antibiotic-impregnated irrigation and topical vancomycin may help reduce the possibility of postoperative infection. Closure is performed using a standard multilayered technique.

26.2.5 Complications

Complications associated with open reduction and internal fixation of thoracic fractures include wound infection, nerve injury or spinal cord injury, pneumothorax, vascular injury, cerebrospinal fluid (CSF) leak, hematoma, screw or rod breakage, and late complications, such as pseudarthrosis or proximal junctional kyphosis or failure. The liberal use of antibiotic-impregnated irrigation and topical vancomycin in the wound can help reduce the possibility of infection. CSF leak can be addressed primarily or with dural substitutes or sealants, and we generally leave a subfascial Jackson–Pratt drain to reduce the risk of postoperative hematoma or seroma formation. Mean arterial pressure should be kept elevated to allow for adequate spinal cord perfusion. Furthermore, intraoperative neural monitoring can help assess the functional integrity of the neural elements.

26.3 Percutaneous

26.3.1 Indications

During the past decade, a host of improvements have been made in minimally invasive spine surgery (MIS), and these improvements have subsequently led to an increase in the treatment of patients with thoracic spine fractures using percutaneous techniques. Although the use of MIS techniques in the management of spinal trauma must be weighed against the established and validated open conventional treatment, emerging evidence supports the use of MIS in select cases.[7,8]

Fluoroscopy-assisted pedicle screw insertion is associated with a decrease in pedicle wall disruption compared with the disruption that occurs in open surgery; however, it is also associated with increased radiation exposure for both the patient and the surgeon.[5] Furthermore, the advantages of percutaneous pedicle screw fixation include the preservation of the posterior paraspinal muscles, decreased blood loss, shorter operating times, decreased risk of postoperative infection, and shorter hospital stays and rehabilitation. However, the disadvantages of MIS fixation of traumatic thoracic fractures, in addition to increased radiation exposure, include the inability to achieve decompression of the spinal canal and limitations in the ability to perform adequate arthrodesis.

With an open posterior approach, there is an obligate need to detach and aggressively retract the paraspinal musculature. Doing so results in both muscle denervation and devascularization, with subsequent muscular atrophy. In addition to the increased blood loss and the need for blood transfusions, the increased postoperative pain associated with an open posterior approach leads to a delay in recovery and postoperative mobilization, resulting in increased hospital stays and an increased likelihood of prolonged rehabilitation.[9]

26.3.2 MIS Technique

As with the open approach, general endotracheal intubation is preferable for patients undergoing MIS. The patient is positioned prone on a Jackson table or a radiolucent operating room table, which allows for an unobstructed view during surgery. All pressure points and bony prominences are padded to avoid pressure ulcers and skin tears. The anterior chest wall should also have enough space to allow for adequate ventilation throughout the operation.

Neuromonitoring is critical, and we recommend the use of SSEPs of both the upper and lower extremities, as well as MEPs. AP or lateral fluoroscopy is used much more extensively in percutaneous fixation, and thus the surgeon must wear protective clothing (e.g., a leaded apron) to reduce the risk of exposure. As in the open techniques, after patient positioning, SSEPs can be used in conjunction with MEPs to verify spinal alignment and to rule out compression of the spinal cord, especially in patients with gross spinal instability or retropulsed fragments that could migrate after positioning or during the operation. Once again, the MIS approach is generally not used in patients who have possible retropulsed fragments or hematomas, as these cannot be adequately addressed during MIS fixation.

Localization is performed using AP and lateral fluoroscopy. It is prudent to verify the alignment of the vertebral body end plates when localizing each vertebral level. Lateral fluoroscopy can be difficult to use in localization, most often in the upper thoracic spine due to thoracic kyphosis and the angle of the ribs, but also in obese patients, osteoporotic patients, and those with severe deformities of the spine. The minimally invasive technique allows bypass of an extensive open incision, and a small stab incision can be made instead just lateral to midline, followed by use of a tubular retractor or a Jamshidi needle with a beveled tip. AP fluoroscopy can help determine how lateral to place the stab incision, and lateral fluoroscopy can also assist in rostral or caudal trajectory determination. The beveled tip of the Jamshidi needle is usually medialized after targeting the tip on the lateral pedicle edge with the assistance of AP fluoroscopy. As the pedicle is further cannulated, the depth should be 15 to 20 mm at the medial edge of the pedicle on AP fluoroscopy. After the cannula is advanced sufficiently into the vertebral body, a Kirschner wire is placed to allow removal of the Jamshidi needle, followed by tapping of the pedicle, and

placement of an appropriately sized screw. Frequent AP and lateral fluoroscopy is recommended to ensure proper placement of all instrumentation. In patients with osteoporotic bone, PMMA injection through fenestrated cannulated screws can add some additional stability in fixation, although this technique has not been scientifically validated.

Although less common, a mini-open technique can also be used unilaterally, to allow for an extended approach to perform a laminotomy, a laminectomy, a costotransversectomy, or even a transpedicular decompression. After completion of pedicle screw fixation, with or without additional mini-open decompression, bilateral rods can be placed, followed by verification with AP or lateral fluoroscopy. As always, the use of ample antibiotic-impregnated irrigation and topical vancomycin may aid in reducing the postoperative infection. A standard multilayered technique is used for closure.

26.3.3 Complications

MIS outcomes depend largely on the surgeon's technical skills and knowledge of surgical anatomy. In contrast to the view with open approaches, the surrounding anatomy is not well visualized in MIS, given the limited exposure, including the loss of key surgical landmarks. As a result, frequent fluoroscopy is instrumental to avoid complications and to allow operations to proceed efficiently. Complications associated with the use of percutaneous fixation of thoracic spine fractures include infection, nerve injury, spinal cord injury, pneumothorax, vascular injury, CSF leak, hematoma, mechanical or screw or rod breakage, and late complications, such as pseudarthrosis or proximal junctional kyphosis or failure. When a CSF leak is encountered, whether iatrogenic or secondary to the trauma, it substantially limits the technical ability to achieve a durable repair. There are still no well-designed prospective studies that analyze the complication rates of MIS versus those of the open approach.

It is worth noting that, given the inability to perform posterior arthrodesis from an MIS approach, the screws and rods that are implanted act mainly as internal fixators while allowing the fracture to heal biologically over time. Patients who have gross instability or fractures at high risk of nonunion are unlikely to be ideal candidates for an MIS approach to thoracic spine fixation. Furthermore, patients with a significant distraction injury may also not be ideal candidates for an MIS approach, given the limited exposure and challenges in achieving aggressive correction.

26.4 Kyphoplasty

26.4.1 Indications

Percutaneous kyphoplasty is a therapeutic procedure characterized by injection of PMMA into a vertebral body. First described in 1987 in France,[10] this procedure is a minimally invasive approach that can yield good clinical results and low complication rates in properly selected patients. The ideal candidates are patients with subacute or chronic thoracic compression fractures, whose focal pain is secondary to the fractured level. In contrast, patients with acute burst fractures or fragments within the canal are not suitable candidates because the loose fragments of bone are at risk for further retropulsion and worsened canal compromise.

26.4.2 Surgical Technique

Although general endotracheal intubation is preferable, local anesthesia with intravenous conscious sedation can be considered when the purpose of the operation is to address only one level. The patient is positioned prone on a Jackson table or a radiolucent operating room table, thereby allowing an unobstructed view during surgery. All pressure points and bony prominences are padded to reduce the likelihood of pressure ulcers and skin tears. For neuromonitoring, which is critical, we recommend the use of SSEPs of both the upper and lower extremities, as well as MEPs. Accurate localization of the level, and of the location or trajectory of kyphoplasty tools and materials, depends on precise AP and lateral fluoroscopy.

A small stab incision (approximately 0.5 mm) is made just lateral to the midline (approximately 1 cm), followed by use of an 11-gauge Jamshidi needle to cannulate the pedicle under fluoroscopic guidance. The beveled tip of the Jamshidi needle is usually medialized after targeting the tip on the lateral pedicle edge under AP fluoroscopy. As the pedicle is further cannulated, the depth should be 15 to 20 mm at the medial edge of the pedicle on AP fluoroscopy. Once the needle has entered the posterior cortex of the vertebral body, the stylet can be removed with insertion of a hand-operated drill bit. Lateral fluoroscopy should then be used to verify placement, followed by advancement toward the anterior aspect of the vertebral body, 3 to 4 mm posterior to the margin of the anterior cortex. Two deflated balloon tamps are then guided into the cavity, attached to locking syringes with a digital manometer, then inflated slowly with contrast. Under fluoroscopic guidance, the balloon is inflated until the kyphotic deformity is reduced, the tamp reaches the anterior margin, or maximum pressure is reached. The balloon is then deflated, followed by preparation and insertion of the PMMA. The volume of cement fills the cavity, matching, or even just exceeding, the volume of the inflated balloon tamp.

26.4.3 Complications

Percutaneous kyphoplasty is generally considered to be a safe procedure, but potential complications include bleeding, wound infection, allergic reaction, rib fracture, aberrant placement of cement and subsequent pulmonary embolism, nerve root irritation, and spinal cord compression or paralysis.[11,12,13] The rate of complications varies, depending on the series, but can range as high as 10%. Other reported neurologic complications include leakage of PMMA into the epidural venous system and systemic hypotension from monomer toxicity. However, with proper patient selection and careful use of fluoroscopy to ensure safe deployment of the cement, percutaneous kyphoplasty can lead to a high degree of success and patient satisfaction.

References

[1] Singh H, Rahimi SY, Yeh DJ, Floyd D. History of posterior thoracic instrumentation. Neurosurg Focus. 2004; 16(1):E11
[2] Stillerman CB, Gruen JP, Roy R. Thoracic and lumbar fusion: techniques for posterior stabilization. In: Menezes A, Sonntag VKH, eds. Principles of Spinal Surgery. New York, NY: McGraw-Hill; 1996:1199–1224
[3] Greenberg MS, Baaj AA. Handbook of Spine Surgery. 2nd ed. New York, NY: Thieme; 2016
[4] Kim YJ, Lenke LG, Bridwell KH, Cho YS, Riew KD. Free hand pedicle screw placement in the thoracic spine: is it safe? Spine. 2004; 29(3):333–342, discussion 342
[5] Cuartas E, Rasouli A, O'Brien M, Shufflebarger HL. Use of all-pedicle-screw constructs in the treatment of adolescent idiopathic scoliosis. J Am Acad Orthop Surg. 2009; 17(9):550–561
[6] Morales-Avalos R, Leyva-Villegas J, Sánchez-Mejorada G, et al. Age- and gender-related variations in morphometric characteristics of thoracic spine pedicle: a study of 4,800 pedicles. Clin Anat. 2014; 27(3):441–450
[7] McAnany SJ, Overley SC, Kim JS, Baird EO, Qureshi SA, Anderson PA. Open versus minimally invasive fixation techniques for thoracolumbar trauma: a meta-analysis. Global Spine J. 2016; 6(2):186–194
[8] Sun XY, Zhang XN, Hai Y. Percutaneous versus traditional and paraspinal posterior open approaches for treatment of thoracolumbar fractures without neurologic deficit: a meta-analysis. Eur Spine J. 2017; 26(5):1418–1431
[9] Court C, Vincent C. Percutaneous fixation of thoracolumbar fractures: current concepts. Orthop Traumatol Surg Res. 2012; 98(8):900–909
[10] Galibert P, Deramond H, Rosat P, Le Gars D. Preliminary note on the treatment of vertebral angioma by percutaneous acrylic vertebroplasty. Neurochirurgie. 1987; 33(2):166–168
[11] Bernhard J, Heini PF, Villiger PM. Asymptomatic diffuse pulmonary embolism caused by acrylic cement: an unusual complication of percutaneous vertebroplasty. Ann Rheum Dis. 2003; 62(1):85–86
[12] Jang JS, Lee SH, Jung SK. Pulmonary embolism of polymethylmethacrylate after percutaneous vertebroplasty: a report of three cases. Spine. 2002; 27(19):E416–E418
[13] Lee BJ, Lee SR, Yoo TY. Paraplegia as a complication of percutaneous vertebroplasty with polymethylmethacrylate: a case report. Spine. 2002; 27(19):E419–E422

27 Ventral Approaches to the Thoracic Spine for Trauma

Robert Harper and Eric Klineberg

Abstract

A ventral approach to the thoracic spine for trauma may be clinically necessary for fractures that require decompression and/or stabilization that cannot be accomplished through the posterior approach alone. Retropulsion of vertebral body fragments into the canal can cause compression of the spinal cord or thecal sac can cause neurologic injury. A ventral approach allows for direct decompression and visualization of these neural elements, and superior ventral neural decompression more than posterior-only approaches. Significant vertebral body comminution also may require a corpectomy and anterior column support that is best accomplished with ventral access. A low anterior cervical approach provides access to the cervicothoracic junction through traditional anterior cervical interval with the addition of a transsternal, transmanubrial, or transclavicular modifications. Thoracotomy provides wide access for thoracic spine fractures. Mobilization and retraction of the scapula with thoracotomy extends the approach cranially to access upper thoracic fractures. Ventral retroperitoneal dissection with takedown of the diaphragm when performed with caudal thoracotomy joins the thoracic and abdominal cavities to expose thoracolumbar fractures.

Keywords: cervicothoracic fracture, thoracotomy, thoracic fracture, thoracolumbar fracture

Clinical Pearls

- Low anterior cervical approach should be limited to when ventral visualization is critical or if a costotrasversectomy is too difficult, the usual indication is primary en bloc tumor resection.
- Anterior column support in the upper thoracic spine is rarely indicated for fractures due to robust posterior segmental fixation.
- Thoracotomy or thoracoabdominal approaches may be used for thoracic vertebral fractures with spinal canal compromise and neurological deficits.
- A double lumen endotracheal tube is rarely needed for thoracotomy as the inflated lung can easily be retracted, causing less trauma than lung deflation.
- Care must be taken to close the diaphragm if it is reflected during access to the thoracolumbar spine.
- While access to the fractured vertebrae is relatively easy using a minimally invasive surgical approach, instrumentation through these retractors can often be challenging; therefore, a posterior pedicle screw stabilization procedure is often preferred for definitive stabilization.

27.1 Introduction

Thoracic spinal fractures may significantly disrupt the architecture of the spine. The anterior column supports up to 80% of the axial load of the spine (▶ Fig. 27.1a, b). For most fractures of the thoracic spine, posterior stabilization is the preferred approach. Posterior modern instrumentation allows for rigid fixation, fracture reduction, and stabilization of the posterior elements (▶ Fig. 27.1c, d). The ventral approach only becomes clinically necessary in several scenarios wherein the posterior approach prevents sufficient access for either stabilization or decompression. A comminuted vertebral body may necessitate corpectomy and structural bone graft or titanium cage to reestablish the integrity of the anterior column.[1] Retropulsion of the fractured vertebral body fragments into the canal compresses the anterior spinal cord or thecal sac and may cause neurological deficits. Posterior segmental instrumentation and ligamentotaxis is not always sufficient to provide sufficient decompression of the spinal cord. The anterior approach allows for direct decompression and visualization of neural elements (▶ Fig. 27.1e, f). The load sharing classification of spine fractures first introduced by McCormick et al develops a scoring system and provides a rationale to predict the need for anterior, or long posterior stabilization for operative thoracic and thoracolumbar fractures.[2] The key features of the classification are comminution, kyphosis, and amount of spread or separation of the fragments. One to three points, depending on the severity are assigned each for vertebral body comminution, the degree of kyphosis corrected and the apposition of fracture fragments. Fractures that scored seven points or more were found to have an increased risk of failure of the posterior only construct and the need for anterior stabilization. In studies comparing anterior-only versus posterior-only fixation of thoracolumbar fractures, anterior instrumentation demonstrated better maintenance, and correction of angular deformity[3] with greater loss of sagittal correction at follow-up with posterior fixation.[4] In a series of 150 patients with thoracolumbar burst fractures with neurological deficit, Kaneda et al found a fusion rate of 93% with anterior decompression, grafting and instrumentation at a mean of 8 years postoperative. Ninety-five percent of patients in the series improved at least one Frankel grade, with 72% achieving complete neurologic recovery.[5] A multicenter fracture study showed that bladder function improved significantly with anterior versus posterior decompression and fusion.[6] Delayed fracture presentation can interfere with indirect decompression through ligmentotaxis with posterior approach, necessitating anterior approach for hematoma evacuation and direct anterior column stabilization. Generally accepted indications for a ventral approach for spine fractures include retropulsed fragments that reduce the canal by greater than 67% of total area, comminution of the anterior column with associated kyphosis of greater 30%, and a delay in surgery by more than 4 days.[7]

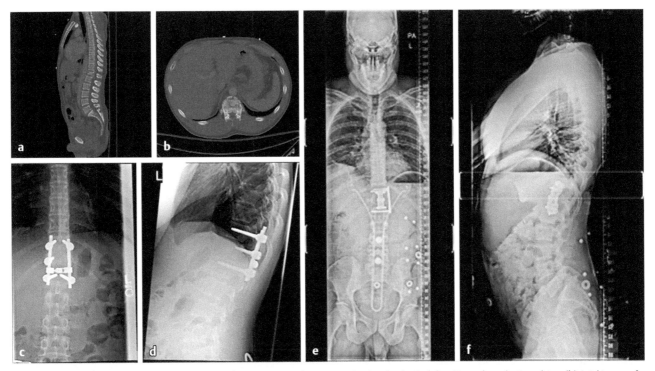

Fig. 27.1 (a) Sagittal CT of a T12 fracture with significant anterior column comminution, kyphotic deformity, and canal retropulsion. (b) Axial image of the fracture with retropulsion of fragments and significant canal compromise. (c) Anterior–posterior radiograph with excellent restoration of height after posterior short segment fixation. (d) Lateral radiograph with excellent restoration of height after posterior short segment fixation. (e) Anterior–posterior radiograph with excellent restoration of height after anterior short segment fixation. (f) Lateral radiograph with excellent restoration of height after anterior short segment fixation.

27.2 Cervicothoracic Spine

The cervicothoracic junction is generally accepted to be the region from C6 to T3. The biomechanical environment involves transition from cervical lordosis to thoracic kyphosis and can be region of high stress during trauma. Fractures of the cervicothoracic junction are uncommon and account for only 2.4 to 4.5% of all spine fractures.[8] As a result, ventral approaches to the upper thoracic spine are most commonly reserved for spinal tumor or debridement of osteomyelitis and discitis. The low anterior cervical approach provides access to C7-T1 vertebra; transsternal and transclavicular modifications can be added to gain access to the T3 vertebra.[9,10] We would suggest the assistance of an ear, nose, and throat specialist and/or cardiothoracic surgical team to facilitate the dissection for fractures requiring sternal splitting approach.

27.2.1 Low Anterior Cervical Approach

The low anterior cervical approach to the ventral thoracic spine begins with supine positioning. The shoulders are retracted by placing a towel roll between the scapulae and the arms are tucked at the sides. The shoulders are then taped to the bed to retract caudally, allowing improved fluoroscopic view of the spine intraoperatively. The head is extended and can be turned away from the desired side of approach. The left-sided approach is often favored due to the more predictable course of the left recurrent laryngeal nerve.[11] Incision is made along the

anterior border of the sternocleidomastoid extending to the suprasternal notch (▶ Fig. 27.2a). The incision is extended along the midsagittal plane of the sternum to the level between the second and third ribs if reaching T2-3. The skin is incised through subcutaneous tissue and the platysma is divided. The manubrial and clavicular insertions of the sternocleidomastoid are identified. The sternocleidomastoid is removed by subperiosteal dissection and reflected laterally. The sternohyoid and sternothyroid muscles are then dissected in similar fashion and reflected medially. If necessary, clavicular osteotomy can be accomplished with saw or osteotome at either the middle or medial third. The sternoclavicular joint is then disarticulated.

Sternum splitting allows for distal extension of the approach. The sternum is exposed subperiosteally. A Gigli or oscillating saw may be used to split the manubrium and proximal sternum longitudinally. A transverse cut is then made in the second and third intercostal space (▶ Fig. 27.2b). Care must be taken not to disarticulate the ribs from the sterum, as this will lead to chronic pain. A self-retaining retractor is used for deeper exposure through the manubrium and sternum. The thymus and retrosternal structures are mobilized bluntly and protected. The trachea and esophagus are then gently retracted medially while the carotid sheath and jugular are retracted laterally. Care should be taken to protect the thoracic duct and the recurrent laryngeal nerve as the prevertebral fascia is dissected to reveal the vertebral bodies from C6 to T3.

Closure begins with sternal wiring or nonabsorbable suturing of the sternum and manubrium. A drain may be placed deep to

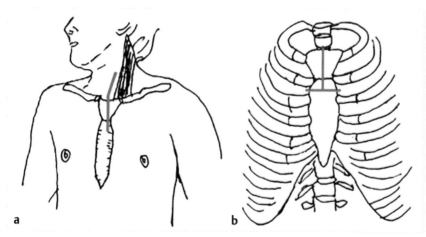

Fig. 27.2 **(a)** Incision is made along the anterior border of the sternocleidomastoid muscle to the sternal notch, then extends longitudinally to the level between the second and third ribs. **(b)** Median sternotomy extends 2 cm distal to the sternal angle with transverse cut in the second intercostal space. (Reproduced with permission from Liu et al.[9])

the sternum. The clavicle is then fixed into placed if removed. The strap muscles and then the sternocleidomastoid is reapproximated to their distal attachments on the clavicle. The platysma and wound are then closed in layered fashion.

27.2.2 Complications

The most frequent complication of the ventral approach to the cervicothoracic junction is dysphagia from esophageal retraction. Injury to the recurrent laryngeal nerve may also occur, causing vocal cord paralysis[12,13] with incidence up to 16.67%. Other complications include sternal/manubrial nonunion, great vessel injury, carotid sheath injury, damage to sympathetic chain, and tracheal/esophageal injury. An infrequent, but serious complication is chyle leak from thoracic duct damage.[9]

27.3 Upper Thoracic Spine

A modified thoracotomy provides excellent access to the upper thoracic spine and is indicated for anterior exposure for fractures from T1 to T4. A double lumen endotracheal intubation may be used for selective lung isolation. Chest tube placement is often required and should be anticipated. Most injuries in this location can be addressed with a costotransversectomy if bony fragments need to be removed from the ventral spinal cord. A contraindication for this procedure is significant lung trauma that would preclude single lung ventilation. The approach also involves the mobilization of the scapula for the approach. A transpleural or retropleural approach can be used for vertebral column access.

27.3.1 Modified Thoracotomy Approach

The patient is positioned in the lateral decubitus position. The laterality of approach is determined by fracture and vertebral level. A right-sided approach avoids the heart, aorta, and great vessels when accessing upper thoracic spine. The arms are abducted and forward flexed. The arm on the operative side can be placed on stacked towels or a padded mayo stand. The knees and elbows are placed into a slightly flexed position to relax any neural tension. A soft roll is placed beneath the axilla. A double lumen endotracheal tube is used for lung isolation. A

hockey stick incision is made from the T1 spinous process along the medial and inferior border of the scapula (▶ Fig. 27.3). The trapezius and latissimus are divided from their attachments and the scapula is rotated superiorly.

The lung may be selectively deflated prior to dissection into the chest. The ribs are counted down internally to the operative level, either the second or third rib. Intraoperative fluoroscopy can be used to verify the location. Subperiosteal dissection is used to free the rib of intercostal muscles. Care is taken to protect the neurovascular bundle that runs along the inferior surface of the rib. A rib cutter is used to resect the rib as far anteromedially and posterolaterally as possible. The resected rib can be used for bone graft for fracture fixation. The sharp ends are smoothed with a rasp and bone wax is applied to the ends.

For the transpleural approach to the spine, the pleural cavity is entered by dividing the endothoracic fascia and parietal pleura in the rib bed. A rib spreader is used for retraction. A malleable retractor with a lap sponge is used for protection of the lung during the approach. The spine is visible at the deep portion of the incision once the pleural cavity is entered. The sympathetic chain, intercostal arteries, and veins are found within the endothoracic fascia overlying the vertebral column.[14] The parietal pleura overlying the vertebral column is incised longitudinally along the axis of the spine. The endothoracic fascia and periosteum are divided sharply. The intervening intercostal arteries and veins are ligated and divided. Full access is the gained to the fractured vertebra and intervertebral disc.

Closure is performed in stepwise fashion beginning with the parietal pleura. The lung is reinflated prior to closure of the chest wall for visual confirmation. The resected rib defect can be closed with wire or nonabsorbable suture taking care to avoid the neurovascular bundle. A chest tube is placed in the ninth intercostal space and set to water seal.

Retropleural thoracotomy as described by McCormick[15] proceeds in similar fashion as transpleural thoracotomy up through the rib resection. However, for a retropleural thoracotomy, the endothoracic fascia is divided in the rib bed, exposing the parietal pleura. The neurovascular bundle inferior to the rib is isolated and protected. The parietal pleura is bluntly dissected from the endothoracic fascia. The exposure is carried down to the level of the rib articulation. The parietal pleura is then dissected to the vertebral column; any tears in the pleura are repaired with suture.

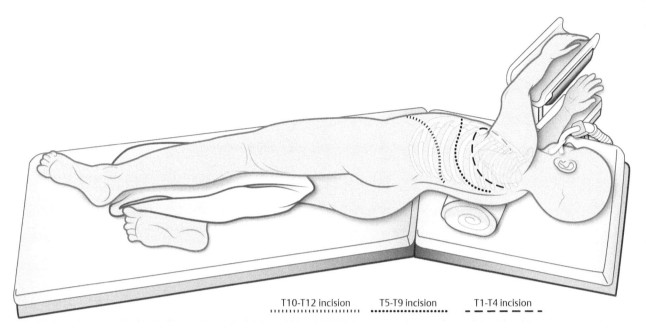

T10-T12 incision ··············· T5-T9 incision ••••••••••••• T1-T4 incision ― ― ― ― ―

Fig. 27.3 A hockey stick incision is made from the T1 spinous process along the medial and inferior border of the scapula. (Reproduced from Operative procedure. In: Ullman J, Raksin P, ed. Atlas of Emergency Neurosurgery. 1st ed. New York, NY: Thieme; 2015.)

Closure for the retropleural approach begins with replacing the endothoracic fascia over the vertebral body. The rib defect is closed with wire or nonabsorbable suture while protecting the neurovascular bundle. No chest tube is necessary if no pleural tears are encountered. A chest tube is necessary in the event of pleural tear, pleural leak, or significant intrathoracic air. Pleural tears can be identified by having the anesthesiologist deliver positive pressure.

27.3.2 Complications

The most common complication is pain from the approach, as well as the significant morbidity from this extended exposure. Postthoracotomy pain syndrome is estimated to occur in 30 to 50% of patients.[16,17] A chest tube is often required and should be anticipated. Lung injury is another rare but serious complication.

27.4 Midthoracic Spine

Thoracotomy is the preferred access to the anterior thoracic spine and is indicated for fractures from T5 to T12. Double lumen endotracheal intubation may be used for selective lung isolation, although the inflated lung can easily be held out of the surgical field, causing less trauma than lung deflation. Contraindication for the procedure is significant lung trauma that precludes single lung ventilation or entry into the chest cavity. As with the approach to the upper thoracic spine, a transpleural or retroplural approach can be made.

27.4.1 Approach

The patient is positioned in the lateral decubitus position. The laterality of approach is determined by fracture and vertebral level. A left-sided approach is usually favored in the midthoracic spine. The vena cava is thin walled and difficult to repair when injured when approaching from the right. The aorta is more tolerant to manipulation when gaining access to the spine. The arms are abducted and forward flexed. The arm on the operative side can be placed on stacked towels or a padded mayo stand. The knees and elbows are placed into a slightly flexed position. A soft roll is placed beneath the axilla. A double lumen endotracheal tube is used for lung isolation.

Incision is made along the rib of the fractured vertebra from the posterior angle of the rib along its curvature to the posterior axillary line (▶ Fig. 27.4a). Incision level is verified with intraoperative fluoroscopy. The skin is incised down through subcutaneous tissue. The latissimus dorsi is identified and divided. The serratus may need to be divided anteriorly depending on level. The lung is selectively deflated prior to dissection into the chest. Subperiosteal dissection is used to free the rib of intercostal muscles. Care is taken to protect the neurovascular bundle that runs along the inferior surface of the rib (▶ Fig. 27.4b). A rib cutter is used to resect the rib as far antermedially and posterolaterally as possible. The resected rib can be used for bone graft in fracture fixation. The sharp ends are smoothed with a rasp and bone wax is applied to the ends.

For the transpleural approach to the spine, the pleural cavity is entered by dividing the endothoracic fascia and parietal pleura in the rib bed. A rib spreader is used for retraction. A malleable retractor with a lap sponge is used for protection of the lung during the approach. The spine and aorta are visible at the deep portion of the incision once the pleural cavity is entered. The parietal pleura overlying the vertebral column is incised longitudinally in the axis of the spine. Segmental vessels are isolated tied off away from the aorta to prevent loosening and bleeding. The endothoracic fascia and periosteum are divided sharply. The intervening intercostal arteries and veins are

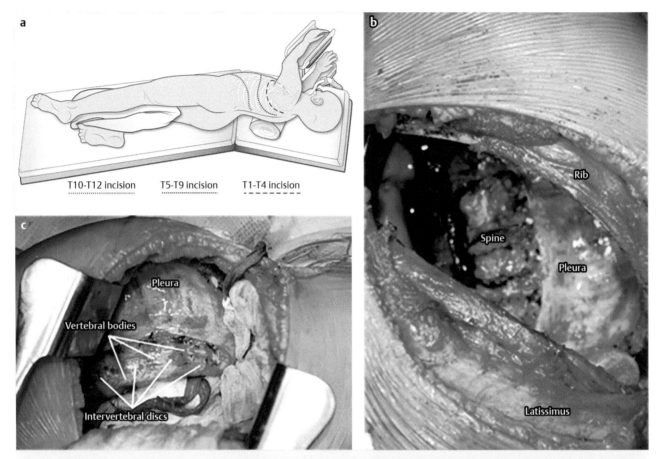

Fig. 27.4 **(a)** Incision is made along the rib to be resected from the posterior angle of the rib to the posterior axillary line. (Reproduced from Operative procedure. In: Ullman J, Raksin P, ed. Atlas of Emergency Neurosurgery. 1st ed. New York, NY: Thieme; 2015.) **(b)** The latissimus is divided and the rib bed is dissected to the level of the pleura. The pleura is divided giving access to the spine in the deep portion of the wound. **(c)** The lungs are protected and the pleura is divided over the vertebral column, providing access to the fractured segment.

ligated and divided. Full access is the gained to the fractured vertebra and intervertebral disc (▶ Fig. 27.4c).

When performing a corpectomy the bone is often deformed and cancellous bleeding can be significant. The easiest way to perform the corpectomy is to first identify the discs at the level above and below and perform as much of a discectomy as possible. Then using a rongeur or osetotome remove the middle third of the vertebral body. The bleeding can be significant until the cancellous bone has been removed. I usually perform this maneuver with rongeur and curettes. Identification of the canal is the next important step. The neural foramen can provide the anatomic location for the thecal sac, and is often more dorsal than you may expect due to the deformity and fracture. Using the foramen as your posterior extent of the vertebral body, resect the bone from the pedicle to foramen so that the edge of the dura is identified. The bone that is compressing the thecal sac can then be pushed into the vertebral defect away from the spinal canal.

Once a intervertebral graft has been chosen, pushing on the posterior elements outside of the surgical field can restore lordosis (or reduce kyphoisis) and allow for a large graft to be placed. Alternatively, an expandable cage can be used to sequentially enlarge and restore normal spinal alignment. Use a graft/device that covers the majority of the endplate to prevent subsidence. Spinal instrumentation may be then placed either anteriorly or posteriorly at this juncture.

Closure is performed in stepwise fashion beginning with the parietal pleura. The lung should be reinflated prior to closure of the chest wall for visual confirmation. The resected rib defect can be closed with wire or nonabsorbable suture taking care to avoid the neurovascular bundle. A chest tube is placed in the ninth intercostal space and set to water seal.

Retropleural thoracotomy as described by McCormick[15] proceeds in similar fashion as transpleural thoracotomy up through the rib resection. In retropleural thoracotomy, the endothoracic fascia is divided in the rib bed, exposing the parietal pleura. The neurovascular bundle inferior to the rib is isolated and protected. The parietal pleura is bluntly dissected from the endothoracic fascia. The exposure is carried down to the level of the rib articulation. The parietal pleura is dissected to the vertebral column; any tears in the pleura are repaired with suture.

Closure for the retropleural approach begins with replacing the endothoracic fascia over the vertebral body. The rib defect is closed with wire or nonabsorbable suture while protecting the neurovascular bundle. No chest tube is necessary if no pleural tears occurred. A chest tube is necessary in the event of pleural tear, pleural leak, or significant intrathoracic air. Pleural tears can be identified by having the anesthesiologist deliver positive pressure.

27.4.2 Complications

Pain is the most frequent complication of thoracotomy. Post-thoracotomy pain syndrome is estimated to occur in 30 to 50% of patients.[16,17] Postthoracotomy pain syndrome can be significant and may persist long after surgery. Pleural tears will require the use of a chest tube postoperatively for the retropleural approach.

27.5 Thoracolumbar Spine

Fractures of the thoracolumbar region are the most common fractures of the spine. This transitional zone from the rigid thoracic spine to the more mobile lumbar spine subjects this location of the spine to high biomechanical stress during trauma. Exposure of the thoracolumbar spine is indicated for access to fractures from T10 to L2 and should be familiar to all spine surgeons. Depending on fracture level, the approach involves mobilization of the diaphragm, entry into the retroperitoneal space and entry into the pleural space. Double lumen endotracheal intubation may be used for selective lung isolation, although the lung is easily retracted without the need for lung deflation. Contraindications to the approach include severe abdominal injury and pulmonary injury. Caution should be used in patients with previous surgery within the retroperitoneum as adhesions may prevent dissection through the retroperitoneal space. A general surgeon or trauma surgeon is often utilized for this approach.

27.5.1 Thoracolumbar Approach

The patient is placed in the lateral decubitus position with external support or beanbag. A left-sided approach is favored in the thoracolumbar region. The liver can inhibit access from the right side and the left side avoids mobilizing the vena cava, which is difficult to repair when injured. The arms are forward flexed with elbows slightly bent; the operative side arm is placed on stacked towels or a mayo stand. A soft roll is placed beneath the axilla. The knees and hips are flexed to relax the psoas muscles. All bony prominences are well padded. The fracture is centered over the break in the table. Lateral flexion at the injured vertebra widens the intercostal spaces to improve exposure and provides distraction to facilitate graft placement.

The operative vertebra is confirmed with intraoperative fluoroscopy. Approach is made two levels cranial to the fractured vertebra. The incision is made obliquely along the curvature of the rib. Incision starts at the posterior angle of the rib and proceeds anteriorly (▶ Fig. 27.5a). The exposure can be extended distally along the lateral border of the rectus muscle for lumbar fractures. Skin is incised through fat and subcutaneous tissue. Electrocautery is used to provide hemostasis as the exposure is deepened. The latissimus is divided or retracted posteriorly. The external oblique is divided and retracted anteriorly. The intercostal muscles are divided subperiosteally off the surface of the rib, taking care to avoid the neurovascular bundle in the inferior border. Rib excision allows for wider exposure and provides autograft material for fixation. Osteotomy is performed at the costochondral junction anteriorly and the costotransverse articulation posteriorly with a rib cutter. The edges are smoothed with a rasp and bone wax is applied for hemostasis.

For fractures at T10 to T11, the diaphragm may be left in place. The lung is selectively deflated. The rib bed is entered and the parietal pleura is identified. A rib spreader is used for retraction. A transpleural or retropleural approach may be taken to reach the vertebral bodies. The lung is gently retracted with wet lap sponge on a malleable retractor.

For transpleural, the parietal pleura is dissected with scissors. The thoracic cavity is entered and the vertebral body is identified at the deep portion of the exposure. The parietal pleura overlies the vessels and sympathetic chain. The aorta and esophagus are evident with left-sided approach. The pleura is split longitudinally. Segmental vessels are tied off and ligated. Dissection of the vertebral body should proceed anteriorly to the anterior longitudinal ligament and posteriorly to the rib articulation. The vertebral body is then exposed for corpectomy.

For retropleural approach, the interval between the endothoracic fascia and the parietal pleura is identified. The interval is bluntly dissected to the level of the vertebral body, proceeding to the anterior longitudinal ligament. The retropleural approach can provide access to as low as the T12 or T11 levels.

For fractures from T12 to L1 (▶ Fig. 27.5b, c), the diaphragm needs to be taken down for exposure of the vertebral bodies. The external oblique, internal oblique, and transverse abdominis muscles are divided at the anterior portion of the incision. The dissection is carried down through the transversalis fascia to the level of the parietal peritoneum. The peritoneum is swept from the inferior surface of the diaphragm down to the crus and the spine. The diaphragm is then ready for release. The muscle is incised circumferentially from the anterior chest wall down to the crus. A 1-cm cuff is left for reapproximation. Tag sutures are left in place for anatomic restoration. The crus is taken down and the diaphragm is retracted anteriorly. The thoracic and abdominal cavities are now joined for exposure of the spine. Access can be achieved through a retropleural/retrocrural exposure. This small triangle can be expanded with use of blunt dilation and provide access to the T12 and L1 levels. For exposure of L1 and L2, the psoas must often be mobilized subperiosteally to avoid injury to the nerve roots. The psoas is then retracted posteriorly to access the vertebral bodies.

When performing a corpectomy the bone is often deformed and the cancellous bleeding can be significant. The easiest way to perform the corpectomy is to first identify the discs at the level above and below and perform as much of a discectomy as possible (▶ Fig. 27.5d). Then using a rongeur or osetotome remove the middle third of the vertebral body. The bleeding can be significant until the cancellous bone has been removed. I perform this maneuver with rongeur and curettes. Identification of the canal is the next important step. The neural foramen can provide the anatomic location for the thecal sac, and is more dorsal then you may expect due to the deformity and fracture. Using the foramen as your posterior extent of the vertebral body, resect the bone from the pedicle to foramen so that the edge of the dura is identified. The bone that is compressing the thecal sac can then be pushed into the vertebral defect.

Once an intervertebral graft has been chosen, pushing on the posterior elements outside of the surgical field can restore lordosis (or reduce kyphoisis) and allow for a large graft to be placed. Alternatively, an expandable cage can be used to sequentially enlarge and restore normal spinal alignment (▶ Fig. 27.5e). Use a graft/device that covers the majority of the

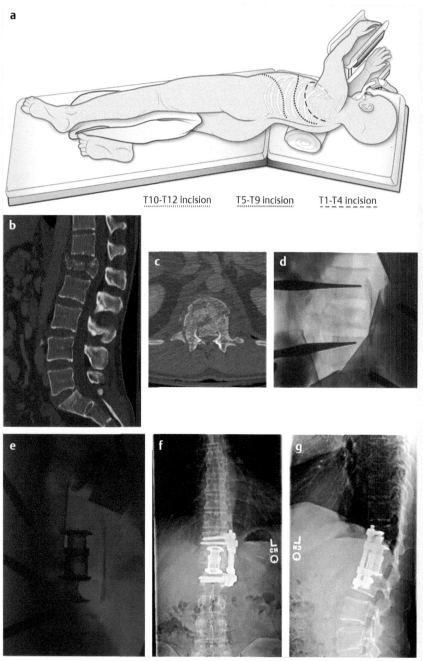

T10-T12 incision   T5-T9 incision   T1-T4 incision

Fig. 27.5 **(a)** The incision is centered over the fracture, starting from the posterior angle of the rib, curving anteriorly. The incision may be carried inferiorly along the rectus. (Reproduced from Operative procedure. In: Ullman J, Raksin P, ed. Atlas of Emergency Neurosurgery. 1st ed. New York, NY: Thieme; 2015.) **(b)** Sagittal CT of comminuted L1 burst fracture with significant canal retropulsion and greater than 50% height loss. **(c)** Axial CT image of L1 burst fracture with canal retropulsion and greater than 67% canal compromise. **(d)** Intraoperative localization of the fractured segment prior to corpectomy for canal decompression and identification of discs prior to discectomy. **(e)** Intraoperative placement of expandable cage for restoration of height and reduction of the kyphotic deformity. **(f)** Anterior–posterior final radiograph after anterior placement of cage and segmental instrumentation. **(g)** Lateral radiograph after anterior placement of cage and segmental instrumentation, with minimal loss of correction 2 years postoperative.

endplate to prevent subsidence. Spinal instrumentation may be then placed either anteriorly or posteriorly at this juncture (▶ Fig. 27.5f, g).

For transpleural access, the lung is inflated prior to closure. The parietal pleura is closed over the spine and at the chest wall. A chest tube is placed. Any tears in the pleura are repaired with a retropleural approach. The diaphragm is reattached with nonabsorbable suture. A retroperitoneal drain may be placed. The abdominal muscles are repaired in layered fashion. The rib defect is closed with wire or nonabsorbable suture while protecting the neurovascular bundle.

27.5.2 Complications

Complications of the procedure include visceral, diaphragmatic, and great vessel damage from the approach.

27.6 Minimally Invasive

There is significant interest in minimally invasive approaches in spine surgery to limit approach-related morbidity and allow faster return to function with less pain. Thoracoscopic assisted minithoracotomy provides minimally invasive access to the ventral thoracic spine for fracture accessed through open thoracotomy. Minithoracotomy is accomplished with specialized retractor systems[18,19] and corpectomy and strut graft placement are performed with thorascopic assistance. Buhren et al found reduced postoperative pain, shorter hospital stay, and earlier functional recovery in patients treated with minimally invasive thoracotomy.[20] Spiegl et al found no approach related complications at 6 years postoperatively using the minimally invasive thoracotomy,[18] while Kossman et al had no intraoperative or postoperative complications related to the approach.[19] The current authors preferred technique does not use the assistance of thoracoscopy, and utilizes a mini thoracotomy via specialized retractor systems that are used primarily for the transpsoas approach. This minimally invasive, retropleural/retrocrural, or transpsoas approach can provide exposure to the ventral thoracolumbar spine for fracture treatment, without the need for thorascopy and with decreased pain and morbidity.

27.6.1 Approach

The patient is placed in the lateral decubitus position with external support or beanbag. A left-sided approach is favored in the thoracolumbar region. The liver can inhibit access from the right side and the left side avoids mobilizing the vena cava which is difficult to repair when injured. The arms are forward flexed with elbows slightly bent; the operative side arm is placed on stacked towels or a mayo stand. A soft roll is placed beneath the axilla. The knees and hips are flexed to relax the psoas muscles. All bony prominences are well padded. The fracture is centered over the break in the table. Lateral flexion at the injured vertebra widens the intercostal spaces to improve exposure and provides distraction to facilitate graft placement.

Fluoroscopy is used to verify the operative level. The anterior and posterior vertebra are drawn on the skin. A longitudinal incision is centered over the bodies and carried down through skin to subcutaneous tissue to the external oblique muscle. The muscle is incised along its fibers and dissection is carried down to the level of the internal oblique fascia. Care should be taken as the approach is continued through the internal oblique and transverse abdominis as the ilioinguinal and iliohypogastric nerves through the muscle layers.

For T10 to T12, a retroperitoneal approach is used, reflecting the parietal pleura anteriorly away from the fractured vertebrae. For T12-L1 a retrocrural approach can be used by developing a plane behind the crus and diaphragm, above the retroperitoneum, and below the retropleural space. For lower fractures from L1 and below,(▶ Fig. 27.6a, b), blunt dissection is carried down through the retroperitoneal fat to the psoas muscle taking care to protect the ureter. For lower thoracolumbar fractures, the diaphragm may be left in place. For fractures at L1 or L2, the crus of the diaphragm will need to be taken down to access the vertebral bodies. For fractures at T11 or T12 an incision is made in the diaphragm to access the vertebral bodies. The psoas fascia is incised longitudinally and the muscle is bluntly dissected to the level of the vertebral body. Care should be taken with the neurovascular structures running through the psoas. the L1-2 contribution to the lumbar plexus emerge at the posterior annulus of the L1-2 disc. The genitofemoral nerve lies within the muscle belly cranial to the L3-4 level and emerges below this level to run on the anterior surface of the muscle. Self-retaining retractors, secured to a table mounted arm provide the working window to the vertebral body. Corpectomy and grafting proceed in standard fashion. Instrumentation may then be placed anteriorly or posteriorly (▶ Fig. 27.6 c, d).

Closure is performed stepwise. The diaphragm is repaired with nonabsorbable suture. A drain may be placed in the retroperitoneal space and the abdominal muscles are closed in layered fashion. Chest tube placement is often needed and should be planned for before the start of the case.

27.6.2 Complications

Transient hip flexion weakness due to manipulation and dissection of the psoas is the most common complication of the approach, but is usually a problem lower in the lumbar spine. Sensory disturbances of the proximal thigh due to retraction and stretch of the nerves of the lumbar plexus can also occur, but again this is usually in the lower lumbar spine. Less common, but more serious complications include, damage to the lumbar plexus through direct injury or prolonged stretch and retraction leading to lower extremity weakness, visceral, and great vessel injury.

27.7 Conclusion

Multiple surgical approaches are available for the surgeon treating spinal fractures. An anterior approach should be considered for fractures with significant comminution or neural compression and when a posterior approach alone is insufficient. While this may be done throughout the spine, typically the anterior approach for fractures is reserved for the thoracolumbar spine. Newer stabilization techniques, via minimal access approaches are now available and may offer some advantages over traditional open approaches. An understanding of the surgical approach and common complications are critical to develop the appropriate surgical plan for the patient.

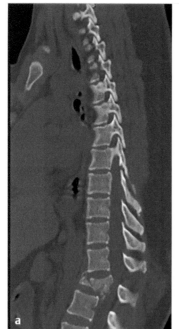

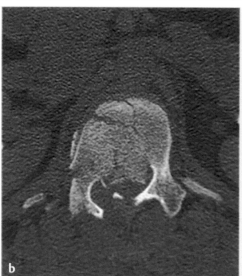

Fig. 27.6 (a) Sagittal CT of an L1 fracture dislocation with significant anterior column comminution, kyphotic deformity, and canal retropulsion. **(b)** Axial image of ► Fig. 27.5b fracture with retropulsion of fragments and significant canal compromise. **(c)** Anterior–posterior radiograph status post MIS corpectomy and graft placement after posterior instrumentation stabilization for the fracture for continued neuro deficits. Complete resolution of those deficits after corpectomy completed. **(d)** Lateral upright radiograph status post MIS corpectomy and graft placement following posterior instrumentation for the fracture.

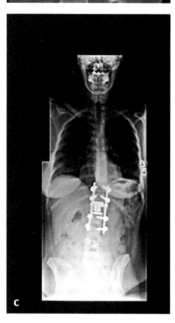

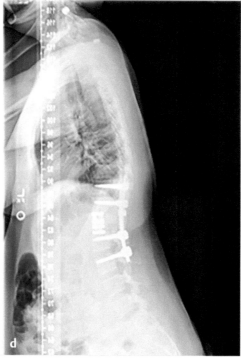

References

[1] Kaneda K, Abumi K, Fujiya M. Burst fractures with neurologic deficits of the thoracolumbar-lumbar spine. Results of anterior decompression and stabilization with anterior instrumentation. Spine. 1984; 9(8):788–795

[2] McCormack T, Karaikovic E, Gaines RW. The load sharing classification of spine fractures. Spine. 1994; 19(15):1741–1744

[3] Hitchon PW, Torner J, Eichholz KM, Beeler SN. Comparison of anterolateral and posterior approaches in the management of thoracolumbar burst fractures. J Neurosurg Spine. 2006; 5(2):117–125

[4] Sasso RC, Renkens K, Hanson D, Reilly T, McGuire RA, Jr, Best NM. Unstable thoracolumbar burst fractures: anterior-only versus short-segment posterior fixation. J Spinal Disord Tech. 2006; 19(4):242–248

[5] Kaneda K, Taneichi H, Abumi K, Hashimoto T, Satoh S, Fujiya M. Anterior decompression and stabilization with the Kaneda device for thoracolumbar burst fractures associated with neurological deficits. J Bone Joint Surg Am. 1997; 79(1):69–83

[6] Gertzbein SD. Scoliosis Research Society. Multicenter spine fracture study. Spine. 1992; 17(5):528–540

[7] McCullen G, Vaccaro AR, Garfin SR. Thoracic and lumbar trauma: rationale for selecting the appropriate fusion technnique. Orthop Clin North Am. 1998; 29 (4):813–828

[8] Amin A, Saifuddin A. Fractures and dislocations of the cervicothoracic junction. J Spinal Disord Tech. 2005; 18(6):499–505

[9] Liu YL, Hao YJ, Li T, Song YM, Wang LM. Trans-upper-sternal approach to the cervicothoracic junction. Clin Orthop Relat Res. 2009; 467(8):2018–2024

[10] Lesoin F, Thomas CE, III, Autricque A, Villette L, Jomin M. A transsternal biclavicular approach to the upper anterior thoracic spine. Surg Neurol. 1986; 26 (3):253–256

[11] Miscusi M, Bellitti A, Peschillo S, Polli FM, Missori P, Delfini R. Does recurrent laryngeal nerve anatomy condition the choice of the side for approaching the anterior cervical spine? J Neurosurg Sci. 2007; 51(2):61–64

[12] Mihir B, Vinod L, Umesh M, Chaudhary K. Anterior instrumentation of the cervicothoracic vertebrae: approach based on clinical and radiologic criteria. Spine. 2006; 31(9):E244–E249

[13] Mulpuri K, LeBlanc JG, Reilly CW, et al. Sternal split approach to the cervico-thoracic junction in children. Spine. 2005; 30(11):E305–E310

[14] McCormick PC. Retropleural approach to the thoracic and thoracolumbar spine. Neurosurgery. 1995; 37(5):908–914

[15] Angevin PD, McCormick PC. Retropleural thoracotomy. Technical note. Neurosurg Focus. 2001; 10(1):ecp1

[16] Mongardon N, Pinton-Gonnet C, Szekely B, Michel-Cherqui M, Dreyfus JF, Fischler M. Assessment of chronic pain after thoracotomy: a 1-year prevalence study. Clin J Pain. 2011; 27(8):677–681

[17] Hetmann F, Kongsgaard UE, Sandvik L, Schou-Bredal I. Prevalence and predictors of persistent post-surgical pain 12 months after thoracotomy. Acta Anaesthesiol Scand. 2015; 59(6):740–748

[18] Spiegl U, Hauck S, Merkel P, Bühren V, Gonschorek O. Six-year outcome of thoracoscopic ventral spondylodesis after unstable incomplete cranial burst fractures of the thoracolumbar junction: ventral versus dorso-ventral strategy. Int Orthop. 2013; 37(6):1113–1120

[19] Kossmann T, Jacobi D, Trentz O. The use of a retractor system (SynFrame) for open, minimal invasive reconstruction of the anterior column of the thoracic and lumbar spine. Eur Spine J. 2001; 10(5):396–402

[20] Bühren V, Beisse R, Potulski M. [Minimally invasive ventral spondylodesis in injuries to the thoracic and lumbar spine]. Chirurg. 1997; 68(11):1076–1084

28 Osteoporotic Compression Fractures

Srikanth R. Boddu, Trong Huynh, Thomas Link, and Athos Patsalides

Abstract

Vertebral compression fractures are pathognomonic of osteoporosis with significant impact on both the individual heath and health care costs. Pain control, correction of kyphosis, prevention of existing fracture worsening, and development of new fractures are the primary goals of treatment. Conventionally, medical management was considered as a first line of treatment. However, with increasing awareness of vertebral augmentation procedures such as vertebroplasty and kyphoplasty, there is paradigm shift toward early surgical intervention with these safe and minimally invasive procedures. In this chapter, we describe the burden of this problem on current health system, risk factors, medical management, and surgical interventions. We discussed the results of vertebroplasty and kyphoplasty trials, potential complications, and concluded with possible future directions. Detailed discussion of osteoporosis and nonosteoporotic vertebral compression fractures (traumatic, myeloma, and metastatic) are beyond the scope of this chapter.

Keywords: vertebral compression fractures, osteoporosis, kyphosis, vertebroplasty, kyphoplasty, polymethylmethacrylate

> **Clinical Pearls**
>
> - Epidemiology and scope of the osteoporotic vertebral fractures.
> - Types of osteoporosis and associated risk factors.
> - Medical management of the osteoporotic fractures.
> - Vertebral augmentation for osteoporotic fractures.
> - Literature review on vertebral augmentation.

28.1 Introduction

Osteoporosis is the leading cause of spine fractures, especially in women over 50 years of age.[1] As defined by the World Health Organization (WHO), osteoporosis is a generalized skeletal disorder of low bone mass and deterioration in its architecture, causing susceptibility to fracture. Approximately 8 million women and 2 million men suffer from osteoporosis while another 34 million with low bone mass are at increased risk for osteoporosis in the United States.[2] Approximately 1.5 million people suffer from an osteoporotic fracture each year and around 700,000 of them are vertebral compression fractures.[1]

28.2 Epidemiology

Vertebral compression fractures affect approximately 25% of all postmenopausal women and nearly 5% of men aged 50 years and above in the United States.[1,3] Vertebral fractures are directly correlated with increasing age and incidence of osteoporosis. The rate of vertebral fractures increases from an annual incidence of 0.9% and prevalence of 5 to 10% among middle-aged women in their 50 s to 60 s, to an incidence of 1.7% and prevalence of greater than 30% among those 80 years and older.[1,3,4] They most commonly occur among Caucasian women and are less common among men and women of African American or Asian ethnicity.[5,6] The actual incidence of vertebral fractures is likely much greater given the large number of vertebral fractures that go undetected, with only a third of vertebral fractures clinically diagnosed.[7] The geriatric (> 65 years) American population in 2014 was estimated as 46 million and was projected to increase over 98 million by 2060, constituting 24% of total population.[8] Geriatric population being the fastest growing segment of the U.S. population, the incidence and prevalence of this age-specific vertebral compression fractures are likely to increase.

28.3 Impact on Health Care

Vertebral compression fractures have a substantial negative impact on the patient's function and quality of life. Approximately 30 to 40% of vertebral compression fracture patients develop disabling pain and/or deformity (kyphosis), resulting in 150,000 hospitalizations annually. In the first year after a painful vertebral fracture, patients require primary care services 14 times greater than the general population.[9] In addition to physical limitations, vertebral compression fractures may produce a psychosocial and emotional burden on the aging person who already faces losses of independent function. The annual U.S. medical cost for vertebral fracture management was estimated at $13.8 billion in 2001 and has likely increased since with the growing elderly population. The total economic cost is also far greater than the cost for acute management given that vertebral fractures can lead to significant long-term morbidity.[10,11]

28.4 Pathophysiology

Bone remodeling is primarily affected by osteoclasts and the osteoblasts. Without estrogen, the osteoclasts are favored and more bone is resorbed than laid down, resulting in thinning of the bone. Therefore, when women reach menopause and their estrogen levels decrease, the rate of bone loss increases to about 2 to 3% per year. After 8 to 10 years, the rate of bone loss returns to the previous rate of 1 and 0.5% per year, respectively. This loss of bone density, particularly after women reach menopause, is one of the primary causes of osteoporosis in women. There are two types of osteoporosis.

28.4.1 Type I Osteoporosis

This is typically seen in postmenopausal women, between the ages of 50 and 70, hence the term "postmenopausal osteoporosis." This is due to significant reduction of estrogen resulting in an increased bone resorption. The process usually results in a reduction of trabecular bone, primarily leads to wrist and vertebral body fractures.

28.4.2 Type II Osteoporosis

This typically affects the elderly population, 70 years and above and women twice as frequently as men. This is also known as "senile osteoporosis," involves a thinning of both the trabecular and cortical bone and often leads to hip and vertebral body fractures.

Osteoporosis may either be a primary problem (types I or II) or may be secondary to another problem. Approximately 20% of women and 40% of men with osteoporosis have a secondary cause of osteoporosis, such as hyperthyroidism or lymphoma. Common causes of secondary osteoporosis are summarized in Box 28.1.

Box 28.1 Causes of secondary osteoporosis

1. **Endocrine disorders**
   - Hypogonadism
   - Cushing's disease
   - Hyperthyroidism
   - Hyperparathyroidism
   - Diabetes mellitus
2. **Marrow disorders**
   - Multiple myeloma
   - Disseminated cancer
   - Chronic alcohol use
   - Lymphoma
3. **Collagen disorders**
   - Osteogenesis imperfecta
   - Marfan syndrome
4. **Gastrointestinal disorders**
   - Malabsorption
   - Malnutrition
5. **Medications**
   - Aluminum antacids
   - Anticonvulsants
   - Chemotherapy
   - Glucocorticoid therapy
   - Thyroid hormone replacement

28.5 Risk Factors

Vertebral compression fractures are recognized as the hallmark of osteoporosis, and many of the risk factors are the same. Risk factors are categorized as those not modifiable and those that are potentially modifiable. **Non-modifiable risk factors** include advanced age, female gender, Caucasian race, presence of dementia, susceptibility to falling, history of fractures in adulthood, and history of fractures in a first-degree relative. Potentially **modifiable risk factors** include being in an abusive situation, alcohol and/or tobacco use, presence of osteoporosis and/or estrogen deficiency, early menopause or bilateral ovariectomy, premenopausal amenorrhea for more than one year, frailty, impaired eyesight, insufficient physical activity, low body weight, and dietary calcium and/or vitamin D deficiency.

28.5.1 Decreased Bone Density

Both osteoporosis and osteopenia are strongly associated with the risk of developing a vertebral fracture, with the risk increasing roughly two times for every standard deviation below average vertebral bone mineral density. Bone density begins to decrease after age 40 for both men and women, and the process is rapidly accelerated in postmenopausal women. WHO defines osteoporosis as T score < -2.5 on dual-energy X-ray absorptiometry (DEXA). Though most commonly found among osteoporotic patients (T < -2.5), vertebral fractures may also occur in up to 18% of women more than 60 years old with osteopenia but not meeting the criteria for osteoporosis (T score > -2.5 but < -1.4). It is estimated that more than a third of postmenopausal vertebral compression fractures occur in osteopenic women who do not meet the criteria for osteoporosis.

28.5.2 Prior Vertebral Osteoporotic Fracture

The risk of developing a vertebral fracture is roughly five times greater if the patient has had a prior fracture, and 20% of osteoporotic postmenopausal women who present with an initial vertebral fracture develop a subsequent vertebral fracture within the year. These patients are also at high risk of developing other significant osteoporotic fractures, such as hip fractures. History of two vertebral compression fractures is the strongest predictor of future vertebral fractures in postmenopausal women. An Australian study over 4,000 men and women reported that after an initial osteoporosis-related fracture, the absolute risk of a subsequent fracture within 10 years of the first was similar in men and women.

28.5.3 Lifestyle and Environmental Factors

In addition to the genetic predisposition, a multitude of lifestyle and environmental factors increase the risk of developing osteoporosis. These include lack of exercise and low body mass index, insufficient dietary calcium, low vitamin D production, glucocorticoid medication, smoking, and excessive alcohol intake. Also, vertebral metastasis, end-stage renal disease and hyperparathyroidism are known predisposing factors for the vertebral compression fractures.

28.6 Sequelae of Osteoporotic Fractures

28.6.1 Height Loss

With the osteoporotic compression fractures, each vertebra tends to lose at least 15–20% of its height. Thus, with successive fractures, the individual may lose a noticeable amount of height. This loss of stature changes the musculature in the back and can cause pain from muscle fatigue that can continue after the bone fracture has healed. Thoracic kyphosis (dowager's hump, or hunched back). The fracture usually occurs in the front of the vertebra and leaves the height at the back of the vertebra unchanged, resulting in a wedge-shaped bone in the spine. With multiple vertebral fractures, as the front of the collapsed vertebrae fuse together, the spine bends forward, causing a kyphotic deformity and hunched over appearance.

28.6.2 Compromised Pulmonary Function

According to a 1998 study there is a significant decrease in the lung function in patients with thoracic vertebral fractures. Each thoracic or upper back fracture causes a 9% loss of vital capacity of the lungs because of progressive kyphosis (*Journal of American Respiratory Disease*).

28.6.3 Bulging Abdomen

As the vertebral fractures cause the patient's spine to shrink in height, the abdominal contents are compressed into less vertical space resulting in crowding of internal organs. As a result, the abdomen can bulge out, causing a pseudo appearance of weight gain.

28.6.4 Gastrointestinal Complaints

The shortened spinal column may also compress the stomach, causing weight loss due to early satiety, constipation, or other problems.

28.6.5 Neck Pain

Patients with severe thoracic kyphosis may be so far hunched forward that they should extend their necks to look forward, which can result in neck pain.

Other sequelae of the vertebral compression fractures include prolonged inactivity, deep venous thrombosis, progressive muscle weakness, loss of independence, emotional and social problems.

28.7 Mortality

The reported mortality in patients with vertebral compression fractures is approximately 15% higher than the age-matched controls. Approximate mortality in these patients is less than mortality from hip fractures at 1 year (15%) and is equal to the mortality from hip fractures at 2 years (20%), and vertebral compression fractures have a decreased 5-year mortality compared to hip fracture patients.[12] The most common cause of premature death was pulmonary disease, emphysema, and pneumonia.

28.8 Clinical Presentation

Only about one-third of vertebral fractures are actually diagnosed because many patients and families regard back pain symptoms as "arthritis" or a normal part of aging. Therefore, compression fracture should be suspected in any patient older than 50 years with acute onset of sudden low back pain. Most patients will remember a specific injury as the cause. In cases of severe osteoporosis, however, the cause of trauma may be simple, such as stepping out of a bathtub, vigorous sneezing, or lifting a trivial object, or the trauma may result from the load caused by muscle contraction. Up to 30% of compression fractures occur while the patient is in bed. In cases of moderate osteoporosis, more force or trauma is required to create a fracture, such as falling off a chair, tripping, or attempting to lift a heavy object.

When symptomatic, patients complain of sudden onset of severe, focal, back pain that may radiate posterolaterally along the intercostal distribution. The vertebral bodies support 80% of the body's weight, so that the pain is typically worse when sitting up, standing, or ambulating, and improved when lying down. This is described as mechanical axial back pain, and can be distinguished through history taking from other etiologies of back pain such as osteoarthritic pain, pathologic pain associated with tumor, and lumbar strain.

Vertebral compression fractures usually occur in the midthoracic or thoracolumbar transition zone of the spine. Though exceedingly rare, occasionally retropulsion of fracture fragments may result in compression of the spinal cord or cauda equina and result in weakness and loss of sensation of the lower extremities or even bowel or bladder incontinence. Depending on the severity and rapidity of deficit onset, this may constitute a surgical emergency.

The loss of height that results from a compression fracture may lead to kyphotic deformity of the spine, especially for multiple compression fractures with significant height loss. This may result in focal or global sagittal imbalance, which may lead to chronic back pain even after the fracture has healed and accelerate the degeneration of adjacent spinal segments. Progressive loss of stature also results in shortening of paraspinal musculature requiring prolonged active contraction for maintenance of posture, resulting in pain from muscle fatigue. This pain may continue long after the acute fracture has healed. The back pain and associated fatigue can severely limit a patient's quality of life and ability to perform activities of daily living. In addition, severe kyphoscoliosis can even lead to a restricted abdominal space, limiting pulmonary vital capacity as well as decreasing nutritional intake, thus compounding patient immobility.

28.9 Diagnostic Imaging

28.9.1 Plain Radiograph

Many imaging studies may be used in the workup of vertebral compression fractures. Plain frontal and lateral radiographs are the initial imaging study obtained for a suspected compression fracture. Findings on plain radiograph such as increased lucency, loss of horizontal trabeculae, and decreased cortical thickness but increased relative opacity of the endplates and vertical trabeculae are suggestive of osteopenia. Comparison to preexisting spine X-rays allows the clinician to diagnose and judge the age of the vertebral fracture.

Radiographically, a decrease in vertebral height of 20% or more, or a decrease of at least 4 mm compared with baseline height is considered positive for compression fracture. Compression fractures may be classified based on the portion of the vertebral body that is affected: wedge-shaped (anterior or posterior) or biconcave. Based on severity of compression fracture (height loss) vertebral compression fractures are graded as: grades I (< 25%), II (25–50%), III (50–75%), and IV (> 75% or vertebra plana). In cases of complete compression fractures there is a reduction in both posterior and anterior height. It is important to image the entire spine because 20 to 30% of vertebral compression fractures are multiple. When multiple, the fractures occur at different levels or in one to five consecutive vertebral bodies. Serial plain radiographs can be used to identify the worsening vertebral compression fractures, especially if one proceeds with conservative, medical management.

28.9.2 Computed Tomography

Noncontrast computed tomography (CT) scan allows for superior characterization of bony anatomy and improved assessment of loss of height, fragment retropulsion, and canal compromise (▶ Fig. 28.1). Noncontrast CT spine is the best study to evaluate intactness of the posterior cortex of the vertebral body, the knowledge of which is vital to prevent retrograde cement leak in to the spinal canal. However, this comes with greater expense and irradiation for the patient. CT scan may also help to distinguish an acute fracture with free air with in the vertebral body from a chronic fracture by the presence of cortication.

28.9.3 Magnetic Resonance Imaging

Magnetic resonance imaging (MRI) is the best study for judging fracture age, as it will show bony edema for an acute fracture (▶ Fig. 28.2). In addition, MRI allows for the evaluation of neural compromise secondary to compression of the spinal cord or nerve roots. MRI short tau inversion recovery sequence will also reveal integrity of the spinal ligamentous complex, which can be important during surgical evaluation of fracture stability. Finally, a postcontrast MRI study will detect a pathologic fracture secondary to an oncologic process. Other, less commonly used imaging studies include bone scan, which will show increased uptake in a fracture.

28.9.4 Dual-energy X-ray Absorptiometry

Spontaneous vertebral compression fractures with minimal force and no history of trauma are typically pathognomonic for osteoporosis. After the diagnosis of a compression fracture on initial imaging, bone density should be assessed by DEXA scan, the gold standard for diagnosis of osteoporosis.[13] The test values are generated by passing low energy X-rays through a target bone (e.g., spine, hip, or wrist). These values when compared to the values of young adult population as baseline generate a "T score." A score above –1 is considered normal; a score between –1 and –2.5 is considered osteopenia; and a score below –2.5 is considered osteoporosis. For each –1 change in T score standard deviation, there is a 2.5 times risk of spine fracture. "Z score" can be generated by comparing to the values of age- and gender-matched control groups as baseline. An unusually high or low Z score may indicate the need for additional tests. According to the National Osteoporosis Foundation, bone mineral density testing is recommended in the following situations:

1. All women over age 65.
2. Postmenopausal women under age 65 who have multiple risk factors.
3. At menopause, if undecided about hormone replacement therapy.
4. Abnormal spine X-rays.
5. Long-term oral steroid use.
6. Hyperparathyroidism (overactive parathyroid gland).

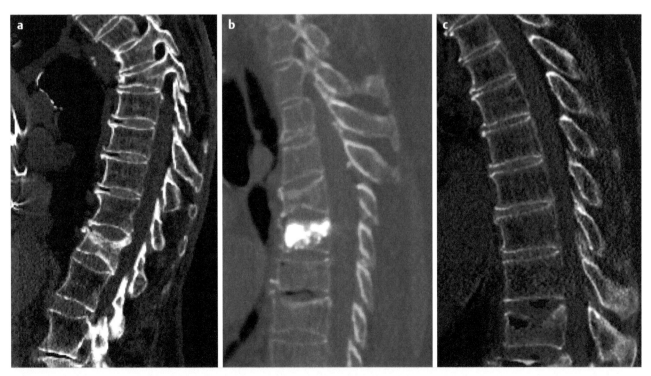

Fig. 28.1 CT demonstration of multiple thoracic compression fractures. (a) Multilevel thoracic compression fractures with associated height loss and kyphotic deformity. (b) Patient with prior kyphoplasty with subsequent new compression fractures above and below prior kyphoplasty. (c) Compression fracture of the lower thoracic vertebra with intraosseous cleft without a kyphotic deformity.

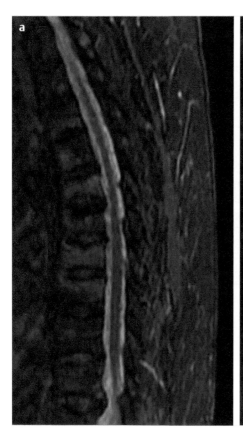
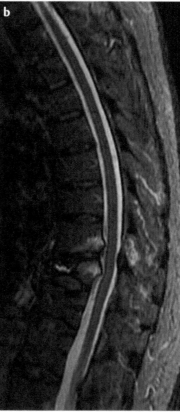

Fig. 28.2 Multiple vertebral compression fractures on sagittal MRI short tau inversion recovery acquisitions. **(a)** Multilevel thoracic compression fractures with no retropulsion or spinal canal compromise. **(b)** Two adjacent vertebral compression fractures involving the lower thoracic spine with mild retropulsion of the posterior cortex at both levels and a fracture cleft with fluid signal in the lower vertebral fracture.

28.9.5 Bone Scan

A nuclear medicine bone scan is useful when surveying the entire skeleton for osteoporotic fractures, especially when symptoms are atypical. It is particularly helpful in diagnosing sacral insufficiency fractures, which are common in osteoporosis but difficult to visualize on radiographs. On bone scan, they appear as increased radiotracer activity in an "H" or "butterfly" pattern across the sacrum. Bone scans also can differentiate between an acute versus healed compression fracture because new fractures will appear "hot."

28.10 Medical Management

Initial management begins with the primary care provider. It is essential to determine if the fracture is stable or unstable. A stable fracture will not be displaced by physiologic forces or movement. Fortunately, compression fractures are normally stable secondary to their impacted nature. Traditional treatment is nonoperative and conservative.[14,15] Conservative management may be attempted for up to 6 weeks. This may involve coordination with other providers including endocrinologists, physical therapists, and possibly pain specialists. Medical therapy should be aimed at pain control, early mobilization with the assistance of bracing and rehabilitation, and improving bone quality with the goal of future fracture prevention.

28.10.1 Pain Control

Following initial evaluation and diagnosis of a vertebral compression fracture, therapy should be aimed at pain control in a manner that avoids prolonged bedrest and allows for early mobilization of the patient. Acute pain control may include nonsteroidal anti-inflammatory drugs (NSAIDs), muscle relaxants, narcotic pain medication, neuropathic pain agents such as tricyclic antidepressants, local analgesic patch, and intercostal nerve blocks, and transcutaneous nerve stimulation units. NSAIDs are often first-line drugs for back pain as they do not have sedating effects. However, NSAIDs have been shown to significantly increase gastrointestinal bleeding in the elderly (evidence level A, randomized controlled trial [RCT]) and an increased risk of cardiac events for patients with hypertension and coronary artery disease and must be used with caution.[16] There is also a theoretical inhibitory effect of NSAIDs on bony healing,[17] though this has not been the case in actual studies. Opioids and muscle relaxants may provide strong relief when NSAIDs are inadequate but have significant sedative effects as well as the risk of dependency needs to be carefully balanced in the geriatric patients. Careful observation of bowel motility and bowel sound is warranted, in the absence of which the patient may require evaluation and treatment for ileus.

28.10.2 Improve Bone Quality

There is now good evidence that diagnosing and treating osteoporosis does indeed reduce the incidence of compression fractures of the spine (evidence level A, RCT). Agents for treating osteoporosis include bisphosphonates, selective estrogen receptor modulators, recombinant parathyroid hormone, and calcitonin. These agents act through either antiresorptive or osteogenic mechanisms. The bisphosphonate alendronate is a first-line medication given its favorable safety profile and efficacy in reducing fracture risk. Hormone replacement therapy may be an option for younger postmenopausal women. Finally, while calcium and vitamin D are insufficient alone in reducing fracture risk, supplementation may be necessary for deficient patients. Follow-up of treatment efficacy may be done with subsequent DEXA scan, though typically a 2-year treatment period is needed before improvement of bone mineral density is detected. Family physicians should take a leadership role in their communities by assessing and addressing those factors that can increase the incidence of vertebral compression fractures in elderly persons, such as inappropriate or overmedication, use of restraints, unsafe home situations, and physical abuse.

Interestingly, several medications for osteoporosis treatment also play a role in acute pain relief. Calcitonin has been found in multiple RCTs to provide pain relief for acute compression fractures.[18] Bisphosphonates have also shown similar improvements in acute pain control. Finally, patients treated with teriparatide (recombinant parathyroid hormone) show decreased back pain, when compared with patients treated with placebo, hormone replacement therapy, or alendronate.

28.10.3 Physical Therapy

Prolonged inactivity should be avoided, especially in elderly patients to minimize the risks of deep venous thrombosis and pulmonary embolism. Physical therapy should assist with early mobilization in the acute phase and prevent further injuries in the long term. As such, the exercises prescribed should have two purposes: (1) strengthening the patient's supportive axial musculature, specifically the spinal extensors and (2) training the patient's proprioceptive reflexes to improve posture and ambulation and decrease the likelihood of future falls.

The erector spinae play a crucial role in the posterior tension band that maintains normal posture, by balancing the biomechanical tendency of the spine to fall forward. This function coincidentally reduces mechanical stress on the vertebral bodies.[19,20] As such, strengthening the spinal extensor muscles will improve lumbar lordosis and posture, thus reducing acute fracture pain as well as chronic back pain associated with kyphotic deformity. This reinforcement is especially important since axial musculature decreases in strength with age, particularly among women, who are most at risk for vertebral fracture. Studies have shown that back extension strength and lumbar mobility are the most important factors for quality of life among postmenopausal osteoporotic women, compared to other relevant factors such as lumbar kyphosis angle and bone mineral density.

While repetitive mechanical loading will stimulate osteogenesis (Wolff's law) and improve patient bone quality, such loading parameters need to be within the physiologic capacity of the compromised bone. The exercise selection and intensity should be tailored toward the individual patient to avoid overstressing the spine and causing new injury. Intense spinal flexion exercise in any form transmits significant force to the intervertebral discs which in geriatric patients with disc degeneration is largely passed on to the vertebral bodies.[20] The risk of further vertebral fracture in postmenopausal osteoporotic women undergoing exercise rehabilitation was 89% with abdominal flexion training compared to only 16% with back extension exercises.[21] Similarly, spinal flexion exercises have shown to reduce some of the protective mechanisms against

back pain. Exercises should focus on strengthening back extension and may include weighted or unweighted prone position extension exercises, isometric contraction of the paraspinal muscles, and careful loading of the upper extremities.

28.10.4 Bracing

Bracing is commonly used for symptomatic management of vertebral fractures. Majority of RCTs examining bracing were based on acute, traumatic burst fractures. As such, there is little consensus on its application for osteoporotic compression fractures. Fractures in the thoracic spine may be treated with thoracolumbar orthoses (TLO) brace. The use of a spinal orthosis maintains neutral spinal alignment and limits flexion, thus reducing axial loading on the fractured vertebra. In addition, the brace allows for less fatigue of the paraspinal musculature and muscle spasm relief. One prospective randomized trial on the 6-month use of a TLO brace for osteoporotic compression fractures found improvement in trunk muscle strength, posture, and body height amongst the treatment group, ultimately with better quality of life and ability to perform activities of daily living.[22,23]

Potential downfalls of a rigid brace include patient discomfort, which may decrease compliance. These patients, typically elderly and frail, are at risk for skin breakdown if the brace edges are not carefully padded. In addition, a brace that is too restrictive may impede the patient's respiratory volume. Finally, with prolonged periods of bracing there is potential for deconditioning and atrophy of the trunk and paraspinal muscles. Many practices including ours have moved away from recommending rigid braces and towards light-weight, soft braces, except in cases of severe deformity.

28.11 Surgical Management

Percutaneous vertebroplasty was developed in France in 1984, designed to reduce the pain and loss of function in patients with vertebral compression fractures. In 1998, the U.S. Food and Drug Administration approved the KyphX inflatable balloon for use in reducing fragility fractures by creating a cavity in the vertebral body and subsequently fill with bone cement leading to the development of kyphoplasty.

Vertebroplasty and kyphoplasty are both minimally invasive surgical procedures for treating osteoporotic fractures where a bone cement is injected directly into the fractured bone.[24,25] Once in position, the cement hardens in about 10 minutes, congealing the fragments of the fractured vertebra and providing immediate stability and pain relief. Kyphoplasty includes an additional step of gently inflating a special balloon prior to injecting the bone cement inside the fractured vertebrae. Kyphoplasty is so named because it often involves the attempt to directly reduce the kyphosis that results from vertebral body collapse. The goal of this step is to restore height to the bone thus reducing deformity of the spine. Most patients return to their normal daily activities after either procedure.

28.11.1 Indications and Contraindications

Patients who do not respond to conservative treatment or who continue to have severe pain may be candidates for surgical management. Vertebroplasty and kyphoplasty are low-risk, minimally invasive, percutaneous procedures performed to treat osteoporotic compression fractures that significantly improve pain relief and physical function. Patients with unremitting pain beyond 6 weeks of conservative management or demonstrated fracture progression on follow-up radiograph, consideration should then be given to a vertebral augmentation procedure. Eligible patients should have significant back pain and tenderness in the fracture area that increases with mechanical axial loading. Factors influencing early intervention with kyphoplasty, that is, within the first 2 weeks of the fracture include:

1. Severe pain that is poorly controlled with pain medication.
2. Severe functional limitations such as inability to stand or walk.
3. Fractures with greater loss of height and angular deformity.
4. Fractures with progressive collapse.
5. Fractures located at the thoracolumbar junction.
6. Multiple fractures (▶ Fig. 28.3).
7. New fracture in a patient with prior old healed compression fractures.

The fracture should be within the acute or subacute phase before it is healed. It is extremely challenging to perform vertebroplasty or kyphoplasty in completely collapsed vertebral bodies, known as vertebra plana. If a CT demonstrates fracture through the posterior wall of the vertebrae, risk of cement extrusion into the spinal canal is greatly increased. An absolute contraindication is bony retropulsion with neurologic compromise, as this may worsen with the injection of cement. In these cases, an open surgical decompression and fixation may be appropriate. Other contraindications include active osteomyelitis of the fracture site or allergies to kyphoplasty cement. Patients should be evaluated for cardiac and pulmonary reserve as they need to tolerate deep sedation or general anesthesia in the prone position, especially during treatment of multiple levels, as both operative time and the risk of pulmonary fat embolism increases.

28.11.2 Procedure

Vertebroplasty involves the fluoroscopically guided transpedicular insertion of a cannulated trochar that is used to inject radiopaque cement, typically polymethylmethacrylate (PMMA) into the fracture. Occasionally in the upper thoracic spine, where the pedicles can be very small, an extrapedicular approach is used with trochar insertion between the medial rib head and lateral edge of the pedicle. The goal is to provide structural support to the compromised trabecular bone and restore lost vertebral height. Typically, a bipedicular approach

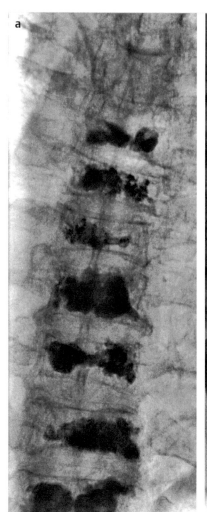
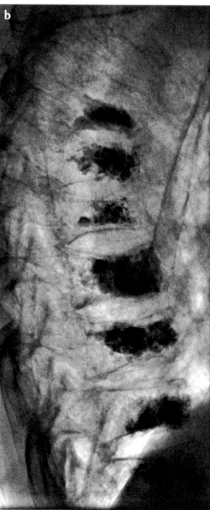

Fig. 28.3 Frontal (a) and lateral (b) projection of the thoracic spine plain radiographs demonstrating multilevel thoracic vertebral compression fractures successfully treated with staged vertebral augmentation, an expected finding in patients with severe osteoporosis.

using two trochars is chosen for more even cement distribution (▶ Fig. 28.4). Unipedicular approach is an alternative to minimize procedural time in challenging patients (▶ Fig. 28.5). Macerator or curved needle is used to facilitate the cement distribution in desired location especially during the Unipedicular approach (▶ Fig. 28.6).

Patient is usually positioned with arms extended overhead for thoracic spine compression fractures or arms positioned to the side for the lumbar spine, to avoid superimposition of the arms over spine in the lateral projection. Ideally, two fluoroscopy machines are used simultaneously around the patient, who is positioned prone, to allow for concurrent frontal (ante-

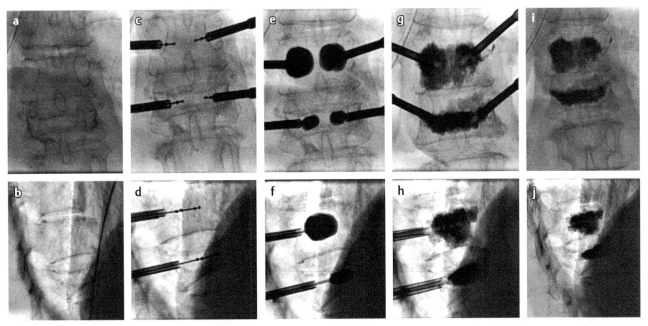

Fig. 28.4 Standard bilateral transpedicular approach for kyphoplasty performed on two adjacent vertebral compression fractures. Frontal and lateral projections demonstrating two adjacent vertebral compression fractures (a,b), trochar and balloon placement (c,d), balloon inflation (e,f), injection of bone cement (g,h). Note the minimal cement leak in to the right paravertebral vein (i,j).

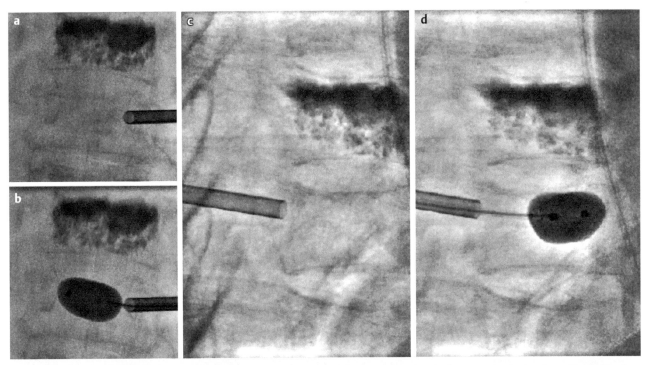

Fig. 28.5 Frontal (a) and lateral (c) projections of right unipedicular approach for the adjacent vertebral compression fracture in a patient with prior kyphoplasty. (b) Single inflatable balloon passed across the midline in the frontal and (d) lateral projections.

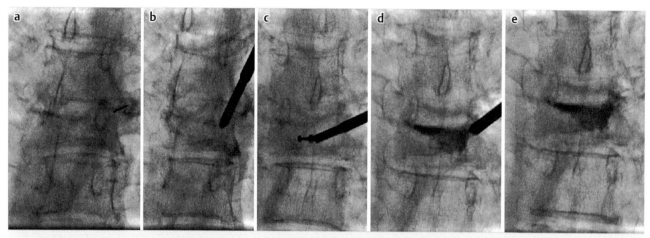

Fig. 28.6 Frontal projection of right unipedicular approach for kyphoplasty demonstrating needle localization **(a)**, trochar insertion **(b)**, macerator to cross-midline **(c)**, and injection of bone cement **(d, e)**.

rior–posterior) and lateral images. This saves time and reduces the chance of contamination by avoiding the need for frequent fluoroscopy repositioning. Preprocedural antibiotic loading dose with 2 gm of intravenous Cefazolin or 600 mg intravenous Clindamycin is our standard practice to minimize the risk of infection. Accurate localization of vertebral compression fracture and correlation with preoperative CT/MRI is vital. Identification of the thoracolumbar variations such as nonrib bearing thoracic vertebrae, lumbarization of the sacral vertebrae or sacralization of the lumbar vertebrae is critical in accurate localization of target compression fracture. A good starting anterior–posterior image, with lined up endplates and clearly outlined pedicles along with a lateral projection with superimposed bilateral pedicles is crucial for preprocedural localization and serves as a baseline image. Contralateral frontal oblique projection demonstrating the widening of the pedicel and better visualization of the costovertebral joints in frontal view helps to better distinguish the transpedicular approach from the extrapedicular approach when introducing the trochars. Frontal oblique projection is used for medial–lateral placement and lateral projection is used for the superior–inferior positioning for initial docking and subsequent advancement of the trochars. Subsequently both straight frontal and lateral images are used to guide the advancement of the trochar into the collapsed vertebral body, avoid medial or lateral breaches, and determine the final depth. Typically, the trochars are advanced in to the anterior half of the vertebral bodies for the vertebroplasty or positioned in the posterior third of the vertebral body for the kyphoplasty. We routinely perform bone biopsy in our patients via the trochars to confirm benign osseous pathology and to exclude an occult malignancy.

Kyphoplasty adds an additional step prior to the cement injection. After trochar insertion and manual drill into the anterior vertebral body, an inflatable balloon tamp is threaded into the fracture and expanded. The purpose of this step is to compact the cancellous bone and create an expanded cavity for cement injection. This plays a significant role in restoring vertebral body height. The extent of inflation is determined by monitoring pressure, inflated volume, and appearance of the balloon and vertebral body on fluoroscopy. Pressure should not

exceed a maximum of 300 psi and is usually kept less than 220 psi. Maximum volume inflation ranges from 4 to 6 mL. During the inflation process sequential images are taken to monitor appropriate expansion of the balloon, ensuring adequate contact with, but avoiding violation of, the cortical endplates. Once the inflation cavity has been created, radiopaque cement is sequentially injected in incremental volumes. It is necessary to take multiple images during injection to ensure that there is adequate cavity filling and no cement retropulsion into the spinal canal.

28.11.3 Potential Complications

Typically, vertebral augmentation is performed as an outpatient procedure and is well tolerated. Patients may experience relief of their back pain within 24 hours of the procedure. The overall reported complication rates are particularly low in cases of osteoporotic compression fractures (< 4%), but increase for oncologic fractures, though symptomatic complications remain less than 10%. The incidence of **cement extravasation** (▶ Fig. 28.7) into the spinal canal or neural foramen is rare (0.4–4%) and often asymptomatic or transient, but it is important to recognize when this occurs, as it may result in painful radiculopathy and weakness. If high enough to affect the spinal cord or conus medullaris, it may even cause paraparesis, which constitutes an emergency and requires surgical decompression. Cement may also extravasate into the paraspinal musculature, which is typically asymptomatic, but on extremely rare instances may enter the venous system and result in **pulmonary embolism**.[26] Finally, **adjacent vertebral fractures** may develop next to the augmented vertebral body.[27,28] Hadley et al[29] have speculated that this is due to increased loading on the adjacent levels secondary to stiffness of the augmented body. Bench studies on treated bone have shown that inserting PMMA does not change the stiffness of the bone, but human studies have not been done. Recent meta-analysis by Zhan et al confirmed no additional risk of adjacent vertebral fractures in patients with prior vertebral augmentation procedures.[30] Osteoporosis is a chronic, progressive disease and the patients who have

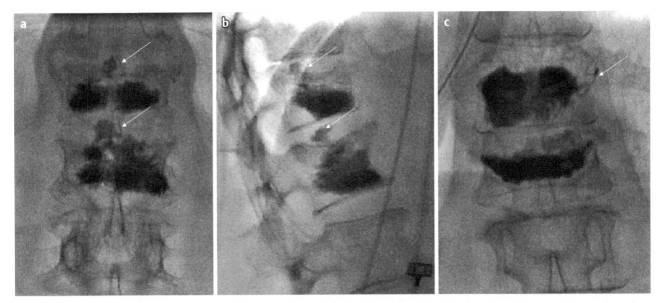

Fig. 28.7 Frontal **(a)** and lateral **(b)** projections demonstrating the bone cement leakage into the adjacent intervertebral discs (*white arrows*) and cement leakage into the right paravertebral vein **(c)** (*white arrow*).

sustained fractures from osteoporosis are at an increased risk for additional fractures due to the loss of bone strength caused by osteoporosis.

28.11.4 Treatment Outcomes

Kyphoplasty and vertebroplasty are safe and effective and are designed to reduce pain, prevent further collapse of the vertebra, and restore the patient's mobility. There is 95% improvement in pain and significant improvement in function following treatment by either of these percutaneous techniques. Kyphoplasty offers the additional advantage of realigning the spinal column and regaining height of the fractured vertebra, which may help decrease the pulmonary, gastrointestinal, and early morbidity consequences related to these fractures.[31] Kyphoplasty improves height of the fractured vertebra, and improves kyphosis by over 50%, if performed within 3 months from the onset of the fracture (onset of pain). There is some height improvement, though not as marked, along with 95% clinical improvement, if the procedure is performed after 3 months.[32]

Despite large number of studies to examine the efficacy of vertebral augmentation compared to optimal medical management, there remains significant controversy.[33,34,35,36] Overall, there are a greater number of studies on vertebroplasty than kyphoplasty given its longer history. McGirt et al[37] published a 20-year review of all vertebral augmentation outcome studies in 2009, including 74 studies of (one level I) of vertebroplasty for osteoporotic compression fractures, 35 kyphoplasty studies for osteoporotic fractures, and 18 studies for tumor-related fractures, which were all level IV studies. The authors found level I evidence that vertebroplasty provides superior pain control over medical management in the first 2 weeks, and levels II to III evidence that within the first 3 months there are superior outcomes in analgesic use, disability, and general health, and finally levels II to III evidence that by 2 years there is a similar level of pain control and physical function. With regards to

kyphoplasty, there were levels II to III evidence of improvement in daily activity, physical function, and pain control at 6 months, compared to medical management.

VERTOS Trial

VERTOS is the first RCT[38] with a limited group of 34 patients reports only on short-term results, evaluated the short-term clinical outcome of patients with painful osteoporotic vertebral compression fracture treated with percutaneous vertebroplasty with patients treated with optimal pain medication (OPM). Long-term results could not be obtained due to the cross-over of many patients from the OPM group to the percutaneous vertebroplasty group already after a 2-week follow-up. VERTOS confirmed significantly better immediate pain relief, improvement of mobility, function and stature after percutaneous vertebroplasty compared to OPM in patients with subacute or chronic osteoporotic vertebral compression fractures.

Subsequently, two double-blind RCTs by Buchbinder et al[39] and by Kallmes et al[40] involved comparisons between vertebroplasty and sham procedure groups rather than the usual comparison group of medical managements. The authors of both studies reported no difference in pain control or function between the groups, from 1-week to 6-month follow-up in one study and 1-month follow-up in the other. They suggested that the benefits of vertebroplasty in prior trials were secondary to a procedural placebo effect. These studies have been the subject of criticism, focusing on their low enrollment numbers (78 and 131 patients), low volume and infrequent rate of vertebroplasty performed at the centers over a prolonged time interval, lack of clear inclusion criteria specifying patients with mechanical axial back pain, and inadequate volume of cement injection. In contradistinction, two open label randomized trials of vertebral augmentation, the VERTOS II trial of vertebroplasty and FREE trial of kyphoplasty, showed efficacy for both techniques compared to conservative management.

FREE Trial

The Fracture Reduction Evaluation (FREE) trial,[41] is a 2-year RCT comparing balloon kyphoplasty and nonsurgical care for treating spinal fractures which enrolled 300 patients with one to three acute vertebral fractures were at 21 sites in 8 countries. Around 149 patients were assigned to receive balloon kyphoplasty while 151 patients were randomized to nonsurgical treatment. Patients in the kyphoplasty group also received some amount of nonsurgical care. As appropriate, patients in both groups were also prescribed calcium and vitamin D supplements and osteoporosis treatment medications such as bisphosphonates. Most kyphoplasty procedures were done under general anesthesia.

The study concluded that the patients treated with balloon kyphoplasty had significantly better outcomes in terms of pain reduction, quality of life, function and mobility both initially, at one month, and throughout the first 12 months after treatment, compared to nonsurgical care. There was no difference in the overall frequency of adverse events between the kyphoplasty and control (nonsurgical care) groups. No procedure-related mortality was reported. The possible increased risk of subsequent fractures after balloon kyphoplasty is unclear from the results of this study. While the numerical rate of additional fractures over time was higher in the kyphoplasty group (33 vs. 25% in the control group at 12 months), the difference was not statistically significant.

VERTOS II Trial

VERTOS II[42] is an open-label randomized trial aimed to clarify whether vertebroplasty has additional value compared with optimum pain treatment in patients with acute vertebral fractures. The trial enrolled 202 patients with acute osteoporotic vertebral compression fractures and persistent pain. The trail confirmed that the percutaneous vertebroplasty is effective and safe with pain relief after vertebroplasty is immediate and sustained for at least a year, and is significantly greater than that achieved with conservative treatment, at an acceptable cost.

Considering conflicting results from prior RCTs, two sham-controlled studies showed no benefit of percutaneous vertebroplasty while an unmasked but controlled RCT (VERTOS II and FREE trials) found effective pain relief at acceptable costs, further efforts were made to address the debate of vertebral augmentation. Because masked trials constitute a higher level of evidence than open label trials, it was necessary to prove the efficacy of vertebroplasty within a masked trial format.

VAPOUR Trial

The VAPOUR is multicenter RCT[43] (vertebroplasty for acute painful osteoporotic fractures) used the same trial methodology as the previous masked trials but with selection criteria: numeric rating scale (NRS) pain $\geq 7/10$, pain duration < 6 weeks, MRI evidence of recent fracture, and both hospital inpatients and outpatients included. Study involved randomization of 120 patients with a mean cement volume was 7.5 cc (compared to 2.7 cc in previous sham trials). The primary endpoint was the proportion of patients with low NRS pain scores ($< 4/10$) at 14 days, which was achieved in a significantly greater proportion of patients in the vertebroplasty group compared with the control group (44 vs. 21%; between-group difference: 23%; $p = 0.011$) and the advantage in this outcome for vertebroplasty remained similar at every data collection time point to 6 months, with a maximum between-group difference at 4 weeks of 33%. The positive secondary outcomes in the vertebroplasty group include: lower mean NRS pain score at every time point, Roland–Morris Disability score was lower from one month to 6 months, analgesic use was lower at 3 and 6 months, median duration of hospitalization was lower by 5.5 days, and fractured vertebral body height was 36% greater than placebo at 6 months. The reduction in hospital stay shows the procedure to be cost effective. Subgroup analysis of the primary endpoint showed significantly greater benefit in the thoracolumbar segment (T11–L2) than in the thoracic (T5–T10) or lumbar (L3–L5) segments ($p = 0.001$).

One ongoing study that may shed light on the unsettled debate of vertebral augmentation in acute painful vertebral compression fractures is the VERTOS IV trial,[44] a nonindustry supported, prospective RCT of 180 patients that compares vertebroplasty to sham procedure, but uses the strict inclusion criteria of the VERTOS II trial. The objective of this study is to compare pain relief after percutaneous vertebroplasty with a sham intervention in selected patients with an acute osteoporotic vertebral compression fractures using the same strict inclusion criteria as in VERTOS II. Secondary outcome measures are back pain related disability and quality of life.

28.12 Future Directions

Increased physician and patient awareness on vertebral augmentation procedures is essential for better utilization of this safe and minimally invasive procedure. Decision on vertebral augmentation should be tailored to the individual patients based on their clinical presentation, quality of life and comorbidities. Innovation of increased viscosity cement can provide improved control over the vertebral cement injection and prevent inadvertent cement leakage into the spinal canal and paravertebral veins. Vertebral augmentation can be performed in conjunction with radiofrequency ablation of in patients with secondary osteoporosis from the marrow disorders such as multiple myeloma. Vertebral augmentation in combination with radiofrequency ablation and stereotactic radiation may evolve into an effective palliative strategy for painful pathological vertebral compression fractures.

References

[1] Ensrud KE, Schousboe JT. Clinical practice. Vertebral fractures. N Engl J Med. 2011; 364(17):1634–1642

[2] Cooper C. Epidemiology and public health impact of osteoporosis. Baillieres Clin Rheumatol. 1993; 7(3):459–477

[3] Melton LJ, III, Lane AW, Cooper C, Eastell R, O'Fallon WM, Riggs BL. Prevalence and incidence of vertebral deformities. Osteoporos Int. 1993; 3(3):113–119

[4] Nevitt MC, Cummings SR, Stone KL, et al. Risk factors for a first-incident radiographic vertebral fracture in women > or = 65 years of age: the study of osteoporotic fractures. J Bone Miner Res. 2005; 20(1):131–140

[5] Cauley JA, Palermo L, Vogt M, et al. Prevalent vertebral fractures in black women and white women. J Bone Miner Res. 2008; 23(9):1458–1467

[6] Ling X, Cummings SR, Mingwei Q, et al. Vertebral fractures in Beijing, China: the Beijing Osteoporosis Project. J Bone Miner Res. 2000; 15(10):2019–2025

[7] Fink HA, Milavetz DL, Palermo L, et al. Fracture Intervention Trial Research Group. What proportion of incident radiographic vertebral deformities is

clinically diagnosed and vice versa? J Bone Miner Res. 2005; 20(7):1216–1222

[8] Mather M. Fact Sheet: Aging in the United States. Available at: http://www.prb.org/Publications/Media-Guides/2016/aging-unitedstates-fact-sheet.aspx

[9] Lindsay R, Silverman SL, Cooper C, et al. Risk of new vertebral fracture in the year following a fracture. JAMA. 2001; 285(3):320–323

[10] Etzioni DA, Liu JH, Maggard MA, Ko CY. The aging population and its impact on the surgery workforce. Ann Surg. 2003; 238(2):170–177

[11] Dolan P, Torgerson DJ. The cost of treating osteoporotic fractures in the United Kingdom female population. Osteoporos Int. 1998; 8(6):611–617

[12] Cooper C, Atkinson EJ, Jacobsen SJ, O'Fallon WM, Melton LJ, III. Population-based study of survival after osteoporotic fractures. Am J Epidemiol. 1993; 137(9):1001–1005

[13] Jergas M, Genant HK. Spinal and femoral DXA for the assessment of spinal osteoporosis. Calcif Tissue Int. 1997; 61(5):351–357

[14] Longo UG, Loppini M, Denaro L, Maffulli N, Denaro V. Conservative management of patients with an osteoporotic vertebral fracture: a review of the literature. J Bone Joint Surg Br. 2012; 94(2):152–157

[15] Longo UG, Loppini M, Denaro L, Maffulli N, Denaro V. Osteoporotic vertebral fractures: current concepts of conservative care. Br Med Bull. 2012; 102:171–189

[16] Bavry AA, Khaliq A, Gong Y, Handberg EM, Cooper-Dehoff RM, Pepine CJ. Harmful effects of NSAIDs among patients with hypertension and coronary artery disease. Am J Med. 2011; 124(7):614–620

[17] Dodwell ER, Latorre JG, Parisini E, et al. NSAID exposure and risk of nonunion: a meta-analysis of case-control and cohort studies. Calcif Tissue Int. 2010; 87(3):193–202

[18] Knopp JA, Diner BM, Blitz M, Lyritis GP, Rowe BH. Calcitonin for treating acute pain of osteoporotic vertebral compression fractures: a systematic review of randomized, controlled trials. Osteoporos Int. 2005; 16(10):1281–1290

[19] Sinaki M. Critical appraisal of physical rehabilitation measures after osteoporotic vertebral fracture. Osteoporos Int. 2003; 14(9):773–779

[20] Sinaki M. The role of physical activity in bone health: a new hypothesis to reduce risk of vertebral fracture. Phys Med Rehabil Clin N Am. 2007; 18(3):593–608, xi–xii

[21] Sinaki M, Itoi E, Wahner HW, et al. Stronger back muscles reduce the incidence of vertebral fractures: a prospective 10 year follow-up of postmenopausal women. Bone. 2002; 30(6):836–841

[22] Pfeifer M, Begerow B, Minne HW. Effects of a new spinal orthosis on posture, trunk strength, and quality of life in women with postmenopausal osteoporosis: a randomized trial. Am J Phys Med Rehabil. 2004; 83(3):177–186

[23] Tuong NH, Dansereau J, Maurais G, Herrera R. Three-dimensional evaluation of lumbar orthosis effects on spinal behavior. J Rehabil Res Dev. 1998; 35(1):34–42

[24] Gangi A, Guth S, Imbert JP, Marin H, Dietemann JL. Percutaneous vertebroplasty: indications, technique, and results. Radiographics. 2003; 23(2):e10

[25] Truumees E, Hilibrand A, Vaccaro AR. Percutaneous vertebral augmentation. Spine J. 2004; 4(2):218–229

[26] Kim YJ, Lee JW, Park KW, et al. Pulmonary cement embolism after percutaneous vertebroplasty in osteoporotic vertebral compression fractures: incidence, characteristics, and risk factors. Radiology. 2009; 251(1):250–259

[27] Spross C, Aghayev E, Kocher R, Röder C, Forster T, Kuelling FA. Incidence and risk factors for early adjacent vertebral fractures after balloon kyphoplasty for osteoporotic fractures: analysis of the SWISSspine registry. Eur Spine J. 2014; 23(6):1332–1338

[28] Lin EP, Ekholm S, Hiwatashi A, Westesson P-L. Vertebroplasty: cement leakage into the disc increases the risk of new fracture of adjacent vertebral body. AJNR Am J Neuroradiol. 2004; 25(2):175–180

[29] Hadley C, Awan OA, Zoarski GH. Biomechanics of vertebral bone augmentation. Neuroimaging Clin N Am. 2010; 20(2):159–167

[30] Zhan Y, Jiang J, Liao H, Tan H, Yang K. Risk factors for cement leakage after vertebroplasty or kyphoplasty: a meta-analysis of published evidence. World Neurosurg. 2017; 101:633–642

[31] Garfin SR, Yuan HA, Reiley MA. New technologies in spine: kyphoplasty and vertebroplasty for the treatment of painful osteoporotic compression fractures. Spine. 2001; 26(14):1511–1515

[32] Taylor RS, Fritzell P, Taylor RJ. Balloon kyphoplasty in the management of vertebral compression fractures: an updated systematic review and meta-analysis. Eur Spine J. 2007; 16(8):1085–1100

[33] Van Meirhaeghe J, Bastian L, Boonen S, Ranstam J, Tillman JB, Wardlaw D, FREE investigators. A randomized trial of balloon kyphoplasty and nonsurgical management for treating acute vertebral compression fractures: vertebral body kyphosis correction and surgical parameters. Spine. 2013; 38(12):971–983

[34] Boonen S, Van Meirhaeghe J, Bastian L, et al. Balloon kyphoplasty for the treatment of acute vertebral compression fractures: 2-year results from a randomized trial. J Bone Miner Res. 2011; 26(7):1627–1637

[35] Chen AT, Cohen DB, Skolasky RL. Impact of nonoperative treatment, vertebroplasty, and kyphoplasty on survival and morbidity after vertebral compression fracture in the medicare population. J Bone Joint Surg Am. 2013; 95(19):1729–1736

[36] Anderson PA, Froyshteter AB, Tontz WL, Jr. Meta-analysis of vertebral augmentation compared with conservative treatment for osteoporotic spinal fractures. J Bone Miner Res. 2013; 28(2):372–382

[37] Wong CC, McGirt MJ. Vertebral compression fractures: a review of current management and multimodal therapy. J Multidiscip Healthc. 2013; 6:205–214

[38] Voormolen MHJ, Mali WPTM, Lohle PNM, et al. Percutaneous vertebroplasty compared with optimal pain medication treatment: short-term clinical outcome of patients with subacute or chronic painful osteoporotic vertebral compression fractures. The VERTOS study. AJNR Am J Neuroradiol. 2007; 28(3):555–560

[39] Buchbinder R, Osborne RH, Ebeling PR, et al. A randomized trial of vertebroplasty for painful osteoporotic vertebral fractures. N Engl J Med. 2009; 361(6):557–568

[40] Kallmes DF, Comstock BA, Heagerty PJ, et al. A randomized trial of vertebroplasty for osteoporotic spinal fractures. N Engl J Med. 2009; 361(6):569–579

[41] Wardlaw D, Cummings SR, Van Meirhaeghe J, et al. Efficacy and safety of balloon kyphoplasty compared with non-surgical care for vertebral compression fracture (FREE): a randomised controlled trial. Lancet. 2009; 373(9668):1016–1024

[42] Klazen CAH, Lohle PNM, de Vries J, et al. Vertebroplasty versus conservative treatment in acute osteoporotic vertebral compression fractures (Vertos II): an open-label randomised trial. Lancet. 2010; 376(9746):1085–1092

[43] Clark W, Bird P, Gonski P, et al. Safety and efficacy of vertebroplasty for acute painful osteoporotic fractures (VAPOUR): a multicentre, randomised, double-blind, placebo-controlled trial. Lancet. 2016; 388(10052):1408–1416

[44] Firanescu C, Lohle PN, de Vries J, et al. VERTOS IV study group. A randomised sham controlled trial of vertebroplasty for painful acute osteoporotic vertebral fractures (VERTOS IV). Trials. 2011; 12:93

Part VII

Further Topics

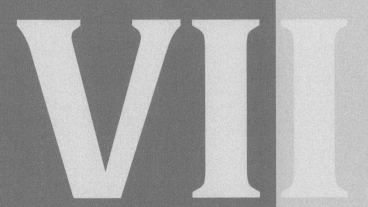

29 Idiopathic Spinal Cord Herniation

Randall J. Hlubek and Jay D. Turner

Abstract

Idiopathic spinal cord herniation (ISCH) is a relatively rare disorder causing patients to present with thoracic myelopathy. The disorder is characterized by herniation of the spinal cord through a ventral dural defect. Diagnostic workup should include magnetic resonance imaging (MRI) of the thoracic spine, which typically reveals anterior displacement and kinking of the spinal cord. Computed tomography myelography is useful in distinguishing between ISCH and an arachnoid cyst. The goals of operative management are to halt progressive neurologic decline and preserve spinal cord function. Two main surgical strategies are used to treat patients with ISCH. The first technique involves repairing the defect primarily, either with sutures or with a dural patch. The second technique consists of widening the dural defect. Postoperative improvement in motor function can be expected in 68% of all cases, stabilization of neurologic function in 19% of all cases, and neurologic deterioration in 7%. Close postoperative clinical follow-up is recommended to monitor patients for possible spinal cord tethering or reherniation.

Keywords: dural defect, idiopathic spinal cord herniation, myelopathy, thoracic spinal cord herniation, thoracic spine

Clinical Pearls

- Magnetic resonance imaging is critical to the diagnosis of idiopathic spinal cord herniation, and findings typically include anterior displacement of the spinal cord, with kinking or beaking.
- Before ventral intradural exploration, bilateral dentate ligament release is recommended to detether the spinal cord, which allows it to be manipulated more safely.
- Close postoperative clinical follow-up is recommended to monitor patients for possible spinal cord tethering or reherniation.

29.1 Introduction

Idiopathic spinal cord herniation (ISCH) is a relatively rare disorder that was first described in 1974 by Wortzman et al.[1] The disorder is characterized by herniation of the spinal cord through a ventral dural defect. Strangulation of the spinal cord occurs because of the constricting edges of the dural defect, which typically leads to progressive myelopathic symptoms. The rarity of ISCH has made it challenging to elicit the incidence, natural history, and optimal treatment of the disease. Groen et al[2] performed a meta-analysis of 126 case reports to better characterize this disorder. The mean age of patients was 51 years, and women were more affected than men, with a male-to-female ratio of 1:1.8. In this meta-analysis, ISCH was most typically found between the T3 and T7 levels and never occurred in the cervical or lumbar region. Brown–Séquard syndrome was present in 66%

of the patients, paraparesis in 30%, isolated sensory deficit in 3%, and isolated motor deficit in 1%. The anatomic proximity between the corticospinal tracts and anterior horn of the spinal cord and the ventral dural defect likely underlies the predisposition for motor deficits.

29.2 Pathogenesis

The etiology of the dural defect and the spinal cord herniation is unknown, but there are several mechanisms proposed in the medical literature. Intraoperative findings by Watanabe et al[3] and Nakazawa et al[4] of a cavity formed by duplicated membranes led them to hypothesize that a congenital duplication of the dura matter is partly the cause of ISCH.[3,4] Alternative theories include acquisition of a dural defect secondary to trauma, degenerative disc herniation,[5] inflammatory process,[6] and pressure-induced erosion from an intradural arachnoid cyst.[7] Chronic cerebrospinal fluid (CSF) pulsations and negative extradural thoracic pressure likely contribute to the gradual displacement of a portion of the spinal cord through the dural defect.[8] Adhesions then form between the defect of the dural edges and the herniated segment of the spinal cord, leading to progressive strangulation of the cord (▶ Fig. 29.1).

29.3 Diagnostic Workup

Magnetic resonance imaging (MRI) is critical to the diagnosis of ISCH, as evidenced by the paucity of cases reported in the literature prior to 1990. MRI findings typically include anterior displacement of the spinal cord, with kinking or beaking (▶ Fig. 29.2). Spinal cord atrophy and T2 signal change may also be seen on MRI. The most common misdiagnosis of ISCH is an intradural arachnoid cyst; however, there are subtle differences between the two on MRI that will aid in diagnosis. Higher kink angles and the disappearance of CSF ventral to the spinal cord are findings that favor ISCH, whereas vertebral scalloping and alterations in CSF flow are suggestive of an arachnoid cyst.[9]

Computed tomography myelography is another imaging modality used to differentiate between ISCH and an arachnoid cyst. Visualization of the dural defect with contrast or visualization of the spinal cord herniation through the defect may be observed (▶ Fig. 29.3). A lack of contrast filling dorsal to the spinal cord suggests a loculated arachnoid cyst.

29.4 Operative Management

Although there are reports of nonoperative management and spontaneous resolution of ISCH,[9] there is a general consensus that symptomatic ISCH warrants operative intervention. The purpose of operative management is to halt progressive neurologic decline and preserve function. Most operative techniques described in published reports are performed via a posterior approach. The goals of surgery are to reduce the herniated spinal cord and prevent recurrence of herniation. There are two

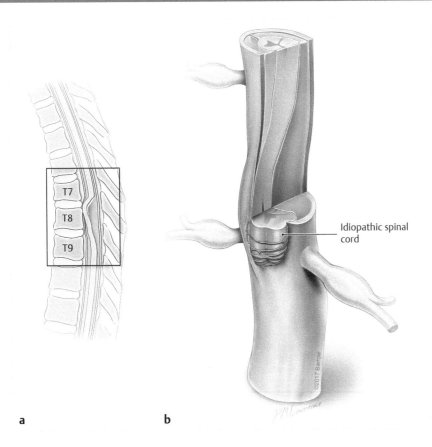

Fig. 29.1 Illustration depicting idiopathic spinal cord herniation and the beaking of the spinal cord on **(a)** a sagittal view and **(b)** strangulation of the spinal cord by the edges of the dural defect on an oblique view. (Used with permission from Barrow Neurological Institute, Phoenix, Arizona.)

Idiopathic spinal cord

T7
T8
T9

a   b

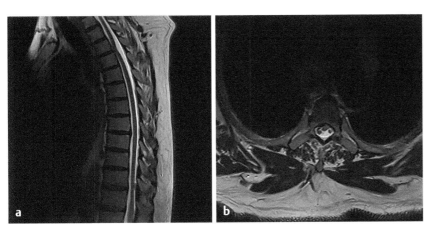

Fig. 29.2 Preoperative **(a)** sagittal and **(b)** axial T2-weighted magnetic resonance images demonstrating the anterior herniation of the thoracic spinal cord at the level of the disc space, with beaking of the spinal cord. (Used with permission from Barrow Neurological Institute, Phoenix, Arizona.)

main strategies to achieving these goals. The first is to repair the defect primarily with sutures or a dural patch.[8] The second strategy is to widen the dural defect.[3] Proponents of the latter technique believe that widening the defect relieves the strangulation with less manipulation of the spinal cord, compared with repairing the defect with sutures or a patch. Critics of this technique believe that closure of the dural defect is necessary to prevent reherniation, reduce the spinal cord to its natural position, and restore normal CSF flow. There is insufficient evidence to suggest that one strategy is superior to the other; however, the preference at our institution is to repair the defect when feasible.

Neuromonitoring with somatosensory evoked potentials and motor evoked potentials (MEPs) is essential for the surgical treatment of ISCH. Manipulation of the densely adherent herniated cord has been associated with new postoperative neurologic deficits. Novak et al[10] identified new deficits in 22 (12.6%) of 175 reported cases. They documented two cases in which severe and long-lasting deterioration of motor function was prevented by the use of MEP during the surgical treatment of patients with ISCH. MEP monitoring allows for intraoperative detection of neurologic dysfunction related to manipulation of the corticospinal tracts near the ventral dural defect and may help prevent postoperative deficits.

Maintaining adequate spinal cord perfusion via systemic hypertension is also recommended for preventing ischemic changes in the spinal cord, particularly when the spinal cord is being manipulated during the intradural portion of the surgical

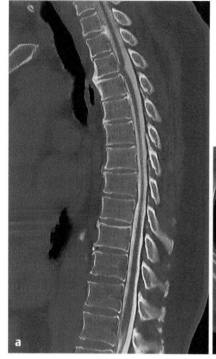

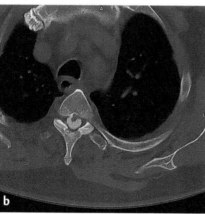

Fig. 29.3 Preoperative (a) sagittal and (b) axial computed tomography myelogram demonstrating communication of the contrast dorsal to the spinal cord with no evidence of arachnoid cyst. (Used with permission from Barrow Neurological Institute, Phoenix, Arizona.)

procedure. At our institution, we target mean arterial pressure to be more than 85 mm Hg. Hypoperfusion is hypothesized to be present in the strangulated portion of the spinal cord due to the compromise of the anterior spinal artery. Maintaining an elevated systemic blood pressure minimizes the risk of spinal cord infarction while the spinal cord is being manipulated.

At our institution, we typically perform a standard midline exposure and laminectomy or laminoplasty centered over the level of interest. Microscopic technique is used to open the dura in either the midline or paramedian if the dural defect is eccentric to one side. A microvac is often placed in the epidural space to continuously aspirate CSF and maintain a clear surgical field. Before ventral exploration and repair, bilateral dentate ligament release is recommended to detether the spinal cord, which allows for safer manipulation of the spinal cord. After the dentate ligament is divided, the stump that remains attached to the spinal cord can be used to manipulate the cord without directly contacting the neural elements. Dissection is then carried down to the ventral dural defect. Arachnoid adhesions between the dural edges of the defect and the herniated cord are lysed. The spinal cord is then gently reduced from the defect, which may be widened and repaired primarily with sutures or which may be repaired by placing a patch over the defect. Our preference is to perform primary repair of the defect whenever possible. Manipulation of the dentate ligament allows the spinal cord to be gently rotated away from the defect and provides room to repair the dura with sutures (▶ Fig. 29.4). If primary repair is not feasible, then we prefer to use a bovine pericardium intradural sling to cover the defect circumferentially and prevent reherniation (▶ Fig. 29.5). The use of a resorbable dural substitute is not recommended because of the possible risk of reherniation when the material has resorbed. Postoperative MRI is typically performed to establish a new radiographic baseline.

29.5 Clinical Outcomes

Groen et al[2] conducted a meta-analysis that revealed postoperative improvement in motor function in 68% of all cases, stabilization of neurologic function in 19%, and permanent neurologic deterioration in 7%. Close postoperative clinical follow-up is recommended to monitor for possible spinal cord tethering or reherniation. MRI is recommended if any new neurologic symptoms develop. The risk of recurrence and long-term clinical outcomes are currently unknown because of the lack of long-term follow-up reported in the literature.

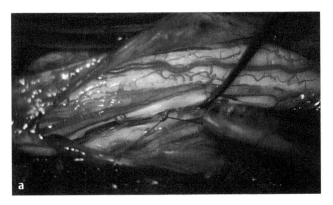

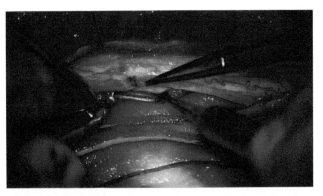

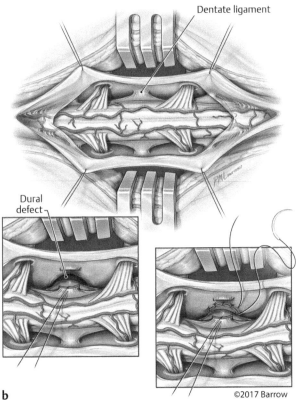

Fig. 29.5 Intraoperative photograph demonstrating the placement of a bovine pericardium intradural sling to cover the defect circumferentially and prevent reherniation. (Used with permission from Barrow Neurological Institute, Phoenix, Arizona.)

Fig. 29.4 **(a)** Intraoperative photograph demonstrating the ventral dural defect. **(b)** Illustration depicting manipulation of the dentate ligament to allow for visualization of the dural defect and primary repair. (Used with permission from Barrow Neurological Institute, Phoenix, Arizona.)

References

[1] Wortzman G, Tasker RR, Rewcastle NB, Richardson JC, Pearson FG. Spontaneous incarcerated herniation of the spinal cord into a vertebral body: a unique cause of paraplegia. Case report. J Neurosurg. 1974; 41(5):631–635

[2] Groen RJ, Middel B, Meilof JF, et al. Operative treatment of anterior thoracic spinal cord herniation: three new cases and an individual patient data meta-analysis of 126 case reports. Neurosurgery. 2009; 64(3) Suppl:ons145–ons159, discussion ons159–ons160

[3] Watanabe M, Chiba K, Matsumoto M, Maruiwa H, Fujimura Y, Toyama Y. Surgical management of idiopathic spinal cord herniation: a review of nine cases treated by the enlargement of the dural defect. J Neurosurg. 2001; 95(2) Suppl:169–172

[4] Nakazawa H, Toyama Y, Satomi K, Fujimura Y, Hirabayashi K. Idiopathic spinal cord herniation. Report of two cases and review of the literature. Spine. 1993; 18(14):2138–2141

[5] Hausmann ON, Moseley IF. Idiopathic dural herniation of the thoracic spinal cord. Neuroradiology. 1996; 38(6):503–510

[6] Najjar MW, Baeesa SS, Lingawi SS. Idiopathic spinal cord herniation: a new theory of pathogenesis. Surg Neurol. 2004; 62(2):161–170, discussion 170–171

[7] Isu T, Iizuka T, Iwasaki Y, Nagashima M, Akino M, Abe H. Spinal cord herniation associated with an intradural spinal arachnoid cyst diagnosed by magnetic resonance imaging. Neurosurgery. 1991; 29(1):137–139

[8] Hawasli AH, Ray WZ, Wright NM. Symptomatic thoracic spinal cord herniation: case series and technical report. Neurosurgery. 2014; 10 Suppl 3:E498–E504, discussion E504

[9] Samuel N, Goldstein CL, Santaguida C, Fehlings MG. Spontaneous resolution of idiopathic thoracic spinal cord herniation: case report. J Neurosurg Spine. 2015; 23(3):306–308

[10] Novak K, Widhalm G, de Camargo AB, et al. The value of intraoperative motor evoked potential monitoring during surgical intervention for thoracic idiopathic spinal cord herniation. J Neurosurg Spine. 2012; 16(2):114–126

30 Intraoperative Neuromonitoring During Thoracic Spine and Spinal Cord Surgery

Ronald Emerson

Abstract

Somatosensory evoked potentials (SSEPs) and motor evoked potentials (MEPs) are employed for spinal cord monitoring during thoracic spine and spinal surgery. SSEPs directly monitor dorsal column function and MEPs directly monitor pyramidal tract function. As spinal cord injury commonly affects both systems, concurrent monitoring of both modalities affords important redundancy while enabling detection of injury insolated to either system. SSEPs may be performed continually throughout surgery, but since each SSEP consists of the average of the brain's response to several hundred stimuli acquired over several minutes, detection of injury by SSEPs is necessarily delayed. MEPs recorded from muscle require no averaging and results are instantaneous. However, since they are performed intermittently, the frequency and timing of MEP testing must be sufficient to detect injury in a timely manner.

Anesthetic management is critical to SSEPs and MEP monitoring. The cortical component of SSEPs is suppressed by most common anesthetic agents. Small changes in anesthetic dose can result in large changes in SSEPs, so it is desirable that stable anesthesia be maintained, and necessary that changes be communicated. The same considerations apply to MEPs recorded from muscle. MEPs are often even more sensitive to anesthetic agents; total intravenous anesthetic is commonly recommended, although balanced anesthesia, including a low dose of volatile inhalational agent, has been reported to be similarly effective in most patients.

Traditionally, monitoring has focused on "critical periods" during surgery, for example, following correction of a spinal deformity. It is now recognized that best practice often entails monitoring throughout the entire procedure.

Keywords: intraoperative neuromonitoring, somatosensory evoked potentials, motor evoked potentials, M-waves, D-waves, anesthetic fade

Clinical Pearls

- Intraoperative neurophysiological monitoring using both motor evoked potentials (MEPs) and somatosensory evoked potentials (SSEPs) enables detection of injury restricted to either motor or sensory pathways. Since spinal cord injury during thoracic spine surgery commonly affects both systems, monitoring both provided added *safety through redundancy*.
- SSEP monitoring should include both cortical and brainstem signals. Cortical SSEPs are the easier to record and less susceptible to interference, but are often affected by anesthetic agents. Brainstem SSEPs, although more difficult to record, are unaffected by anesthetics.
- MEPs are safe. Tongue bites and patient movement are the primary risks.

- MEPs should be recorded with sufficient frequency both to detect injury in a timely manner and also to allow for reassessment of the "baseline" in light of increasing suppression by anesthetics over time, even at constant doses.

30.1 Introduction

Intraoperative neurophysiological monitoring (IONM) serves to detect and to reduce the risk of neurological injury during spine surgery. Somatosensory evoked potential (SSEP) monitoring of spinal cord function was first introduced in the late 1970s.[1] Its effectiveness was subsequently demonstrated in a study of 1,168 scoliosis surgeries at the Royal Orthopedic Hospital, where it was reported to have zero false negatives and a technical failure rate of only 2.2%. The authors suggested that SSEP monitoring was superior to, and should probably replace, the Stagnara wake-up test.[2,3] The utility of SSEP monitoring was firmly established by the mid-1990s, when a large multicenter study revealed a nearly threefold reduction in incidence of severe postoperative neurological deficits following scoliosis surgery when IONM was employed.[4]

Although uncommon, false negatives did occur. This is not surprising, as SSEPs directly monitor the function of the dorsal column sensory pathways of the spinal cord, and serve only as surrogates for the integrity of other pathways. SSEPs are, in fact, generally effective surrogates for "global" cord function because injury due to blunt trauma, compression and ischemia, is usually widespread, affecting multiple pathways.[5,6,7,8] Nonetheless, injury sparing the dorsal columns will go undetected by SSEP monitoring.[9] SSEP monitoring can also fail for technical reasons related, for example, to interference from electrical noise and muscle activity, or to the effects of anesthetic agents; in some cases, baseline pathology may render SSEP monitoring impossible.

Motor evoked potentials (MEPs) elicited by transcranial electrical simulation, initially described in 1980,[10] are directly dependent on corticospinal tract integrity and are more direct monitors of motor function. MEP monitoring is widely employed, along with SSEP monitoring, during surgery that places the spinal cord at risk. The concurrent use of MEP and SSEP monitoring not only permits detection of injury restricted to either motor or somatosensory systems, but also provides an important level of added safety through redundancy. If, for example, MEPs are transiently abolished by a bolus of an anesthetic agent, or SSEPs become unmonitorable due to electrical noise or muscle artifact, monitoring can continue using the other, uncompromised, modality. Additionally, MEP and SSEP monitoring can be complementary, responding with differing sensitivities and speeds to changes in anesthetics and blood pressure, and to spinal cord injury.

30.2 Somatosensory Evoked Potentials

SSEPs are recorded at the scalp following peripheral nerve stimulation—usually the median or ulnar nerves in the upper extremity and tibial or common peroneal nerves in the lower extremity. Subdermal needle electrodes are commonly used for both stimulation and for recording. Subdermal corkscrew type electrodes or surface electroencephalography (EEG) electrodes, secured with collodion, may also be used for recording. Stick-on surface electrodes may be used for stimulation, but are, in general, less reliable. Median SSEPs are usually larger signals, and therefore are easier to record, than ulnar SSEPs, but ulnar SSEPs can provide information about injury below C6 that would not be detected by median SSEPs. They can also be more sensitive to brachial plexus stretch injuries related to patient positioning. Tibial nerve SSEPs are generally higher amplitude and more robust than peroneal SSEPs, and produce much less patient movement. Nonetheless, common peroneal SSEPs are useful in patients in whom tibal SSEPs are not monitorable, for example, due to peripheral neuropathy or ankle edema.

Recording electrodes are placed at specific scalp locations, which correspond to the topography of the electrical fields generated by the somatosensory cortex. In addition to cortically generated signals, scalp electrodes also detect signals that are generated in the brainstem and conducted to the scalp through the cranial contents. SSEPs are recorded using differential amplifiers that *amplify the voltage difference* between two inputs. This allows for selective recording of tiny neurophysiological signals in the presence of electrical noise, such as power main frequency noise radiated by OR equipment (e.g., blood warmers, electrically powered tables and operating microscopes), by eliminating the noise signals seen equally by both amplifier inputs. Differential amplifiers also allows for selective recording of focally recorded, cortically generated, SSEPs by electronically subtracting the widely distributed brainstem signals that are equally detected in both input electrodes. SSEPs are tiny signals, 1 to 2 orders of magnitude smaller than the EEG; typically, responses to several hundred stimuli must be averaged over several minutes to record an SSEP waveform. When the SSEP signal is particularly small, or the electrical environment is noisy, more time is required.

Both cortical and brainstem signals are used for SSEP monitoring. Both provide equivalent information regarding spinal cord integrity, but are affected differently by noise and anesthetic agents. Brainstem SSEP signals are resistant to anesthetic effects, but they are more easily contaminated by electrical noise and interference from muscle activity. They may also be difficult to record in patients with preexisting myelopathies. Cortical SSEPs are less vulnerable to noise contamination but they are more susceptible to attenuation by anesthetic drugs.

30.2.1 Brainstem SSEPs

Brainstem SSEPs can be recorded from any scalp electrode, using a neck electrode as an "inactive" reference. A common misconception is that the neck electrode detects cervical evoked potential signals; indeed, SSEPs recorded using a cervical reference are commonly, but incorrectly, termed "cervical" SSEPs. (A small signal is, in fact, generated by the gray matter of the cervical enlargement following upper extremity stimulation, but its contribution to SSEP monitoring is negligible.) Upper and lower extremity brainstem SSEPs appear quite similar, each consisting of a prominent positivity, reflecting activation of the caudal medial lemniscus, followed by a longer duration negative signal generated in the rostral brainstem (▶ Fig. 30.1). They differ principally in latency following stimulation, reflecting the greater length of sensory pathways from the leg.

30.2.2 Cortical SSEPs

Upper extremity cortical SSEPs (▶ Fig. 30.2) appear as a negative signal detected by an electrode over the contralateral centroparietal scalp, at CP3 or CP4 scalp locations[11] referred to an electrode elsewhere on the scalp to remove noise and subcortically generated SSEP signals. (Throughout this chapter, CP3 and CP4 refer to left and right centroparietal locations, C3 and C4 are slightly anterior to CP3 and CP4, and C1 and C2 are mesial to C3 and C4. CPz is a midline position just posterior to the scalp vertex. Fpz a *frontopolar* scalp location. These positions are defined precisely in the American Clinical Neurophysiology Society electrode nomenclature guideline.[11]) The scalp region where the cortical SSEP is largest can be small, and careful electrode placement is necessary. Several channels, using different

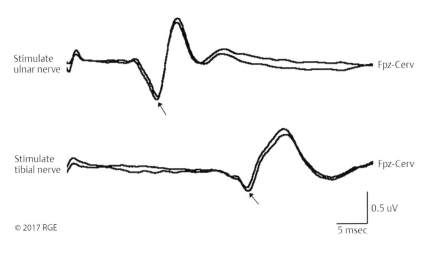

Fig. 30.1 Brainstem SSEPs recorded following ulnar (upper trace) and tibial (lower trace) nerve stimulation. The positive (downward going) peaks denoted by arrows correspond to signals generated in the caudal portion of the medial lemniscus. These are generally the most reliable brainstem SSEP signals for monitoring. Cerv corresponds to a cervical reference electrode.

Stimulate ulnar nerve — Fpz-Cerv

Stimulate tibial nerve — Fpz-Cerv

0.5 uV

5 msec

© 2017 RGE

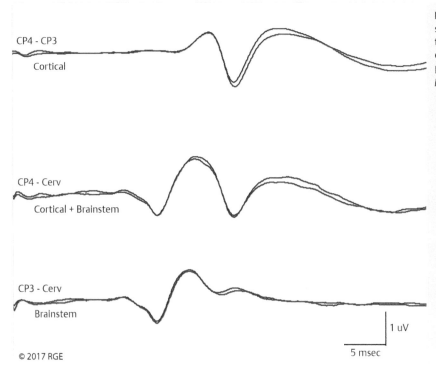

Fig. 30.2 Cortical SSEP to left ulnar nerve stimulation (top trace) is recorded using a "scalp-to-scalp" bipolar derivation CP4 to CP3, to effectively electronically subtract the brainstem potential (CP3-Cerv) from the composite cortical *plus* brainstem potential (CP4-Cerv).

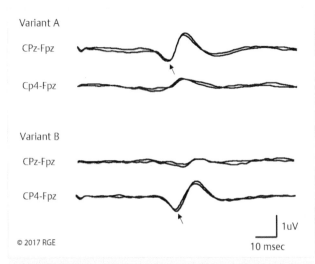

Fig. 30.3 The scalp location of the cortical SSEP to tibial nerve stimulation varies considerably among normal individuals. At one extreme, shown in variant A, a prominent positive signal (*arrow*) is recorded at the vertex, with very little lateral spread. At the other extreme, shown in variant B, a prominent positivity (*arrow*) is recorded over the scalp *ipsilateral* to the stimulated limb, and very little is recorded at the vertex.

electrode pairs, may be used and the channel producing the best recording selected for monitoring.

Lower extremity cortical SSEPs are somewhat more complicated because their scalp topography differs considerably among normal individual. In some patients, lower extremity cortical SSEPs appear as a positivity at the scalp vertex, while in others they consist of a centroparietal positivity *ipsilateral* to

the stimulated leg, accompanied by a contralateral negativity, and very little or nothing recorded from the vertex (▶ Fig. 30.3). In most patients, lower extremity cortical SSEP scalp topography lies somewhere between these two extremes. Accordingly, it is essential that at least two different channels be devoted to detecting lower extremity cortical SSEPs; the channel proving the most robust recording is selected for monitoring.

In addition, when possible, it is helpful to record from electrodes over Erb's point and in the popliteal fossa to detect the SSEP signals distal to the region at risk of surgically related injury. Erb's point and popliteal fossa recordings provide important controls, and help to distinguish loss of SSEPs due to a surgically related cause from loss due to failure of stimulation.

30.2.3 Anesthetic Effects

The halogenated inhalational agents (e.g., isoflurane, sevoflurane, and desflurane) and nitrous oxide attenuate cortical SSEPs.[12,13] Their combined effects are synergistic, that is, SSEP attenuation produced by nitrous oxide along with a halogenated agent is greater than the sum of their effects when used separately.[13,14] Young children and infants can be especially sensitive.[15] Importantly, not only is the degree of SSEP depression dose dependent, but the effect can be nonlinear, so that a small increase in dose can produce a large drop in cortical SSEP amplitude.[16] Moreover, remarkable interpatient variability is encountered (▶ Fig. 30.4). Although most commonly used intravenous agents (i.e., propofol, benzodiazepines, opioids) also have some depressant effects on cortical SSEPs, these are relatively minor.[12,17,18] Dexmedetomidine does not appear to depress cortical SSEPs.[19]

Brainstem SSEPs are essentially unaffected by clinically relevant concentrations of anesthetic agents. Neuromuscular

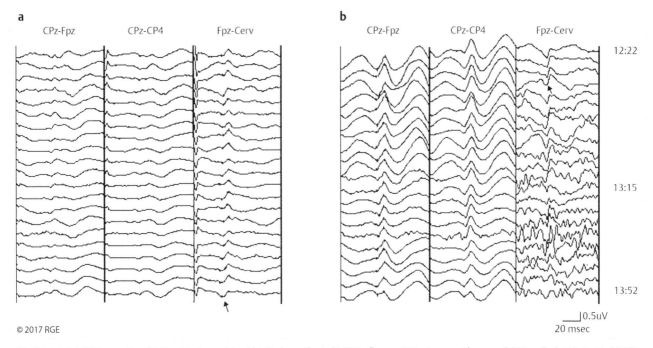

Fig. 30.4 (a,b) SSEPs monitored in 2 patients receiving identical anesthesia (0.5% isoflurane, 50% nitrous oxide, propofol 35 ug/kg/min). Cortical SSEPs (CPz-Fpz and CPz-CP4 channels) are markedly attenuated in patient A, but are well preserved in patient B. Brainstem SSEPs are (arrows in Fpz-Cerv channel) are unaffected in both patients. In patient A, brainstem SSEPs are suitable for monitoring; in patient B, brainstem SSEPs are obscured by muscle artifact after 13:15.

blocking (NMB) agents do not affect the amplitudes or latencies of SSEPs, but they can substantially facilitate SSEP recording by eliminating contamination from electrical interference generated by muscle activity.

30.2.4 Interpretation

The standard "alarm criteria" for SSEP change is a 50% drop in amplitude or a 10% increase in latency compared to baseline.[20] Spinal cord injury most commonly results in loss of SSEP amplitude and deterioration of SSEP waveform morphology, resulting respectively from conduction block and desynchronization of conduction in dorsal column axons. Latency changes are generally less prominent. Since cortical SSEPs are greatly influenced by anesthetic drugs, it is important that baselines be set after stable maintenance anesthesia is achieved, and readjusted following any changes. Further, over hours, cortical SSEPs often gradually increase in latency and decrease in amplitude.[21] This effect, known as "anesthetic fade," must be distinguished from SSEP changes due to clinically significant events. The standard "50/10" warning criteria are empirically based, and best serve as guides, rather than strict thresholds for detection of injury. Further, in practice, trial-to-trial variability and unavoidable contamination by noise and artifact can make 40 and 60% amplitude changes difficult to distinguish meaningfully. A better approach is for the surgeon to be notified when a new, sudden drop in amplitude or deterioration of wave-shape occurs that exceeds that expected based on prior signal variability observed during the case, even if the amplitude change appears less than 50%. This approach can permit more timely alerts and more accurate identification of the cause of SSEP changes.[22]

30.3 Motor Evoked Potentials

MEPs are monitored by stimulating the motor cortex and recording from either the spinal cord or from muscle. A single, brief, transcranial electrical stimulus produces a volley of pyramidal tract activity—a prominent D-wave resulting from *direct* activation of pyramidal cell axons followed by a series of smaller I-waves produced *indirectly* through transsynaptic activation of pyramidal cells by cortical interneurons.[23] A single stimulus is usually insufficient to elicit a response from muscle (M-wave) under general anesthesia. Rather, M-waves are generated using trains of several stimuli, one to several milliseconds apart. Each stimulus in the train produces a D-wave and perhaps several I-waves. Together, they summate temporally at alpha motor neurons in the lumbar and cervical enlargements of the spinal cord, causing the motor neurons to fire and generate an M-wave (▶ Fig. 30.5).[24] M-wave recording can be further enhanced by delivery of two trains, separated by typically 10 or 20 ms. The first train likely acts through segmental and suprasegmental polysynaptic facilitatory mechanisms to reduce postsynaptic membrane polarization, preparing spinal cord alpha motor neurons to more readily reach threshold and fire in response to the second train (▶ Fig. 30.6).[25]

Commonly monitored arm and leg muscles contain several hundred overlapping regions, each 5 to 10 mm in diameter, innervated by a single spinal cord alpha motor neuron. An alpha motor neuron along with the family of muscle fiber it innervates is known as a motor unit. The M-wave is a composite of action potentials generated by activated motor units with muscle fibers close to recording electrodes. An M-wave thus

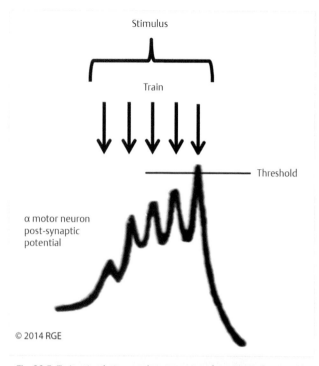

Fig. 30.5 Train stimulation produces a series of propagated corticospinal tract action potentials (D-waves or I-waves). These post-synaptic potentials temporally summate until the alpha motor neurons reach threshold and fires, leading to the generation of an M-wave.

reflects contributions from only a small percentage of the total number of motor units in a given muscle.[26]

30.3.1 M-Wave Motor Evoked Potentials

Subdermal needle or corkscrew electrodes are used for stimulation. Interhemispheric stimulation is typically employed with electrodes placed at, or just anterior to the C3 and C4 scalp locations, or more medially at C1 and C2. The former are generally more effective, but also produce more jaw movement. M-wave MEPs (mMEPs) are maximal on the side contralateral to the anode; electrode polarity is switched to monitor both sides. Alternatively, a midline electrode arrangement may be used, with a vertex anode and frontal cathode. With this arrangement, both legs are stimulated simultaneously, but upper extremity mMEPs are more difficult to obtain.[27,28]

In contrast to SSEPs, which are small and require averaging to resolve, mMEPs are orders of magnitude larger and do not require averaging. However—and also in contrast to SSEPs—mMEPs can be quite variable from one trial to the next. Spontaneous fluctuations in spinal cord motor pool excitability lead to somewhat mercurial behavior of individual motor neurons and correspondingly varying morphologies of the composite M-wave waveform (▶ Fig. 30.7). Further, the small number of motor units contributing the mMEP, each of which fires in an all-or-none manner, leads to nonlinearity in the relationship

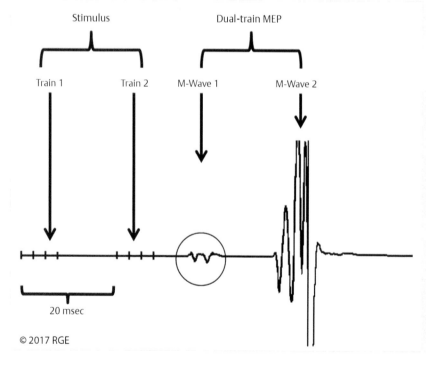

Fig. 30.6 Dual train facilitation of mMEPs. mMEPs are elicited by two stimulus trains, separated typically by 10 to 20 msec. In this example, each train generates an M-wave, but the second is much larger and more complex than the first.

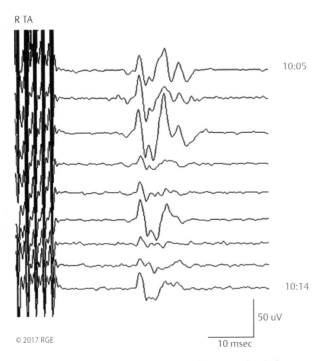

© 2017 RGE

Fig. 30.7 Trial-to-trial variability of mMEPs shown in right tibialis anterior (R TA).

between stimulus intensity and MEP amplitude. When trial to trial variability is pronounced, several mMEP trials are needed to properly assess the overall response.[27,29]

The lateral corticospinal tract is a small, compact, bundle carrying a disproportionately large number of pyramidal axons originating from the correspondingly large sections of the cortical motor homunculus that innervate distal muscles requiring fine control. These muscles produce the most robust and easily elicited mMEPs. For that reason, muscles such as abductor pollicis brevis, first dorsal interosseus and abductor digiti minimi in the upper extremity, and tibial anterior and abductor hallucis in the lower, are routinely monitored. For spinal cord monitoring, they serve as *proxies* for motor function in the monitored limb. Spinal cord injury is often detected sooner by mMEPs than by SSEPs, both because mMEPs are often inherently more sensitive to spinal cord injury, and also because mMEPs require no averaging, thereby permitting immediate feedback to the surgeon. SSEPs, in contrast, require averaging over one or more minutes and thus provide delayed feedback (▶ Fig. 30.8). mMEPs from specific muscles, including anal sphincter and proximal limb muscles, can also be monitored for assessing nerve root function, but as discussed further on, nerve root monitoring using mMEPs is more difficult and can be less reliable than spinal cord monitoring.

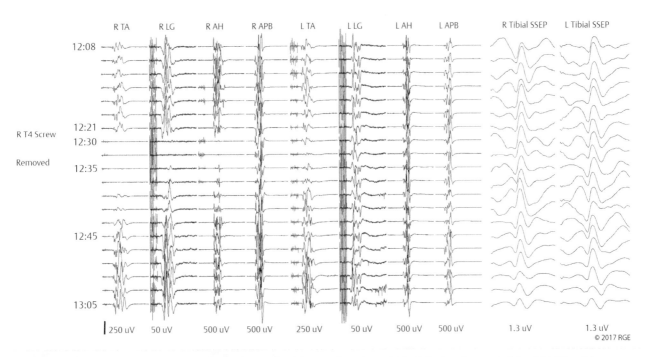

Fig. 30.8 mMEP and SSEP monitoring in a 15-year-old girl with adolescent idiopathic scoliosis. Following placement of the right T4 pedicle screw, mMEPs were lost in right tibialis anterior (R TA), lateral gastrocnemius (R LG), and abductor hallucis (R AH). mMEPs were also attenuated in left tibialis anterior (L TA). mMEPs in abductor pollicis brevis (APB) remain unchanged bilaterally. A medial breech was confirmed on X-ray. Upon removal of the screw, mMEPs quickly returned and regained baseline morphologies after about 10 minutes. Note that no changes were seen in left and right SSEPs, shown respectively in CP4-CPz and CP3-CPz derivations. Sweep durations are 120 msec for MEPs, 100 msec for SSEPs.

30.3.2 D-Wave Motor Evoked Potentials

Stimulating electrodes for D-wave MEP (dMEP) monitoring are the same as for mMEPs. Recording electrodes are placed over the spinal cord, either epidurally or subdurally. In contrast to the rather complex physiology underlying with M-wave generation, dependent on temporal summation and facilitation and requiring one or more stimulus trains, D-waves require only a single transcranial electrical stimulus and are direct measures of corticospinal tract conduction.[29] Since no synapses are involved, D-waves are relatively anesthetic resistant. In contrast to the relatively unstable, nonlinear behavior the mMEPs, dMEPs are very stable. D-wave amplitude reflects the number of pyramidal tract axons activated, and varies linearly with stimulus intensity until plateauing. D-wave amplitude diminishes as the recording site is moved distally, corresponding to the decreased numbers of pyramidal axons in the distal pyramidal tract. D-waves are not readily lateralized and are difficult to record below about T10. They cannot be recorded from the lumbosacral spine and, of course, cannot detect injury to lumbar cord gray matter. D-waves are quickly recorded, and generally require averaging of only a small number of responses to resolve clearly.[27,29]

dMEPs are not monitored routinely during spinal surgery because of difficulty with stable electrode placement and the dependency of D-wave amplitude on electrode position. Changes in electrode position relative to the spinal cord, for example during derotation, can result in spurious changes in recorded D-wave amplitude, leading both to false negative and false positive monitoring results.[30]

D-wave monitoring is useful during intramedullary spinal cord tumor (IMSCT) surgery, where M-wave loss generally precedes loss of D-waves. When loss of M-waves is accompanied by preservation of D-wave amplitude over 50% of baseline, postoperative motor deficits can be expected to be transient. Greater D-wave loss is associated with permanent motor deficits. Accordingly, during IMSCT surgery, D-wave monitoring can allow surgery to proceed past the point of M-wave loss, allowing for more extensive tumor resection (▶ Fig. 30.9).[31,32,33]

30.3.3 Safety Considerations

The major risks of MEP monitoring relate to tongue bite and patient movement. In one series of over 18,000 cases monitored using mMEPs, 25 tongue lacerations were reported, although the authors speculated that additional minor instances of tongue bite might have occurred that went undocumented. Four cases required suturing; the remainder was self-limited. No movement-related injuries occurred. Tongue bite results from strong contractions of temporalis and masseter muscles following transcranial electrical stimulation. Placement of soft bite-blocks (e.g., rolled gauze) to prevent contact between the teeth and the tongue reduces, but does not entirely eliminate, the risk. Patient movement during MEP testing is often unavoidable, although it is often possible to reduce movement by appropriate adjustment of stimulation parameters and stimulating electrode placement. It is essential that MEP stimulation be coordinated with the surgeon so that, for example, surgical instruments are not close to neural structures at the time of stimulation.[34]

Elevated intracranial pressure, skull defects, cerebral lesions, implanted device and a history of epilepsy were initially considered to be relative contraindications to MEP monitoring.[35] However, related complications have not been demonstrated, and at many centers these conditions no longer preclude MEP monitoring.[34,36,37]

MEP stimulation can theoretically produce seizures. Transcranial electrical stimulation has indeed been reported to produce brief afterdischarges (seizure-like EEG discharges),[38] but clinical seizures related to MEP stimulation, if they occur, are very rare. A review of 15,000 published and unpublished cases involving MEP monitoring mentions five seizures, three which appear to be potentially related to MEP stimulation.[35] No seizures were reported in a separate series of 18,862 cases of spine surgery monitored using MEPs at a single institution, including 35 patients with a history of epilepsy. The authors concluded that the risk of seizures triggered by MEP stimulation during spine surgery is negligible.[34] Although employed at some centers, the role of continuous EEG recording during MEP monitoring has not been established.

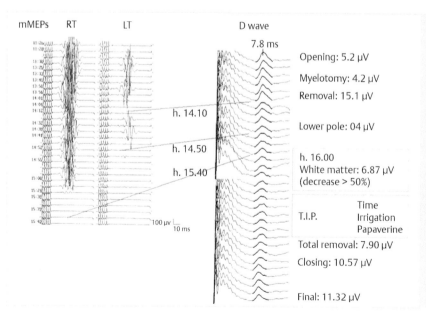

Fig. 30.9 mMEP and dMEP monitoring during removal of a T3-6 ependymoma. mMEPs are shown from right (RT) and left (LT) tibialis anterior muscles. D-Waves were recorded from an epidural catheter electrode inserted below T6. mMEPs were lost on the left at 14:50, and bilaterally at 15:38. D-wave at 15:40 was decreased by 65%, but after surgical pause for about 20 minutes, warm irrigation and local infusion of papaverine, D-wave amplitude increased to over 50% of baseline. Surgery continued with total removal of the tumor. The patient awoke without motor deficits. (Reproduced with permission from Sala F, Lanteri P, Bricolo A. Motor evoked potential monitoring for spinal cord and brain stem surgery. *Adv Tech Stand Neurosurg* 2004;29:133–169, Fig. 15a.)

30.3.4 Anesthesia

mMEP monitoring is affected critically by anesthetic management. M-waves are generally more sensitive than cortical SSEPs to the effects of anesthetic agents, which depress both cortically generated I-waves and spinal cord motor neuron excitability.[39,40] While D-waves are largely unaffected by anesthetic drugs, D-wave monitoring during IMSCT surgery is usually performed in conjunction with M-wave monitoring.[32]

M-waves are particularly sensitive to both the volatile inhalational agent (e.g., isoflurane, sevoflurane, and desflurane) and nitrous oxide.[17,39,41] M-waves are relatively less affected by propofol, although it, too, can suppress M-wave at high doses.[17,42,43]

Total intravenous anesthesia (TIVA), using propofol along with an opioid, is often suggested as the preferred anesthetic regimen for use with in MEP monitoring.[27,32,44] Ketamine and lidocaine may be added to reduce propofol requirements, without significantly affecting M-wave monitoring.[45,46] Dexmedetomidine may be similarly be added, although it does attenuate M-waves at higher doses.[47] High doses of fentanyl, sufentanil and alfentanil can also attenuate M-waves[48]; remifentanil has little affect.[49]

Although TIVA is often recommended for use in conjunction with mMEP monitoring, many anesthesiologists prefer to use balanced anesthesia, for example, a lower dose of propofol along with a low concentration of a volatile inhalational agent, for reasons including concern for delayed emergence, opioid tolerance and the possibility of accidental awareness.[50] A recent retrospective study of 156 patients receiving either TIVA (propofol plus opioid) or balanced anesthesia (1/2 MAC sevoflurane along with a lower dose of propofol or opioid) found that although MEPs were unobtainable in a small number of patients receiving sevoflurane, in the remainder there was no difference in M-wave amplitudes or trial-to-trial variability between the two groups.[16]

mMEPs can be remarkably sensitive to changes in anesthetic doses. It is common for a bolus of propofol, for example, to abolish MEPs transiently. Although opioids generally have minimal effect on M-waves, a large bolus of fentanyl, for example, can have a similar effect. For that reason, stable anesthesia is ideal, and changes must be communicated and correlated with monitoring findings. Changes are best avoided at times when monitoring is critical.

NMB agents are generally avoided during MEP monitoring. Partial NMB can be useful, however, for reducing patient movement, improving SSEP quality, and possibly reducing the severity and frequency of tongue bite injuries. In neurologically normal patients, MEP monitoring has been successfully performed with two to four twitches on train-of-four (TOF) testing.[51,52] Partial neuromuscular blockade, may, however increase mMEP trail-to-trial variability, and be incompatible with mMEP monitoring in neurologically abnormal patients.[34,51] In our experience, a very low dose vecuronium infusion, titrated to produce three to four twitches on TOF testing, can substantially improve SSEP signals (especially brainstem signals), while not interfering with mMEP recording. If employed, it is essential to monitor and to control carefully the degree of blockade.[34,51,53] Boluses of NMB agents should be avoided, as even a small bolus can transiently attenuate or abolish M-waves.

30.3.5 Interpretation

Interpretation of mMEPs is somewhat more complex than interpretation of SSEPs, and there is no firm agreement regarding alarm criteria. Proposed criteria include "presence-or-absence" of responses, various percent drops in amplitude, decreases in waveform duration and complexity, and increase in required stimulation intensity.[54] The difficulty in establishing firm criteria relates both the nature of the M-wave itself, that is, a composite of asynchronous actions potentials recorded from a small number of motor units in varying proximity to the recording electrodes, as well as, the at times pronounced, trial-to-trial variability of M-waves produced by identical sequential stimuli.

While commonly used, the "presence-or-absence" criteria suffers from the limitation that, without recording D-waves, the severity of the injury is impossible to gauge once M-waves are lost. Accordingly, it seems prudent that the surgeon be notified earlier, before the occurrence of potentially catastrophic injury. A 50% amplitude alarm criteria would likely result in excessive false positives. The American Clinical Neurophysiology society therefore recognizes 75 to 90% amplitude drop a more appropriate alarm threshold.[37]

In practice, since deterioration of an MEP reflects dropout of motor units contributing to the aggregate M-wave waveform, amplitude loss is usually accompanied by less easily quantifiable, but readily recognizable changes, including loss of waveform complexity and shortening of aggregate waveform duration. Occasionally, however, there can be prominent loss of waveform complexity, with only a single, simple high amplitude component remaining perhaps reflecting activity in a single motor unit proximate to the recording electrode. MEP interpretation therefore optimally entails assessment of waveform morphology, including but not limited to amplitude, and notification of the surgeon when the appearance of recorded waveform differs substantially from those previously observed, after consideration of baseline trial-to-trial variability. The aforementioned 75 to 90% amplitude threshold serves as a useful guide.

As discussed earlier, distal muscles, in particular abductor pollicis brevis, first dorsal interosseus, tibial anterior and abductor hallucis, are commonly monitored as proxies for pyramidal tract function during spinal cord monitoring. They are used because they generally exhibit the most robust, easily elicited M-wave responses. For thoracic surgery, upper extremity muscles are recorded as controls, affected by systemic and anesthetic factors, but outside of the region at risk for surgically related injury. In the author's experience, it is often useful to include other "higher-threshold" lower extremity muscle as well, as M-waves from these muscles are commonly lost first, providing early warning of compromise.

Since MEPs are performed intermittently, it is important that frequency and timing of MEP testing be adequate to detect spinal cord injury in a timely manner. Additionally, like SSEPs, mMEP often exhibit anesthetic fade. Deterioration of mMEPs over time, despite constant anesthesia, can be pronounced, for reasons perhaps related to underlying complex physiology and nonlinearities of anesthetic effects. This, along with the inherent trial-to-trial variability of M-wave responses, makes it important the mMEPS be measured at sufficiently frequent intervals to recognize expected, noninjury related changes in the MEP "baseline" over time, and to properly distinguish these from changes due to surgically related events.

When surgery extends above or below the thoracic spine, it is important to consider that M-wave loss may reflect *nerve root* injury rather than spinal cord injury. Use of MEPs for assessment of nerve root function is more difficult and less reliable than for assessment of spinal cord function. It is more heavily reliant on trial-to-trial consistency of responses from single muscles, and is limited by multi-radicular innervation of individual muscles that can limit the likelihood of detecting the loss of input from a single root.[55] These constraints notwithstanding, MEPs can be useful for detecting of nerve root injury (▶ Fig. 30.10), and the possibility of root injury should be considered in the appropriate settings.

During IMSCT surgery, if both mMEPs and dMEPs are monitored, surgery may progress past the loss of mMEPs provided that D-wave amplitude loss is less than 50%. Under such circumstances, while a post-operative motor deficit is likely, recovery within weeks is expected.[32]

30.4 Spontaneous Electromyography

Spontaneous, or "free-run," electromyography (EMG) monitoring is employed routinely during lumbar and cervical surgeries for the purpose of detecting nerve root irritation and injury. Characteristic "neurotonic" EMG discharges are produced in innervated muscles by mechanical impact to nerve or nerve root, and serve as real-time indicators of potential nerve injury. While perhaps less well recognized, mechanical injury to thoracic spinal cord can produce similarly appearing suprasegmentally-generated EMG discharges (SEDs) in lower extremity muscles. In one series, "severe" SEDs, defined as trains lasting over one half second, with varying discharge frequencies > 5 Hz, commonly preceded loss of MEPs in cases where injury was attributable to mechanical impact rather than other causes (e.g., hypoperfusion).[56] Since free-run EMG is monitored continually in real time, monitoring for SEDs during thoracic spine and cord surgery can serve a useful complement to MEP monitoring, which necessarily is intermittent. Anesthetic requirements, and concerns related to NMB agents, are identical to those for MEP monitoring, since generation of SEDs relies on the function of both alpha motor neurons in the lumbar enlargement and on the integrity of the neuromuscular junction.

30.5 Duration of Monitoring

In the past, it was common practice for monitoring to focus on "critical periods," for example the 20 minutes following correction of a spinal deformity. It is now recognized that, particularly in the case of spinal deformity surgery, cord injury with loss of monitored signals can occur at any point during the surgery,

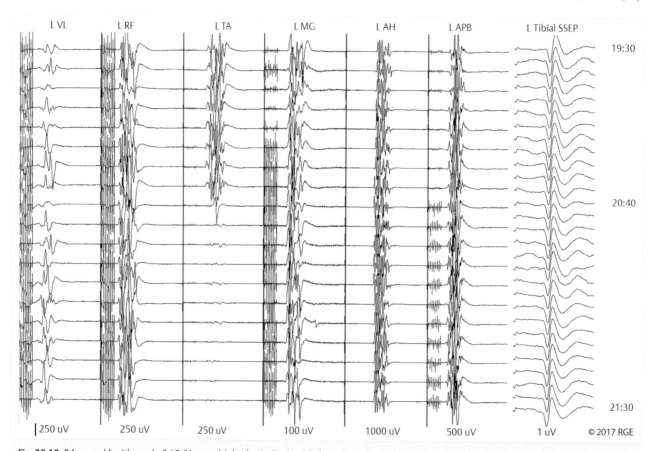

Fig. 30.10 54-year-old with grade 3 L5-S1 spondylolesthesis. During L5 decompression, mMEPs are lost in left tibials anterior (LTA). mMEPs in other muscles remain unchanged, as do SSEPs (CP4–CPz). The patient awoke with a left foot drop that recovered substantially over one month's time. Sweep durations are 120 msec for MEPs, 100 msec for SSEPs.

from positioning through closing. Accordingly, it is often appropriate that monitoring continue throughout the entire procedures, including during closure.[57]

30.6 Example Case

▸ Fig. 30.11a to ▸ Fig. 30.11i show IOMN "screen captures" at multiple times during scoliosis surgery in a 12-year-old girl, and depict serial changes in MEPs and SSEP during several attempts at correction. The procedure was performed using TIVA, with propofol and fentanyl, along with partial neuromuscular blockade titrated to produce 3 twitches on TOF testing.

At baseline (▸ Fig. 30.11a, 9:56), well-formed brainstem (*arrow*) and cortical (*asterisk*) SSEPs are present, along with MEPs.

Following correction and placement of the second rod (▸ Fig. 30.11b, 16:05), SSEPs remain stable, but left lower extremity MEPs are lost. MEPs are lost as well from a single muscle on the right lower extremity (vastus lateralis). As discussed earlier, recording from multiple muscles for spinal cord monitoring not only provides redundancy in case one recording channel fails for technical reasons, but higher threshold, more

difficult to stimulate muscles, are often lost first, providing an early warning of deterioration. Five minutes later (▸ Fig. 30.11c, 16:10) rods have been removed. MEPs are now absent bilaterally, but SSEPs remain unchanged from baseline.

Only after another several minutes (▸ Fig. 30.11d, 16:13) do SSEPs become attenuated. MEPs remain absent. MEPs generally detect spinal cord compromise quicker than SSEPs, both because they are more sensitive to cord injury, and because more time is required for the SSEP averaging process.

Within several minutes (▸ Fig. 30.11e, 16:21) both MEPs and SSEPs have returned. Three superimposed, sequentially recorded, SSEP tracing are shown; the first acquired tracing (*arrows*) shows responses that are notably smaller than the subsequent two recordings.

Following reinsertion of rods, reshaped to achieve less correction, MEPs are again lost bilaterally and SSEPs remain unchanged (▸ Fig. 30.11f, 16:49). With rod removal, MEPs return (▸ Fig. 30.11g, 17:03). On the left, improvement of the SSEP is seen over time, with the first of three superimposed traces showing the smallest response (*arrows*, cortical SSEP; *asterisk*, brainstem SSEP).

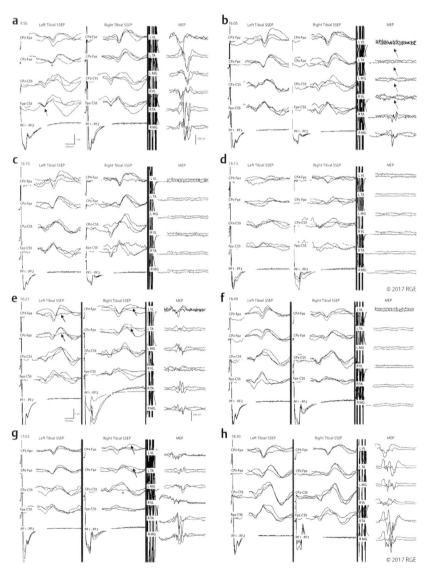

Fig. 30.11 (a–h) A series of "screen captures" during posterior instrumentation for correction of scoliosis surgery in a 12-year-old girl (see text for details). Each figure shows three superimposed sets of tibial SSEP and two sets of lower extremity mMEPS from vastus lateralis (VL), tibialis anterior (TA) and medial gastrocnemius (LG) muscles. Upper extremity controls (ulnar SSEPs and abductor pollicis brevis MEPs) are not shown, but remained unchanged during the case. The SC5 electrode is positioned over the fifth cervical vertebra; PF1 and PF2 refer to electrodes in the popliteal fossa of the stimulated leg.

Finally, rods are adjusted to produce still less correction and reinserted. MEPs and SEP remain stable (▶ Fig. 30.11h). The patient awoke with intact spinal cord function.

References

[1] Nash CL, Jr, Lorig RA, Schatzinger LA, Brown RH. Spinal cord monitoring during operative treatment of the spine. Clin Orthop Relat Res. 1977(126):100–105

[2] Vauzelle C, Stagnara P, Jouvinroux P. Functional monitoring of spinal cord activity during spinal surgery. Clin Orthop Relat Res. 1973(93):173–178

[3] Forbes HJ, Allen PW, Waller CS, et al. Spinal cord monitoring in scoliosis surgery. Experience with 1168 cases. J Bone Joint Surg Br. 1991; 73(3):487–491

[4] Nuwer MR, Dawson EG, Carlson LG, Kanim LE, Sherman JE. Somatosensory evoked potential spinal cord monitoring reduces neurologic deficits after scoliosis surgery: results of a large multicenter survey. Electroencephalogr Clin Neurophysiol. 1995; 96(1):6–11

[5] Deecke L, Tator CH. Neurophysiological assessment of afferent and efferent conduction in the injured spinal cord of monkeys. J Neurosurg. 1973; 39(1):65–74

[6] Baskin DS, Simpson RK, Jr. Corticomotor and somatosensory evoked potential evaluation of acute spinal cord injury in the rat. Neurosurgery. 1987; 20(6):871–877

[7] Shiau JS, Zappulla RA, Nieves J. The effect of graded spinal cord injury on the extrapyramidal and pyramidal motor evoked potentials of the rat. Neurosurgery. 1992; 30(1):76–84

[8] Machida M, Weinstein SL, Imamura Y, et al. Compound muscle action potentials and spinal evoked potentials in experimental spine maneuver. Spine. 1989; 14(7):687–691

[9] Ben-David B, Haller G, Taylor P. Anterior spinal fusion complicated by paraplegia. A case report of a false-negative somatosensory-evoked potential. Spine. 1987; 12(6):536–539

[10] Merton PA, Morton HB. Stimulation of the cerebral cortex in the intact human subject. Nature. 1980; 285(5762):227

[11] Acharya JN, Hani A, Cheek J, Thirumala P, Tsuchida TN. American Clinical Neurophysiology Society Guideline 2: Guidelines for Standard Electrode Position Nomenclature. J Clin Neurophysiol. 2016; 33(4):308–311

[12] Sloan TB, Heyer EJ. Anesthesia for intraoperative neurophysiologic monitoring of the spinal cord. J Clin Neurophysiol. 2002; 19(5):430–443

[13] Clapcich AJ, Emerson RG, Roye DP, Jr, et al. The effects of propofol, small-dose isoflurane, and nitrous oxide on cortical somatosensory evoked potential and bispectral index monitoring in adolescents undergoing spinal fusion. Anesth Analg. 2004; 99(5):1334–1340

[14] Sloan T, Sloan H, Rogers J. Nitrous oxide and isoflurane are synergistic with respect to amplitude and latency effects on sensory evoked potentials. J Clin Monit Comput. 2010; 24(2):113–123

[15] Harper CM, Nelson KR. Intraoperative electrophysiological monitoring in children. J Clin Neurophysiol. 1992; 9(3):342–356

[16] Sloan TB, Toleikis JR, Toleikis SC, Koht A. Intraoperative neurophysiological monitoring during spine surgery with total intravenous anesthesia or balanced anesthesia with 3% desflurane. J Clin Monit Comput. 2015; 29(1):77–85

[17] Chen Z. The effects of isoflurane and propofol on intraoperative neurophysiological monitoring during spinal surgery. J Clin Monit Comput. 2004; 18(4):303–308

[18] Kalkman CJ, Leyssius AT, Bovill JG. Influence of high-dose opioid anesthesia on posterior tibial nerve somatosensory cortical evoked potentials: effects of fentanyl, sufentanil, and alfentanil. J Cardiothorac Anesth. 1988; 2(6):758–764

[19] Tobias JD, Goble TJ, Bates G, Anderson JT, Hoernschemeyer DG. Effects of dexmedetomidine on intraoperative motor and somatosensory evoked potential monitoring during spinal surgery in adolescents. Paediatr Anaesth. 2008; 18(11):1082–1088

[20] Society ACN. Guideline 11B: Recommended standards for intraoperative monitoring of somatosensory evoked potentials. ACNS. Available at: http://www.acns.org/pdf/guidelines/Guideline-11B.pdf. Accessed 6/1/2017

[21] Kalkman CJ, ten Brink SA, Been HD, Bovill JG. Variability of somatosensory cortical evoked potentials during spinal surgery. Effects of anesthetic technique and high-pass digital filtering. Spine. 1991; 16(8):924–929

[22] Moller AR. Intraoperative Neurophysiologic Monitoring. 2 ed. Totowa, NJ: Humana Press; 2006:13–15

[23] Amassian VE, Stewart M, Quirk GJ, Rosenthal JL. Physiological basis of motor effects of a transient stimulus to cerebral cortex. Neurosurgery. 1987; 20(1):74–93

[24] Jones SJ, Harrison R, Koh KF, Mendoza N, Crockard HA. Motor evoked potential monitoring during spinal surgery: responses of distal limb muscles to transcranial cortical stimulation with pulse trains. Electroencephalogr Clin Neurophysiol. 1996; 100(5):375–383

[25] Journée HL, Polak HE, De Kleuver M. Conditioning stimulation techniques for enhancement of transcranially elicited evoked motor responses. Neurophysiol Clin. 2007; 37(6):423–430

[26] Macdonald DB, Stigsby B, Al Homoud I, Abalkhail T, Mokeem A. Utility of motor evoked potentials for intraoperative nerve root monitoring. J Clin Neurophysiol. 2012; 29(2):118–125

[27] Macdonald DB. Intraoperative motor evoked potential monitoring: overview and update. J Clin Monit Comput. 2006; 20(5):347–377

[28] Szelényi A, Kothbauer KF, Deletis V. Transcranial electric stimulation for intraoperative motor evoked potential monitoring: Stimulation parameters and electrode montages. Clin Neurophysiol. 2007; 118(7):1586–1595

[29] Amassian VE. Animal and human motor system neurophysiology related to intraoperative monitoring. In: Deletis V, Shils J, eds. Neurophysiology in neurosurgery. San Diego, CA: Academic Press; 2002:3–23

[30] Ulkatan S, Neuwirth M, Bitan F, Minardi C, Kokoszka A, Deletis V. Monitoring of scoliosis surgery with epidurally recorded motor evoked potentials (D wave) revealed false results. Clin Neurophysiol. 2006; 117(9):2093–2101

[31] Sala F, Lanteri P, Bricolo A. Motor evoked potential monitoring for spinal cord and brain stem surgery. Adv Tech Stand Neurosurg. 2004; 29:133–169

[32] Sala F, Palandri G, Basso E, et al. Motor evoked potential monitoring improves outcome after surgery for intramedullary spinal cord tumors: a historical control study. Neurosurgery. 2006; 58(6):1129–1143, discussion 1129–1143

[33] Deletis V, Sala F. Intraoperative neurophysiological monitoring of the spinal cord during spinal cord and spine surgery: a review focus on the corticospinal tracts. Clin Neurophysiol. 2008; 119(2):248–264

[34] Schwartz DM, Sestokas AK, Dormans JP, et al. Transcranial electric motor evoked potential monitoring during spine surgery: is it safe? Spine. 2011; 36(13):1046–1049

[35] MacDonald DB. Safety of intraoperative transcranial electrical stimulation motor evoked potential monitoring. J Clin Neurophysiol. 2002; 19(5):416–429

[36] MacDonald DB, Deletis V. Safety issues during surgical monitoring. In: Nuwer MR, ed. Handbook of Clinical Neurophysiology. Amsterdam: Elsevier; 2008:882–898

[37] Legatt AD, Emerson RG, Epstein CM, et al. ACNS guideline: transcranial electrical stimulation motor evoked potential monitoring. J Clin Neurophysiol. 2016; 33(1):42–50

[38] Kobylarz EJ, Bilsky MH, Sandhu SK, Avila EA, Victor JD. Monitoring of electroencephalography during transcranial electrical motor evoked potentials. Epilepsia. 2005; 46 Suppl. 8:309–310

[39] Zentner J, Albrecht T, Heuser D. Influence of halothane, enflurane, and isoflurane on motor evoked potentials. Neurosurgery. 1992; 31(2):298–305

[40] Burke D, Hicks R, Stephen J, Woodforth I, Crawford M. Assessment of corticospinal and somatosensory conduction simultaneously during scoliosis surgery. Electroencephalogr Clin Neurophysiol. 1992; 85(6):388–396

[41] Zentner J, Ebner A. Nitrous oxide suppresses the electromyographic response evoked by electrical stimulation of the motor cortex. Neurosurgery. 1989; 24(1):60–62

[42] Scheufler KM, Reinacher PC, Blumrich W, Zentner J, Priebe HJ. The modifying effects of stimulation pattern and propofol plasma concentration on motor-evoked potentials. Anesth Analg. 2005; 100(2):440–447

[43] Nathan N, Tabaraud F, Lacroix F, et al. Influence of propofol concentrations on multipulse transcranial motor evoked potentials. Br J Anaesth. 2003; 91(4):493–497

[44] Sutter M, Eggspuehler A, Muller A, Dvorak J. Multimodal intraoperative monitoring: an overview and proposal of methodology based on 1,017 cases. Eur Spine J. 2007; 16 Suppl 2:S153–S161

[45] Zaarour C, Engelhardt T, Strantzas S, Pehora C, Lewis S, Crawford MW. Effect of low-dose ketamine on voltage requirement for transcranial electrical motor evoked potentials in children. Spine. 2007; 32(22):E627–E630

[46] Sloan TB, Mongan P, Lyda C, Koht A. Lidocaine infusion adjunct to total intravenous anesthesia reduces the total dose of propofol during intraoperative neurophysiological monitoring. J Clin Monit Comput. 2014; 28(2):139–147

[47] Mahmoud M, Sadhasivam S, Salisbury S, et al. Susceptibility of transcranial electric motor-evoked potentials to varying targeted blood levels of dexmedetomidine during spine surgery. Anesthesiology. 2010; 112(6):1364–1373

[48] Thees C, Scheufler KM, Nadstawek J, et al. Influence of fentanyl, alfentanil, and sufentanil on motor evoked potentials. J Neurosurg Anesthesiol. 1999; 11 (2):112–118

[49] Scheufler KM, Zentner J. Total intravenous anesthesia for intraoperative monitoring of the motor pathways: an integral view combining clinical and experimental data. J Neurosurg. 2002; 96(3):571–579

[50] Padit J, Cook T. Accidental Awareness During General Anesthesia in the United Kingdom and Ireland. 2014. Available at: http://www.nationalaudit-projects.org.uk/NAP5report. Accessed April 28, 2017

[51] Sloan TB. Muscle relaxant use during intraoperative neurophysiologic monitoring. J Clin Monit Comput. 2013; 27(1):35–46

[52] Adams DC, Emerson RG, Heyer EJ, et al. Monitoring of intraoperative motor-evoked potentials under conditions of controlled neuromuscular blockade. Anesth Analg. 1993; 77(5):913–918

[53] Sloan T. Anesthesia and intraoperative neurophysiological monitoring in children. Childs Nerv Syst. 2010; 26(2):227–235

[54] Langeloo DD, Journée HL, de Kleuver M, Grotenhuis JA. Criteria for transcranial electrical motor evoked potential monitoring during spinal deformity surgery: a review and discussion of the literature. Neurophysiol Clin. 2007; 37 (6):431–439

[55] Lyon R, Gibson A, Burch S, Lieberman J. Increases in voltage may produce false-negatives when using transcranial motor evoked potentials to detect an isolated nerve root injury. J Clin Monit Comput. 2010; 24(6):441–448

[56] Skinner SA, Transfeldt EE, Mehbod AA, Mullan JC, Perra JH. Electromyography detects mechanically-induced suprasegmental spinal motor tract injury: review of decompression at spinal cord level. Clin Neurophysiol. 2009; 120(4):754–764

[57] Kamerlink JR, Errico T, Xavier S, et al. Major intraoperative neurologic monitoring deficits in consecutive pediatric and adult spinal deformity patients at one institution. Spine. 2010; 35(2):240–245

31 Neuronavigation for Complex Thoracic Spine Surgery

Ana Luís, Rodrigo Navarro-Ramirez, Jonathan Nakhla, Christoph Wipplinger, and Roger Härtl

Abstract

The management of spinal pathology was greatly influenced by the advent of spinal instrumentation, which allowed for treatment of more complex spinal disorders, while maintaining or restoring stability and alignment. Regardless of the complexity of the operation, anatomical region, level of training and comfort level of the individual surgeon, image navigation techniques in spinal procedures can be an asset in addition to a thorough understanding of the anatomy and the surgical technique. Their use is associated with: higher accuracy for instrumentation placement (which is particularly important for complex thoracic spine surgery where there is a much lower margin of error because of spinal anatomy and the surrounding structures) and avoidance of wrong-level surgery. Image navigation techniques are particularly relevant in procedures that lack open visualization, such as in minimally invasive spinal surgery.

Keywords: navigation, thoracic spine surgery, screw accuracy

Clinical Pearls

- The use of neuronavigation in the thoracic spine is associated with higher accuracy for instrumentation placement.
- Because of the spinal anatomy, thoracic instrumentation has a much lower margin of error.
- Despite its advantages, intraoperative navigation does not substitute for the need to know the anatomy.
- Especially in minimally invasive spinal surgery where anatomical landmarks are limited, it is critical to verify anatomical landmarks with navigation at every crucial step (e.g., screw placement and drill utilization).
- Neuronavigation is a practical and reliable tool and is especially useful for intraoperative localization of pathologies, for example, on thoracic spine tumors.

31.1 Introduction

The advent of spinal instrumentation and the development and use of screw-based fixation devices greatly influenced the management of spinal disorders, allowing for treatment of more complex spinal pathology while maintaining or restoring spinal stability and alignment.[1,2,3]

As spinal procedures progressed and became more complex, it became crucial to minimize the injuries associated with incorrectly positioned implants and screws that, when misplaced can cause spinal, nerve roots and vascular injuries as well as dural tears with cerebrospinal fluid leakage.[2,3]

Pedicle screw-based instrumentation remains one of the strongest posterior fixation techniques for the thoracolumbar spine and it is the standard procedure for treatment of thoracic spine disease. By traversing all three columns of the vertebrae, pedicle screws can rigidly stabilize both the ventral and dorsal aspects of the spine and the rigidity of pedicle fixation allows for the incorporation of fewer normal motion segments to achieve stabilization of an abnormal level. Furthermore, pedicle screw fixation does not require intact dorsal elements and so it can be used after a laminectomy or traumatic disruption of laminae, spinous processes and/or facets.[4]

However, in comparison with the lumbar spine, in the thoracic spine there is admittedly a much lower margin of error, as errant screws are capable of injuring the spinal cord and other structures intimately related to the vertebrae, including the thoracic pleura, esophagus and intercostal and segmental vessels. Other structures within the thoracic cavity at potential risk include the thoracic duct, azygous vein, inferior vena cava, and aorta.

Moreover, wide variations in diameters and angles of thoracic pedicles, depending on the thoracic level, have been documented in anatomical studies. Therefore, placement of thoracic pedicle screws can be even more challenging, as pedicle angles and attachment to the vertebrae tends to be more anatomically varied in the thoracic spine, especially at the middle thoracic levels, which have the narrowest pedicles and a closer proximity between the medial pedicle wall and the spinal cord. Minor deviations in the starting point or angulation can result in marked malpositioning of the screw.[5] The smallest pedicle is typically found at T4 and its diameter can be as small as 4.5 mm and the largest pedicle is usually T11 or T12, with about 8 mm diameter.[6,7] The risk of malpositioned screws is even higher in spinal deformities where vertebral anatomy can vary even more widely.[8,9]

The classical technique for pedicle screw insertion is the "free-hand" pedicle screw insertion and is essentially a blind technique where adequate screw placement depends on correct identification of anatomical landmarks, surgeon experience, and reproducible technique.[10]

As such, early on, the learning curve associated with usage of this technique became apparent, leading to increased surgeon usage of image-assisted techniques. The technology used to acquire imaging for intraoperative navigation has evolved from the discovery of X-rays in the late 19th century to the highly sophisticated intraoperative computed tomography (CT)-based navigation tools used today.[3,11,12] Before the advent of spinal image guidance, surgeons relied on their knowledge of anatomy, complemented with the preoperatively image examinations and intraoperative imaging such as serial radiographs and later on fluoroscopy. Although plain radiography is still used by some surgeons to assist localizing the skin incision, determining the proper anatomical level, and confirming satisfactory position of the spinal implants prior to closure. Unfortunately, conventional radiography processing is time consuming and only static images can be acquired. Therefore, instantaneous positional information regarding instrument position within the surgical field cannot be obtained.

Fluoroscopy, namely C-arm fluoroscopy, addressed some of the disadvantages of plain radiography. Hence, spine surgeons started to use this tool as their primary mean of intraoperative navigation. This technique allows real-time imaging when used continuously (e.g., to obtain immediate updates of an instrument's position), or it can be used to acquire multiple static images in succession.[13] One of its main shortcomings is the potential for significant occupational radiation exposure, especially when continuous fluoroscopy is used.[14,15] The surgeon is at particular risk due to their close proximity to the fluoroscope and the patterns of radiation scatter. Also, when using a single fluoroscope, images can only be obtained in a single plane at a time. When simultaneous biplanar fluoroscopy is needed, two independent C-arms are required for intraoperative navigation, which can create some create ergonomic constraints that hinder access to the surgical field and potential for breeches in sterility.[13] Furthermore, this technique provides only two-dimensional imaging of complex three-dimensional structures, leaving to the surgeon extrapolate the third dimension based on his/her interpretation of the images and the knowledge of pertinent surgical anatomy.[12] This conventional intraoperative imaging cannot provide the axial plane, which is for most screw procedures, a critical plane to confirm precise screw placement.[12] Fluoroscopy is used so often during pedicle screw placement that it has been referred to as the "conventional" method, perhaps reflecting its almost expected usage when attempting to employ free-hand techniques.

The conventional techniques used for pedicle screw insertion are based on anatomical landmarks either without image guidance ("free-hand technique") or with fluoroscopic guidance in a lateral, anterior–posterior, or oblique ventrodorsal projection.[16]

In order to help the surgeon obtain optimal thoracic screw placement, different entry points, screws trajectories, and insertion techniques have been described.[7,8,17,18,19,20,21,22] However, those are not discussed in this chapter, as it focuses on the landmarks relevant to applying navigation techniques.

In vivo and in vitro studies, in which free-hand technique and fluoroscopy-guided techniques have been used, report thoracic pedicle misplacement rates, from 3 to 55%.[8,23] Even experienced surgeons misdirect the screws medially in 5% and inferolaterally in 15% of the cases, using fluoroscopic imaging.[5]

The accuracy is achieved by surgeon's expertise and familiarity with the surgical anatomy and is greatly facilitated through intraoperative imaging. This is especially pertinent when the surgeon needs to be precisely oriented to that part of the spinal anatomy that is not exposed in the surgical field. This is the case when using minimally invasive spinal surgery (MISS) procedures, when the visualization based on anatomical reference points that can be used as a basis for orientation and implant placement is not available.[2,12,24]

Computer-assisted spine surgery (CAS) is a computer-based technology that links spine image, acquired by conventional techniques, such as fluoroscopy and CT, with an accurate representation of intraoperative anatomy.[25,26] This gives the surgeon the ability to manipulate multiplanar CT or fluoroscopic images during the surgical procedure in order to gain a greater degree of orientation to the nonvisualized spinal anatomy and, therefore enhancing the accuracy of spine surgery, of upmost importance during spinal instrumentations. It can also minimize the surgical team's exposure to radiation.

Navigation has been questioned in terms of accuracy, namely concerning pedicle screw insertion, and it has shown to attain high accuracy (> 95–99%)[23,27,28,29,30,31,32,33,34,35,36] in comparison

with free-hand and/or fluoroscopy-based techniques and a lower rate of screw-related complications.[29,30] Especially the latest navigation technology set-ups seem to have virtually eliminated the need for reoperation for screw malposition, as they allow for intraoperative confirmation of implant positioning.[37] Furthermore, the navigation techniques allows for decreased radiation exposure for the surgical team and operating room (OR) staff.[38,39]

31.1.1 Historical Perspective on Image-guided Spinal Navigation

The image-guided spinal navigation, or CAS, evolved from the principles of stereotaxic, which consists in localizing a specific point in space through the use of three-dimensional coordinates combined with optoelectronic position sensing techniques.[2,11,40] The technology behind this was initially developed for intracranial neurosurgical procedures. At the beginning, stereotaxic demanded the use of an external frame attached to the patient's head and even so, the procedures were associated with a certain degree of inaccuracy, mainly due to the movement of brain structures during retraction and resection of brain tissue (*brain shift*).[11] Applying the same principles to spinal surgeries was more challenging both because an external frame was unpractical and of the lack of anatomical constancy in a moving spine. Furthermore, the skin and underlying soft tissue are mobile relative to the spinal column and it was therefore necessary to use bony landmarks for registration, what requires an extensive and meticulous surgical exposure.[41]

Even though the use of intraoperative navigation was not initially compatible with spinal anatomy, there was great demand for this technology among spine surgeons who felt that navigation would be especially useful in situations where spinal implants were placed without direct visualization, such as placement of pedicle screws.[41]

With the evolution of computer-based technologies in the 1990s appeared the frameless navigation technology, raising the possibility of using stereotaxic on other different procedures, namely, spinal navigation.[11] Brodwater and Roberts, in 1993,[42] published the first attempted transition from intracranial to spinal surgery, using an image-guided microscope and skin surface fiducial markers for registration. However, these markers were subject to movement in reference to the underlying spinal anatomy, resulting in significant navigation inaccuracy.[12]

Kalfas et al[25,26] and Nolte et al[40,43] demonstrated feasibility of using navigational technology to improve accuracy of lumbar pedicle screws insertion and Foley et al[44] described the use of easily distinguishable anatomical landmarks on the posterior aspect of the spine as fiducial points, in conjunction with a dynamic reference array that was fixed to the spine, partially solving the issue of inaccuracy. With the evolution of spinal navigation, the necessity of intraoperative imaging became increasingly important to provide accurate registration of the spine to the navigation system. And, the most recent intraoperative CT-based image-guided (CT) navigation has improved, including localization, real-time navigation, phantom trajectory prediction, and better definition of bony and soft tissues.[28,45,46]

31.1.2 Principals of Image-guided Spinal Navigation

The initial step in integrating CAS with any type of spinal procedure is the acquisition of multiple successive images of the region of interest, a process that may be accomplished with either fluoroscopy or CT.[47] The CAS or image guidance technology is available in a variety of setups which may be differentiated according to the manner in which these images are captured, processed, and presented to the surgeon.[47] Usually, the elements that compose a navigation system are: (1) a system for image acquisition that allows tracking of specialized instruments in relation to a single or multiple reference points attached to suitable anatomical landmarks and (2) a computer workstation that reconfigures this data set into a series of multiplanar images that are displayed on a monitor along with the relative position of any instrumentation within the operative field.[47]

Image Acquisition

Usually, the elements that allow image acquisition consist of a two-camera optical localizer that interfaces with the image-processing computer workstation through emission of infrared light to the operative field or an electromagnetic registration system. Passive reflective spheres placed in a hand-held navigation tool serve as the connection between the surgeon and the computer workstation. These passive reflectors can also be attached to the traditional surgical instruments like the drill guide, a tap, or a pedicle screwdriver. In order to accurately calculate the position of the instruments in the surgical field and the anatomical points, where the tip of the instruments is resting, the spacing and positioning of the passive reflectors on each navigational probe or customized trackable surgical instrument are programmed into the computer workstation. In fact, after the infrared light is transmitted toward the operative field and is reflected to the optical localizer by the passive reflectors, the information is conveyed to the computer workstation, allowing the calculation of the spatial location by matching spinal image data (CT or fluoroscopic images) to its corresponding surgical anatomy.[2,3]

Registration System

The accurate translation of spatial information into detailed renderings of spinal anatomy necessitates a stable frame of reference that enables the computer-assisted system to calculate the relative positioning of instruments within the surgical field in all three dimensions. This process of establishing a relation between the "real" coordinate system, as defined by the patient's array, and the "virtual" coordinate system of the imaging data is called registration. Different registration techniques can be applied.[11,12]

Point Matching Registration Technique

Several anatomical points are selected in CT and MRI data set and in the corresponding anatomy. These points have to be selected for each spinal level to be instrumented. Any anatomical landmark that can be identified both preoperatively and intraoperatively can be used as a reference point. Examples of these frequent points are the tip of a spinous or transverse process or the apex of a facet joint. After selecting one of these points in the CT image data, the tip of the navigation tool is placed onto the corresponding point in the surgical field, with reflective spheres on the tool handle aimed toward the camera. Infrared light from the camera is reflected off the spheres toward the camera and into the computer, which calculates the spatial position of the probe's tip and the anatomical structure it is resting on. This effectively "links" the point selected in the image data with the point selected in the surgical field. If a minimum of three points are registered, when the probe is placed on any other point in the surgical field, the corresponding point in the image data set will be identified on the computer workstation. The disadvantage of this technique is that any error on the part of the surgeon in selecting the specific anatomical point in the surgical field will result in varying degrees of navigational inaccuracy. This paired point protocol can also be performed in conjunction with surface matching.[12]

Another method of registration is CT–fluoroscopy matching. This technique is used sometimes, when the navigation system is preoperatively CT based. When using this technique, the preoperative CT is matched with intraoperative two-dimensional fluoroscopy images of the spine, which are taken from different angles of the patient.[48]

Surface Matching Registration Technique

Surface matching is a supplementary registration technique in which the surgeon randomly selects multiple anatomical points on the exposed posterior elements to provide supplementary topographic data. This technique does not preclude prior selection of the points in the image set, although several discrete points in both the image data set and the surgical field are frequently needed to improve the accuracy of surface mapping. The positional information of these points is transferred to the workstation, and a topographic map of the selected anatomy is created and "matched" to the patient's image set. The concomitant use of the point-to-point and surface matching approaches was shown to result in a significantly lower mean registration error compared with that of paired point matching alone for the insertion of pedicle screws.[12]

Automated Registration

Automated registration is performed without any input from the surgeon and with less potential for registration error. It can be performed only when the image data are acquired intraoperatively. This technique involves attaching a reference frame with reflective spheres to some site in the exposed spinal anatomy or, in lumbar surgery, to the iliac crest. A second reference frame is built into the intraoperative CT imaging scanner or fluoroscope. As the intraoperative images are acquired, the two reference frames allow registration to occur without the need for the surgeon's input. The CT scanner or fluoroscope can then be removed, and real-time navigation of up to five separate spinal levels is performed.[2,47,49]

Tracking System

The image guided navigation systems use either optical or electromagnetic tracking systems.[47]

Optical Tracking

As previously mentioned, with the optical systems, a source produces a series of pulsed beam, that is, infrared light, which is passively reflected off the spheres on the surgical instruments and afterward is captured by a specialized camera—or the camera may detect the infrared light that is actively emitted by an array of diodes that are fixed to the instruments and to any number of reference points. The positional information obtained from this infrared signal is merged with the reference data that was previously acquired during the anatomical registration process, allowing specific location of the instrument to be identified in space and displayed on multiplanar images of the spine. The use of infrared wavelengths minimizes the distortion that may be caused by any surrounding metal or electrical fields present within the OR, but the successful function of the optical system depends on a clear "line of sight" between the tracking device and the surgical field. The reflective array integral to all optical tracking systems increases the size and weight of these specialized instruments, which may make them more unwieldy for the surgeon to handle. It has also been suggested in the anesthesia literature that this infrared technology may interfere with pulse oximetry monitoring during the case.

Electromagnetic Registration Systems

These systems have been developed as another method for tracking the location of instruments during surgical navigation to address the disadvantages of optical devices, namely the need of a clear "line of sight" between the tracking device and the passive signal emitters (reflective spheres) in the surgical field.[50] This may restrict the operator's normal range of movement and thus limit the intuitive handling of the instruments. Moreover, the trackers needed for optical systems with active and passive reflectors are attached to the instruments and the operation areas in order to be referenced and have anatomical and ergonomic disadvantages. Also, the instruments used are significantly larger and heavier, resulting in poorer ergonomics and handling for the operator.

In the electromagnetic registration systems, three orthogonal electromagnetic fields are generated by a transmitter attached to a fixed anatomical reference point, such as a spinous process. The positional data of these instruments are collected by a receiver and integrated to facilitate navigation. Since a line of sight is not required, the surgeon and the nursing staff are able to work freely within the operative field. However, electromagnetic registration image guidance may be compromised by metal artifacts, including surgical implants, as well as by any electromagnetic fields originating from other equipment in the OR, such as monopolar electrocautery, electrocardiogram monitoring, and cell phones. Given the limited area of these electromagnetic registration fields, the transmitter may also need to be repeatedly transferred to additional anatomical structures to obtain sufficient tracking information for multilevel procedures.[47,51]

31.1.3 Types of Navigational Systems

As highlighted in ▶ Fig. 31.1, the two main types of navigation systems are intraoperative-based image and preoperative-based image.

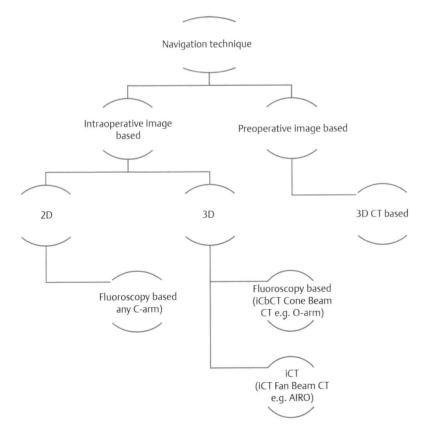

Fig. 31.1 A diagram showing the differences between intraoperative and preoperative navigation systems.

The two primary options for intraoperative imaging of the spine are still radiography and fluoroscopy. C-arm fluoroscopy remains a low cost and widely available mode of intraoperative image acquisition and allows for rapid and serial visualization of two-dimensional images in real time.[13]

Nonetheless, the past three decades of image-guided spine surgery have witnessed the development of multiple modalities for intraoperative imaging and navigation. The ultimate utility of these technologies depends on critical appraisal of the unique advantages and disadvantages of each system.[12,41]

Computer-Based Tomography/Preoperative (CT)-Based Navigation

The first available mode of intraoperative navigation was this modality. This technique uses preoperative thin-slice scans and one of the several registration processes to create a data set, which forms the basis for intraoperative navigation. In fact, prior to the surgery, a two-dimensional thin-cut CT through the region of interest that is obtained and uploaded to a workstation where it creates a virtual three-dimensional reconstruction that can be used for planning the surgery simulates the implants. On this preoperative reconstruction, anatomical landmarks are selected for intraoperative registration.[41,48]

However, preoperative CT scans are acquired with the patient in a supine position, while during surgery patients are usually in the prone position. The resulting vertebral shift and realignment create a risk for navigation errors. Therefore, to account for shifting anatomy during surgery, each level must be registered separately to accurately plan and perform the surgery.[13,52] One significant disadvantage of CT-based guidance systems is the need for surgeon-dependent registration of anatomical landmarks on preoperative CT images and the corresponding anatomy of the patient intraoperatively. In addition, extensive bony exposure is required for adequate registration and it may be difficult to identify landmarks for registration in patients with prior laminectomies.[13,41]

During navigation, the surgeon is presented with reformatted CT images on virtual three-dimensional multiplanar image reconstructions, along with the selected screw entry point and trajectory superimposed on the images. This information updates in real time, as adjustments are made to the selected trajectory in the surgical field.[53]

The disadvantages of this technology includes increased radiation exposure to the patient preoperatively.[13]

Intraoperative Image-Based Navigation

Intraoperative-based navigation systems eliminate the need for surgeon-dependent registration step because the system is automatically registered during the acquisition of images intraoperatively. Thus, the need for spinal exposure for point matching is obviated. Furthermore, in this setting, as images are obtained after patient positioning, they are an accurate representation of vertebral anatomy at the time of surgery.[49]

Two-Dimensional Fluoroscopy-Based Navigation

"Virtual fluoroscopy" or two-dimensional fluoroscopy-based navigation is a strategy that combines a standard two-dimensional C-arm with a computer navigation system. It uses a standard anterior–posterior and lateral image of the spinal anatomy acquired immediately before the start of the procedure.[53] Registration is performed automatically with a reference frame attached to the C-arm.[41] A series of fluoroscopy images in anterior–posterior, lateral, and sometimes the pedicle oblique view are acquired with a reference frame attached to a stable anatomical landmark, often a spinous process in the vicinity of the vertebrae that will be operated. These images are transferred to the navigation workstation and this data set is used to navigate implants on the virtual anatomy viewed on the screen. An infrared camera aimed at the reference arc and navigation tools allows continuous recognition of the navigation tools in relation to the relevant anatomy. A continuous "line of sight" must be kept among the infrared camera, the reference arc, and the navigation tools. The accuracy of the system will be maintained as long as the stability of the reference arc is maintained, motion segments do not change their position compared to acquired images, and the navigation tools are kept in line with the desired trajectory. Therefore, fluoroscopy-based navigation allows a completely automatic registration of the spine, correction of image distortion, and reduction of radiation exposure to the staff, yet is limited to two-dimensional projection images. The risk of navigation errors is increased and the abnormal axial anatomy is more likely to remain unrecognized, as it does not provide three-dimensional visualization of the spinal anatomy during navigation. Errors may also be greater in cases of poor bone quality, excess intra-abdominal gas, morbid obesity, spinal deformity, prior surgery, and congenital anomalies. Furthermore, image resolution is typically best in the center of the field and any structures around the periphery may appear distorted secondary to parallax, so to maintain the accuracy of navigation across several spinal segments the process of data acquisition and anatomical registration may need to be repeated several times.[13,41,49]

In summary, two-dimensional navigation provides an easier learning curve for surgeons who are familiar and very comfortable with conventional anterior–posterior–lateral fluoroscopy. It is readily available and is easily incorporated into the workflow when using devices or techniques that require real-time X-ray control and fluoroscopy to be brought into surgery. Such procedures include cement injection in vertebroplasty procedures, kyphoplasty procedures, or while using K-wires. Two-dimensional navigation can also be applied in situations that require frequent radiographic updates because of anatomy changes during surgery, such as translumbar discectomy and fusion procedures like extraforaminal lumbar interbody fusion (ELIF) where the cage placement and its relationship between vertebrae requires X-ray exposure. In these situations, two-dimensional navigation (NAV) will not eliminate the need for fluoroscopy, but can significantly reduce the need of continuous X-ray and will help improve the workflow. For example, two-dimensional NAV reduces the operative time and the risk of intraoperative contamination because the C-arm does not need to be continually repositioned during the case. This strategy is also preferable to preoperative CT-based navigation, which necessitates a suitable preoperative CT that must be matched to the corresponding anatomical structures by a manual registration process before proceeding with navigation.

This navigational system is a relatively inexpensive system (compared to three-dimensional navigation) that combines the benefits of navigation with affordable purchasing and

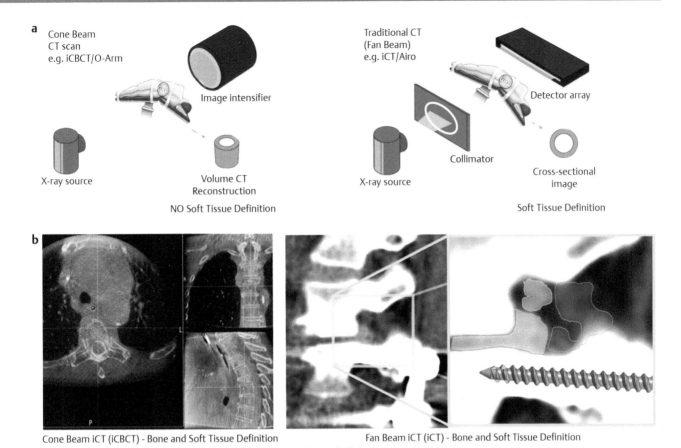

Fig. 31.2 Workstation screen demonstrating a fluoroscopic navigational system.
(a) Standard anteroposterior and lateral views are provided with superimposed simulation to determine the ideal pedicle entry point, trajectory, and the appropriate pedicle screw size. **(b)** Simulation to determine the ideal medial/lateral trajectory in order to avoid medial pedicle violation initially a pedicle screw is simulated that is no longer than the pedicle. If this short, simulated screw does not breach the medial border of the pedicle on the anteroposterior view and seems to be in perfect medial/lateral position, simulation is extended until the desired screw length is achieved. (Reproduced with permission from Njoku et al.[54])

maintenance costs, which can be of utmost importance when there are economic and infrastructural challenges. We have encouraged the use of navigation technologies whenever possible. We advocate the use of navigation whenever possible. During our annual mission in Tanzania, we effectively helped implement potable hardware and two-dimensional navigation system in a hospital that had no prior experiences of using such equipment (▸ Fig. 31.2).[54]

Three-Dimensional Fluoroscopy-Based Navigation

First system to appear was the three-dimensional fluoroscopy. It uses an isocentric C-arm fluoroscope to generate a three-dimensional data set intraoperatively that can be used for surgical navigation when combined with an image-guidance system. The fluoroscope obtains multiple images during an automated 190-degree rotation around the patient and these images are automatically reconstructed into multiplanar axial, coronal, and sagittal anatomical views.[41]

The cone beam CT (cbCT) technology was then developed. This is a modality where the high-resolution three-dimensional view is acquired from the "spin" of a cone-shaped X-ray beam around

the patient to a flat panel detector.[27,42] Embodiments of cbCT include fixed-room C-arms, mobile C-arms, mobile U-arms, and mobile O-arms.[43] The multiple images generated by the spin are processed into the three-dimensional volumetric data set (axial, sagittal, and coronal anatomical CT-like views).[27,44] These reformatted images have less quality than the conventional CT imaging and are superior to isocentric C-arm imaging.

Similar to two-dimensional fluoroscopy-based navigation, cbCT-based navigation systems perform automatic registration and eliminate the error caused by the anatomical shift of scanning the patient in the surgical position.[45] The main disadvantage of cbCT compared to intraoperative CT-based navigation, apart from the quality of the image, is that only several levels can be visualized at a time, depending on the scan volume per "spin." This is particularly relevant for large deformity surgeries where the entire surgical site cannot be included within one "spin," and the cbCT device must be recentered.[27]

At the end of surgery, if the accuracy of the hardware needs to be checked, the axial reconstituted can be obtained right away to confirm the accurate placement of the hardware in all three planes (i.e., axial, coronal, and sagittal).[27]

Intraoperative exposure to radiation is of concern to both patients and the surgical team. When using this navigational system, the acquisition of three-dimensional images of the surgical field is done while the surgical team and OR staff leave the room or stands behind a lead shield, and thus is removed from radiation exposure. However, this technique implies higher radiation for the patient.[46,47]

Intraoperative CT Scan Navigation

Intraoperative CT navigation technology uses a portable CT scanner that translates in the rostral to caudal axis over the patient. The intraoperative CT navigation workstation registers the patient's anatomy and creates three-dimensional images. These images allow for navigated instrumentation and for intraoperative planning throughout the procedure (e.g., one can plan the accurate measurement of the implants).[41]

The intraoperative CT computer-guided navigation technique affords immediate survey of screw/implants position and intraoperative revision.[55]

The quality of the image (same as a diagnostic CT scanner for bone and soft tissue) and an extended scan volume that eliminates the need to recenter the device even in large deformity

cases are other advantages of intraoperative CT. First generation of intraoperative CT scanners presented with several drawbacks, which includes high cost; inferior ergonomics, as they used to be permanently installed intraoperative CT scanners in a single dedicated OR; less flexibility due to requirements for specialized operating tables; small intraoperative CT gantry opening (e.g., making it impossible for obese patients); and increased preparation time.[41,56] The latest generation of full-fledged intraoperative CT imaging and navigation overcame some of the previous mentioned limitations, as it became portable, with its own table, a small footprint, and a bigger-sized gantry opening, but with a slim gantry. Nonetheless, the cost shortcoming remains (▶ Fig. 31.3).[33,56]

However, similar to what happens with cbCT, although the OR staff is not exposed to radiation, the technique entails a higher radiation for the patient.[41]

Robotic Navigation

Robotic navigation is the one of the most recent developments in spinal navigation.

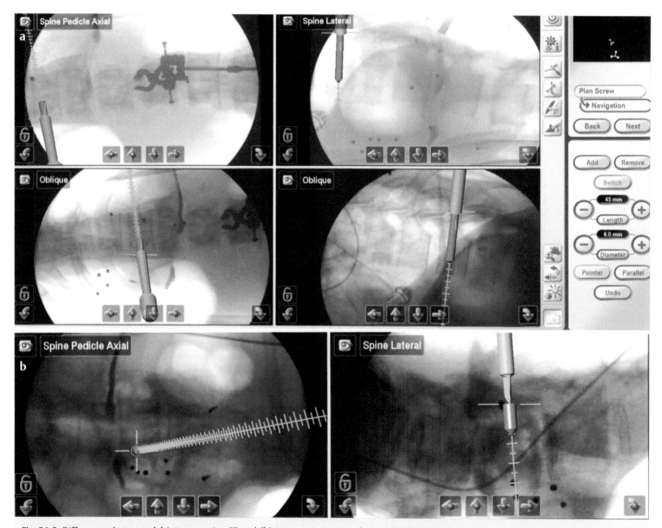

Fig. 31.3 Differences between **(a)** intraoperative CT and **(b)** intraoperative cone beam CT. Workstation screen demonstrating a fluoroscopic navigational system. Although intraoperative CT and cone beam CT bear some similarities in the nature of the images they produce, they are inherently different imaging modalities. Intraoperative cone beam CT is classified as a mobile X-ray system and uses a cone beam configuration, whereas intraoperative CT is classified as a true or conventional CT scanner that uses a fan beam configuration.

On a specially designed graphic user interface with specific software, the surgeon uses preoperatively acquired CT images to plan the trajectory of the screws.

And intraoperatively fluoroscopic images (anterior–posterior and lateral views) are obtained in order to facilitate automated registration. During navigation, the robotic arm moves into the appropriate position to guide screw insertion accurately along the appropriate trajectory.[2] Intraoperative image intensifier X-rays, with targeting devices, are then matched with the CT-based virtual images, as well as the surgeon's plan. A clamp is attached to the spinous process, or a minimally invasive frame is mounted on the iliac crest and on a spinous process. The miniature robot is then attached to the clamp and/or frame. On the basis of combined CT scan and image intensifier data, the robot aligns itself to the desired entry point and trajectory, as dictated by the surgeon's preoperative plan.[24]

Studies report that procedures using robotic surgery have found high levels of accuracy for implant placements. The downside of robotic surgery includes the fact that active tracking is not possible, and that implant accuracy can only be checked after surgery via a CT scan.[24]

31.2 Navigation in Thoracic Spine Surgery—Tips, Pearls, and Workflow Model

Although three-dimensional navigation seems to increase instrumentation accuracy and reduce surgeon's exposure to radiation,[57] its implementation into the clinical practice has been challenged by its costs and by the surgeon's concerns about increased operative time, ease of use, integration into the surgical flow, and safety.[33]

In 2013, Härtl et al[58] published a global survey on the use of computer-aided spine surgery that provided interesting data on the use of spinal navigation. In this survey, approximately 80% of the respondents were favorable to the use of spinal navigation. However, despite its widespread availability, only 11% of spine surgeons in North America and Europe used navigation. The routine users of navigation mentioned its accuracy, the potential of making complex surgeries safer, and minimizing radiation exposure as advantages. The nonusers indicated lack of equipment and high costs as the most important reason not to use navigation, as well as inadequate training and increased OR time.

It has been proposed that the reason navigation system might prolong the overall operative time is the time needed for OR setup and navigation workflow, as well as the time required to scan and register the patient intraoperatively. As a matter of fact, it has been observed that even when the overall OR time is prolonged, time per screw insertion is shorter due to quicker identification of bony anatomy.[59,60] Also, the use of the new-generation navigation settings requires less scanning and registration time.[61]

Hence, application of step-by-step guidelines might overcome potential delays related to the OR setup and workflow with intraoperative image-guided navigation, making it more efficient, reproducible, and decreasing the overall OR time.[33,56,62,63,64]

Every navigation system has its own characteristics and, consequently, the workflow, pearls, and pitfalls vary according to the navigation system being used. At our institution, different systems have been used over time, a journey of transition from conventional fluoroscopy to cone beam three-dimensional navigation, and lastly to three-dimensional intraoperative CT navigation in a process that has proven to be effective and perfectly applicable to any clinical practice. Also, we have introduced the concept of *total navigation*, implying the use of intraoperative CT navigation in the steps of surgery as an attempt to eliminate the radiation exposure for the surgical staff, to eliminate K-wires for instrumentation,[65] and to eliminate pedicle probe.

The elimination of K-wires represents a major improvement in this setting. Usually, the systems that use three-dimensional navigation for percutaneous screw placement work via K-wires and require separate navigation of multiple instruments, such as the drill guide, awl, tap and, finally, the screw. The idea behind the creation of a navigated guide tube was reducing the number of instruments that need to be navigated and the potential risks associated with the K-wires (i.e., they can break or bend during the procedure and pose risk of visceral or vascular injuries). This navigated tube is attached to a reference array and is used to determine the ideal pedicle trajectory, an appropriated-sized pedicle screw is simulated using the navigation software, and the navigated tube is gently impacted so that the teeth would hold onto the bony anatomy. A drill, tap, and, finally, a pedicle screw without screw head can be inserted through this guide tube (▶ Fig. 31.4).[65]

We present the tips, pearls, and workflow used at our institution applied to three-dimensional intraoperative CT, as published by Navarro-Ramirez et al[33] (▶ Table 31.1).

31.2.1 Surgical Workflow Pearls

As the concern with learning curve and deceleration of the surgical workflow appears to be one of the major drawbacks, limiting its applicability, we present an example of workflow, for a portable intraoperative CT navigation, that in our practice enhances the safety and accuracy and diminishes (almost eliminates) radiation exposure to the staff (▶ Table 31.2).[33]

31.2.2 Operating Room Setup

The intraoperative CT-guided NAV includes the Airo CT scanner, an image-guidance system, an infrared tracking camera navigation system (Brainlab Curve, Brainlab AG), and a patient reference array (Brainlab AG). The design of the Airo CT scanner comprises of large gantry opening (107 cm) with a slim gantry (30.5 × 38 cm) and a small footprint (1.5 m²). The suspension-controlled electrical drive system allows the machinery to be moved around the OR. A mobile, radiolucent carbon fiber table (Trumpf TruSystem 7500, TRUMPF Inc., Farmington, CT) was attached to the gantry during surgery. Airo and Curve systems were connected to an automatic image-transfer device and an image-patient coregistration that assisted in navigation. Precalibrated or manually calibrated instruments could be used with navigation for enhanced workflow.

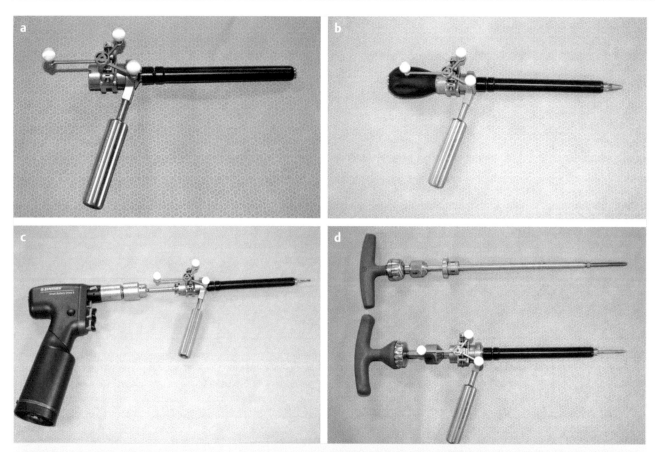

Fig. 31.4 (a) The navigated guide tube comprises a 170-mm-long tube with a 10-mm outer diameter and 8.3-mm cannulation and handle. An interface for attachment to an infrared reference array positioned on a 270 degrees rotatable collar on the proximal end to allow flexible positioning of the guide tube with respect to the navigation camera. **(b–d)** A drill, tap, and finally a pedicle screw without screw head can be inserted through this guide tube. (*Continued*)

Table 31.1 Tips to improve accuracy of intraopeartive CT-guided navigation in thoracic spine surgery[33]

Draping	• Securing the patient with tape to the OR table minimizes tissue movement • Tape across the chest and hips and laterally from the patient's side downward
Intraoperative scan	• Includes anatomical landmarks, allowing accurate determination of the index level/pathology • Obtain intraoperative CT immediately before it is actually needed (sometimes after the anatomical structures have been exposed, e.g., posterior cervical cases, this minimizes the chances of shift and inaccuracies caused by surgical manipulation)
Verification of accuracy	• Verify anatomical landmarks with navigation at every crucial step (e.g., screw placement and drill utilization), especially in MISS where landmarks are limited. • Constantly compare position and tactile feedback of the navigated instrument during surgery • Reflective markers should not be contaminated
Master the anatomy	• Intraoperative navigation does not substitute for the need to know the anatomy
Prevent excessive movement	• Throughout the procedure, confirm stable placement and avoid hitting the array during surgery • Avoid pressure, mechanical impact (with hammers or mallet), or movements • Use a battery-driven drill to prepare screw holes and avoid Jamshidi needles
"Hands-off test"	• After full insertion of the tap into the pedicle, let go of the instrument • If the screw simulation on the navigation screen demonstrates an adequately positioned screw in the pedicle without breach, this usually confirms a well-placed screw trajectory. (This test should be avoided in patients with poor bone quality and in the cervical spine)
Neuromonitoring	• Intraoperative neuromonitoring and screw stimulation with a cutoff of approximately 9 m Amp
Verification of position	• Intraoperative CT scan after implantation of instrumentation/implants to verify desired position and accuracy

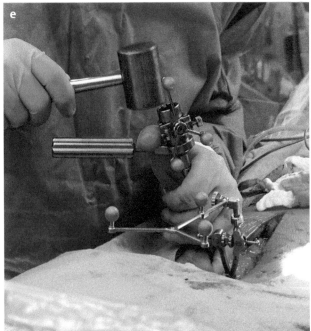
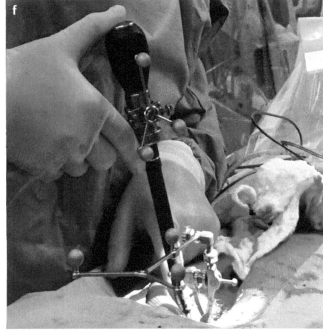
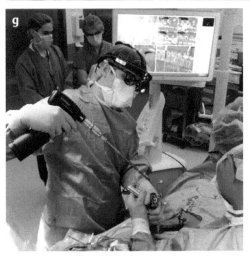
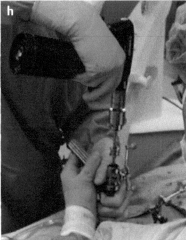
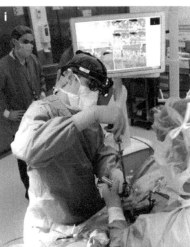

Fig. 31.4 (*Continued*) **(e, f)** A tissue protection sleeve and a trocar are made of PEEK material and facilitate percutaneous placement of the guide tube. **(g–i)** The navigated guide tube is used to determine the ideal pedicle trajectory, the tube is gently impacted a drill, tap and finally a pedicle screw without screw head are inserted through this guide tube.

31.2.3 Setup of Intraoperative CT NAV for Total Navigation

1. Before surgery, the intraoperative CT NAV is positioned parallel to the rail system and the gantry, facing anesthesia (▶ Fig. 31.5).
2. After the patient is anesthetized on a transport bed parallel to the gantry, the gantry of the portable intraoperative CT system is rotated perpendicular to the rails into the scanning position.
3. Hereafter, a Trumpf carbon fiber tabletop with a T3 frame is connected to the Trumpf column on the integrated rail system.

4. Intubation and insertion of the needle electrodes for electromyographic monitoring are conducted, followed by flipping the patient onto the T3 frame.
5. The patient is positioned and taped to the table. Adequate taping is important because it minimizes anatomical displacement, especially in obese patients. Care must be taken not to tape too tightly in order to avoid skin necrosis or pressure points.
6. The gantry is located on the cranial side of the patient and all cables (e.g., Bovie, suction, and electromyography monitoring) are let through the gantry.
7. While the intraoperative CT scanner is running, the surgical staff leaves the room and thus avoids unnecessary radiation exposure (▶ Fig. 31.5).

Table 31.2 Advantages and disadvantages of the different navigational systems[5]

	Fluoroscopy	Two-dimensional fluoroscopy NAV	Three-dimensional cbCT	Three-dimensional intraoperative CT	Three-dimensional preoperative CT
Major advantage	Only true real-time imaging modality	Navigation may be performed using images acquired intraoperatively in the surgical position. Automatic registration is possible	Three-dimensional images may be acquired during surgery and used for navigation	Higher resolution imaging and extended scan volume when compared to cbCT	Preoperative CT may be coupled to intraoperative navigation system
Need for intraoperative image acquisition?	Yes	Yes	Yes	Yes	No
Requires additional preoperative imaging?	No	No	No	No	Yes
Need for reregistration for multiple level Surgeries?	No	No	No	No	Yes
Real-time image?	Yes	Yes (if needed)	Yes (if needed)	No	No
Screw accuracy	◆◆	◆◆	◆◆◆◆	◆◆◆◆	◆◆◆
Bone quality image	◆◆	◆◆	◆◆◆◆	◆◆◆◆	◆◆◆◆
Soft-tissue quality image	–	–	◆	◆◆◆	◆◆◆◆
Surgical team's radiation exposure	◆◆◆◆	◆◆◆	–	–	–
Patient's radiation exposure	◆◆	◆	◆◆◆	◆◆◆◆	◆◆◆◆ (pre- ± postoperative)
Cost	◆	◆◆	◆◆◆◆	◆◆◆◆	◆◆◆
Level of expertise	◆	◆◆◆	◆◆◆◆	◆◆◆◆	◆◆◆
Hardware limitations (need for specific devices)	No	No	Yes	Yes	Yes

Abbreviations: cbCT, cone beam CT; CT, computed tomography.

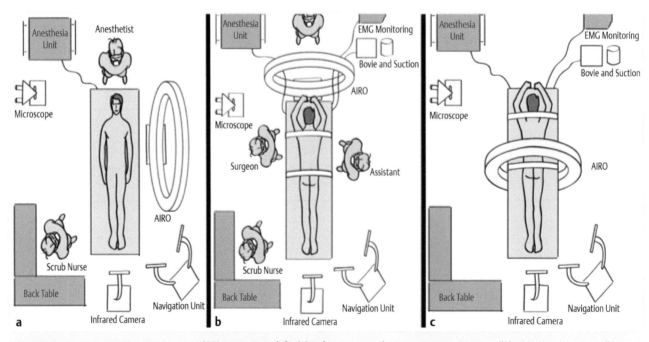

Fig. 31.5 Intraoperative CT operating room (OR) setup. **From left: (a)** Before surgery, the intraoperative CT is parallel with the rail system. **(b)** Intraoperative OR suite setup. The patient is face down with arms up for a lumbar procedure (note: arms should be placed down at the side for cervical surgery). It is important to lead all anesthesia, electromyography, Bovie, and suction cords through the gantry of the intraoperative CT. Cloth tape is applied across the chest and hips and laterally from the patient's side downwards in order to minimize tissue movement and shifting during surgery. **(c)** OR suite setup when taking intraoperative CT scans of the patient. All personnel leave the room while the intraoperative CT is in use.

31.2.4 Workflow for Lower Thoracic Spinal Surgery with Pedicle Screw Instrumentation[33]

1. For lower thoracic cases, that is, if the pathology is from T12 to pelvis, a two-pin fixator is attached to the patient's pelvis using two 3-mm Schanz pins and the reference array is connected to the two-pin fixator and tightened; if the pathology is from C3 to T11, the reference array is clamped to the spinous process (one or two levels cranially or caudally to the index level). The reference array may also be clamped to the table with the patient adequately immobilized with tape for localization only (e.g., intradural tumor and thoracic disc herniation).
2. For the preoperative scan, two half sheets are draped around the incision site and the region of interest is marked on the drape.
3. An infrared camera is positioned toward the reference array and reflective markers on the gantry.
4. All personnel leave the OR before a radiology technician initializes the scan via a remote control. This method eliminates the surgical staff's exposure to X-ray radiation.
5. After the scan, the images are automatically transferred to the NAV.
6. The site of incision and its proper trajectory are identified with a pointer. In open cases, accuracy is confirmed by palpation of anatomical landmarks (i.e., spinous or transverse process at several levels). In MISS, the tip of a transverse process or the costotransverse joint is used to verify the accuracy.
7. For MISS cases, a drill guide tube[65] is calibrated and placed at the desired entry point through a small skin and fascial incision. The use of a navigated guide tube streamlines the workflow by eliminating K-wires and the need to navigate multiple instruments (point–drill–tap–screw). The navigated guide tube is used for drilling, tapping, and screw placement.
8. A power drill with a 3.2-mm fluted drill bit is then used to prepare the entry point, followed by tapping the pedicle. Drill and tap only go in 35 mm. Make sure this is not too deep in the thoracic spine—in that case it can be adjusted to a shorter distance.
9. The desired screw is now inserted through the navigated guide tube. The screw is then stimulated; we use at threshold above 9 mA for acceptance of the screw position.
10. In cases requiring additional decompression and placement of a cage, the following steps are taken: bone graft can be harvested from the iliac crest, and the pointer can be used for best localization of appropriate iliac crest bone. When a tubular retractor is placed for decompression and facetectomy, the fascial incision for the tubular retractor is determined with navigation. The fascial incision is typically 2 to 3 cm medially to the fascial incision required for screw placement. The pointer identifies the inferior edge of the lamina and facet joint. Over a series of tubular dilators, the retractor is then placed and adequate exposure of the anatomy is again confirmed with the navigated pointer. The decompression and facetectomy are performed under the microscope and can also be done with the assistance of

navigation. Navigation at this point will also be helpful to determine, for example, the localization of the pedicle, disc space, and trajectory of the disc space. We then use navigation to determine the trajectory of the discectomy and cage placement.
11. After placement of the cage, a control CT scan is obtained. On the basis of this CT scan, the length of the rods can be determined with navigation or directly from the computer screen.

31.2.5 Workflow for Localization of Spinal Pathology[33]

Accurate and efficient intraoperative localization of spinal cord lesions is crucial to patient safety and to maximize clinical outcomes. This is especially challenging in the thoracic spine, where a combination of factors such as patient's size, scapular shadows, decreased bone density (e.g., osteoporosis) makes accurate intraoperative visualization of the bony anatomy difficult with standard radiographs or fluoroscopy. In such cases, surgeons may use preoperative marking (e.g., gold, polymethyl methacrylate cement) in order to identify the correct thoracic level on the intraoperative imaging.[66,67] Even if wrong-level surgery has a rare occurrence (0.04–5.3%), it is not without potential adverse consequences to the patient and the surgeon. According to a survey of spine surgeons in the North American Spine Society, 68% have performed a wrong-level operation at least once in their career.

Navigation is a practical and reliable tool, as well as a very useful one for intraoperative localization (e.g., on thoracic spine tumors).

1. The patient is placed in either prone or supine position and secured to the table using cloth tape, as described in the lumbar total navigation workflow.
2. The reference array is placed and secured to the table or with a Mayfield head-holder, depending on the anatomical region of interest.
3. For the preoperative scan, two half sheets are draped around the incision site and the region of interest is marked on the drape.
4. An infrared camera is positioned toward the reference array and reflective markers on the gantry.
5. All personnel left the OR before a radiology technician initializes the scan via a remote control. This eliminated the X-ray exposure for the surgical staff.
6. After the scan, the images are automatically transferred to the NAV.
7. The site of incision and its proper trajectory are identified with a pointer. In open cases, accuracy could be confirmed by palpation of anatomical landmarks (i.e., spinous transverse process at several levels). In MISS, the tip of a transverse process is used to verify accuracy.
8. Displacement of anatomical structures must be taken into consideration, and rescanning or anatomical landmark confirmation may be necessary, especially when treating intradural spine tumors.
9. A final CT is obtained in those cases where permanent hardware is implanted, especially in occipitocervical instrumentation.

Apart from the localization (incision planning, tubular retractor placement, extent of laminectomy, index level, spinal tumor, and thoracic disc herniation), intraoperative CT navigation can also be used for measuring instruments (screws, rod, and cage size) and assessing neural decompression.[33]

31.2.6 Examples of Clinical Application

Case 1: Intradural Extramedullary Tumor Resection

A 47-year-old patient presented with right upper superficial abdominal pain and right-sided mid-lower back pain that started 4 years ago. The pain has been progressively worse and is now at 8 to 10 on a visual analog scale.

In ▶ Fig. 31.6, we can see first the diagnostic studies, images, how the navigation was used for localization and real-time orientation and for accurate placement of pedicle screws above and below the indexed level, due to the destabilizing effect of the approach.

Case 2: Thoracic Corpectomy and Instrumentation

A 78-year-old female presented with a 4-month history of back pain and bilateral leg pain and weakness that suddenly got worse 2 weeks before her admission. ▶ Fig. 31.7 illustrates a pathological fracture. The patient was taken to the OR and a T12 navigation-aided corpectomy and fusion was performed.

31.3 Potential Advantages and Disadvantages of Computer Assisted Surgery

Potential advantages of CAS:
- Improves accuracy of instrumentation placement and optimizes the size of instrumentation used.
- Reduces radiation exposure to surgeons and the staff.
- Enables less-invasive approaches through smaller access.
- Allows preoperative planning of instrumentation size and trajectories and osteotomy procedures.
- Allows verification of screw accuracy intraoperatively (true intraoperative CT scanners or intraoperative portable cbCT systems).
- Minimizes the risks of wrong-level surgery.
- Decreases reoperation rate.

Potential disadvantages of CAS:
- The learning curve associated with the technologies for the surgeon and the OR staff could be significant.
- Upfront costs of the capital equipment.
- Interruption of surgical "flow."
- Additional equipment and footprint in the OR.
- Lack of scientific data supporting its clinical benefit.
- Limited imaging quality and field of view with mobile three-dimensional imaging devices currently in the market.
- Potential increase in OR time.
- Potential line of sight limitations for optical systems.

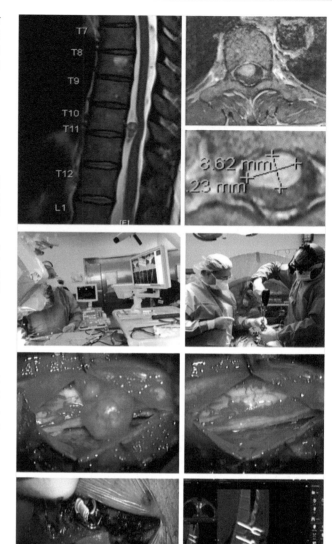

Fig. 31.6 Workflow with intraoperative CT navigation for the resection of a thoracic intradural extramedullary tumor. **Top line:** T1 and T2 MRI images of localization and size of the tumor. **Second line:** localization and navigated pedicle screw placement. **Third line:** intraoperative photographs of exposed tumor (left) and spinal cord post resection (right). **Fourth line:** intraoperative photograph (left) and intraoperative CT image of the pedicle screws above and below the index level (right).

- Concerns about accuracy and interference with metallic instruments using electromagnetic navigation systems.

31.4 Future Developments

We envision the use of navigation in the thoracic spine not only for localization, but also for future merging of robotic surgery and spinal navigation. It must first be proven safe, and once this is accomplished, thoracic spinal surgeries may be done in a semiautomatic mode with high fidelity and safety.

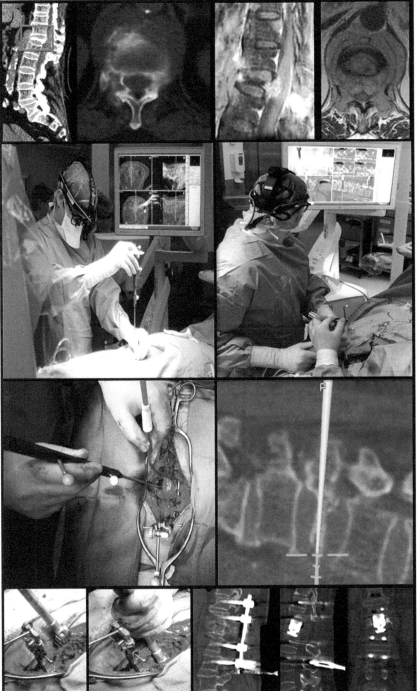

Fig. 31.7 **Top line:** CT scan (left) and MRI scan (right) of a T12 vertebral body fracture with spinal cord compression. **Second line:** intraoperative CT navigated localization of the affected segment. **Third line:** navigation post corpectomy. **Fourth line:** navigated instrumentation (left two images) and post-instrumentation intraoperative CT scan (right three images).

References

[1] Malhotra D, Kalb S, Rodriguez-Martinez N, et al. Instrumentation of the posterior thoracolumbar spine: from wires to pedicle screws. Neurosurgery. 2014; 10 Suppl 4:497–504, discussion 505

[2] Kalfas IH. Image-Guided Spinal Navigation: Principles and Clinical Applications, in Minimally Invasive Spine Surgery: A Practical Guide to Anatomy and Techniques. In: Ozgur B, Benzel E, Garfin S, eds. New York, NY: Springer; 2009:7–22

[3] Kalfas IH. Minimally Invasive Spine Surgery: A Practical Guide to Anatomy and Techniques. In: Ozgur B, Benzel E, Garfin S, eds. 1st ed. New York, NY: Springer; 2012

[4] Mullin JZ, Walsh K, Benzel E. Dorsal thoracic and lumbar screw fixation and pedicle fixation techniques. In: Benzel's Spine Surgery. Elsevier; 2017:717–728.e3

[5] Mirza SK, Wiggins GC, Kuntz C, IV, et al. Accuracy of thoracic vertebral body screw placement using standard fluoroscopy, fluoroscopic image guidance, and computed tomographic image guidance: a cadaver study. Spine. 2003; 28 (4):402–413

[6] Karapinar L, Erel N, Ozturk H, Altay T, Kaya A. Pedicle screw placement with a free hand technique in thoracolumbar spine: is it safe? J Spinal Disord Tech. 2008; 21(1):63–67

[7] Hartl R, T, heodore N, Dickman CA, Sonntag VKH. Technique of thoracic pedicle screw fixation for trauma. Oper Tech Neurosurg. 2004; 7:22–30

[8] Perna F, Borghi R, Pilla F, Stefanini N, Mazzotti A, Chehrassan M. Pedicle screw insertion techniques: an update and review of the literature. Musculoskelet Surg. 2016; 100(3):165–169

[9] Luther N, Iorgulescu JB, Geannette C, et al. Comparison of navigated versus non-navigated pedicle screw placement in 260 patients and 1434 screws: screw accuracy, screw size, and the complexity of surgery. J Spinal Disord Tech. 2015; 28(5):E298–E303

[10] Puvanesarajah V, Liauw JA, Lo SF, Lina IA, Witham TF. Techniques and accuracy of thoracolumbar pedicle screw placement. World J Orthop. 2014; 5(2): 112–123

[11] Mezger U, Jendrewski C, Bartels M. Navigation in surgery. Langenbecks Arch Surg. 2013; 398(4):501–514

[12] Kalfas IH. Image-guided spinal navigation: application to spinal metastases. Neurosurg Focus. 2001; 11(6):e5

[13] Holly LT. Image-guided spinal surgery. Int J Med Robot. 2006; 2(1):7–15

[14] Sanders R, Koval KJ, DiPasquale T, Schmelling G, Stenzler S, Ross E. Exposure of the orthopaedic surgeon to radiation. J Bone Joint Surg Am. 1993; 75(3): 326–330

[15] Rampersaud YR, Foley KT, Shen AC, Williams S, Solomito M. Radiation exposure to the spine surgeon during fluoroscopically assisted pedicle screw insertion. Spine. 2000; 25(20):2637–2645

[16] Hahn P, Oezdemir S, Komp M, et al. Navigation of pedicle screws in the thoracic spine with a new electromagnetic navigation system: a human cadaver study. BioMed Res Int. 2015; 2015:183586

[17] Avila MJ, Baaj AA. Freehand thoracic pedicle screw placement: review of existing strategies and a step-by-step guide using uniform landmarks for all levels. Cureus. 2016; 8(2):e501

[18] Kim YJ, Lenke LG, Bridwell KH, Cho YS, Riew KD. Free hand pedicle screw placement in the thoracic spine: is it safe? Spine. 2004; 29(3):333–342, discussion 342

[19] Kim YJ, Lenke LG. Thoracic pedicle screw placement: free-hand technique. Neurol India. 2005; 53(4):512–519

[20] Gaines RW, Jr. The use of pedicle-screw internal fixation for the operative treatment of spinal disorders. J Bone Joint Surg Am. 2000; 82(10):1458–1476

[21] Vialle R, Zeller R, Gaines RW. The "slide technique": an improvement on the "funnel technique" for safe pedicle screw placement in the thoracic spine. Eur Spine J. 2014; 23 Suppl 4:S452–S456

[22] Zindrick MR, Wiltse LL, Doornik A, et al. Analysis of the morphometric characteristics of the thoracic and lumbar pedicles. Spine. 1987; 12(2):160–166

[23] Gelalis ID, Paschos NK, Pakos EE, et al. Accuracy of pedicle screw placement: a systematic review of prospective in vivo studies comparing free hand, fluoroscopy guidance and navigation techniques. Eur Spine J. 2012; 21(2):247–255

[24] Härtl R., Korge A. Minimally Invasive Spine Surgery:Techniques, Evidence, and Controversies. 1st ed. Stuttgart: Thieme; 2012

[25] Kalfas IH, Kormos DW, Murphy MA, et al. Application of frameless stereotaxy to pedicle screw fixation of the spine. J Neurosurg. 1995; 83(4):641–647

[26] Murphy MA, McKenzie RL, Kormos DW, Kalfas IH. Frameless stereotaxis for the insertion of lumbar pedicle screws. J Clin Neurosci. 1994; 1(4):257–260

[27] Allam Y, Silbermann J, Riese F, Greiner-Perth R. Computer tomography assessment of pedicle screw placement in thoracic spine: comparison between free hand and a generic 3D-based navigation techniques. Eur Spine J. 2013; 22(3):648–653

[28] Tian NF, Huang QS, Zhou P, et al. Pedicle screw insertion accuracy with different assisted methods: a systematic review and meta-analysis of comparative studies. Eur Spine J. 2011; 20(6):846–859

[29] Rivkin MA, Yocom SS. Thoracolumbar instrumentation with CT-guided navigation (O-arm) in 270 consecutive patients: accuracy rates and lessons learned. Neurosurg Focus. 2014; 36(3):E7

[30] Aoude AA, Fortin M, Figueiredo R, Jarzem P, Ouellet J, Weber MH. Methods to determine pedicle screw placement accuracy in spine surgery: a systematic review. Eur Spine J. 2015; 24(5):990–1004

[31] Kotani Y, Abumi K, Ito M, et al. Accuracy analysis of pedicle screw placement in posterior scoliosis surgery: comparison between conventional fluoroscopic and computer-assisted technique. Spine. 2007; 32(14):1543–1550

[32] Laine T, Lund T, Ylikoski M, Lohikoski J, Schlenzka D. Accuracy of pedicle screw insertion with and without computer assistance: a randomised controlled clinical study in 100 consecutive patients. Eur Spine J. 2000; 9(3): 235–240

[33] Navarro-Ramirez R, et al. Total navigation in spine surgery; a concise guide to eliminate fluoroscopy using a portable intraoperative-CT 3D navigation system. World Neurosurg. 2017; 100:325:335

[34] Shin MH, Ryu KS, Park CK. Accuracy and Safety in Pedicle Screw Placement in the Thoracic and Lumbar Spines : Comparison Study between Conventional C-Arm Fluoroscopy and Navigation Coupled with O-Arm® Guided Methods. J Korean Neurosurg Soc. 2012; 52(3):204–209

[35] Van de Kelft E, Costa F, Van der Planken D, Schils F. A prospective multicenter registry on the accuracy of pedicle screw placement in the thoracic, lumbar, and sacral levels with the use of the O-arm imaging system and StealthStation Navigation. Spine. 2012; 37(25):E1580–E1587

[36] Scheufler KM, Franke J, Eckardt A, Dohmen H. Accuracy of image-guided pedicle screw placement using intraoperative computed tomography-based navigation with automated referencing, part I: cervicothoracic spine. Neurosurgery. 2011; 69(4):782–795, discussion 795

[37] Santos ER, Sembrano JN, Yson SC, Polly DW, Jr. Comparison of open and percutaneous lumbar pedicle screw revision rate using 3D image guidance and intraoperative CT. Orthopedics. 2015; 38(2):e129–e134

[38] Cho MS, et al. Inducing differentiation of neural progenitors from human embryonic stem cells with high efficiency and purity comprises the use of selected media and physical methods. Jeil Pharmaceutical Co., Ltd.; 2008

[39] Drazin D, Liu JC, Acosta FL, Jr. CT navigated lateral interbody fusion. J Clin Neurosci. 2013; 20(10):1438–1441

[40] Nolte LP, Zamorano L, Visarius H, et al. Clinical evaluation of a system for precision enhancement in spine surgery. Clin Biomech (Bristol, Avon). 1995; 10 (6):293–303

[41] Karhade AV, Vasudeva VS, Pompeu YA, Lu Y. Image guided spine surgery: available technology and future potential. Austin Neurosurg Open Access.; 3 (1):1043

[42] Brodwater BK, Roberts DW, Nakajima T, Friets EM, Strohbehn JW. Extracranial application of the frameless stereotactic operating microscope: experience with lumbar spine. Neurosurgery. 1993; 32(2):209–213, discussion 213

[43] Nolte L, Zamorano L, Arm E, et al. Image-guided computer-assisted spine surgery: a pilot study on pedicle screw fixation. Stereotact Funct Neurosurg. 1996; 66(1–3):108–117

[44] Foley KT, Smith MM. Image-guided spine surgery. Neurosurg Clin N Am. 1996; 7(2):171–186

[45] Wood MJ, McMillen J. The surgical learning curve and accuracy of minimally invasive lumbar pedicle screw placement using CT-based computer-assisted navigation plus continuous electromyography monitoring—a retrospective review of 627 screws in 150 patients. Int J Spine Surg. 2014; 8:8

[46] Larson AN, Polly DW, Jr, Guidera KJ, et al. The accuracy of navigation and 3D image-guided placement for the placement of pedicle screws in congenital spine deformity. J Pediatr Orthop. 2012; 32(6):e23–e29

[47] Patel AA, Whang PG, Vaccaro AR. Overview of Computer-Assisted Image-Guided Surgery of the Spine. Semin Spine Surg. 2008; 20(3):186–194

[48] Ringel F, et al. Navigation, robotics, and intraoperative imaging in spinal surgery. In: Advances and Technical Standards in Neurosurgery: Volume 41. Schramm J, ed. Cham: Springer International Publishing; 2014:3–22

[49] Acosta FL, Jr, Thompson TL, Campbell S, Weinstein PR, Ames CP. Use of intraoperative isocentric C-arm 3D fluoroscopy for sextant percutaneous pedicle screw placement: case report and review of the literature. Spine J. 2005; 5 (3):339–343

[50] Hedrick MH, Fraser JK. Processing regenerative cells from adipose tissue for placement in patient suffering from e.g. liver disorder involves separating, concentrating, and manipulating regenerative cells for enhancement of therapeutic effects. 2008, Cytori Therapeutics Inc

[51] Hahn P, Oezdemir S, Komp M, et al. A new electromagnetic navigation system for pedicle screws placement: a human cadaver study at the lumbar spine. PLoS One. 2015; 10(7):e0133708

[52] Papadopoulos EC, Girardi FP, Sama A, Sandhu HS, Cammisa FP, Jr. Accuracy of single-time, multilevel registration in image-guided spinal surgery. Spine J. 2005; 5(3):263–267, discussion 268

[53] Kalfas IH. Benzel's Spine Surgery—193 Intraoperative Imaging of the Spine. 4th ed. Elsevier; 2017

[54] Njoku I, Wanin O, Assey A, et al. Minimally invasive 2D navigation-assisted treatment of thoracolumbar spinal fractures in East Africa: a case report. Cureus. 2016; 8(2):e507

[55] Lee MH, et al. Feasibility of intra-operative computed tomography navigation system for pedicle screw insertion of the thoraco-lumbar spine. J Spinal Disord Tech. 2013; 26(5):E183–E187

[56] Hecht N, Kamphuis M, Czabanka M, et al. Accuracy and workflow of navigated spinal instrumentation with the mobile AIRO(®) CT scanner. Eur Spine J. 2016; 25(3):716–723

[57] Slomczykowski M, Roberto M, Schneeberger P, Ozdoba C, Vock P. Radiation dose for pedicle screw insertion. Fluoroscopic method versus computer-assisted surgery. Spine. 1999; 24(10):975–982, discussion 983

[58] Härtl R, Lam KS, Wang J, Korge A, Kandziora F, Audigé L. Worldwide survey on the use of navigation in spine surgery. World Neurosurg. 2013; 79(1):162–172

[59] Khanna AR, Yanamadala V, Coumans JV. Effect of intraoperative navigation on operative time in 1-level lumbar fusion surgery. J Clin Neurosci. 2016; 32:72–76

[60] Meng XT, Guan XF, Zhang HL, He SS. Computer navigation versus fluoroscopy-guided navigation for thoracic pedicle screw placement: a meta-analysis. Neurosurg Rev. 2016; 39(3):385–391

[61] Kotani T, Akazawa T, Sakuma T, et al. Accuracy of pedicle screw placement in scoliosis surgery: a comparison between conventional computed tomography-based and o-arm-based navigation techniques. Asian Spine J. 2014; 8(3):331–338

[62] Kim TT, Johnson JP, Pashman R, Drazin D. Minimally invasive spinal surgery with intraoperative image-guided navigation. BioMed Res Int. 2016; 2016:5716235

[63] Lian X, Navarro-Ramirez R, Berlin C, et al. Total 3D Airo® navigation for minimally invasive transforaminal lumbar interbody fusion. BioMed Res Int. 2016; 2016:5027340

[64] Rahmathulla G, Nottmeier EW, Pirris SM, Deen HG, Pichelmann MA. Intraoperative image-guided spinal navigation: technical pitfalls and their avoidance. Neurosurg Focus. 2014; 36(3):E3

[65] Shin BJ, Njoku IU, Tsiouris AJ, Härtl R. Navigated guide tube for the placement of mini-open pedicle screws using stereotactic 3D navigation without the use of K-wires: technical note. J Neurosurg Spine. 2013; 18(2):178–183

[66] Hsu W, Sciubba DM, Sasson AD, et al. Intraoperative localization of thoracic spine level with preoperative percutaneous placement of intravertebral polymethylmethacrylate. J Spinal Disord Tech. 2008; 21(1):72–75

[67] Macki M, Bydon M, McGovern K, et al. Gold fiducials are a unique marker for localization in the thoracic spine: a cost comparison with percutaneous vertebroplasty. Neurol Res. 2014; 36(10):925–927

Index